ALLERGIC DISEASES – HIGHLIGHTS IN THE CLINIC, MECHANISMS AND TREATMENT

Edited by **Celso Pereira**

Allergic Diseases – Highlights in the Clinic, Mechanisms and Treatment
Edited by Celso Pereira

Published by InTech
Janeza Trdine 9, 51000 Rijeka, Croatia

Publishing Process Manager Molly Kaliman

Technical Editor Teodora Smiljanic

Cover Designer InTech Design Team

Additional hard copies can be obtained from orders@intechopen.com

Allergic Diseases – Highlights in the Clinic, Mechanisms and Treatment,
Edited by Celso Pereira
p. cm.
ISBN 978-953-51-0227-4

For EU product safety concerns:
IN TECH d.o.o., Prolaz Marije Krucifikse Kozulić 3, 51000 Rijeka, Croatia,
info@intechopen.com or visit our website at intechopen.com.

Meet the editor

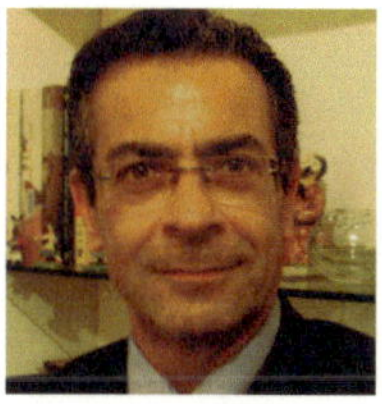

Prof Celso Pereira is currently a graduated specialist in Immuno-allergy at Coimbra's Universitary Hospital Centre, at Coimbra, Portugal. He is also the present elected president of the Immunoallergy Board of the Portuguese Medical Association. His main activities include clinical practice, education (pre and post graduate) and clinical and laboratorial research. He is member of national committee for vaccination. His scientific interests include the participation and development of several research projects, but now have focused his interest in the mechanisms of allergy and specific immunotherape has edited two scientific books, and has more than 90 scientific publications including book chapters, and scientific papers. He published over 300 abstracts related to the research projects developed and presented at scientific events. He was also honored with 31 scientific awards. He was responsible for the first subcutaneous application of latex immunotherapy and for the first long term sublingual native Pru p3 desensitization. During his Iberian Chapter Presidency of the Latin-American Allergy, Asthma and Immunology Society he coordinated an international multicentre study focusing aeroallergen sensitization in the Iberian Peninsula. He is an associate editor of 4 scientific Journals related to Allergy and Clinical Immunology. He has been participating in the organization of scientific meetings and actively collaborates with the scientific committees of diverse Medical Scientific Societies.

Contents

Preface XI

Part 1 Allergens, Inflammation and Basic Mechanisms 1

Chapter 1 **New Challenges for Old Diseases: The Impact of -Omics Technologies in the Understanding of Allergic Diseases 3**
Blanca Cárdaba, Miriam Aguerri, David Calzada and Carlos Lahoz

Chapter 2 **Expression of the Histamine H_4 Receptor in Human Tissue 31**
Katsunori Yamaura, Masahiko Suzuki, Takao Namiki and Koichi Ueno

Chapter 3 **The Type I and Type II Receptor Complexes for IL-4 and IL-13 Differentially Regulate Allergic Lung Inflammation 43**
Nicola M. Heller, Preeta Dasgupta, Nicolas J. Dorsey, Svetlana P. Chapoval and Achsah D. Keegan

Chapter 4 **Enzymatic and Chemical Modifications of Food Allergens 83**
Dragana Stanić-Vučinić and Tanja Ćirković Veličković

Chapter 5 **Characterization of Seafood Proteins Causing Allergic Diseases 107**
Anas M. Abdel Rahman, Robert J. Helleur, Mohamed F. Jeebhay and Andreas L. Lopata

Chapter 6 **Birch Pollen-Related Food Allergy: An Excellent Disease Model to Understand the Relevance of Immunological Cross-Reactivity for Allergy 141**
Brinda Subbarayal, Marija Geroldinger-Simic and Barbara Bohle

Part 2 Clinical Allergy 165

Chapter 7 **Anaphylaxis: Etiology, Clinical Manifestations, Diagnosis and Management 167**
Aslı Gelincik and Suna Büyüköztürk

Chapter 8 **Allergic Airway Inflammation 195**
Gabriel Morán, Claudio Henriquez and Hugo Folch

Chapter 9 **Asthma and Sensitization Pattern in Children 209**
Ute Langen

Chapter 10 **Wheezing Infant 231**
Yukinori Yoshida, Tomoshige Matsumoto, Makoto Kameda, Tomoki Nishikido, Isamu Takamatsu and Satoru Doi

Chapter 11 **Comorbidities of Allergic Rhinitis 239**
Doo Hee Han and Chae-Seo Rhee

Chapter 12 **Allergy and Benign Lesions of the Vocal Cord Mucosa 255**
Alenka Kravos

Chapter 13 **Drug Hypersensitivity 261**
María L. Sanz, Cristobalina Mayorga, Ruben Martínez-Aranguren and Pedro M. Gamboa

Chapter 14 **Diagnosis and Management of Cows' Milk Protein Allergy in Infants 279**
Elisabeth De Greef, Gigi Veereman-Wauters, Thierry Devreker, Bruno Hauser and Yvan Vandenplas

Chapter 15 **Natural Rubber Latex Allergy 289**
Ana Maria Sell and Jeane Eliete Laguila Visentainer

Part 3 Specific Aspects of Allergic Diseases 311

Chapter 16 **Psychological Factors in Asthma and Psychoeducational Interventions 313**
Lia Fernandes

Chapter 17 **Obesity, Diet, Exercise and Asthma in Children 339**
Luis Garcia-Marcos and Manuel Sanchez-Solis

Chapter 18 **Asthma and Health Related Quality of Life in Childhood and Adolescence 365**
Esther Hafkamp-de Groen and Hein Raat

Part 4 Treatment Strategies 373

Chapter 19 **Specific Immunotherapy and Central Immune System 375**
Celso Pereira, Graça Loureiro, Beatriz Tavares and Filomena Botelho

Chapter 20 **β_2-Adrenoceptor Agonists and Allergic Disease: The Enhancing Effect of β_2-Adrenoceptor Agonists on Cytokine-Induced TSLP Production by Human Lung Tissue Cells 403**
Akio Matsuda and Kyoko Futamura

Chapter 21 **Microbiota and Allergy: From Dysbiosis to Probiotics 413**
Anne-Judith Waligora-Dupriet and Marie-José Butel

Chapter 22 **Natural Products and Dermatological Hypersensitivity Diseases 435**
Clayton MacDonald and Marianna Kulka

Chapter 23 **Preventive Phytotherapy of Anaphylaxis and Allergic Reactions 461**
Elaine A. Cruz, Michelle F. Muzitano, Sonia S. Costa and Bartira Rossi-Bergmann

Chapter 24 ***Cissampelos sympodialis* (Menispermaceae): A Novel Phytotherapic Weapon Against Allergic Diseases? 477**
M.R. Piuvezam, C.R. Bezerra-Santos, P.T. Bozza, C. Bandeira-Melo, G. Vieira and H.F. Costa

Chapter 25 **Derived Products of Helminth in the Treatment of Inflammation, Allergic Reactions and Anaphylaxis 499**
C.A. Araujo and M.F. Macedo-Soares

Chapter 26 **Parasite-Derived Proteins Inhibit Allergic Specific Th2 Response 531**
Hak Sun Yu

Chapter 27 **Pharmaceutical Treatment of Asthma Symptoms in Elite Athletes – Doping or Therapy 545**
Jimmi Elers and Vibeke Backer

Preface

The clinical and basic science of allergic disease is moving and evolving so rapidly that it is nearly impossible to keep up full of information regarding the news mechanisms, signalling cell markers, cellular plasticity and expression, biological mediators targets or molecular and genetic discovers aspects related to the allergy. Moreover the systemic impact of this pathology determines the complexity of the more recent evidence demonstrates that the rapid regulation of central immune organs in clinical response of the mucosa to the allergen or offending agent. The enormous diversity clinical, etiologic, pathogenic, diagnose and therapy is not possible to develop in a sustainable way in this book all forms of allergic diseases present in the clinic.

Therefore, this book tried to incorporate into its own matrix the crucial issues that are recent contributions to learning less frequent topics, with very promising therapy approaches. So the aim and the project was at the final the scope of the title "Allergic diseases - highlights in the clinic, mechanisms and treatment", since it would not be possible to materialize a project that seeks to be a formal Medical Treaty covering the full breadth and complexity of allergy. Nevertheless, this book provides an accurate and current learning of many clinical issues.

The quality and scientific preciseness of the authors coming from several countries, does much to give strength to the whole book, especially as it reflects local and regional realities that characterize the diversity of expression allergic. In fact, the etiology and clinical response of allergic patient is very different, depending on the location, habits, socio-economic conditions and even the specific interests of key lines of investigation developed that the authors have incorporated into the chapters, but always guided by higher values of accuracy.

The basic and clinical aspects of allergic disease were described, namely concepts of innate and adaptive immune response, systemic and localized immune-mediated allergic disease, including recent update on pathogenesis. The clinical aspects were also subject and comprehensive developed and described, affecting different organ systems, particularly the anaphylaxis the main severe form of allergy.

This book will provide a valuable reference text in allergy and immunology not only for primary care physicians which are the first interfaces for an overall higher prevalent pathology, but also for residents in training as well for specialists. The chapters develop themes with enormous depth and expertise, supported by updated references, and often illustrated with personal research of great interest to further key points of clinical investigation. Our understanding of the inflammatory process in allergic disease is clearly defined in many of these chapters, as is the application of science to clinical treatment. The technologies enrolled in the genetic approach were also described as well highlight the tools for molecular study of allergy.

Overall the allergy is a sustained process of chronic inflammation why aspects of quality of life and the contribution and understanding of the psychological dimension, emotional and psychiatric naturally had to be enrolled in this book.

The chapters on treatment modalities and new strategies bring the latest concepts on the use of actual and very promising researches based on the better understanding of the mechanism of the allergic disease. Each of these topics is as current as possible and written by a leader in the field. Clinicians will all benefit from these reviews.

The effort and dedication of the authors in the time expended in the writing of the different chapters is fully demonstrated by the final quality of this project. To them goes my greatest of gratitude.

I am particularly indebted to Drs Graça Loureiro, Beatriz Tavares, Daniel Machado and Prof A Segorbe Luís, from Immunoallergy Departement of Coimbra University Hospital Center who willingly assisted me in the review and in the scientific discussion of some fundamental aspects that have benefited the final version. The preparation of this edition for publication depends heavily on the excellent professional secretarial work of Ms Molly Kaliman, Publishing Process Manager. Of course a special thanks to the Intech-Open Access Publisher who had honored me with that feat challenge. I am exceedingly grateful to my family and all those who are close to me for successfully enduring this ordeal yet again.

In my humble opinion, "Allergic diseases - highlights in the clinic, mechanisms and treatment" represents a shining example of a productive international collaboration among colleagues, and the information inserted in this book should conduct to an improved health care for patients with allergic diseases which are the essence of our work.

Celso Pereira, PhD, MD
Immunoallergology
Coimbra University Hospital Center, Coimbra
Portugal

Part 1

Allergens, Inflammation and Basic Mechanisms

1

New Challenges for Old Diseases: The Impact of -Omics Technologies in the Understanding of Allergic Diseases

Blanca Cárdaba[1,2], Miriam Aguerri[1], David Calzada[1] and Carlos Lahoz[1,2]
[1]*Immunology Department, IIS-Fundación Jiménez Díaz, Madrid,*
[2]*CIBER de Enfermedades Respiratorias, CIBERES,*
Spain

1. Introduction

Allergic diseases are an adverse reaction of the immune system against otherwise innocuous substances and are characterized by their high complexity. Patients can be asymptomatic or their involvement could be as severe as asthma. The complex nature of the phenotypes involved seems to point to genetic and environmental factors implication.

Familiar aggregation or genetic implication in the development of these diseases is well reported, and experts seem to agree that atopic diseases affect homozygotic twins more than dizigotic twins (Ownby, 1990, Duffy et al., 1990).

Allergic diseases are characterized by a Th2 inflammatory response involving several possible modulator factors (genetics and environmental factors), subject-related or antigen-related modulators such as adjuvants, solubility in the microenvironment of mucosa, size of the sensitization agent, mucosa permeability, viral infections, and the greater or lesser ability of effectors cells to liberate mediators.

Other factors include atmospheric pollution, exposure to tobacco, lifestyle-related diet and hygiene habits and maternal effects. The interaction between these factors produces the clinical picture of allergic disease.

Great advances have been performed in the understanding, diagnosis and treatment of these diseases but the search of specific protective or risk biomarkers is an unsolved field.

Since completion of the human genome project a rapid progress in genetics and bioinformatics have enabled the development of multiple tools as well as a large public databases, which include genetic and genomic data linked to clinical health data. The scientific revolution represented by the description of the human genome was largely facilitated by the use of DNA microarray technology, which made it possible to build a catalog of all genes within a given organism. The human genome project found that humans have an average of between 20,000 and 25,000 protein-coding genes (IHGSC, 2004). In addition, genetic variability between individuals is approximately 1% (Venter et al., 2001), suggesting that interactions between genes, proteins and the environment contribute to differences in human phenotype, maintenance of health and susceptibility to disease. On the other hand, the emergence of gene expression microarray technology in the mid-1990s has enabled genome-wide measurement of gene expression in a single experiment. This is turn

has allowed for significant advances in our understanding of gene expression, regulation, and function and continues to serve as an important tool in basic science research. This novel technology was subsequently extended from molecular genetics to proteomics, allowing the start of the Human Proteome Project, designed to determine protein function as essential elements in diagnosis and treatment.
Mainly, the genome project has fundamentally changed the way in which we approach questions in biology. The technology that the genome project has enabled, rather than the data it has produced, has induced the most profound impact on our conduct of biological research. In particular, functional genomics approaches, suchs as DNA microarrays, proteomics and metabolomics have greatly increased the rate at which we can generate data on biological systems allowing us, to begin to observe on a molecular level the holistic response of an organism to a particular stimulus (Quackenbush, 2006).
In this review, will be summarize the principle of these new methodologies and the impact of omics-techniques, mainly genomic-transcriptomics (analysis of single nucleotide polymorphisms or gene-expression) and proteomic (identification and quantification of proteins), in the knowledge of different aspects of allergy diseases (diagnosis, screening, monitoring of treatment, protective or risk biomarkers and drug development) and the advance to define the personalized and molecular medicine in this complex kind of diseases.

2. High-throughput technologies: "Omics approaches" review

During the last decade, high-throughput technologies including genomic, transcriptomic, epigenomic, and proteomic have been applied to further our understanding of molecular pathogenesis of heterogeneous disease, and to develop strategies that aim to improve the management of patients. These approaches called omics should lead to sensitive, specific and non-invasive methods for early diagnosis, and facilitate the prediction of response to therapy and outcome, as well as the identification of potential novel therapeutic targets (Ocak et al., 2009).
Omics approaches to the study of complex biological systems with potential applications to molecular medicine are attracting great interest in clinical as well as in basic biological research. Genomics, transcriptomics and proteomics are characterized by the lack of an *a priori* definition of scope, and this gives sufficient leeway for investigators (a) to discern all at once a globally altered pattern of gene/protein expression and (b) to examine the complex interactions that regulate entire biological processes (Silvestri et al., 2011). All classes of biological compounds, from genes through mRNA to proteins and metabolites, can be analyzed by the respective "omic" approaches, namely, genomics (Study of genomes and the complete collection of genes that they contain), transcriptomics (or functional genomics, attempts to analyze patterns of gene expression and to correlate the patterns with the underlying biology), epigenomic (the large-scale study of epigenetic modifications), proteomics (examine the collection of proteins to determine how, when and where they are expressed) or metabolomics (or metabonomics, is a large-scale approach to characterize and to quantify the compounds involved in cellular processes in a single assay to derive metabolic profiles). Such an "omic" approach leads to a broader view of the biological system, including the pathology of diseases.
Two popular platforms in "omics" are DNA microarray, which measure messenger RNA transcript levels, and proteomic analyses, which identify and quantify proteins. Because of their intrinsic strengths and weaknesses, no single approach can fully unravel the

complexities of fundamental biological events. However, an appropriate combination of different tools could lead to integrative analyses that would furnish new insights not accessible through one-dimensional datasets (Silvestri et al., 2011). Indeed, while the data obtained from genomics may explain the disposition of diseases (i.e., increasing risk of acquiring a certain disease), several other mechanisms that are not gene mediated may be involved in the onset of disease.

Genomic studies were the first to move this field forward by providing novel insights into the molecular biology of cancer by generating candidate biomarkers of disease progression. Epigenetic regulation by DNA methylation and histone modifications modulate chromatin structure and, in turn, either activate or silence gene expression. Proteomic approaches critically complement these molecular studies, as the phenotype is determined by proteins and cannot be predicted by genomics or transcriptomics alone. Indeed, expression levels of proteins are commonly subject to post-transcriptional modifications that may modify their functions.

Moreover, a single gene can be processed to result in several different mRNAs or proteins, which directly determine different cellular functions. Genomic and proteomic data analyses have proven to be essential for an understanding of the underlying factors involved in human disease and for the discovery of diagnostic biomarkers, as well as for the provision of further insights into signalling molecules.

Therefore, while genomics/transcriptomics enables assessments of all potential information, proteomics enables us to assess the programs that are actually executed, and metabolomics will mostly display the results of such executions.

In the postgenomic era, functional analysis of genes and their products constitutes a novel and powerful approach since the expression levels of multiple genes and proteins can thereby be analyzed simultaneously, in both health and disease. Among the techniques used in functional genomics, both DNA microarrays and classical and ongoing proteomic approaches hold great promise for the study of complex biological systems and have applications in molecular medicine. These technologies allow high-throughput analysis as they are complementary to each other, and they may lead to a better understanding of the regulatory events involved in physiological, and disease, processes.

2.1 Genomic

Genomic provides us with platforms to measure quantitatively the essential elements (genes) of the cell and includes haplotyping and single nucleotide polymorphism detection. Is the study of an organism's entire genome. Some of the most important of the related technologies are high-throughput capillary sequencing and single-nucleotide polymorphism (SNP) arrays.

2.1.1 Global genome sequencing

This method has made major improvements from gel-based sequencing to automated reading of the four nucleotides (TGCA) (Wheeler et al., 2008, Wang J et al., 2008, Levy et al., 2007), by sequencing-by-synthesis technology that binds short fragments of DNA to small beads that are dropped into wells in a fibreoptic chip. The DNA adds another molecule to its chain and the sequencer identifies the molecule used, indicating which base is next in the sequence. Although the assemble of these pieces of DNA is a major challenge and may require multiple runs through a sequencer before assembling all the sequence, the use of

capillary electrophoresis instead of a gel, has allowed the automation DNA loading system, leading to and increase in throughput and higher speeds.
The systematic re-sequencing of genes tumours has provided in cancer field a rich source of clinically relevant information increasing the discovery of critical mutations as has been revised by Ocak et al., 2009.

2.1.2 SNP arrays

These arrays allow accurate measurement of specific loss of heterozygosity in a high-throughput manner with the possibility to identify patterns of allelic imbalance and small regions of copy number alterations, with potential prognosis and diagnostic utilities. They are synthesised by photolithography and contain up to 40 separate oligonucleotide probes for each SNP locus, with up 2 million SNP loci formats. After DNA labelling and hybridisation, fluorescence intensities are measured for each allele of each SNP.
This methodology is mainly used in the genome-wide association studies (GWASs) using case-control or case-only approaches. GWAS approaches are based on the ability to rapidly analyze genetic variants (mainly single nucleotide polymorphisms [SNPs], usually with a high degree of heterozygosity) across the whole genome to determine which genetic variants are associated with disease susceptibility (case-control studies) or which are associated with measures of disease severity or response to treatment (ie, pharmacogenetics; case-only studies). GWASs are also performed in families, especially trios, which are defined as an affected child with genotyping from both parents (eg, the National Heart, Lung, and Blood Institute [NHLBI]'s Childhood Asthma Management Program study identified *PDE4* (Himes et al., 2009) as an asthma susceptibility gene) but it is generally easier to ascertain and characterize a large number of unrelated cases and control subjects than to study multiple family members (Meyers, 2010).
The basic principle of a GWAS is straightforward: the frequency of each genetic variant is compared between cases (ie, subjects with the disease under investigation) and control subjects without the disease. A statistically significant increased frequency in cases compared with control subjects provides evidence that the genetic variant is related to disease susceptibility. Because many genetic variants (SNPs) are tested (usually 300,000 to 1 million), adjustment for multiple testing is required; for example, in the National Institutes of Health catalog of GWAS results, only those with P values of 5×10^{-8} or less are included in their chromosomal map of association results from many common diseases (www.genome.gov/GWAS).
The results from GWASs are the first step. Replication studies are necessary, and meta-analyses are useful to determine the importance of these variants in multiple populations.

2.2 Transcriptomic

Transcriptomic afford information about the expression of individual genes at the messenger RNA (mRNA) levels.
Is the study of global analysis of gene expression or transcriptome, the complete set of mRNA transcript produced by the genome. The most common related high-throughput technologies are gene expression arrays or microRNA (miRNA) expression arrays.

2.2.1 Gene expression arrays

This methodology derivate from two families of technologies: the first for nucleic acid detection and the second for the development of multiplex solid-phase assays (Patel A,

2008). The technique for detection of specific nucleic acid sequences by hybridization of labels nucleic acid sequences to known sequences immobilized on a solid support was developed initially for DNA detection (Southern, 1975), adapted for messenger RNA detection (Alwine et al., 1977) (Northern blot), and modified for placing the detection reagent (antibody or nucleic acid probe) on the solid support and leave the analyte in the liquid phase (eg, reverse Northern blot, dot blot)(Catt et al.,1966, Engvall et al., 2005, Kafatos et al., 1979).

The next significant technological development was the description of a system for detecting multiple analytes via the use of microspots (Ekins et al, 1990, 1999). Each microspot would contain a capture antibody to bind the analyte if present. A second antibody would be used to detect the presence of bound sensor antibody. If labelled fluorescently with different fluorophores, the ratio of fluorescence intensity between bound and unbound sensor antibody could be determined by laser scanning confocal microscopy, and with appropriate standards, this could be used to precisely quantify the amount of a given analyte. These were in essence the microarrays bases, the microspots, the bound detection reagent and the fluorescent readout.

However, several new technologies and information resources were required, mainly related with the improvement in the platforms, with the use of impermeable support materials (smaller amount of probe material), the increase of information from probes used for each target (derived from sequencing projects), system for detection of small amounts of labelled nucleic acid bound to complementary probes on small spots via confocal or non-confocal laser scanning techniques, and especially image analysis and data analysis techniques, that represent a significant challenge given the large number of variables, which has led to multiple approaches for microarrays data analysis (Patel A, 2008).

These arrays mostly make use of matrix-bound probes to which processed mRNA templates of the analysed specimens will hybridise. Two major types of arrays have been developed: oligonucleotide (use short oligonucleotides synthesised on the array matrix) and cDNA arrays (employs probes of copy-DNA).

There are two basic approaches to generate microarray data (Quackenbush, 2006). In a two-color array, two samples of RNA, each labelled with a different dye, are simultaneously hybridized to the array. Such an assay compares paired samples and reports expression as the logarithms of the ratio of RNA in a query sample to that in a control sample. For single-colour arrays, such as the GeneChip (Affymetrix), each sample is labelled and individually incubated with an array. After non-hybridized material in the sample is removed by washing, the level of expression of each gene is reported as a single fluorescence intensity that represents an estimated level of gene expression. Regardless of the approach or technique, the data used in all subsequent analyses are expression measures for each gene in each sample. Following hybridisation of a pre-processed and fluorescently labelled mRNA sample, the arrays are scanned and transcript abundance is measured as a direct correlate of signal intensity. After data normalisation, data can be analysed using a virtually unlimited array of computational and statistical methods. Normalization and filtering transformations must be carefully applied, because they can have a profound effect on the results. Different methods of statistical analysis applied to the same data set may produce different (but usually overlapping) sets of significant genes.

To ease interpretation of the results of multiple hybridizations, elements of the data in a matrix are often rendered in colour, which indicates the level of expression of each gene in each sample and yields a visual representation of gene-expression patterns in the sample being analyzed. In the most common approach, the colours used for the genes are based on the log-ratio for each sample measured as compared with a control sample : close to zero in black, values greater than zero in red (indicating up-regulated genes) and those with negative values in green (down-regulated genes). The intensity of each element, as compared with the intensities of others, indicates the relative expression of the gene that the element represents.

After the appropriate data have been recorded, normalized and filtered and a means of measuring similarity has been chosen, a variety of approaches are available for further analysis. These approaches are generally grouped into two types: supervised and unsupervised methods. Supervised methods depend on prior knowledge about the samples in order to search for genes that correlate with a diseases state, and they are useful for classification studies and can yield gene sets or signatures of genes that can distinguish between *a priori* defined subsets of samples. Unsupervised methods disregard prior knowledge and can be useful for identifying subgroups of samples that may represent unrecognized disease states. This method allow self-organisation of data matrices, group samples (or genes, or both), according to similarity of expression profiles features. This approached can help identify subgroups of samples not known *a priori* that are characterised by a typical transcriptional signature.

In order to minimise the risk of over fitting the predictive signature, such approaches typically involve validation of the predictor in a separate dataset or by splitting the original dataset into a learning and test set. In the latter case, the predictor is built using the learning set and then validated in the test set.

The discovery of biomarker signatures or panels for diagnosis by non-invasive methods is crucial for some diseases, as lung cancer, reason why these methodologies are very important. Soon after microarrays were introduced, many researchers realized with this technique could be used to find new subclasses in diseases states (Alon et al., 1999, Perou et al., 1999) and identify biological markers (biomarkers) associated with disease (Moch et al., 1999) and that even the expression patterns of genes could be used to distinguish subclasses of disease (Khan et al., 1998, Goiub et al., 1999, Bloom et al .,2004).

Many early studies focused an unsupervised approach to data-mining, such as hierarchical clustering for class discovery, because such studies take an unbiased approach to searching for subgroups in the data. The analysis was useful in lymphoma (Alizadeh et al., 2000) for identifying two subclasses related to a different stage of B-cell differentiation and showed the distinct clinical progress.

Other kind of studies (Golub et al., 1999) showed that microarray-expression profiles can be used to classify disease states. This kind of studies made clear that disease classification according to expression profiles will be come an important area of application for microarrays, proteomics, metabolomics and other high-throughput genomic techniques. The question is whether a pattern can be found that can be used to distinguish biological samples on the basis of some inherent property.

As will be remarked in the specific paragraph, this is one of the high-throughput methodologies more used in allergy diseases studies and with more interesting advances.

2.2.2 miRNA expression arrays

miRNAs are single-stranded, small (18 to 24 nucleotides in length), noncoding RNAs that negatively regulate gene expression by binding to and modulating the translation of specific mRNAs. It is estimated that miRNAs may be responsible for regulating the expression of nearly one-third of the human genome. Each miRNA appears to regulate the translation of multiple genes, and many genes appear to be regulated by multiple miRNAs. The methodology is like gene expression arrays by using arrays with up to 1300 distinct probes of eight to nine nucleotides (Ocak et al., 2009).

Although is estimated that miRNAs may be responsible for regulating the expression of nearly one-third of the human genome, few studies have explored their relevance to the pathogenesis of diseases and specifically in lung diseases (review in Serge et al., 2009). However, miRNA may be considered as potential therapeutic targets, as regulators of gene transcription and protein production and their study could be very useful for understanding human health and disease.

2.3 Epigenomics

The field of epigenetic has emerged to explain how cells with the same DNA can differentiate into alternative cell types and how a phenotype can be passed from one cell to its daughter cells (Baye et al., 2010). Unlike genetic alterations, which are permanent and usually affect all cells, epigenetic modifications are cell type specific and epigenetic regulation of immune system occurs at many levels, including T cells (Locksley, 2009, Wells, 2009). Epigenetic effects on gene expression can persist even after removal of the inducing agent and can be passed on through mitosis to subsequent cell generations, constituting a heritable change (Baye et al., 2010). The role of epigenetic in diseases, and specifically in allergic diseases is becoming increasingly evident (review in Kumar et al., 2009).

Recent development of epigenomic or the large-scale study by high-troughput/genome wide detection of epigenetic modifications, as heritable changes in gene expression without DNA sequence alterations, mainly DNA methylation and histone post-translational modification, should bring out more data relevant to allergic diseases.

Different techniques coupled to high-throughput technologies are available for the detection of DNA methylation, based on the ability to distinguish cytosine from 5-methylcytosine in the DNA sequence. To study histone modifications, there is a microarray platform of chromatin immuno-precipitation-on chip that allow the assessment of chromatin states.

It should be very interesting to know how genetics, environmental factors and epigenetics regulate each other for understanding the molecular events that underlie complex diseases such allergy diseases.

2.4 Proteomics

Is the large-scale study of proteins, particularly their structure and function. Proteomics focuses on determination of individual protein concentrations present in the biological sample being investigated, whereas functional proteomic determines constituent protein-protein, protein-DNA, and protein-RNA interactions and their resulting complexes.

Proteins are excellent targets in disease diagnostics, prognostics, and therapeutics. Consequently, proteomic approaches (such as two-dimensional gel electrophoresis (2D-E), two-dimensional liquid chromatography (2-DL), and mass spectrometry (MS), which allow the simultaneous measurement and comparison of the expression levels of hundreds of proteins, represent powerful tools for (a) the discovery of novel hormone/drug targets and biomarkers and (b) studies of cellular metabolisms and protein expression (Righetti et al., 2004, Vlahou et al., 2005). Increasingly, proteomic techniques are being adopted to solve

analytical problems and obtain a more comprehensive identification and characterization of molecular events associated with pathophysiological conditions.
Several high-throughput technologies have been developed and a brief summary of the main technological characteristics is exposed.

2.4.1 Two-dimensional gel electrophoresis

This technique relies on polyacrilamide gels that separate proteins based first on their charge and then on their molecular weight. Gel are scanned with laser densitometers and analysed with software allowing the semiquantitative visualisation of >500-1000 proteins per gel (Bergman et al., 2000). Individual protein spots of interest can be digested into peptides for sequence analysis by mass spectrometry (MS). A modification of this technique is the differential in gel-electrophoresis (DIGE), used to compare two protein mixtures on the same gel, using different fluorescent dyes, mixed together and run on the same gel (Patton, 2002). Identical proteins from the two pools co-migrate and are independently detected by quantitative fluorometry. Differentially expressed proteins of interest are identified by alterations in the ratios of the two fluorescent signals.

2.4.2 Matrix-assisted laser desorption ionisation time-of-flight MS (MALDI-TOF MS)

Is a high-throughput technique that analyses with high sensitivity and specificity proteins expressed in complex biological mixtures, such as serum, urine and tissues (Caprioli et al., 1997, Farmer et al., 1991). It requires sample co-crystallisation with a matrix that absorbs laser energy and subsequently ejects and ionises molecules into the gas phase. Ions are accelerated from the ion source by a fixed potential difference and travel a fixed-length, field-free distance before reaching the detector. The time taken by each ion permits its characterization. This methodology has been extensively applied to proteomic profiling of biological specimens.

2.4.3 Liquid chromatography tandem MS

This technique combines high-performance liquid chromatography (LC) with electrospray ionisation MS, ionising and vaporising proteins from liquid solutions. The shotgun proteomic analysis platform uses digestion of the sample with site-specific proteases, multidimensional separation of peptides by strong cation exchange chromatography (Link et al., 1999, Wolters et al., 2001, Cargile et al., 2004, Essader et al., 2005), followed by reverse phase LC separation coupled directly to a tandem MS instrument (MS/MS). The most abundant peptides are sequentially selected for MS/MS analyses. Resulting fragments ions are analysed in a MS scan and based on their molecular weight, the peptide sequence can be derived (Liebler, 2004). Through comparisons with predicted sequences of same nominal mass in databases, peptides are identified and the proteins from which they came are deduced.

2.4.4 Protein arrays

This is an efficient way of simultaneously analysing multiple samples or proteins in a high-throughput manner. There are two main forms: 1. Forward-phase arrays where hundreds of specifics antibodies are arrayed on a glass slide and one complex protein sample could be analysed for expression levels of post-translational modifications of hundreds of proteins in a single experiments. 2. Reverse-phase arrays, where hundreds of proteins (natural or recombinants) are placed on glass slides and probed with a single sample.

Post-translational modifications of proteins, such as phosphorylation, glycosilation and proteolytic processing, are common events and have the potential to significantly modify protein functions as well as confer cellular or tissue specificity. Since these modifications are reversible, drugs inhibiting these modifications are developed and hold great promise for some therapies as lung cancer therapy. Proteomics strategies have an important role by allowing not only the identification of post-translational modifications, but also the quantification and monitoring of the changes induced by their regulators.

2.5 Other complementary technologies

2.5.1 Pharmacogenomics

Is an emerging area of biomedical research, strongly influenced by growing availability of genomic databases, high-throughput genomic technologies, bioinformatics tools and artificial computational modelling approaches. Pharmacogenomics offers a new tool for the discovery of new targets for drugs development purposes, and for the individual variation in drug response. One main area is the discovery of new drugs and drug targets with molecular genetic, genomic or even bioinformatics methods and the other is the study of how genomic differences influence the variability in patient´ responses to drugs. Genes that have been found implicated in the disease are potential new drug targets and several pharmacological investigations are underway to utilize these new discoveries (Szalai et al., 2008).

2.5.2 Immunoinformatics, or computional immunology

Is an emerging area that provides fundamental methodologies in the study of immunomics, that is, immune-related, genomics and proteomics. The integrations of immune informatics with system biology approach made lead to a better understanding of immune related diseases at various system levels.

The information about genetic diversity of the immune system may help define patient's subgroups for individualized vaccine or drug development. Cellular pathways and host immune-pathogens interactions have a crucial impact on disease pathogenesis and immunogen design. Epigenetic studies may help understand how environmental change influence complex immuno diseases such as allergy. High-throughput technologies enable the measurements and catalogue of genes, proteins, interactions, and behaviour. Such perception may contribute to the understanding of the interaction network among humans, vaccines and drug, to enable new insights of diseases and therapeutic responses.

Bioinformatics plays an indispensable role in designing experiments, so as high-throughput studies, and helping to establish and test hypothesis trough data analyses. This essential task in drug discovery and in development cannot be accomplished with traditional approaches alone (Yang, 2010).

System biology studies the interactions among biological elements toward the understanding of diseases at the system level (Yang, 2005). The combination of bioinformatics and systems biology approach can lead to a better understanding of immune-related diseases (Rapin et al., 2006).

With the comprehensive examination of structures, functions, and relationships between them at the molecular level, we can scale at the higher level to gain a more complete view of how the immune system work and interact with other systems.

The understanding of changes in molecular and cellular pathways and interactions can be useful for finding new drug, target and designing effective drugs. These pathways are potential targets for developing novel therapeutics.

On the other hand, the structure-function analysis includes the examination of how sequence variants such as polymorphisms may have functional influences. Studies of transcription factors, functional motifs, 2D and 3D structure may help with the identification of epitopes and design of vaccines. These studies may shed light on the mechanisms of cellular pathways and protein-protein interactions. Advances in high-throughput analysis may greatly enhance such investigations.

The perception at these points may contribute to the understanding of the interaction networks among humans, vaccines, drugs, and the environment and enable new insights of disease mechanisms and therapeutic responses. The integration of all of the information at various systems levels may ultimately lead to the development of optimized vaccines and drugs tailored to individualized prevention and treatment.

3. Omics approach in allergy diseases

Our knowledge of how genetic variation between subjects determines susceptibility, severity and response to treatment has expanded considerably, providing intriguing insights into the pathophysiology of these multifactorial disorders. The picture is complex but our understanding is exponentially increasing in the last years thanks to new technologies and bioinformatics tools.

3.1 Genetic and genomic studies in allergy

During the last 20 years many efforts were realized in order to identify protective factors that could increase the tolerance against allergens. The main objective of multiple investigations was to identify potential risk factors in the environment and to identify "allergy genes".

Classically there were two main approaches for searching genes related with asthma/allergy diseases: analysis of candidate genes or genome-wide screening, looking for new disease loci or genes (Ober & Hofman., 2006, Risk et al., 1996, Cárdaba et al., 1993, Carlson et al., 2004, Vercelli, 2008, Holloway et al., 2010). Population genetic studies like association studies and linkage analysis have played major roles in identification of several causative genes. Population genetic studies could be either hypothesis driven, which is the case in candidate gene studies, or with no prior hypothesis such as linkage studies. In candidate gene studies, genes are selected from the pathways shown or expected to play role in allergy disease pathogenesis. The advantage of this approach is that candidate genes have biological plausibility and often display known functional consequences that have potentially implications for the disease. Disadvantage is the limitations to discovery novel genes. Candidate gene studies could be based on allele frequency differences between affected and non-affected individuals (case-control studies) or based on transmission distortion or disequilibrium of allele(s) as in family based association studies (Cárdaba et al., 2000, Cárdaba et al., 2002). Candidate genes are supposed to have high sensitivity to detect alleles or variants playing minor role in disease pathogenesis (Risk et al., 1996). Numerous association studies have been published (Vercelli, 2008, Ober &Hofman, 2006, Llanes et al., 2009.), there are almost 1,000 studies that examine polymorphisms in several hundred genes including those involved an innate immunity (TLRs, *CD14*, *CARD15*, etc,), inflammation (e.g. various cytokines, chemokines, etc.), lung function, growth and development (*TGFB1*, *ADRB2*, *NOS1* and *SPINK5*, etc.) and genes implicated as modifiers of responses to environmental exposures (*GSTM*1, *GSTP1*, *GSTT1*). Few candidate genes have been consistently replicated: 54 genes in 2-5 independent samples, 15 genes in 6-10 independent samples and 10 genes in >10 independent samples (Ober &Hofman, 2006).

Linkage studies are usually carried out to identify novel disease loci/genes by genotyping evenly markers in the entire genome, in large extended families. Approximately 20 genome-wide linkage screens have been reported in different study populations to identify chromosomal regions linked to asthma/atopy and one or more allergy-phenotypic feature (Sleiman & Hakonarson, 2010). The lack of statistically power, differences in study design, and genetic differences in the populations studied could be the reason for low reproducibility of results. However, some chromosomal region demonstrated consisted linkage and contained genes biologically relevant in allergy, such as the cytokine cluster on chromosome 5q, *FcεRI-β* on 11q, *IFN-γ* and *STAT6* on 12q, and *IL4R-α* on 16p. Linkage studies followed by positional cloning have identified novel genes which may influence susceptibility to asthma, including *ADAM33, DPP10, PHF11 and GPRA* (Sleiman &Hakonarson, 2010).

Up to now, despite significant findings regarding susceptibility regions and genes in some cases, these studies have still resulted in only a very limited understanding of asthma and allergic diseases. Some of the reasons for the failure to replicate the detection of particular loci across studies and for the modest contribution of each of these susceptibility loci might relate to heterogeneity factors between studies that might be difficult to detect and take into account in small-scale studies (Von Mutius, 2004). However, there are some essential points that are well established by scientific community, as to recognize that few genes might have independent effects, as is typical for Mendelian diseases. It has become clear that the pathogenesis of complex polygenic disorders is dependent on multilayered gene-environment interactions over time, in a model well described by Hersey (2004). Nonetheless, the approaches that have been used to find susceptibility genes, either through linkage or association studies, have for the most part considered one gene at a time. Despite this overly simplistic modelling of asthma and atopy genetics, many important discoveries have been made (Ober, 2005, Blumenthal, 2005).

However, most recently, this kind of studies has been revolutionized by array-based SNP genotyping technologies and the characterization of millions of SNP variants in the human genome. This has made possible the simultaneous determination of the genotype of >500,000 SNPs throughout the genome of a subject. This has allowed the use of genome-wide, hyphotesis-independent association studies that do not require the recruitment and phenotyping of large family-based samples and achieve greater statistically power for the same number of subjects. Genome wide association studies (GWASs) have become feasible in large cohorts of patients and controls. Using this approach, there are many evidences for genetic variants involved in different diseases (Sleiman &Hakonarson, 2010).

GWAS approaches are based on the ability to rapidly analyze genetic variants (mainly single nucleotide polymorphisms (SNPs), usually with a high degree of heterozygosity) across the whole genome to determine which genetic variants are associated with disease susceptibility (case-control studies) or which are associated with measures of disease severity or response to treatment (ie, pharmacogenetics; case-only studies). GWASs are also performed in families, especially trios, which are defined as an affected child with genotyping from both parents but it is generally easier to ascertain and characterize a large number of unrelated cases and control subjects than to study multiple family members (Meyers, 2010). GWASs allows the identification of disease genes with only modest increases in risk, a severe limitation in linkage studies and the very type of genes one expects for common disorders.

To date, several GWASs have been performed with great success in allergic diseases, such as asthma, eczema, and allergic sensitization (Holloway et al., 2010). In mid-2007 the first application of GWA to bronchial asthma was the description of a novel asthma susceptibility locus contains the ORM1-like 3 (*ORMDL3*) and Gasdermin like (*GSDML*) genes on chromosome 17q12-21.1 (Moffatt et al., 2007). Importantly, subsequent studies have replicated the association between variation in the chromosome 17q21 region and asthma in ethnically diverse populations (Leung et al., 2009, Bisgaard et al., 2009, Wu et al., 2010, Galanter et al., 2008, Tavendale et al., 2008). Further allergy-related phenotypes susceptibility genes have been discovered by GWAS as chromosome 5q12 at the region of the phosphodiesterase 4D (*PDE4D)* (Himes et al., 2009) involved in way smooth muscle concentration, an association with asthma and chromosome 1, at the region of *DENND1B* (gene that encodes for a protein that interact s with the TNF-α receptor) (Sleiman & Hakonarson , 2010). Using GWASs significant evidences were observed for asthma association and several genes as *DPP10* (Mathias et al., 2010), *TGFB1, IL1RL1 and CYFIP2* (Wu et al., 2010). In addition six studies have been reported (Sleiman & Hakonarson, 2010) using quantitative triat loci as intermediate phenotypes. A promoter SNP in the *CHI3L1*gene that encodes the chitinase-like protein (YKL-40) was shown to be a major determinant of elevated serum protein, being associated with asthma, bronchial responsiveness and pulmonary function (Ober et al., 2008), *FCERA1A* and *RAD50* genes were associated with IgE levels and increased risk of asthma and atopic eczema (Weidinger et al., 2008), blood eosinophil counts was associated with five loci reached significance, one of which, *IL1RL1* was also associated with asthma in a collection of different populations (Gudbjartsson et al., 2009).

Finally, two large meta-analysis of lung function identified 11 candidate genes/regions. The first (Hancock et al., 2010) found that genes in the *INTS12-GSTCD-NPNT* region were associated with FEV_1, and 8 genes (*HHIP, GPR126, ADAM19, AGER-PPT2, FAM13A, PTCH1, P1D1 and HTR4*) were associated with FEV_1/forced vital capacity ratios. The second (Repapi et al., 2010) identified 4 genes (*HHIP, GSTCD, TNS1* and *HTR4*) associated with FEV_1 and 3 loci (*HHIP, NOTCH4-AGER-PPT2, and THSD4)* associated with FEV_1/forced vital capacity ratios. The important question is to research the relationship among these regions and allergy-related phenotypes.

In conclusion, with the recent advances in genotyping technology and the information provided by Human Genome and International HapMap projects, our ability to locate the genes underlying complex diseases has been dramatically improved. The results from GWASs are the first step. Replication studies are necessary, and meta-analyses are useful to determine the importance of these variants in multiple populations. However, in allergic diseases, environmental factors influence gene regulation/expression for that, gene-environment interactions could be critical in these diseases (Cárdaba et al., 2007). In fact, in the last four years there has been an increase in the research of this field (review in Vercelli, 2010b) and although the gene-environment interactions known to date have been identified through hypothesis-driven research and candidate gene approaches, several efforts are doing in order to develop novel analytical methods at allowing efficient testing for gene-environment interactions in GWASs (Murcray et al., 2009, Chatterjee et al., 2009, Vineis et al., 2008). These studies could be a new era of gene-environment-wide interaction studies (GEWIS) (Khoury &Wacholder, 2009) that may change our understanding of gene-environment interactions and their impact on complex disease susceptibility (Vercelli, 2010).

It is possible to group the genes identified until now as contributing to allergic disease into 4 broad groups (Holloway et al., 2010): First, there is a group of genes that are identified are involved directly modulating response to environmental exposures. The second major group includes many of the genes identified by hypothesis-independent genome-wide approaches and is a group of genes involved in maintaining the integrity of the epithelial barrier at the mucosal surface and signalling to the immune system after environmental exposure. The third group are those that regulate the immune response, the TH1/TH2 differentiation and effector functions, and others that might regulate the level of inflammation that occurs at the end organ for allergic disease.
Finally, given the large amount of GWAS data available for many diseases, the results can be interrogated across studies to determine whether the same genes are being observed in different diseases, even if there is not known relationship between the diseases. After analysis of GWAS results from across 118 studies (Johnson & O´Donnell, 2009) evidence for the MHC region on chromosome 6 was observed across many studies, and genes involved in cell adhesion, signal transduction, and protein phosporilation were the most likely to be observed in different diseases entities. This bioinformatics approach can be useful for identifying potential similarities between disease processes that can be investigated further (Meyers, 2010).
Anyway, functional biologic studies to understand the role of the identified genes, genetic variants and interactions are crucial to further our understanding of disease pathogenesis.

3.2 Analysis of gene-expression or transcriptomic in allergic diseases

Because microarray analysis is a more mature technique than the other approaches and because of the relative ease of working with nucleic acids, microarray remain the -omics technique that is most likely to have early applications in diagnosis or prognosis.
One of the most popular omic-approach for disease gene identification has been the analysis of gene-expression by microarrays, which take advantage of the fact that transcript of various genes (until all the genome) can be assayed at large scale simultaneously (Rolph et al., 2006). Using both human subjects and animal models a number of studies have identified novel genes/pathways or validated others that play important role in asthma pathogenesis and may have therapeutic potentials (Rolph et al., 2006). Combined with animal models this technology has played pivotal role in identification of genes/molecules involved in complex diseases. Animal models are suitable as confounding factors can be better controlled and tissue samples can be harvested sufficiently with easy. Also, identical genetic background of the inbred animal strains allow for dissection of environmental factors in influencing gene regulation in different pathological conditions (Kumar & Ghosh, 2009).
DNA microarrays can be used to compare differential gene-expression between control and case or patients before and after treatment, in order to find new genes and disease mechanisms and to define molecular signatures that can be useful in the diagnosis or classification of the disease and specific treatments. Major applications of this methodology have been related with cancer disease or single-genes disorders but in complex disorders, as allergic diseases, the number of studies is lower and only in the last years, this field is giving some interesting results.
The first review of microarray technology in allergic diseases (Benson et al., 2004), described how some pioneers works identified differentially expressed genes between patient and

controls in allergic rhinitis or atopic dermatitis and how in a study of asthma, a combination of genes was showed to more accurately discriminate between the asthmatics and healthy controls than IgE (Brutsche et al., 2002). But most importantly, the authors remarked the distinctive characteristic of microarrays to identify whole groups of functionally related genes, rather than individuals, and the effects of specific cytokines relevant to allergy, as for example, the finding that a TH2 cytokine as IL-13, induce distinct transcriptional programs in different kind of cells (Lee et al., 2001), as well as pathways (Benson et al., 2002, Zimmermann et al., 2003).

Most recently, interesting advances in allergic diseases has been associated with microarray studies. I would like to emphasis three major kinds of advances: Firstly the finding and verification of differentially expressed genes, with the description of many potential biomarkers and/or therapeutic targets that are still being validated, evaluated and explored with no clinical diagnostic or therapeutic benefit to date (Hansel et al., 2008, Sääf AM et al., 2008, Izuhara & Saito, 2006, Kuperman et al., 2005, Rolph et al., 2006, Tyner et al., 2006, Ricciardolo et al., 2005, Hansel & Diette, 2007, Woodruff et al., 2007, Hakonarson et al., 2005, Jones et al., 2009) but with a high potential. Secondly, the possibility to find molecular signatures associated with clinical subphenotypes, as has been demonstrated in asthma where at least two distinct molecular phenotypes defined by degree of TH2 inflammation were described (Woodruff et al., 2009). Interestingly, non-Th2–driven asthma represents a significant proportion of patients and responds poorly to current therapies. Most recently, gene expression patterns of TH2 inflammation and intercellular communication have been described in asthmatic airways (Choy et al., 2011). These results suggest that a predominant pattern of differential gene expression in asthma is related to TH2-driven airway inflammation; however, this pathway is linked to a large number of other factors associated with aspects of airway pathophysiology. An unsolved question is whether TH2 inflammation is a cause or a consequence of the extended network of inflammatory and regulatory factors described as implicated. And finally, and interesting field is the possibility to discover dysregulated pathways by the analysis of modules that include tightly interacting genes, usually functional related genes. This approach was recently used to identify an inhibitory role for IL7R in allergic inflammation (Mobini et al., 2009). The gene expression profiles can be used to identify key regulatory networks, to identify novel potential candidate genes, and to define phenotypes, which can then serve as quantitative traits for genetic studies (Baye et al., 2010). An integrated genetic/genomic approach allows the mapping of the genetic factors that underpin individual differences in quantitative levels of expression. ArrayExpress and Gene Expression Omnibus are the two major public data repository for experimental microarray data with multiple gene annotations, including gene symbol, GO terms and disease associations. Integration of molecular and functional information it is necessary and the bioiformatic is an area essential for advancing in this field. With this integration, using publicly available gene expression datasets from multiple sources and tools a functional and regulatory map of asthma (Novershther et al., 2008) was described.

An entire field of biology (Systems Biology) has emerged, with the goal of unravelling the complex networks of cells and signals underlying all biological processes. This ongoing exploration should lead to better tools to help us interpret gene expression microarray data and will ultimately allow us to leverage this technology in the diagnosis and treatment of diseases.

3.3 Use of protein microarrays in allergy

DNA microarrays are limited to provide information on the identity or amount or RNA or DNA present in a sample. Translational products of genes can not be analyzed on such arrays and, therefore, require the use of polypeptide-based array. Most drug targets are proteins, therefore, protein and peptides microarrays are set to have an important impact on drug discovery. An important challenge when producing protein microarrays is maintaining functionality, such as post-transcriptional modifications and phosporylation.

Due to the improvement in proteomics methodologies, several important proteomic applications have been used in allergy diseases (revised by Lucas, 2010). Basic research microarray technology has been used for the study of interactions among allergenic proteins, immunoglobulins and T cell receptors, with a view to developing genetic modifications which can yield hypoallergenic variants of plant proteins (Singh et al., 1999). Microarrays have been applied in the investigation of clonal diversity (Pinilla et al., 1999) and immune response heterogeneity among patients (Sheffler et al., 2005) and to establish the clinical correlations between antibody diversity and the allergic manifestations (Beyer et al., 2003, Chatschatee et al., 2001,). Microarray technology has been shown to be very useful for mapping and characterising allergenic epitopes (Lin et al., 2009). An example is represented by cow's milk allergens with differentiation between IgE and IgG4 patterns for sequential epitopes of alpha (s1)-, alpha (s2)-, beta-and kappa-caseins and beta-lactoglobulin in reactive patients and tolerant individuals (Cerecedo et al., 2008).

But one of the most important applications of proteomic in the allergy field is the microarray of allergic components that offer the possibility to study hundreds of allergenic components (recombinant or purified) in a single test, and using a very small amount of serum sample. This kind of studies or allergenic component-resolved diagnosis (CDR) microarrays, afford an image of patient sensitisation at molecular level, allowing the identification of the potential disease-eliciting molecules. This analysis led to the development of a new concept in allergy diagnosis: molecular diagnosis (Ferrer et al., 2009, Lindholm et al., 2006). Performance characteristics for allergens so far tested are comparable with the diagnostic tests currently used (Janh-Smith et al., 2003, Wohrl et al., 2006, Ott et al., 2008, Ebo et al., 2010).

One of the most important utility of molecular diagnosis in allergy is its ability to reveal the allergens to which patients are sensitized, including primary or species-specific allergens and markers of cross-reactivity to proteins with similar protein structures may help to evaluate the risk of reaction on exposure to different allergen sources (Sastre, 2010).

Using microarray-based testing makes it possible to determine the IgE reactivity profile of a patient and assess their clinical pattern. The whole profile can give complementary information to the results achieved by single allergen components or extract-based testing. *In vitro* test results should always be evaluated together with the clinical history, because allergen sensitization does not necessarily imply a clinical reaction. The use of a predefined large number of allergen components in microarray systems can facilitate this task, although such an approach puts greater demands on interpretation.

The use of IgE epitope mapping of allergens using microarray-based immunoassay will probably be the next step in development (Lin et al., 2009).

Another area of research looks to establish whether information from molecular medicine can provide an indication as to the chances of tolerance development or if the allergy will be persistent. Molecular medicine can also be a support tool for adapting treatment strategy to the particularities of each patient in a timely manner, open the possibility of personalizing

the actions to be taken, as include targeted allergen exposure reduction advice, selection of suitable allergens for specific immunotherapy (SIT) or the need to perform food challenges.
Although the fundamental role of two-dimensional gel electrophoresis combined with other proteomics techniques in the characterization of allergens, other proteomic approach as SELDI-TOF-MS has been useful for discovering biomarkers in asthma-related inflammation and remodelling, in a mice model (Calvo et al., 2009) and recently, the use of LC-MS/MS analysis combined with genomic expression analyses has been described for identifying novel potential markers of glucocorticoids treatment in intermittent allergic rhinitis (Wang et al., 2011).

4. Conclusions

In the last few years, our knowledge about of the human genome improved considerable. Still we are very far from the total understanding of the genomic background of complex diseases, but the news high-throughput technologies together with other complementary tools, as bioinfomatic, have contributed to highly increase our understanding of these complex disorders, and most importantly, have produced a change in the focusing of biological studies. The concept of biological systems open a broader, integrated view of biological system will yield a more complete understanding of disease, providing improved tools for identifying prognostic, diagnostic, biomarkers and treatment.
However, we need many efforts before to design effective intervention in these diseases. New approaches and access to high quality, well-annotated datasets that will allow us to gain insight into novel process that we can associate with biological outcomes such as disease are needed. Microarray themselves provide only testable hypotheses, not firm conclusions, and validating is necessary. This complexity is reflect of the large number of new genes (and new splice variants and the expanding classes of noncoding RNAs) discovered by the ongoing sequencing of genomes and transcripts. Complicating this is the lack of information on molecular interactions; genes expression can only measure gene transcription, not translation, and certainly not the complex regulatory pathways and interactions leading to the array result, a snapshot of one sample at one moment. This leads to the current state of gene expression microarray data in asthma/allergy, where although many differentially expressed genes have been found and verify potential biomarkers and/or therapeutic targets are still being validated, evaluated and explored with no clinical diagnostic or therapeutic benefit to date. Molecular phenotyping of diseases, using technologies such as gene expression microarrays, has the potential to provide insights into the phenotypic heterogeneity of disease and the identification of associated biomarkers as well as strategies to select patients with an increased potential to respond to molecularly targeted therapies. However, the efficacy of molecularly targeted therapies in a clinical setting depends on both appropriate patient selection and appropriate outcome selection.
We need to understand individual gene-gene, gene-protein, and protein-protein network interactions in human health and disease. An understanding of these networks should enable the opportunity to diagnose disease before it is clinically manifest or to define the targeted to be regulated.
However, some areas have been considerable improvement with the high-throughput methodologies. Some microarray applications, as allergenic component microarrays offer an elegant way to avoid the problem of allergen standardisation and false polysensitisation. The possibility of determining specific IgE antibodies against multiple recombinants and

purified natural allergen components has allowed for the development of Molecular Diagnosis. This novel diagnostic technology is minimally invasive, makes use of small sample volumes, offers quantitative results, and constitutes a multianalytic test, thus facilitating its incorporation to clinical use. This technology opens the door to personalised medical practice, by allowing diagnosis and planning at molecular level, specific for each patient, with a known and balanced dosing of standardised allergens for immunotherapy. Molecular Diagnosis can be a support tool for reaching appropriate and timely clinical decisions on patients, which afford clinicians the possibility of individualizing the actions taken.

In conclusion, although the advances in the understanding of molecular basis of allergic diseases have been highly improved by new "omics-approaches" and the potential it is undoubted, due to the complexity of this kind of diseases, many efforts before to design effective intervention are needed. These kinds of studies highlight the importance of understanding the underlying basis of heterogeneity in disease and the relationships between targeted pathways and in vivo patophysiology for developing strategies to identify patient populations with maximal potential benefit from molecularly targeted therapies. Besides, many other concepts as well as missing heritability (study of rare variants or minor allele frequency) gene-environment interactions, epigenetic effects, and well-defined consistent phenotypes across large population sets should be analyzed. Although the future is very promising and we have made great advances, still there is a long way to walk.

5. Acknowledgment

We are grateful to the F.I.S. FJD-UTE (CP05/0183), "Incorporación de Investigadores al SNS" Program, for financial support.

Funding sources: Supported in part by research grants CP05/00183, PI07/0024, PI10/0025 and CIBERES (ISCIII, 0013) from the Fondo de Investigación Sanitaria (Ministerio de Sanidad y Consumo, Spain). M. Aguerri and D. Calzada are supported by Fundación Conchita Rábago, Madrid, Spain.

6. References

Alizadeh, A.A.; Eisen, M.B.; Davis, R.H.; Ma, C. ; lossos, I.S. ; Rosenwald, A. ; Boldrick, J.C.; Sabet, H.; Tran, T.; Yu, X.; Powell, J.I.; Yang, L.; Marti, G.E.; Moore, T.; Hudson, J.Jr; lu, L.; Lewis, D.B.; Tibshirani, R.; Sherlock, G.; Chan, W.C.; Greiner, T.C.; Weisenburguer, D.D.; Armitage, J.O.; Warnke, R.; Levy, R.; Wilson, W.; Grever, M.R.; Byrd, J.C.; Botstein, D.; Brown, P.O. & Staudt, L.M. (2000). Distinct types of diffuse large B-cell lymphoma identified by gene expression profiling. *Nature*, Vol. 403, No. 6769 (Feb 2000), pp. (503-511) , ISSN 0028-0836

Alon, U.; Barkai, N. ; Notterman, D.A. ; Gish, K. ; Ybarra, S. ;Mack, D..& Levine, A.J.(1999). Broad patterns of gene expression revealed by clustering analysis of tumor and normal colon tissues probed by oligonucleotide arrays. *Proc Natl Acad Sci USA* ,No. 96 (Jun 1999), pp. (6745-6750), ISSN 0027-8424

Alwine, JC.; Kemp, DJ. & Stark, GR. (1977). Method for detection of specific RNAs in agarose gels by transfer to diazobenzyloxymethyl-paper and hybridization with

DNA probes. *Proc Natl Acad Sci U S A*, Vol.74, No.12, (December 1977), pp.5350-5354, ISSN 1091-6490.

Baye, TM., Martín, LJ& Hershey, GKH. (2010). Application of genetic/genomic approaches to allergic disorders. *J Allergy Clin Immunol*, Vol.126, pp 425-436.

Benson, M.; Olsson, M.; Rudemo, M.; Wennergren, G. & Cardell, LO. (2004). Pros and cons of microarray technology in allergy research. *Clin Exp Allergy*, Vol.34, No.7, (July 2004), pp.1001-1006, IISN 0954-7894.

Bergman, AC. ; Benjamin, T. ; Alaiya, A. ; Waltham, M. ; Sakaguchi, K. ; Franzen, B. ; Linder, S. ; Bergman, T. ; Auer, G.; Appella, E.; Wirth, PJ. & Jörnvall, H.(2000). Identification of gel-separated tumor markers proteins by mass spectrometry. *Electrophoresis*, Vol. 21, No. 3 (Feb 2000), pp. (679-686), ISSN 0173-0835

Beyer, K.; Ellman-Grunther, L.; Jarvinen, KM.; Wood, RA.; Hourihane, J & Sampson, HA. (2003). Measurement of peptide-specific IgE as an additional tool in identifying patients with clinical reactivity to peanuts. *J Allergy Clin Immunol*, Vol.112, No.1, (July 2003), pp.202-207, IISN 0091-6749.

Bisgaard, H.; Bønnelykke, K.; Sleiman, PM.; Brasholt, M.; Chawes, B.; Kreiner-Møller, E.; Stage, M.; Kim, C.; Tavendale, R.; Baty, F.; Pipper, CB.; Palmer, CN. & Hakonarsson, H.(2009). Chromosome 17q21 gene variants are associated with asthma and exacerbations but not atopy in early childhood. *Am J Respir Crit Care Med*, Vol.179, No.3, (February 2009), pp.179-185, IISN 1073-449X.

Bloom, G. ; Yang, IV ; Boulware, D. ; Kwong, K.Y.; Coppola, D.; Eschrich, S.; Quackenbush, J. & Yeatman, T.J.(2004). Multi-platform, multi-site, microarraybased human tumor classification. *Am J Pathol* , Vol. 164, No. 1 (Jan 2004), pp. (9-16), ISSN 0002-9440

Blumenthal, MN. (2005). The role of genetics in the development of asthma and atopy. *Curr Opin Allergy Clin Immunol* Vol. 5, No.2, (April 2005), pp141-145.

Brutsche, MH.; Joos, L.; Carlen Brutsche, IE.; Bissinger, R.; Tamm, M.; Custovic, A. & Woodcock, A.(2002). Array-based diagnostic gene-expression score for atopy and asthma. *J Allergy Clin Immunol*, Vol.109, No.2, (February 2002), pp.271-273, IISN 0091-6749.

Calvo, FQ.; Fillet, M.; de Seny, D.; Meuwis, MA.; Maree, R.; Crahay, C.; Paulissen, G.; Rocks, N.; Gueders, M.; Wehenkel, L.; Merville, MP.; Louis, R.; Foidart, JM.; Noël, A. & Cataldo, D. (2009). Biomarker discovery in asthma-related inflammation and remodeling. *Proteomics*, Vol.9, No.8, (April 2009), pp.2163-2170, IISN 1615-9853.

Caprioli, RM.; Farmer, TB.; Gile, J.(1997). Molecular imaging of biological samples: localization of pepetides and proteins using MALDI_TOF MS. *Anal Chem*, Vol. 69, No. 23 (Dec 1997), pp. (4751-476), ISSN 0003-2700

Cárdaba, B.; Vilches, C.; Martín, E.; de Andrés, B.; del Pozo, V.; Hernández, D.; Gallardo, S.; Fernández, JC.; Villalba, M.; Rodríguez, R.; Basomba, A.; Kreisler, M.; Palomino, P. & Lahoz, C. (1993). DR7 and DQ2 are associated with IgE response to the main antigen of Olive pollen (Ole e I) in allergic patients. *Human Immunol*, Vol. 38, No 4, pp. (293-299). ISSN: 0198-8859.

Cárdaba, B.; Cortegano, I.; Florido, F.; Arrieta, I.; Aceituno, E.; del Pozo, V.; Gallardo, S.; Rojo, M.; Palomino, P & Lahoz, C. (2000). Genetic restritions in olive pollen allergy. *J Allergy Clin Immunol*. Vol. 105, No 2, pp. (292-298). ISSN: 0091-6749.

Cárdaba, B.; Cortegano, I.; Florido, F.; Civantos, E.; del Pozo, V.; Gallardo, S.; Rojo, M.; Palomino, P & Lahoz, C. (2002). Update in the understanding of genetic predisposition to olive pollen sensitization. *Allergy*. Vol. 57, S71, pp. (41-46). ISSN: 1398-9995.

Cárdaba, B.; Llanes, E.; Chacártegui, M.; Sastre, B.; López, E.; Mollá, R.; del Pozo, V.; Florido, F.; Quiralte, J.; Palomino, P & Lahoz, C. (2007). Modulation of Allergic Response by gene-environment interaction: Olive pollen allergy. *J Invest Allergy Clin Immunol.* Vol. 17, No 1, pp. (83-87). ISSN: 1018-9068.

Cargile, BJ.; Bundy, JL. & Stephenson, JL Jr (2004). Potential for false positive identifications from large databases through tandem mass spectrometry. *J Proteome Res*, Vol. 3, No. 5 (Oct 2004), pp. (1082-1085), ISSM *1535-3893.*

Carlson, CS.; Eberle, MA.; Kruglyak, L. & Nickerson, DA. (2004). Mapping complex disease loci in whole-genome association studies. *Nature*. Vol. 429, pp446-452.

Catt, K.; Niall, HD. & Tregear, GW. (1966). Solid-phase radioimmunoassay of human growth hormone. *J Lab Clin MedBiochem J*, Vol.70, No.5, (November 1967), pp.820-830, ISSN 0264-6021.

Cerecedo, I.; Zamora, J.; Shreffler, WG.; Lin, J.; Bardina, L.; Dieguez, MC.; Wang, J.; Muriel, A.; de la Hoz, B & Sampson, HA. (2008). Mapping of the IgE and IgG4 sequential epitopes of milk allergens with a peptide microarray-based immunoassay. *J Allergy Clin Immunol*, Vol.122, No.3, (September 2008), pp.589-594, IISN 0091-6749.

Chatchatee, P.; Järvinen, KM.; Bardina, L.; Vila, L.; Beyer, K. & Sampson, HA. (2001). Identification of IgE and IgG binding epitopes on beta- and kappa-casein in cow's milk allergic patients. *Clin Exp Allergy*, Vol.31, No.8, (August 2001), pp.1256-1262, IISN 54-7894.

Chatterjee ,N. & Wacholder, S. (2009). Invited commentary: efficient testing of gene-environment interaction. *Am J Epidemiol*, Vol.169, No.2, (January 2009), pp. 231-233, IISN 0002-9262.

Choy, DF.; Modrek, B.; Abbas, AR.; Kummerfeld, S.; Clark, HF.; Wu, LC.; Fedorowicz, G.; L *J Immunol*, Vol.186, No.3, (February 2011), pp.1861-1869, IISN 0022-1767.

Duffy, DL.; Martin, NG.; Battistutta, D; Hopper, JL. & Mathews, JD. (1990). Genetics of asthma and hay fever in Australian twins. *Am Rev Respir Dis.*, Vol.142, No.6 Pt 1, (December 1990), pp.1351-1358, IISN 0003-0805.

Ebo, DG.; Hagendorens, MM.; De Knop, KJ; Verweij, MM.; Bridts, CH.; De Clerck, LS. & Stevens, WJ. Component.resolved diagnosis from latex allergy by microarray. *Clin Exp Allergy*, Vol. 40, No. 2 (Feb 2010), pp. (349-358), ISSN 0954-4538

Ekins, R.; Chu, F & Biggart, E. (1990). Multispot, multianalyte, immunoassay. *Ann Biol Clin (Paris)*, Vol.48, No.9, pp.655-666, ISSN 0003-3898.

Ekins, R.; Chu, FW. (1999). Microarrays: their origins and applications. *Trends Biotechnol*, Vol.17, No.6, (June 1999), pp.217-218, ISSN 0167-7799.

Engvall, E. (2005) Perspective on the historical not on EIA/ELISA by Dr. R. M. Lequin. *Clin Chem*, Vol.51, No.12, (December 2005), pp.2225, ISSN 0272-2712.

Essader, AS.; Cargile, BJ. ; Bundy, JL. & Stephenson JL.(2005). A comparison of inmobilized pH gradient isoelectric focusing and strong-cation.exchange chromatography as a first dimension in shotgun proteomics. *Proteomics*, Vol. 5, No. 1 (Jan 2005), pp. (24-34), ISNN *1615-9853*

Farmer, TB.; Caprioli, RM. (1991) Assesting the multimeric states of proteins:studies using laser desorption mass spectrometry. *Biol Mass Spectrometry* , Vol. 20, No. 12 (Dec 1991), pp. (796-800), ISSN 1052-9306

Ferrer, M.; Sanz, ML.; Sastre, J; Bartra, J.; del Cuvillo, A. ; Montoso, J.; Jaurequi, I; Dávila, I.; Mullol, J. & Valero, A. Molecular diagnosis in allergology: application of the microarray technique. *J Investig Allergol Clin Immunol*, Vol. 19, Suppl 1 (2009), pp. (19-24), ISSN 1018-9068.

Galanter ,J.; Choudhry, S.; Eng, C.; Nazario, S.; Rodríguez-Santana, JR.; Casal, J.; Torres-Palacios, A.; Salas, J.; Chapela, R.; Watson, HG.; Meade, K.; LeNoir, M.; Rodríguez-Cintrón, W.; Avila, PC. & Burchard EG.(2008). ORMDL3 gene is associated with asthma in three ethnically diverse populations. *Am J Respir Crit Care Med*, Vol177, No.11, (June 2008), pp.1194-2000, IISN 1073-449X.

Golub, TR.; Slonim, DK.; Tamayo, P.; Huard, C.; Gaasenbeek, M.; Mesirov, J.P.; Coller, H.; Loh, M.L.; Howning, J.R.; Caligiuri, M.A.;Bloomfield, C.D. & Lander, E.S.(1999). Molecular classification of cancer:class discovery and class prediction by gene expression monitoring. *Science*, Vol. 286, No. 5439 (Oct 1999), pp. (531-537), ISSN 0036-8075

Golub, TR.; Slonim, DK.; Tamayo, P.; Huard, C.; Gaasenbeek, M.; Mesirov, JP.; Coller, H.; Loh ML.; Downing, JR.; Caliqiuri, MA.; Bloomfield, CD. & Lander, ES. (1999). Molecular classification of cancer:class discovery and class prediction by gene expresión monitoring. *Science*, Vol. 286, No. 5439 (Oct 1999), pp. (531-537), ISSN 0036-8075.

Gudbjartsson, DF.; Bjornsdottir, US.; Halapi, E.; Helgadottir, A.; Sulem, P.; Jonsdottir, GM.; Thorleifsson, G.; Helgadottir, H.; Steinthorsdottir, V.; Stefansson, H.; Williams, C.; Hui, J.; Beilby, J.; Warrington, NM.; James, A.; Palmer, LJ.; Koppelman, GH.; Heinzmann, A.; Krueger, M.; Boezen, HM.; Wheatley, A.; Altmuller, J.; Shin, HD.; Uh, ST.; Cheong, HS.; Jonsdottir, B.; Gislason, D.; Park, CS.; Rasmussen, LM.; Porsbjerg, C.; Hansen, JW.; Backer, V.; Werge, T.; Janson, C.; Jönsson, UB.; Ng, MC.; Chan, J.; So, WY.; Ma, R.; Shah, SH.; Granger, CB.; Quyyumi, AA.; Levey, AI.; Vaccarino, V.; Reilly, MP.; Rader, DJ.; Williams, MJ.; van Rij, AM.; Jones, GT.; Trabetti, E.; Malerba, G.; Pignatti, PF.; Boner, A.; Pescollderungg, L.; Girelli, D.; Olivieri, O.; Martinelli, N.; Ludviksson, BR.; Ludviksdottir, D.; Eyjolfsson, GI.; Arnar, D.; Thorgeirsson, G.; Deichmann, K.; Thompson, PJ.; Wjst, M.; Hall, IP.; Postma, DS.; Gislason, T.; Gulcher, J.; Kong, A.; Jonsdottir, I.; Thorsteinsdottir, U. & Stefansson, K. Sequence variants affecting eosinophil numbers associate with asthma and myocardial infarction. (2009). *Nat Genet,* Vol.41, No.3, (March 2009), pp.342-347, IISN 1061-4036.

Hakonarson, H.; Bjornsdottir, US.; Halapi, E.; Bradfield, J.; Zink, F.; Mouy, M.; Helgadottir, H.; Gudmundsdottir, AS.; Andrason, H.; Adalsteinsdottir, AE; Kristjansson, K; Birkisson, I; Arnason. T.; Andresdottir, M.; Gislason, D.; Gislason, T.; Gulcher, JR. & Stefansson, K. (2005). Profiling of genes expressed in peripheral blood mononuclear cells predicts glucocorticoid sensivity in asthma patients. *Proc Natl Acad Sci U S A*. Vol.102, No.41, (October 2005), pp.14789, ISSN 0027-8424.

Hancock, DB.; Eijgelsheim, M.; Wilk, JB.; Gharib, SA.; Loehr, LR.; Marciante, KD.; Franceschini, N.; van Durme, YM.; Chen, TH.; Barr, RG.; Schabath, MB.; Couper,

DJ.; Brusselle, GG.; Psaty, BM.; van Duijn, CM.; Rotter, JI.; Uitterlinden, AG.; Hofman, A.; Punjabi, NM.; Rivadeneira, F.; Morrison, AC.; Enright, PL.; North, KE.; Heckbert, SR.; Lumley, T.; Stricker, BH.; O'Connor, GT. & London, SJ. (2010). Meta-analyses of genome-wide association studies identify multiple loci associated with pulmonary function. *Nat Genet*, Vol.42, No.1, (January 2010), pp.45-52, IISN 1061-4036.

Hansel, NN.; Cheadle, C.; Diette, GB.; Wright, J.; Thompson, KM.; Barnes, KC. & Georas, SN. (2008), Analysis of CD4+ T-cell gene expression in allergic subjects using two different microarray platforms. *Allergy,* Vol.63, No.3, (March 2008), pp.366-369, IISN 0105-4538.

Hansel, NN. & Diette, GB. (2007). Gene expression profiling in human asthma. *Proc Am Thorac Soc*, Vol.4, (June 2006), pp.32-36, ISSN 1546-3222.

Hersey, KG. (2004). Is it all in our genes?. The "mite-y" truth. *J Allergy Clin Immunol,* Vol.113, pp392-394. IISN 0091-6749.

Himes BE, Hunninghake GM, Baurley JW, Rafaels NM, Sleiman P, Strachan DP et al. (2009). Genome-wide associations analysis identifies PDE4D as an asthma-susceptibility gene. *Am J Hum Genet*, Vol.84, pp581-93.

Holloway, JW.; Yang, IA. & Holgate, ST. (2010). Genetics of allergic disease. *J Allergy Clin Immunol, Vol.125*, ppS81-94.

International Human Genome Sequencing Consortium (IHGSC). (2004). Finish the euchromatic sequence of the human genome. *Nature*, Vol.431, pp931-945.

Izuhara, K.; Saito H. (2006). Microarray-based identification of novel biomarkers in asthma. *Allergol Int*, Vol.55, No.4, (December 2006), pp.361-367, IISN 1323-8930.

Janh-Schmid, B.; Harranegg, C.; Hiller, R.; Bohle, B.; Ebner, C.; Scheiner, O. & Mueller, MW. (2003). Allergen microarray: comparison of microarray: comparison of microarray using recombinant allergens with conventional diagnosis methods to detect allergen-specific serum immunoglobulin. *Clin Exp Allergy,* Vol. 33, No. 10 (Oct 2003), pp. 1443-1449, ISSN 0954-7894.

Johnson, AD. & O'Donnell, CJ. (2009). An open access database of genome-wide association results. *BMC Med Genet,* Vol.10, (January 2009), pp.6, IISN 1471-2350.

Jones, SM.; Pons, L.; Roberts, JL.; Scurlock, AM.; Perry, TT.; Kulis, M.; Shreffler, WG.; Steele, P.; Henry, KA.; Adair, M.; Francis, JM.; Durham, S.; Vickery, BP.; Zhong, X. & Burks, AW. (2009). Clinical efficacy and immune regulation with peanut oral immunotherapy. *J Allergy Clin Immunol,* Vol.124, No.2, (August 2009), pp.292-300, IISN 0091-6749.

Kafatos, FC.; Jones, CW. & Efstratiadis, A. (1979). Determination of nucleic acid sequence homologies and relative concentrations by a dot hybridization procedure. *Nucleic Acids Res*, Vol.7, No.6, (November 1979), pp.1541-1552, ISSN 0305-1048.

Khan, J.; Simon, R.; Bittner, M.; Chen, Y.; Leighton, SB.; Pohida, T.; Smith, PD.; Jiang, Y.; Gooden, GC.; Trent, JM. & Meltzer, PS. (1998), *Cancer Res,* Vol.58, No.22, (November 1998), pp.5009-5013, IISN 1533-0346.

Khoury, MJ. & Wacholder, S. (2009). Invited commentary: from genome-wide association studies to gene-environment-wide interaction studies--challenges and opportunities. *Am J Epidemiol,* Vol.169, No.2, (January 2009), pp.227-230, IISN 0002-9262.

Kumar, A. & Ghosh, B. (2009). Genetics of asthma; a molecular biologist perspective. *Clin Mol Allergy*, Vol.7, pp1-9.

Kuperman, DA.; Lewis, CC.; Woodruff, PG.; Rodriguez, MW.; Yang, YH.; Dolganov, GM.; Fahy, JV. &, Erle, DJ. (2005). Dissecting asthma using focused transgenic modeling and functional genomics. *J Allergy Clin Immunol*, Vol.116, No.2, (August 2005), pp.305-311, IISN 0091-6749

Llanes, E.; Quiralte, J.; López, E.; Sastre, B.; Chacártegui, M.; del Pozo, V.; Palomino P.; Lahoz, C & Cárdaba, B. (2009). Analysis of polymorphisms in olive pollen allergy: IL13, IL4RA, IL5 and β_2Adrenergic Receptor genes. *Int Archives Allergy Clin Immunol*. Vol. 148, pp.(228-238). ISSN: 1010-2438.

Levy, S.; Sutton, G. ; Ng, PC. ;Feuk, L. ; Halpern, AL .; Walenz, BP.;Axelrod, N.; Huang, J.; Kirkness, EF.; Denisov, G.; Lin, Y.; MacDonald, JR.; Pang AW.; Shago, M.; Stockwell, TB.; Tsiamouri, A.; Bafna, V.; Bansal, V.; Kratitz, SA.; Busam, DA.; Beeson, KY.; McIntosh, TC.; Remigton, KA.; Abril, JF.; Grill, J.; Borman, J; Rogers, YH.; Frazier, ME.; Scherer, SW.; Strausberg, RL. & Venter, JC.(2007). The diploid genome sequence of an individual human. *PLos Biol*, Vol 5, No 10 (Sep 2007), pp. e254, ISSN *1545-7885*

Lee, JH.; Kaminski, N.; Dolganov, G.; Grunig, G.; Koth, L.; Solomon, C.; Erle, DJ. & Sheppard, D. (2001). Interleukin-13 induces dramatically different transcriptional programs in three human airway cell types. *Am J Respir Cell Mol Biol*, Vol.25, No.4, (October 2001), pp.474-485, IISN 1044-1549.

Leung, TF.; Sy, HY.; Ng, MC.; Chan, IH.; Wong, GW.; Tang, NL.; Waye, MM. & Lam, CW. (2009). Asthma and atopy are associated with chromosome 17q21 markers in Chinese children. *Allergy*, Vol.64, No.4, (April 2009), pp.621-628, IISN 0105-4538.

Lidholm, J.; Ballmer-Weber, BK.; Mari, A. & Vieths, S.(2006). Component-resolved diagnostics in food allergy. *Curr Opin Allergy Clin Immunol*, Vol. 6, No. 3 (Jun 2006), pp. (234-240), ISSN 1528-4050

Liebler, DC.(2004). Shotgun mass spec goes independent. *Nat Methods* , Vol. 1, No. 1 (Oct 2004), pp.(16-17), ISSN 1548-7091.

Lin, J.; Bardina, L. & Shreffler, WG. (2009). Microarrayed allergen molecules for diagnostics of allergy. *Methods Mol Biol*, Vol.524, pp.259-272, IISN 1064-3745.

Lin, J.; Bardina, L.; Shreffler, WG, Andreae, DA.; Ge, Y.; Wang, J.; Bruni, FM.; Fu, Z.; Han, Y. & Sampson, HA.(2009). Development of a novel peptide microarray for large-scale epitope mapping of food allergens. *J Allergy Clin Immunol*, Vol. 124, No. 2 (Aug 2009), pp. (315-322), ISSN 0091-6749

Link, AJ.; Eng, J.; Schieltz, DM.; Carmack, E.; Mize, GJ.; Morris, DR.; Garvik, BM. & Yates, JR. 3rd. (1999). Direct analysis of protein complexes using mass spectrometry. *Nat Biotechnol* 1999, Vol. 17, No. 7 (Jul 1999), pp.(676-682), ISSN *1087-0156*.

Locksley, R.M. (2009). Mine lives: plasticity among T helper cell subsets. *J Exp Med*. Vol. 206, pp 1643-1646.

Lucas, J.M. (2010).Microarrays: Molecular allergology and nanotechnology for personalized medicine, *Allergol Immunopathol (Madr)*, Vol.38, No.4, (August 2010), pp. 217-233, ISSN 0301-0546.

Meyers, D.A. (2010). Genetics of asthma and allergy: What have we learned?. *J Allergy Clin Immunol*, Vol. 126, pp.439-446.

Mobini, R.; Andersson, BA.; Erjefält, J.; Hahn-Zoric, M.; Langston, MA.; Perkins, AD.; Cardell, LO. & Benson, M. (2009). A module-based analytical strategy to identify novel disease-associated genes shows an inhibitory role for interleukin 7 Receptor in allergic inflammation. *BMC Syst Biol*, Vol.12, No.3, (February 2009), pp.19, IISN 1752-0509.

Moch, H.; Schraml, P.; Bubendorf, L.; Mirlacher, M.; Kononen, J.;Gasser, T.; Mihatsch, M.J.; Kallioniemi, O.P. & Sauter, G.(1999). Identification of prognostic parameters for renal cell carnicoma by cDNA arrays and cell chips. *Verh Dtsch Ges Pathol*, No. 83 (1999), pp. (225-232), ISSN 0070-4113.

Moffatt, M,; Kabesch, M.; Liang, L.; Dixon, AL.; Strachan, D.; Heath, S.; et al. (2007). Genetic variants regulating ORMDL3 expression contribute to the risk of childhood asthma. *Nature*, Vol. 448, pp470-473.

Murcray, CE.; Lewinger, JP. & Gauderman, WJ. (2009). Gene-environment interaction in genome-wide association studies. *Am J Epidemiol*, Vol.169, No.2, (January 2009), pp.219-226, IISN 0002-9262.

Novershtern, N.; Itzhaki, Z.; Manor, O.; Friedman, N. & Kaminski, N. (2008). A functional and regulatory map of asthma. *Am J Respir Cell Mol Biol*, Vol.38, No.3, (March 2008), pp.324-336, IISN 1044-1549.

Ocak, S.;Sos, ML.;Thomas, R.K. & Massion, P.P.(2009). High-throughput molecular analysis in lung cancer:insights into biology and potential clinical applications. *Eur Respir J* , Vol. 34, No. 2 (Aug 2009), pp. (489-506), ISSN 0903-1936.

Ober, C. (2005). Perspectivas on the past decade of asthma genetics. *J Allergy Clin Immunol*, Vol.116, pp274-278.

Ober, C. & Hoffjan S. (2006). Asthma genetics 2006: the long and winding road to gene discovery. *Genes Immun*, Vol:7, No.2, pp95-100.

Ober, C.; Tan, Z.; Sun, Y.; Possick, JD.; Pan, L.; Nicolae, R.; Radford, S.; Parry, RR.; Heinzmann, A.; Deichmann, KA.; Lester, LA.; Gern, JE.; Lemanske, RF Jr.; Nicolae, DL.; Elias, JA. & Chupp, GL. (2008).Effect of variation in CHI3L1 on serum YKL-40 level, risk of asthma, and lung function. *N Engl J Med*, Vol.358, No.16, (April 2008), pp.1682-1691, ISSN 0028-4793.

Ownby, DR. (1990). Environmental factors versus genetic determinants of childhood inhalant allergies. *J Allergy Clin Immunol*, Vol.86, No.3 Pt 1, (September 1990), pp.279-287, IISN 0091-6749.

Ott, H.; Baron, JM.; Heise, R.; Pcklenburg, C; Stanzel, S.; Merk, HF.; Niggemann, B. & Beyer, K. (2008). Clinical usefulness of microaraay-based IgE detection in children with suspected food allergy. *Allergy*, Vol. 63, No. 11 (Nov 2008), pp. (1521-1528), ISSN 0105-4538

Patel AC. (2008). Basic science for the practicing physician: gene expression microarrays. *Ann Allergy Asthma Immunol*, Vol.101, (September 2008), pp.325-332, ISSN 0003-4738.

Patton, WF.(2002). Detection technologies in proteome analysis. *J Chromatogr B Analyt Technol Bioned Life Sci*. No. 771 (May 2002), pp. (3-31), ISSN 1570-0232

Perou, C.M.; Jeffrey, S.S.;van de Rijn, M.; Rees, C.A.; Eisen, MB.; Ross, D.T., Pergamenschikoz, A.; Williams, C.F.; Zhu, S.X.; Lee, J.C.; Lashkari, D.; Shalon, D.; Brown, P.O. & Botstein, D.(1999). Distinctive gene expresión patterns in human mammary epithelial cells and breast cancers. *Proc Natl Acad Sci USA* , Vol. 96, No. 16 (Aug 1999), pp. (9212-9217), ISSN 0027-8424

Pinilla, C.; Martin, R.; Gran, B.; Appel, JR.; Boggiano, C.; Wilson, DB. & Houghten, RA. (1999). Exploring immunological specificity using synthetic peptide combinatorial libraries. *Curr Opin Immunol,* Vol.11, No.2, (April 1999), pp.193-202, IISN 0952-7915.

Quackenbush J (2006). From ´omes to biology. *Animal Genetics,* Vol 37 (Suppl. 1) , pp48-56.

Rapin, N.; Kesmir, C.; Frankild, S.; Nielsen, M.; Lundegaard, C.; Brunak, S. & Lund, O. (2006). Modeling the human immune system by combining bioinformatics and system biology approaches. *J Biol Phys,* Vol.32, (October 2006), pp.335-353, ISSN 0092-0606.

Repapi, E.; Sayers, I.; Wain, LV.; Burton, PR.; Johnson, T.; Obeidat, M.; Zhao, JH.; Ramasamy, A.; Zhai, G.; Vitart, V.; Huffman, JE.; Igl, W.; Albrecht, E.; Deloukas, P.; Henderson, J.; Granell, R.; McArdle, WL.; Rudnicka, AR.; Barroso, I.; Loos, RJ.; Wareham, NJ.; Mustelin, L.; Rantanen, T.; Surakka, I.; Imboden, M.; Wichmann, HE.; Grkovic, I.; Jankovic, S.; Zgaga, L.; Hartikainen, AL.; Peltonen, L.; Gyllensten, U.; Johansson, A.; Zaboli, G.; Campbell, H.; Wild, SH.; Wilson, JF.; Gläser, S.; Homuth, G.; Völzke, H; Mangino, M.; Soranzo, N.; Spector, TD.; Polasek, O.; Rudan, I.; Wright, AF.; Heliövaara, M.; Ripatti, S.; Pouta, A; Naluai, AT.; Olin, AC.; Torén, K.; Cooper, MN.; James, AL.; Palmer, LJ.; Hingorani, AD.; Wannamethee, SG.; Whincup, PH.; Smith, GD.; Ebrahim, S.; McKeever, TM.; Pavord, ID.; MacLeod, AK.; Morris, AD.; Porteous, DJ.; Cooper, C.; Dennison, E.; Shaheen, S.; Karrasch, S.; Schnabel, E.; Schulz, H.; Grallert, H.; Bouatia-Naji, N.; Delplanque, J.; Froguel, P.; Blakey, JD.; Britton, JR.; Morris, RW.; Holloway, JW.; Lawlor, DA.; Hui, J.; Nyberg, F.; Jarvelin, MR.; Jackson, C.; Kähönen, M.; Kaprio, J.; Probst-Hensch, NM.; Koch, B.; Hayward, C.; Evans, DM.; Elliott, P.; Strachan, DP.; Hall, IP. & Tobin, MD. (2010). Genome-wide association study identifies five loci associated with lung function. *Nat Genet,* Vol.42, No.1, (January 2010), pp.36-44, IISN 1061-4036.

Ricciardolo, FL.; Zaagsma, J. & Meurs, H. (2005). The therapeutic potential of drugs targeting the arginase pathway in asthma. *Expert Opin Investig Drugs,* Vol.14, No.10, (October 2005), pp.1221-1231, ISSN 1354-3784.

Righetti, PG.; Castagna, A.; Antonucci, F.; Piubelli, C.; Cecconi, D.; Campostrini, N.; Antonioli, P.; Astner, H. & Hamdan, M.(2004). Critical survey of quantitative proteomics in two-dimensional electrophoretic approaches. *J Chromatogr A,* Vol.1051, No.1-2, (October 2004), pp.3-17, IISN 0021-9673.

Risch, N. & Merikangas, K. (1996). The future of genetic studies of complex human diseases. *Science,* Vol.273, pp1516-1517.

Rolph, MS.; Sisavanh, M.; Liu, SM. & Mckay, CR. (2006). Clues to asthma pathogenic from microarray expression studies. *Pharmacol Ther,* Vol.109, (October 2005), pp.284-294, IISN 0009-9236.

Sääf, AM.; Tengvall-Linder, M.; Chang, HY.; Adler, AS.; Wahlgren, CF.; Scheynius, A.; Nordenskjöld, M. & Bradley, M. (2008). Global expression profiling in atopic eczema reveals reciprocal expression of inflammatory and lipid genes. *PLoS One,* Vol.3, No.12, (December 2008), pp.e4017, IISN 1932-6203.

Sastre, J. (2010). Molecular diagnosis in allergy. Clinical *Et Experimental Allergy*, Vol. 40, No. 10 (Oct 2010), pp. (1442-1460), ISSN *0954-7894*

Schreffer, W.; Lencer, D.; Bardina, L. & Sampson, H. (2005). Epitope mapping by microarray peptide immunoassay and cluster analysis reveals interpatient heterogeneity and a more detailed map. *Clin Immunol*, Vol.116, No.4, (October 2005), pp.893-899, IISN 1521-6616.

Serge, P.; Nana-Sinkam; Hunter, M.; Nuovo, GJ.; Schmittgen, TD.; Gelinas, R.; Galas, D. & Marsh, CB. (2009). Integrating the MicroRNome into the Study of Lung Disease *Am J Respir Crit Care Med*, Vol. 179, No 1 (Jan 2009), pp. (4-10), ISSN 073-449X

Singh, MB.; de Weerd, N. & Bhalla, PL. (1999). Genetically engineered plant allergens with reduced anaphylactic activity. *Int Arch Allergy Immunol*. Vol. 119, No.2, (June 1999), pp.75-85, IISN 1018-2438.

Silvestri, E.; Lombardi, A.; de Lange, P.; Glinni, D.; Senese, R.; Cioffi, F.; Lanni, A.; Goglia, F. & Moreno, M. (2011). Studies of complex biological systems with applications to molecular medicine: the need to integrate transcriptomic and proteomic approaches. *J Biomed Biotechnol*, IISN 1110-7243.

Sleiman, PM. & Hakonarson, H. (2010). Recent advances in the genetics and genomics of asthma and related traits. *Curr Opin Pediatr*, Vol.22, No.3, (June 2010), pp.307-312, IISN 1040-8703.

Southern, EM. (1975). Detection of specific sequences among DNA fragments separated by gel electrophoresis. *J Mol Biol*, Vol.98, No.3, (November 1975), pp. 503-517, ISSN 0022-2836.

Szalai, C.; Ungvári, I.; Pelyhe, L.; Tölgyesy, G. & Falus, a (2008). Asthma from a pharmacogenomic point of view .*British Journal of Pharmacology* , Vol. 153, No. 8 (Apr 2008), pp. (1602-1614), ISSN 0007-1188-

Tavendale, R.; Macgregor, DF.; Mukhopadhyay, S. & Palmer, CN. (2008). A polymorphism controlling ORMDL3 expression is associated with asthma that is poorly controlled by current medications. *J Allergy Clin Immunol*, Vol.121, No.4, (April 2008), pp.860-863, IISN 0091-6749.

Tyner, JW.; Kim, EY.; Ide, K.; Pelletier, MR.; Roswit, WT.; Morton, JD.; Battaile, JT.; Patel, AC.; Patterson, GA.; Castro, M.; Spoor, MS.; You, Y.; Brody, SL. & Holtzman, MJ. (2006). Blocking airway mucous cell metaplasia by inhibiting EGFR antiapoptosis and IL-13 transdifferentation signals. *J Clin Inves*t, Vol.116, No.2, (February 2006), pp.309-321, ISSN 0021-9738.

Venter, JC.; Adams, MD.; Myers, EW.; Li, PW.; Mural, RJ.; Sutton, GG.; Smith, HO.; Yandell, M.; Evans, CA.; Holt RA.; Gocayne, JD.; Amanatides, P.; Ballew, RM.; Huson, DH.; Wortman, JR.; Zhang, Q.; Kodira, CD.; Zheng, XH.; Chen, L.; Skupski, M.; Subramanian, G.; Thomas, PD.; Zhang, J.; Gabor Miklos, GL.; Nelson, C.; Broder, S.; Clark, AG.; Nadeau, J.; McKusick, VA.; Zinder, N.; Levine, AJ.; Roberts, RJ.; Simon, M.; Slayman, C.; Hunkapiller, M.; Bolanos, R.; Delcher, A.; Dew, I.; Fasulo, D; Flanigan, M.; Florea, L.; Halpern, A.; Hannenhalli, S.; Kravitz, S.; Levy, S.; Mobarry, C.; Reinert, K.; Remington, K.; Abu-Threideh, J.; Beasley, E.; Biddick, K.; Bonazzi, V.; Brandon, R.; Cargill, M.; Chandramouliswaran, I.; Charlab, R.; Chaturvedi, K.; Deng, Z.; Di Francesco, V.; Dunn, P.; Eilbeck, K.; Evangelista, C.; Gabrielian, AE.; Gan, W.; Ge, W.; Gong, F.; Gu, Z.; Guan, P.; Heiman, TJ.; Higgins, ME.; Ji, RR.; Ke,

Z.; Ketchum, KA.; Lai, Z.; Lei, Y.; Li, Z.; Li, J.; Liang, Y.; Lin, X.; Lu, F.; Merkulov, GV.; Milshina, N.; Moore, HM.; Naik, AK.; Narayan, VA.; Neelam, B.; Nusskern, D.; Rusch, DB.; Salzberg, S.; Shao, W.; Shue, B.; Sun, J.; Wang, Z.; Wang, A.; Wang, X.; Wang, J.; Wei, M.; Wides, R.; Xiao, C.; Yan, C.; Yao, A.; Ye, J.; Zhan, M.; Zhang, W.; Zhang, H.; Zhao, Q.; Zheng, L.; Zhong, F.; Zhong, W.; Zhu, S.; Zhao, S.; Gilbert, D.; Baumhueter, S.; Spier, G.; Carter, C.; Cravchik, A.; Woodage, T.; Ali, F.; An, H.; Awe, A.; Baldwin, D.; Baden, H.; Barnstead, M.; Barrow, I.; Beeson, K.; Busam, D.; Carver, A.; Center, A.; Cheng, ML.; Curry, L.; Danaher, S.; Davenport, L.; Desilets, R.; Dietz, S.; Dodson, K.; Doup, L.; Ferriera, S.; Garg, N.; Gluecksmann, A.; Hart, B.; Haynes, J.; Haynes, C.; Heiner, C.; Hladun, S.; Hostin, D.; Houck, J.; Howland, T.; Ibegwam, C.; Johnson, J.; Kalush, F.; Kline, L.; Koduru, S.; Love, A.; Mann, F.; May, D.; McCawley, S.; McIntosh, T.; McMullen, I.; Moy, M.; Moy, L.; Murphy, B.; Nelson, K.; Pfannkoch, C.; Pratts, E.; Puri, V.; Qureshi, H.; Reardon, M.; Rodriguez, R.; Rogers, YH.; Romblad, D.; Ruhfel, B.; Scott, R.; Sitter, C.; Smallwood, M.; Stewart, E.; Strong, R.; Suh, E.; Thomas, R.; Tint, NN.; Tse, S.; Vech, C., Wang, G., Wetter, J.; Williams, S.; Williams, M., Windsor, S.; Winn-Deen, E.; Wolfe, K.; Zaveri, J.; Zaveri, K., Abril, JF.; Guigó, R.; Campbell, MJ.; Sjolander, KV.; Karlak, B.; Kejariwal, A.; Mi, H.; Lazareva, B.; Hatton, T.; Narechania, A.; Diemer, K.; Muruganujan, A.; Guo, N.; Sato, S.; Bafna, V.; Istrail, S.; Lippert, R.; Schwartz, R.; Walenz, B.; Yooseph, S.; Allen, D.; Basu, A.; Baxendale, J.; Blick, L.; Caminha, M.; Carnes-Stine, J.; Caulk, P.; Chiang, YH.; Coyne, M.; Dahlke, C.; Mays, A.; Dombroski, M.; Donnelly, M.; Ely, D.; Esparham, S.; Fosler, C.; Gire, H.; Glanowski, S.; Glasser, K.; Glodek, A.; Gorokhov, M.; Graham, K.; Gropman, B.; Harris, M.; Heil, J.; Henderson, S.; Hoover, J.; Jennings, D.; Jordan, C.; Jordan, J.; Kasha, J.; Kagan, L.; Kraft, C.; Levitsky, A.; Lewis, M.; Liu, X.; Lopez, J.; Ma, D.; Majoros, W.; McDaniel, J.; Murphy, S.; Newman, M.; Nguyen, T.; Nguyen, N.; Nodell, M.; Pan, S.; Peck, J.; Peterson, M.; Rowe, W.; Sanders, R.; Scott, J.; Simpson, M.; Smith, T.; Sprague, A.; Stockwell, T., Turner, R.; Venter, E.; Wang, M.; Wen, M.; Wu, D.; Wu, M.; Xia, A.; Zandieh, A. & Zhu, X. (2001) The sequence of the human genome. *Science*, Vol.291, No.5507, (February 2001), pp.1304-1351, IISN 0036-8075.

Vercelli, D. (2008). Discovering susceptiblility genes for asthma and allergy. *Nat Rev Immunol*, Vol. 8, No.3, pp169-182.

Vercelli, D. a (2010). Genetics and biology of asthma 2010: La´ci darem la mano. *J Allergy Clin Immunol,* Vol 125, pp347-348.

Vercelli, D. b (2010). Gene-environment interactions in asthma and allergy : the end of the beginning?. *Curr Opin Allergy Immunol,* Vol. 10, (April 2010), pp.145-148, IISN 1528-4050.

Vineis, P.; Brennan, P.; Canzian, F.; Ioannidis, JP.; Matullo, G.; Ritchie, M.; Stromberg, U.; Taioli, E. & Thompson, J. (2008). Expectations and challenges stemming from genome-wide association studies. *Mutagenesis,* Vol.23, No.6, (November 2008), pp.439-444, IISN 0267-8357.

Vlahou,A. & Fountoulakis, M. (2005). Proteomic approaches in the search for disease biomarkers, J *Chromatogr B Analyt Technol Biomed Life Sci.*, Vol.814, No.1, (January 2005), pp.11-19, IISN 1570-0232.

Von Mutius, E. (2004). Influences in allergy: Epidemiology and the environment. *J Allergy Clin Immunol,* Vol.113, pp373-379.

Wang, J.; Wang, W.; Li, R.; Li, Y.; Tian, G.; Goodman, L.; Fan, W.; Zhang, J.; Li, J.; Zhang, J.; Guo, Y.; Feng, B.; Li, H.; Lu, Y.; Fang, X.; Liang, H.; Du, Z.; Li, D.; Zhao, Y.; Hu, Y.; Yang, Z.; Zheng, H.; Hellmann, I.; Inouye, M.; Pool, J.; Yi, X.; Zhao, J.; Duan, J.; Zhou, Y.; Qin, J.; Ma, L.; Li, G.; Yang, Z.; Zhang, G.; Yang, B.; Yu, C.; Liang, F.; Li, W.; Li, S.; Li, D.; Ni, P.; Ruan, J.; Li, Q.; Zhu, H.; Liu, D.; Lu, Z.; Li, N.; Guo, G.; Zhang, J.; Ye, J.; Fang, L.; Hao, Q.; Chen, Q.; Liang, Y.; Su, Y.; San, A.; Ping, C.; Yang, S.; Chen, F.; Li, L.; Zhou, K.; Zheng, H.; Ren, Y.; Yang, L.; Gao, Y.; Yang, G.; Li, Z.; Feng, X.; Kristiansen, K.; Wong, GK.; Nielsen, R.; Durbin, R.; Bolund, L.; Zhang, X.; Li, S. & Yang, H.(2008). The diploid genome sequence of an Asian individual human. *Nature* , Vol. 456, No. 7218 (Nov 2008), pp. (60-65), ISSN 0028-0836.

Wang,H.; Chavali, S.; Mobini, R.; Muraro, A.; Barbon, F.; Boldrin, D.; Aberg, N. & Benson, M. (2011). A pathway-based approach to find novel markers of local glucocorticoid treatment in intermittent allergic rhinitis. *Allergy,* Vol.66, No.1, (January 2011), pp.132-140, IISN 0105-4538.

Weidinger, S.; Gieger, C.; Rodriguez, E.; Baurecht, H.; Mempel, M.; Klopp, N.; Gohlke, H.; Wagenpfeil, S.; Ollert, M.; Ring, J.; Behrendt, H.; Heinrich, J.; Novak, N.; Bieber, T.; Krämer, U.; Berdel, D.; von Berg, A.; Bauer, CP.; Herbarth, O.; Koletzko, S.; Prokisch, H.; Mehta, D.; Meitinger, T.; Depner, M.; von Mutius, E.; Liang, L.; Moffatt, M.; Cookson, W.; Kabesch, M.; Wichmann, HE. & Illig, T. (2008). Genome-wide scan on total serum IgE levels identifies FCER1A as novel susceptibility locus. *PLoS Genet,* Vol.4, No.8, (August 2008), pp.e1000166, IISN 1553-7390.

Wells, A.D. (2009). New insights into the molecular basis of T cell anergy: anergy factors, avoidance sensors, and epigenetic imprinting. *J Immunol.* Vol.182, pp7331-7341.

Wheeler, D.A.; Srinivasan, M.; Egholm, M.; Shen, Y.; Chen, L.; McGuire, A.; He, W.; Chen, Y.J.; Makhijani, V.; Roth, G.T.; Gomes, X.; Tartaro, K.; Niazi, F.; Turcotte, C.L.; Irvyk, G.P.; Lupski, J.R.; Chinault, C.; Song, X.Z.; Liu, Y.; Yuan, Y.;Nazareth, L.; Oin, X.; Muzny, D.M.; Margulies, M.; Weinstock, G.M.; Gibbs, R.A. & Rothberg, J.M.(2008). The complete genome o fan individual by massively parallel DNA sequencing. *Nature,* Vol. 452, No. 7189 (Apr 2008), pp. (872-876), IISN 0028-0836.

Wohrl, S.; Vigl, K.; Zehetmayer, S; Hiller, R.; Jarisch, R.; Prinz, M.; Stingl. G. & Kopp, T. (2006). The performance of a component-based allergen microarray in clinical practice. *Allergy,* Vol. 61, No. 5 (May 2006), pp. (633-639), ISSN 0105-4538

Wolters, DA.; Washburn, MP. & Yates JR 3rd.(2001). An automated multidimensional protein identification technology for shotgun proteomics. *Anal Chem* , Vol. 73, No. 23 (Dec 2001), pp. (5683-5690), ISSM 0003-2700

Woodruff, PG.; Boushey, HA.; Dolganov, GM.; Woodruff, PG.; Boushey, HA.; Dolganov, GM.; Barker, CS.; Yang, YH.; Donnelly, S.; Ellwanger, A.; Sidhu, SS.; Dao-Pick, TP.; Pantoja, C.; Erle, DJ.; Yamamoto, KR. & Fahy, JV. (2007). Genome-wide profiling identifies epithelial cell genes associated with asthma and with treatment response to corticosteroids. *Proc Natl Acad Sci U S A,* Vol.104, No.40, (October 2007), pp.15858-15863, ISSN 0027-8424.

Woodruff, PG.; Modrek, B.; Choy, DF.; Jia, G.; Abbas, AR.; Ellwanger, A.; Koth, LL.; Arron, JR. & Fahy, JV. (2009). T-helper type 2-driven inflammation defines major subphenotypes of asthma. *Am J Respir Crit Care Med,* Vol.180, No.5, (September 2009), pp.388-395, IISN 1073-449X.

Wu, H.; Romieu, I.; Sienra-Monge, JJ.; Li, H.; del Rio-Navarro, BE. & London, SJ. (2009). Genetic variation in ORM1-like 3 (ORMDL3) and gasdermin-like (GSDML) and childhood asthma. *Allergy,* Vol.64, No., (April 2009), pp.629-635, ISSN 0105-4538.

Wu, H.; Romieu, I.; Shi, M.; Hancock, DB.; Li, H.; Sienra-Monge, JJ.; Chiu, GY.; Xu, H.; del Rio-Navarro, BE. & London SJ. (2010). Evaluation of candidate genes in a genome-wide association study of childhood asthma in Mexicans. *J Allergy Clin Immunol,* Vol.125, No.2, (February 2010), pp.321-327, IISN 0091-6749.

Yan, Q. (2005). Pharmacogenomics and systems biology of membrane transports. *Mol Biotechnol,* Vol.29, No.1, (January 2005), pp.75-88, ISSN 1073-6085

Yan Q. (2010). Immunoinformatics and Systems Biology Methods for Personalized Medicine. *Methods Mol Biol,* Vol 662, pp203-220. ISSN 1064-3745.

Zimmermann, N.; King, NE.; Laporte, J.; Yang, M.; Mishra, A.; Pope, SM.; Muntel, EE.; Witte, DP.; Pegg, AA.; Foster, PS.; Hamid, Q. & Rothenberg, ME. (2003). Dissection of experimental asthma with DNA microarray analysis identifies arginase in asthma pathogenesis. *J Clin Invest,* Vol.111, No.12, (June 2003), pp.1863-74, ISSN 0021-9738.

2

Expression of the Histamine H_4 Receptor in Human Tissue

Katsunori Yamaura[1], Masahiko Suzuki[2], Takao Namiki[3] and Koichi Ueno[1,4]
[1]*Department of Geriatric Pharmacology and Therapeutics, Graduate School of Pharmaceutical Sciences,*
[2]*Research Center for Frontier Medical Engineering,*
[3]*Department of Japanese-Oriental "KAMPO" Medicine, Graduate School of Medicine,*
[4]*Center for Preventive Medical Science, Chiba University, Japan*

1. Introduction

The histamine H_4 receptor (H_4R) is the most recently identified of the four histamine receptors (H_1R–H_4R), and belongs to the same G-protein-coupled receptor (GPCR) family. The amino acid sequence of H_4R shares approximately 26%, 27%, and 58% homology with H_1R, H_2R, and H_3R, respectively, in the transmembrane regions (Nguyen et al., 2001). Furthermore, H_4R couples to Gi/o proteins and shows 10^3- to 10^4-fold higher ligand affinity than H_1R and H_2R (Thurmond et al., 2008).

Several organs express H_4R, and immune tissues such as the spleen, thymus, bone marrow, and leukocytes have a wide range of expression levels (Oda et al., 2000). It has been reported that chemotaxis of mast cells and eosinophils is stimulated by histamine via H_4R; the receptor is therefore attractive as a new target of research into allergic diseases (de Esch et al., 2005).

2. Expression of H_4R in synovial tissue in rheumatoid arthritis

A role for histamine has been implicated in rheumatoid arthritis (RA). RA consists mainly of synovial tissue inflammation that may be dispersed throughout the body, but its molecular etiology remains unclear. Macrophage infiltration and excessive formation of fibroblasts cause a variety of cytokines to be secreted from synovial membranes in patients with RA, and this in turn stimulates osteolytic activity (Sweeney & Firestein, 2004). There is evidence of a significant increase in histamine concentration in synovial samples from patients with RA (Frewin et al., 1986). These observations suggest a potentially significant role of H_4R in the cause, progression, and treatment of RA.

The presence of H_1R and H_2R in human synovial cell culture (HSCC) has been clearly shown by ligand-binding experiments (Nagata, 1991). However, there has been no definitive evidence or conclusive reports of the similar presence of H_3R or H_4R. Therefore, utilizing our expertise in reverse transcription polymerase chain reaction (RT-PCR) techniques, we examined the H_4R-specific mRNA expression in HSCC obtained from 11 RA patients who underwent artificial knee-replacement surgery (Ikawa et al., 2005).

After excising the synovial membrane specimen under aseptic conditions, the sample was treated with collagenase and trypsin solution to separate it into single cells. The cells were cultured for 2 weeks in medium containing fetal bovine serum. When the culture reached confluence, the cells were harvested and all RNA extracted. Analysis of the expression of the 4 subtypes of histamine receptor-specific mRNA in 2 patients with RA (RA1 and RA2) by RT-PCR showed that, under the experimental conditions, H_1R-, H_2R-, and H_4R-specific mRNAs were expressed, but H_3R-specific mRNA was not (Fig. 1). Expression of H_4R-specific mRNA was confirmed in all 11 samples (RA1–RA11; Fig. 2). Notably, the intensity of the separated H_4R-specific mRNA bands varied considerably from one sample to another, suggesting differences in cellular concentrations of H_4R between patients.

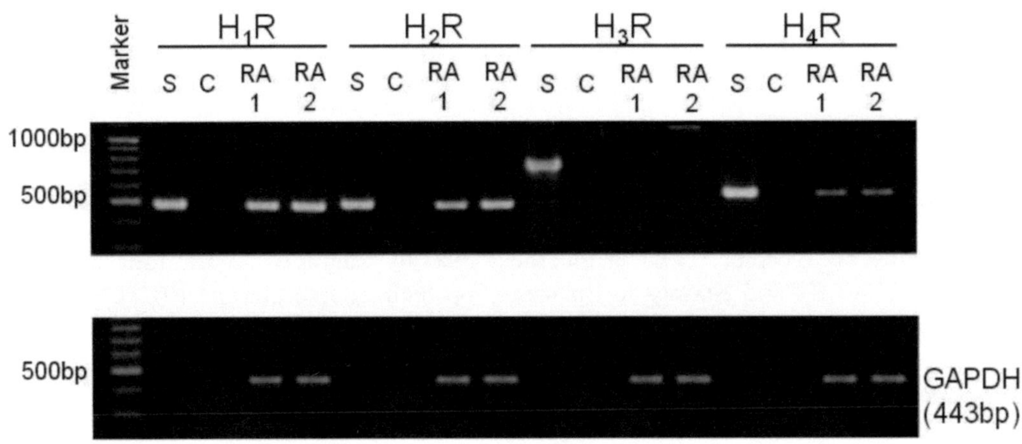

Fig. 1. Expression of mRNAs specific to 4 subtypes of histamine receptor (H_1R, H_2R, H_3R, and H_4R) in HSCC from 2 patients with RA. The gel was loaded with 5 µL of amplified products. A 100-bp DNA ladder was used as a molecular weight marker. S: standard; C: control; samples from 2 RA patients, RA1 and RA2. Figure reprinted with permission from the Pharmaceutical Society of Japan.

Inflamed synoviocytes consist of 3 cell types: (1) macrophage-like cells; (2) fibroblast-like cells; and (3) dendritic cells (Tanaka, 2005). High levels of lymphocyte infiltration have been observed in RA compared to other types of arthritis (Fonseca et al., 2005). A variety of cell types such as macrophage-like cells, dendritic cells, and granulocytes have also been identified in the human RA synovium. As H_4R has been reported to be present in immune cells, expression of H_4R mRNA seems most likely to occur in cells derived from the hematopoietic system, such as macrophage-like or dendritic cells from synovial sites. Consequently, we examined the protein expression levels of H_4R in RA HSCC, and used fluorescence immunoassays (Ohki et al., 2007) to determine the types of the cells in which expression occurred by identifying co-expression of cell type-specific human proteins: PH and CD55 for fibroblast-like cells; CD68 and CD163 for macrophage-like cells; and CD1a and CD208 for dendritic cells.

First, we examined the expression patterns of prolyl-4-hydroxylase (PH) (red) and CD68 (green) using 2 morphologically distinct cell types we identified in our HSCC: fibroblast-like and macrophage-like cells. In similar experiments, no expression of human dendritic cell markers (either CD1a or CD208) was detectable. Subsequent assays for fibroblast and macrophage markers showed that human H_4R protein is expressed in both fibroblast-like and macrophage-like cells in RA synovial tissues (Fig. 3 and Fig. 4). Others have also reported identification of H_4R in synovial tissue of patients with RA (Grzybowska-Kowalczyk et al., 2007).

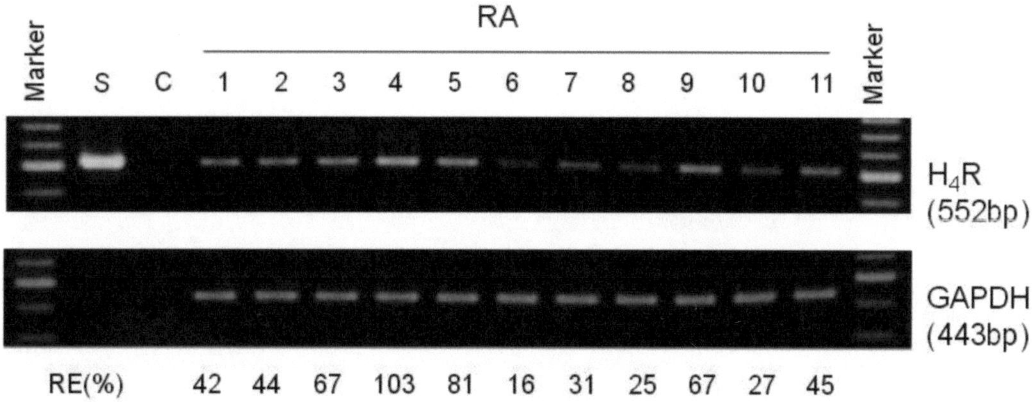

Fig. 2. Expression of H_4R-specific mRNA in HSCC from 11 RA patients. The gel was loaded with 5 μL of amplified products. A 100-bp DNA ladder was used as a molecular weight marker. S: standard; C: control; RE: relative expression; sample from 11 different RA patients, RA1 to RA11. RE of mRNA was calculated by normalizing the separated sample intensity value, taking that of the corresponding internal control (GAPDH) as 100%. Intensity values were measured using an image analyzer (IX81, OLYMPUS). Figure reprinted with permission from the Pharmaceutical Society of Japan.

Next, we focused attention on the expression of H_4R mRNA in synovial tissues, and serum matrix metalloproteinase-3 (MMP-3) concentration in RA. We found a significant negative correlation between H_4R expression in synovial tissues and serum MMP-3 concentration, but no correlation between MMP-3 and H_1R or H_2R (Yamaura et al., 2011). These observations suggest that H_4R is a potential target of novel pharmacotherapeutic agents for RA, and H_4R functional analysis may be useful in developing such treatments.

In addition, we detected H_4R expression in human cartilage chondrocytes and in a murine chondrocytic cell line, ATDC5 (Yamaura et al., in press). Further work is needed to determine the expression mechanism and function of H_4R on chondrocytes.

3. Expression of H_4R in human skin

Following detection of H_4R expression in synovial tissue, we also analyzed H_4R expression in human epidermal tissue (Yamaura et al., 2009) and fibroblast cell cultures (Ikawa et al., 2008). Our immunoassays revealed that H_4R is expressed in both human epidermal tissues and dermal fibroblasts.

Keratinocytes are the major constituent of the epidermis. We found that immunohistochemical staining showed strong H_4R expression in keratin (K)10-positive differentiated keratinocytes in the prickle cell and granular layers of the epidermis (Fig. 5a). By contrast, H_4R was weakly expressed in K14-positive proliferating keratinocytes in the basal layer (Fig. 5b).

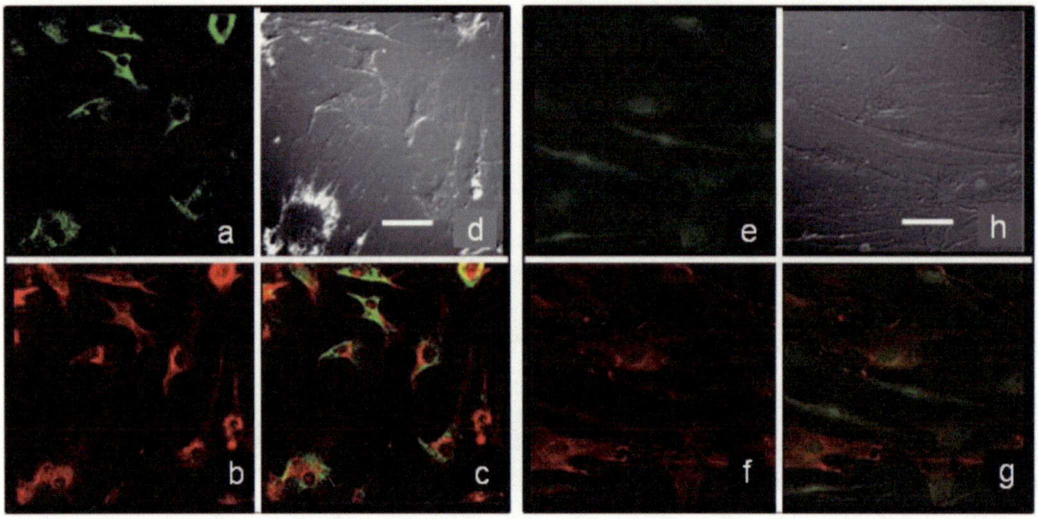

Fig. 3. Co-expression of H_4R protein with fibroblast-specific marker proteins. (a) Mouse anti-PH followed by Cy2-conjugated anti-mouse (green); (b) rabbit anti-H_4R followed by Cy3-conjugated anti-rabbit (red); (c) superposition of a on b; (d) Nomarski phase contrast microscopy image (NPCMI); (e) rabbit anti-H_4R followed by Cy2-conjugated anti-rabbit (green); (f) mouse anti-CD55 followed by Cy3-conjugated anti-mouse (red); (g) superposition of e on f; (h) NPCMI. Scale bar: 50 μm. Figure reproduced with permission from the Pharmaceutical Society of Japan.

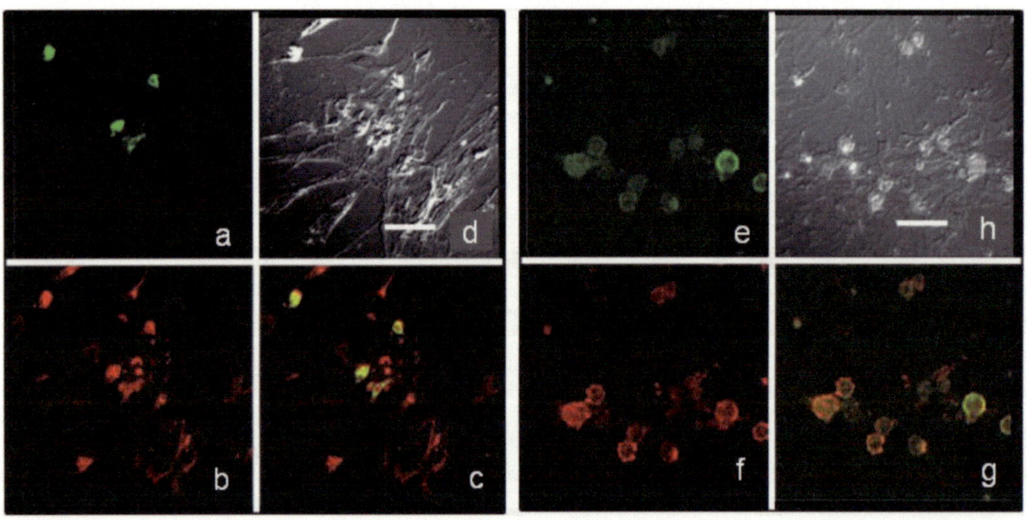

Fig. 4. Co-expression of H_4R protein with macrophage-specific marker proteins.(a) Mouse anti-CD68 followed by Cy2-conjugated anti-mouse (green); (b) rabbit anti-H_4R followed by Cy3-conjugated anti-rabbit (red); (c) superposition of a on b; (d) NPCMI; (e) mouse anti-CD163 followed by Cy2-conjugated anti-mouse (green); (f) rabbit anti-H_4R followed by Cy3-conjugated anti-rabbit (red); (g) superposition of e on f; (h) NPCMI. Scale bar: 50 μm. Figure reproduced with permission from the Pharmaceutical Society of Japan.

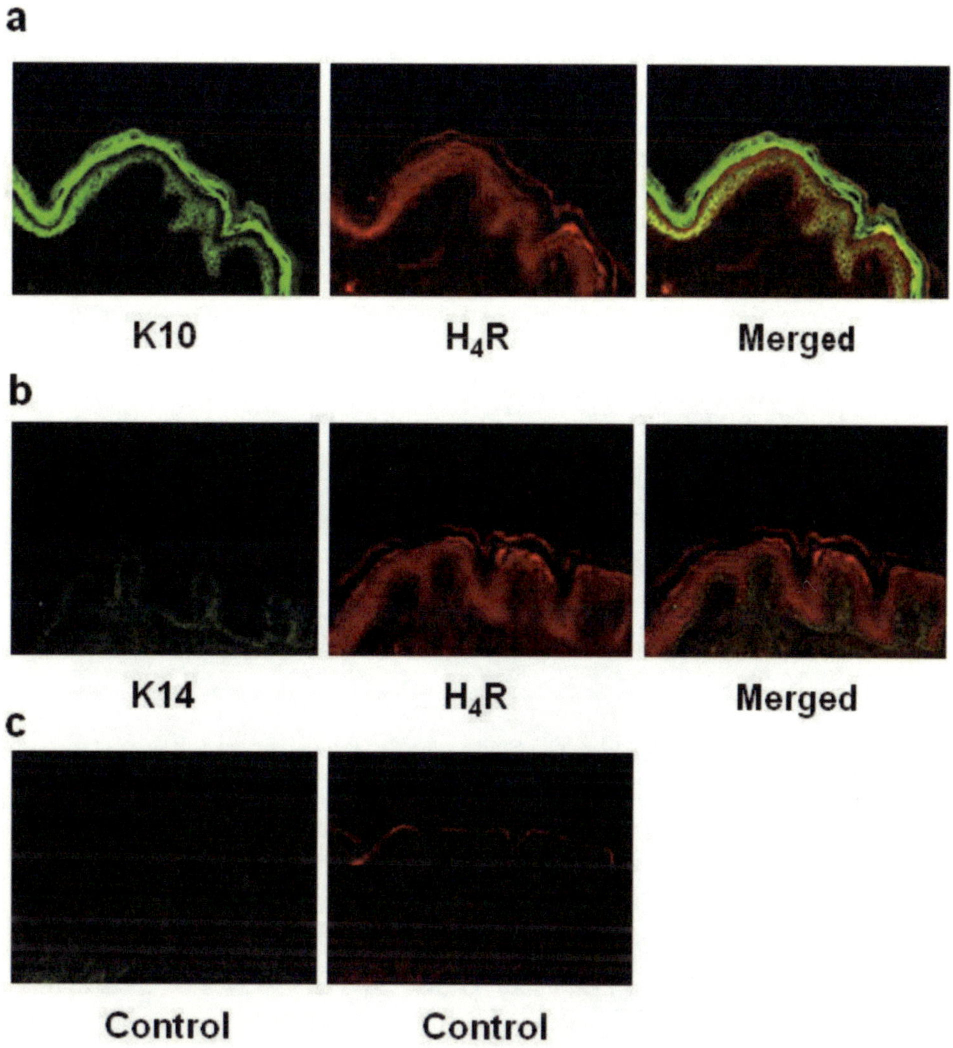

Fig. 5. H_4R expression in human epidermal tissues. Double immunofluorescence staining of human epidermal tissues with anti-human H_4R antibody followed by Cy2-conjugated anti-rabbit secondary antibody (red), and anti-K10 (a) or anti-K14 (b) antibody followed by Cy2-conjugated anti-mouse secondary antibody (green). (c) For the negative control, tissues were only exposed to the secondary antibody. Figure reprinted with permission from the Japanese Society of Toxicology.

Keratinization is the result of keratinocytes dividing in the basal lamina and moving to the upper layer as they mature. K10 is expressed in keratinocytes in the early stages following differentiation, whereas K14 is expressed in undifferentiated keratinocytes. Accordingly, our results suggest that keratinocytes increase expression of H_4R following differentiation; however, further work is necessary to determine the expression mechanism and the physiological role of the receptors.

Increased H_4R expression has been reported in $CD4^+$ T cells of patients with atopic dermatitis (Gutzmer et al., 2009), and skin mast cells have been shown to express H_4R (Lippert et al., 2004). These findings suggest that dermal cells may play an important role, via H_4R, in skin disorders. Dermal fibroblasts are a major component of the dermis. When the skin is damaged, they perform important roles including production of extracellular matrix molecules such as collagens. We have demonstrated the expression of H_4R in human dermal fibroblast cells using immunohistochemical staining (Fig. 6). Furthermore, Western blot analysis showed enhancement of the expression level of H_4R in dermal fibroblasts by stimulation with dexamethasone (Fig. 7).

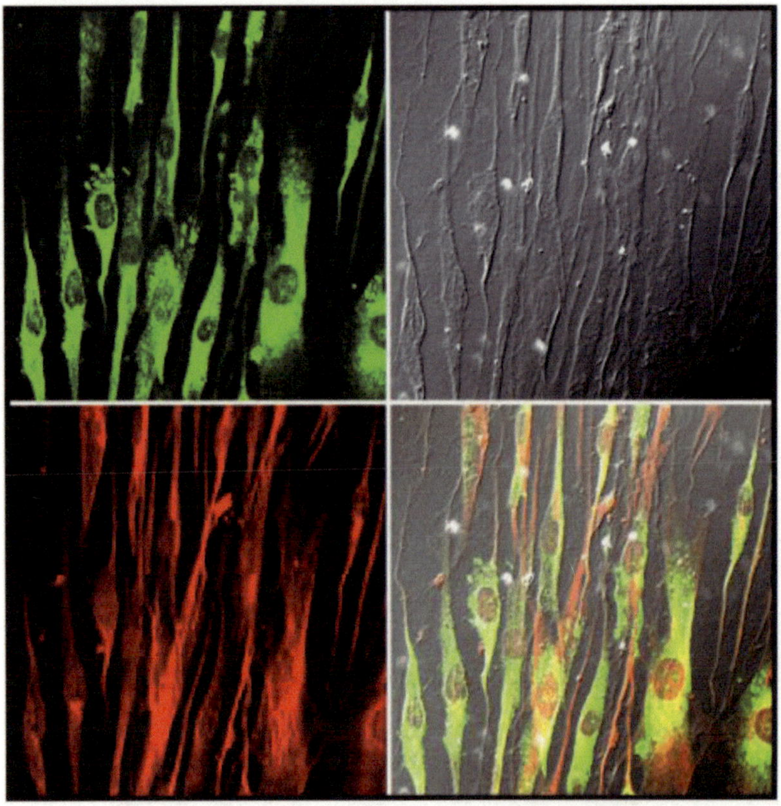

Fig. 6. Expression of H_4R on human dermal fibroblasts.Double immunofluorescence staining of dermal fibroblast cells treated with anti-human PH antibody followed by Cy2-conjugated anti-mouse secondary antibody (green), and anti-human H_4R antibody followed by Cy3-conjugated anti-rabbit secondary antibody (red). Magnification x 400. Figure reprinted with permission from the Japanese Society of Toxicology.

Ohnishi et al. (2008) reported that the levels of leukotriene B_4 receptor 1, which belongs to the GPCR family, were up-regulated by dexamethasone. This suggests that H_4R, which is part of the same family, may be up-regulated by dexamethasone too. This up-regulation of H_4R expression might be associated with itching that occurs as a rebound phenomenon after withdrawal of high-dose topical glucocorticoids. We confirmed that significant enhancement of pruritus occurred after chronic topical application of dexamethasone in mice (Yamaura et al., 2011). However, further study is needed to investigate the relationship between the expression of H_4R in skin and pruritus, which are both enhanced by dexamethasone.

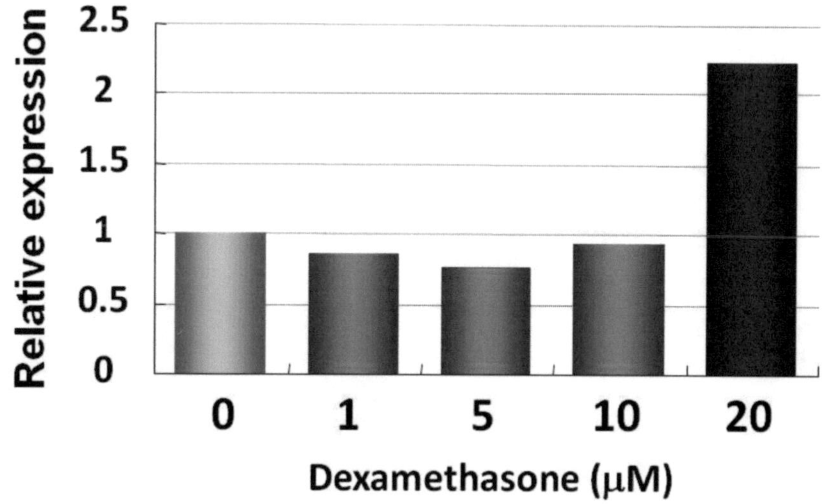

Fig. 7. Effects of dexamethasone on H_4R protein expression in human dermal fibroblast cell cultures. Expression of H_4R was analyzed by Western blot analysis. Protein levels of H_4R were normalized to the corresponding β-actin protein levels. The mean value of the non-treatment group was set to 1.0. Data are expressed as means (n=2–3). Figure reprinted with permission from the Japanese Society of Toxicology.

4. Effect of H_4R antagonists on pruritus model

Chronic pruritus, associated with chronic conditions such as skin, liver, and kidney diseases and metabolic disorders, is a major diagnostic and therapeutic problem and can have a profound impact on the quality of life of patients. Recent studies have raised the possibility that H_4R, in addition to the H_1R, may contribute to histamine-mediated pruritic responses in mice (Bell et al., 2004). Both specific H_4R agonists and histamine were shown to induce pruritic responses which could be blocked by pretreatment with H_4R antagonists; the response was also found to be markedly attenuated in H_4R-deficient mice. We thus examined the effectiveness of selective H_4R antagonists as antipruritic drugs by their effect on histamine H_1R antagonist-resistant acute pruritus induced by substance P in mice.

We investigated the effect of the H_1R antagonist fexofenadine and the H_4R antagonist JNJ7777120 on histamine-induced acute pruritus (Yamaura et al., 2009). Oral administration of fexofenadine caused a slight reduction in scratching, whereas JNJ7777120 showed a significant reduction (Fig. 8). We then examined the effect of these antagonists in substance P-mediated acute pruritus. Fexofenadine showed no reduction in substance P-induced scratching. By contrast, JNJ7777120 at 10 and 30 mg/kg doses reduced substance P-induced scratching in a dose-dependent manner (Fig. 9). Although JNJ7777120 crosses the blood–brain barrier, it does not cause sedation in rodents (Dunford et al., 2007); hence its antipruritic action is not a secondary effect of sedation. The results suggest that H_1R has only limited involvement in histamine-induced pruritus. By contrast, the significant effect of JNJ7777120 suggests that H_4R

has a much greater role. Substance P-induced pruritus is resistant to H_1R antagonists (Togashi et al., 2002); given its occurrence in mast cell-deficient mice (Andoh et al., 2001), histamine from mast cells is unlikely to be involved. The role of H_1R is also thought to be minor, with fexofenadine having no observable effect. However, the suppression of the pruritic response by JNJ7777120 suggests that histamine may act via H_4R rather than H_1R.

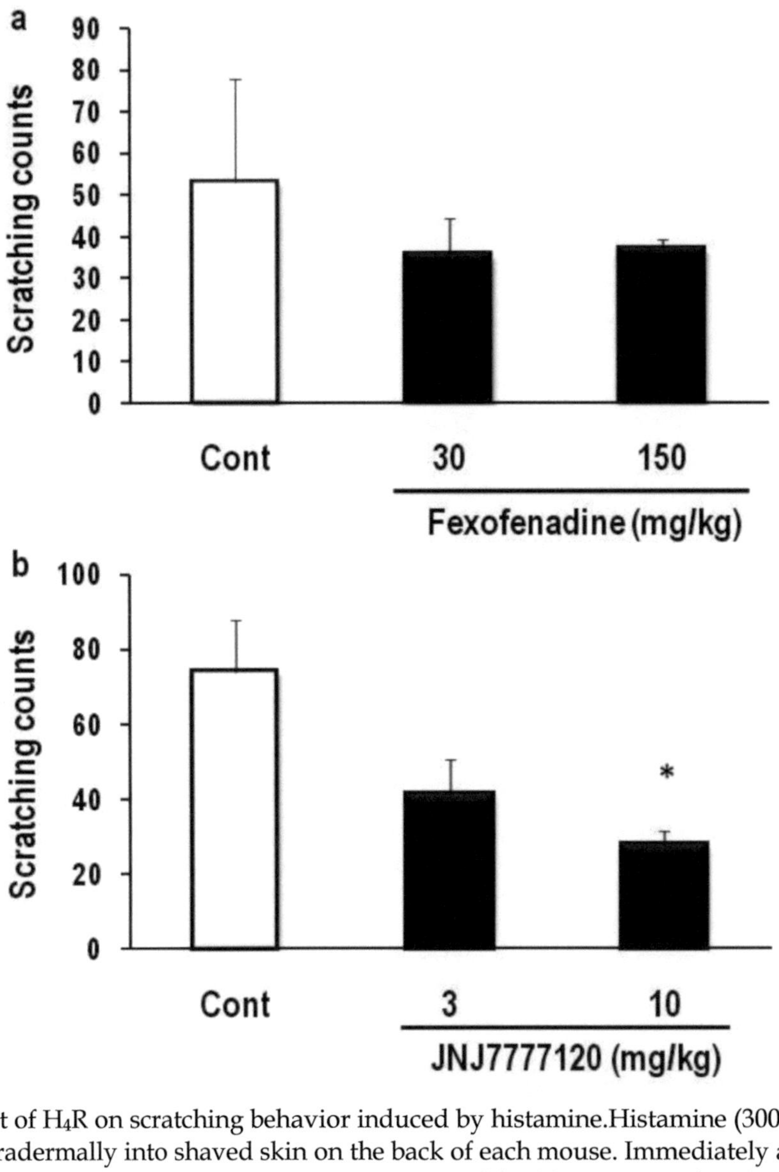

Fig. 8. Effect of H_4R on scratching behavior induced by histamine.Histamine (300 nmol) was injected intradermally into shaved skin on the back of each mouse. Immediately after the injection of pruritogen, scratching events were counted for 30 min using the MicroAct apparatus (Neuroscience Inc., Tokyo, Japan). Fexofenadine (a) or JNJ7777120 (b) was administered orally 20 min before the injection of pruritogen. Values represent the mean ± SEM of four mice. *$p<0.05$ vs. control (Dunnett's multiple comparisons). Figure reprinted with permission from the Japanese Society of Toxicology.

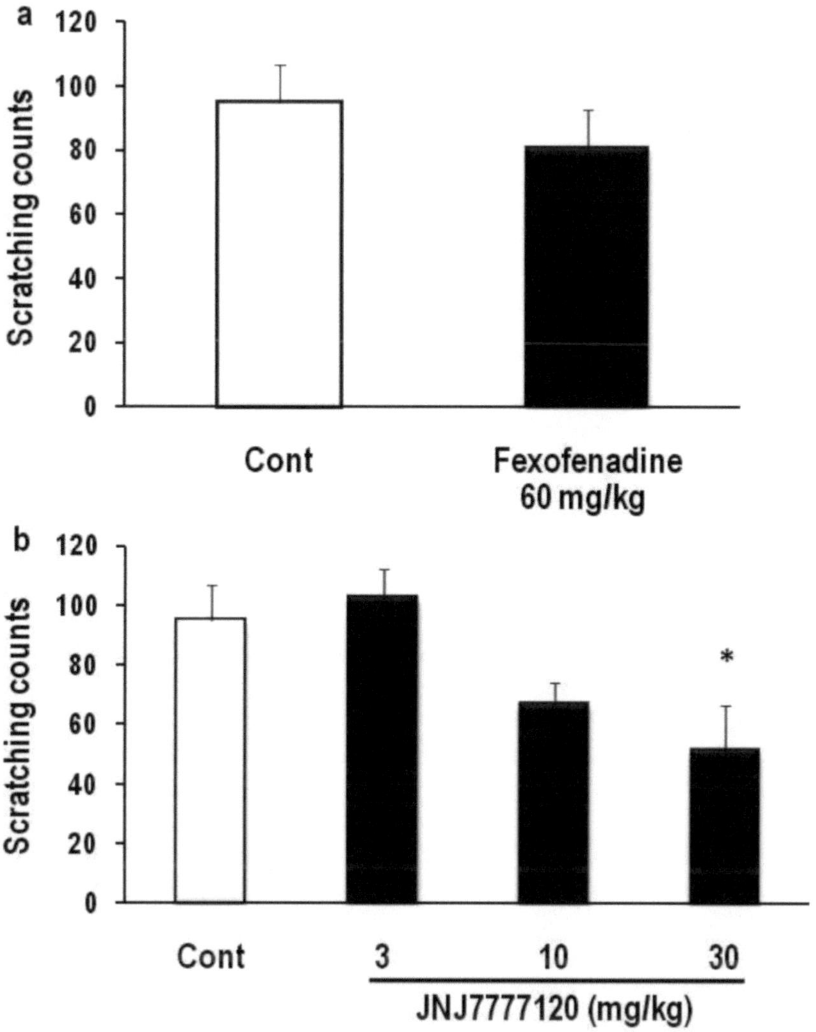

Fig. 9. Effect of H_4R on scratching behavior induced by substance P. Substance P (100 nmol) was injected intradermally into shaved skin on the back of each mouse. Immediately after the injection of pruritogen, scratching events were counted for 30 min using MicroAct. Fexofenadine (a) or JNJ7777120 (b) was administered orally 20 min before the injection of pruritogen. Values represent the mean ± SEM of four mice. *$p<0.05$ vs. control (Dunnett's multiple comparisons). Figure reprinted with permission from the Japanese Society of Toxicology.

Further, we created a chronic itch model in which repeated application of 2,4,6-trinitrochlorobenzene to the back skin of HR-1 mice was seen to elicit frequent scratching behavior at 24 h after challenge. JNJ7777120 at 10 and 30 mg/kg doses reduced this scratching behavior, whereas fexofenadine had no such effect (Suwa et al., 2011). These results suggest that H_4R antagonists may be useful for treatment of H_1R antagonist-resistant chronic pruritus such as atopic dermatitis.

5. Conclusion

We have demonstrated the expression of H_4R in human synovial cells from patients with RA and found a significant negative correlation between H_4R expression in RA synovial tissues and serum MMP-3 concentration. Furthermore, we have shown expression of H_4R in human skin and demonstrated that an H_4R antagonist ameliorates both H_1R antagonist-resistant acute and chronic pruritus. Taken together, these results suggest that histamine H_4R could be a new drug target for therapeutic use in RA or pruritic skin disorders such as atopic dermatitis.

6. Acknowledgment

We thank Johnson & Johnson Pharmaceutical Research & Development, L.L.C., for generously providing JNJ7777120. This research was supported in part by Grants-in-Aid for Scientific Research from the Japan Society for the Promotion of Science.

7. References

Andoh T., Katsube N., Maruyama M., & Kuraishi Y. (2001). Involvement of leukotriene B(4) in substance P-induced itch-associated response in mice. *J. Invest. Dermatol.* 117: 1621-1626, ISSN 0022-202X.

Bell JK., McQueen DS., & Rees JL. (2004). Involvement of histamine H4 and H1 receptors in scratching induced by histamine receptor agonists in Balb C mice. *Br. J. Pharmacol.* 142: 374-380, ISSN 0007-1188.

de Esch IJ., Thurmond RL., Jongejan A., & Leurs R. (2005). The histamine H4 receptor as a new therapeutic target for inflammation. *Trends Pharmacol. Sci.* 26: 462-469, ISSN 0165-6147.

Dunford PJ., Williams KN., Desai PJ., Karlsson L., McQueen D., & Thurmond RL. (2007). Histamine H4 receptor antagonists are superior to traditional antihistamines in the attenuation of experimental pruritus. *J. Allergy Clin. Immunol.* 119: 176-183, ISSN 0091-6749.

Fonseca JE., Cortez-Dias N., Francisco A. Sobral M., Canhão H., Resende C., Castelão W., Macieira C., Sequeira G., Saraiva F., da Silva JA., Carmo-Fonseca M., & Viana Queiroz M. (2005). Inflammatory cell infiltrate and RANKL/OPG expression in rheumatoid synovium: comparison with other inflammatory arthropathies and correlation with outcome. *Clin. Exp. Rheumatol.* 23: 185-192, ISSN 0392-856X.

Frewin DB., Cleland LG., Jonsson JR., & Robertson PW. (1986). Histamine levels in human synovial fluid. *J. Rheumatol.* 13: 13-14, ISSN 0315-162X.

Grzybowska-Kowalczyk A., Wojtecka-Lukasik E., Maslinska D., Gujski M., & Maslinski S. (2007). Distribution pattern of histamine H4 receptor in human synovial tissue from patients with rheumatoid arthritis. *Inflamm. Res.* 56(Suppl 1): S59-S60, ISSN 1023-3830.

Gutzmer R., Mommert S., Gschwandtner M., Zwingmann K., Stark H., & Werfel T. (2009). The histamine H4 receptor is functionally expressed on T(H)2 cells. *J. Allergy Clin. Immunol.* 123: 619-625, ISSN 0091-6749.

Ikawa Y., Suzuki M., Shiono S., Ohki E., Moriya H., Negishi E., & Ueno K. (2005). Histamine H4 receptor expression in human synovial cells obtained from patients suffering from rheumatoid arthritis. *Biol. Pharm. Bull.* 28: 2016-2018, ISSN 0918-6158.

Ikawa Y., Shiba K., Ohki E., Mutoh N., Suzuki M., Sato H., & Ueno K. (2008). Comparative study of histamine H4 receptor expression in human dermal fibroblasts. *J. Toxicol. Sci.* 33: 503-508, ISSN 0388-1350.

Lippert U., Artuc M., Grützkau A., Babina M., Guhl S., Haase I., Blaschke V., Zachmann K., Knosalla M., Middel P., Krüger-Krasagakis S., & Henz BM. (2004). Human skin mast cells express H2 and H4, but not H3 receptors. *J. Invest. Dermatol.* 123: 116-123, ISSN 0022-202X.

Nagata Y. (1991). The role of histamine in human synovial fibroblasts. *Med. J. Kinki Univ.* 16: 117-126 (in Japanese), ISSN 0385-8367.

Nguyen T., Shapiro DA., George SR., Setola V., Lee DK., Cheng R., Rauser L., Lee SP., Lynch KR., Roth BL., & O'Dowd BF. (2001). Discovery of a novel member of the histamine receptor family. *Mol. Pharmacol.* 59:427–433, ISSN 0026-895X.

Oda T., Morikawa N., Saito Y., Masuho Y., & Matsumoto S. (2000). Molecular cloning and characterization of a novel type of histamine receptor preferentially expressed in leukocytes. *J. Biol. Chem.* 275: 36781-36786, ISSN 0021-9258.

Ohnishi H., Miyahara N., Dakhama A., Takeda K., Mathis S., Haribabu B., & Gelfand EW. (2008). Corticosteroids enhance CD8+ T cell-mediated airway hyperresponsiveness and allergic inflammation by upregulating leukotriene B4 receptor 1. *J. Allergy Clin. Immunol.* 121: 864-871, ISSN 0091-6749.

Ohki E., Suzuki M., Aoe T., Ikawa Y., Negishi E., & Ueno K. (2007). Expression of histamine H4 receptor in synovial cells from rheumatoid arthritic patients. *Biol. Pharm. Bull.* 30: 2217-2220, ISSN 0918-6158.

Suwa E., Yamaura K., Oda M., Namiki T., & Ueno K. (2011). Histamine H4 receptor antagonist reduces dermal inflammation and pruritus in a hapten-induced experimental model. *Eur. J. Pharmacol.* 667: 383-388, ISSN 0014-2999.

Sweeney SE., & Firestein GS. (2004). Rheumatoid arthritis: regulation of synovial inflammation. *Int. J. Biochem. Cell Biol.* 36: 372-378, ISSN 1357-2725.

Tanaka M. (2005). Autoimmune abnormality. *Nippon Rinsho* 63(Suppl 1): 80-83 (in Japanese), ISSN 0047-1852.

Togashi Y., Umeuchi H., Okano K., Ando N., Yoshizawa Y., Honda T., Kawamura K., Endoh T., Utsumi J., Kamei J., Tanaka T., & Nagase H. (2002). Antipruritic activity of the kappa-opioid receptor agonist, TRK-820. *Eur. J. Pharmacol.* 435: 259-264, ISSN 0014-2999.

Thurmond RL., Gelfand EW., & Dunford PJ. (2008). The role of histamine H1 and H4 receptors in allergic inflammation: the search for new antihistamines. *Nat. Rev. Drug. Discov.* 7: 41-53, ISSN 1474-1776.

Yamaura K., Oda M., Suwa E., Suzuki M., Sato H., & Ueno K. (2009). Expression of histamine H4 receptor in human epidermal tissues and attenuation of experimental pruritus using H4 receptor antagonist. *J. Toxicol. Sci.* 34: 427-431, ISSN 0388-1350.

Yamaura K., Doi R., Suwa E., & Ueno K. (2011). A novel animal model of pruritus induced by successive application of glucocorticoid to mouse skin. *J. Toxicol. Sci.* 36: 395-401, ISSN 0388-1350.

Yamaura K., Oda M., Suzuki M., & Ueno K. (2011). Lower expression of histamine H(4) receptor in synovial tissues from patients with rheumatoid arthritis compared to those with osteoarthritis. *Rheumatol Int.* Sep 1 (Epub ahead of print), ISSN: 0172-8172

Yamaura K., Akiyama S., & Ueno K. (2011). Increased expression of the histamine H4 receptor subtype in hypertrophic differentiation of chondrogenic ATDC5 cells. *J Cell Biochem.* In press, ISSN 1097-4644.

3

The Type I and Type II Receptor Complexes for IL-4 and IL-13 Differentially Regulate Allergic Lung Inflammation

Nicola M. Heller, Preeta Dasgupta, Nicolas J. Dorsey,
Svetlana P. Chapoval and Achsah D. Keegan
University of Maryland School of Medicine, Baltimore, MD, USA

1. Introduction

Approximately 300 million (M) people worldwide currently suffer from asthma; this number is projected to reach 400M by 2025 (Bahadori, et al., 2009). During the allergic immune response, inhaled allergens first stimulate epithelial cells, basophils, mast cells, and macrophages. This priming leads to the generation of allergen specific T-cells. Atopic asthma is strongly correlated with a robust CD4+ Th2 effector response, which results in elevated levels of the cytokines IL-4, 5, and 13. These cytokines act on multiple cells types to initiate and propagate the hallmark features of asthma such as pulmonary inflammation, periodic narrowing of airways, and mucus hypersecretion. Two of these cytokines, IL-4 and IL-13, share receptor chains and signaling proteins. In this chapter we discuss the cells that produce IL-4 and IL-13 including CD4+ T-cells and cells of the innate immune system, the structure of their receptors, their binding potency and kinetics, and their signal transduction. Furthermore, we present evidence for the differential effects of IL-4 and IL-13 acting via these receptor complexes on features of allergic lung inflammation. Finally, we discuss their contribution to the control of negative regulatory mechanisms that act to suppress allergic inflammation.

2. Cells that produce IL-4 and IL-13

Interleukin-4 and Interleukin-13 are closely related cytokines (Chomarat & Banchereau, 1998) critical to the development of T cell-mediated humoral immune responses, which are associated with allergy and asthma. Both cytokines display many overlapping functions (Chomarat & Banchereau, 1998). However, studies in cytokine-knockout mice and the use of blocking antibodies *in vivo* have shown that IL-4 is a critical cytokine for Th2 development whereas IL-13 plays critical roles in allergic asthmatic response (Grunig, et al., 1998, Wills-Karp, et al., 1998). Both cytokines can be secreted by many cell types but Th2 cells are considered to be the major producers. In this section, we will focus on cells capable of producing either IL-4, or IL-13, or both.

2.1 T cells

Upon antigen receptor stimulation, naive CD4+ T cells can differentiate into several different types, including T helper type 2 cells (Th2) depending on the cytokine milieu present during the priming. IL-4 itself is important for the differentiation of naïve CD4+ T cells into Th2 cells capable of producing large amounts of IL-4, IL-13, and IL-5 (Zhu&Paul, 2008). Recent evidence points to basophils (van Panhuys, et al., 2011), mast cells (Plaut, et al., 1989), natural killer (NK) T cells (Akbari, et al., 2003), and γ/δ T cells (Ferrick, et al., 1995) as early producers of IL-4 in the innate immune response necessary for the optimal priming of the Th2 adaptive response. Therefore, in addition to CD4+ T cells, other T cell subpopulations such as NKT cells and γ/δ T cells are capable of making IL-4.

IL-4 and IL-13 producing NKT cells have been shown to be essential for the development and progression of allergic airway inflammation (Akbari, et al., 2003). NKT cell-deficient (Cd1d1$^{-/-}$) mice showed reduced Th2 responses after allergen challenge including allergic airway inflammation and airway hyperreactivity. The abrogated Th2 response in these mice could be restored by the adoptive transfer of purified NKT cells producing IL-4 and IL-13, but not by IL-4-deficient and IL-13-deficient NKT cells. IL-13 instillation to the mice could restore allergic airway responses. This led the authors to conclude that IL-4 and IL-13 produced by NKT cells potentiate the development of Th2 response in the lung. However, other studies suggest that NKT cells do not play an important role in allergic lung inflammation models (Das, et al., 2006).

Gamma/delta T cells also can differentiate into cells producing Th2 cytokines (Wen, et al., 1998). When WT mice were infected with *Nippostrongylus brasiliensis,* an extracellular parasite known to induce Th2 responses, γ/δ T cells from these mice produced IL-4 (Ferrick, et al., 1995). The ability of human γ/δ T cells to differentiate into Th2 cytokine producing cells was tested using stimulation of peripheral blood-derived γ/δ T cells with phosphoantigen isopretenyl pyrophosphate (Wesch, et al., 2001). When these cells were stimulated with Ag under Th2 priming conditions, they developed into cells producing IL-4.

CD8+ T cells have been shown to produce IL-4 under specific *in vitro* stimulation (Seder, et al., 1992). When mouse CD8+ T cells were stimulated with immobilized CD3 in the presence of IL-2 and IL-4, they became high IL-4 producers. Moreover, both CD4+ T cells and CD8+ T cells separated from bulk lymph node T cell cultures with anti-CD3 plus IL-2 and IL-4 where equally effective in secretion of IL-4 after restimulation with anti-CD3 plus IL-2. The authors suggested that in certain *in vivo* conditions, CD8+ T cells could be major IL-4 producers. Human CD8+ T cell clones capable of IL-4 secretion were identified previously (Paliard, et al., 1988).

2.2 Granulocytes (Mast cells, basophils, and eosinophils)

Mouse non-T, non-B cells derived from spleen produce IL-4 and IL-13 in response to FcR crosslinkage (Ben-Sasson, et al., 1990). The same phenomenon was described for human bone marrow non-B and non-T cells in response to stimulation through either Fcε or Fcγ receptors (Piccinni, et al., 1991). It has been suggested then that those IL-4-secreting cells could be either mast cells or basophils, or both. Indeed, the ability of mast cells to secrete both cytokines has been reported utilizing human cord blood derived mast cells (Toru, et al., 1998). These cells can generate both cytokines after stimulation with PMA or FcεR crosslinking. However, these cells do not produce Th2 cytokines spontaneously. Similarly, the ability of mouse mast cells to secrete IL-4 and IL-13 in response to specific immunological stimulation has been reported for fetal liver derived mast cell lines, bone marrow derived mast cells, and the mast cell line C1.MC/C57.1 (Brown, et al., 1987, Burd, et al., 1995). Of note, mast cells secrete relatively high IL-13 but low IL-4 levels.

As noted above, basophils were among three major cell populations of IL-4 producers in the lung under inflammatory conditions (Voehringer, et al., 2004). The ability of basophils to secrete both cytokines and other mediators of inflammatory response was extensively reviewed by Min and Paul in 2008 (Min & Paul, 2008). Importantly, it has been shown that peripheral blood basophils in asthmatic patients are the main producers of IL-4 and IL-13 (Schroeder, et al., 1995), suggesting a role in asthma exacerbation. IL-4 was detected in cultures of human basophils treated with diesel exhaust particles (Devouassoux, et al., 2002) suggesting that environmental exposure can predispose basophils to initiate Th2 responses.

Eosinophils can also make IL-4 under certain circumstances. When mice were injected with *Schistosoma mansoni* eggs intraperitoneally, there were high levels of IL-4 in the peritoneal exudate cell cultures (Sabin, et al., 1996). IL-5 and eosinophils were necessary for the observed IL-4 production as suggested from similar experiments using egg-immunized IL-5$^{-/-}$ mice or anti-IL-5 treated mice (Kopf, et al., 1996). Interestingly, these eosinophils were found to produce IL-4 early after immunization. The authors suggested that *Schistosoma mansoni* induced an early IL-5 production by mast cells that attracted eosinophils which, in their turn, produced IL-4 thus stimulating the development of antigen-specific Th2 cells. The ability of eosinophils to make Th2 cytokines was also tested in a more recent study (Voehringer, et al., 2004). The authors characterized IL-4 producing cells in the inflamed lungs by immunohistochemistry, flow cytometry, and microarray in mice with a bicistronic knock-in IL-4 gene linked via internal ribosomal entry site (IRES) with enhanced green fluorescent protein (eGFP). Eosinophils, basophils, and Th2 cells were reported as three cell populations producing IL-4 in these mice.

2.3 Myeloid cells

Macrophages have been shown to produce IL-4 or IL-13 in response to certain stimuli. A strong expression of IL-13 in the lung was observed in the experimental model of particle inhalation-induced inflammation (Kang, et al., 2005). Immunostaining of lung tissues of TiO2-exposed mice demonstrated that alveolar macrophages are major producers of IL-13 and IL-25 in the inflamed lungs (Kang, et al., 2005). It has also been shown that human alveolar macrophages can produce IL-4 (Pouliot, et al., 2005). It has been shown that infectious pathogens including *Francisella tularensis* and respiratory syncitial virus (RSV) induce lung and peritoneal macrophages to produce IL-4 and IL-13 (Shirey, et al. 2008, Shirey, et al., 2010).

3. Receptor structure, ligand binding properties, and signal transduction

3.1 The structure of the IL-4 and IL-13 receptors

IL-4 and IL-13 elicit a wide variety of cellular responses by binding to high affinity receptor complexes expressed on the surface of cells. The IL-4/IL-13 receptor system is complex (**Figure 1**). The IL-4 specific receptor is composed of the IL-4Rα chain paired with the common γ chain, or γC, forming the Type I IL-4 receptor complex. The IL-4Rα chain can also pair with the IL-13Rα1 chain, forming the Type II receptor (**Figure 1**). Type I receptors are activated by the binding of IL-4 to the ligand-binding IL-4Rα chain and Type II receptors can be activated by either IL-4 or IL-13, with the IL-4Rα or IL-13Rα1 acting as the initial ligand-binding chain, respectively. IL-13 can also engage another kind of IL-13 receptor, the IL-13Rα2 chain.

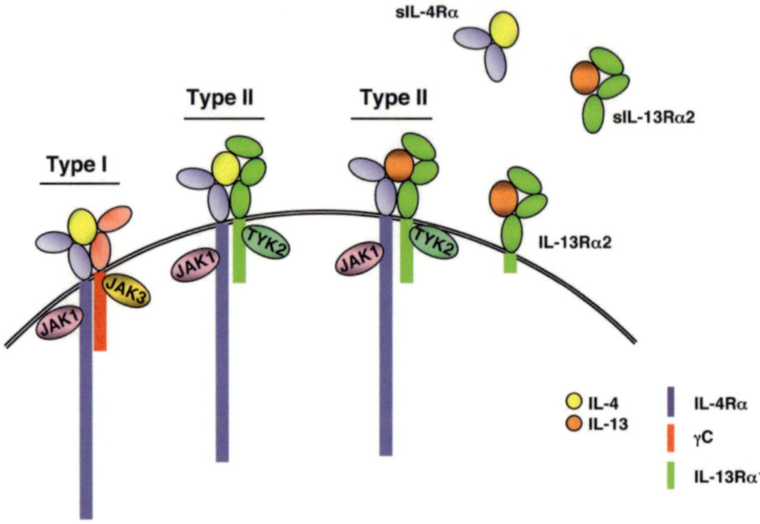

Fig. 1. **The IL-4 and IL-13 Receptor System.** A functional IL-4 receptor is composed of two transmembrane proteins. IL-4Rα chain binds IL-4 with high affinity, leading to dimerization with either common gamma chain (γC) or IL-13Rα1, forming the Type I or Type II receptor complex, respectively. IL-13 binds to IL-13Rα1 with lower affinity, followed by heterodimerization with IL-4Rα to form a high affinity complex. IL-13 also binds to IL-13Rα2 (the so-called "decoy receptor") at the cell surface, or in soluble form, but this interaction fails to activate the JAK/STAT pathway and generally it is thought to be inhibitory. Soluble forms of IL-4Rα (sIL-4Rα), IL-13Rα1 and IL-13Rα2 exist that can also bind ligand. Following ligand binding and heterodimerization, receptor-associated Janus Kinases (JAKs) are activated.

3.1.1 IL-4Rα

The IL-4Rα chain (CD124) is a 140 kDa protein. Human and mouse IL-4 receptors show a broad distribution on hematopoietic and non-hematopoietic cells (Park, et al., 1987, Lowenthal, et al., 1988), generally expressed at low levels (20-4000 receptors per cell).The IL-4Rα cDNAwas cloned from the mouse cytotoxic T-lymphocytic (CTLL-2) cell line (Mosley, et al., 1989) and from the human myeloid cell line, TF-1 (Galizzi, et al., 1990). Sequence analysis demonstrated that the IL-4Rα belongs to the hematopoeitin receptor superfamily. There are two extracellular structural features that characterize this family: type III fibronectin (FN) repeats and a membrane-proximal WSXWS motif.

The 2.3 Å resolution crystal structure of human IL-4 complexed to the extracellular domain of the human IL-4Rα determined the overall shape of the two, linked type III FN-like domains, D1 and D2 (Hage, et al., 1999). Five IL-4Rα peptide loops protrude from these two D domains and interact with IL-4. Binding of IL-4 to IL-4Rα occurs through interaction of IL-4 with two clusters or sites (I and II) within the receptor, with Y183 and D72 at the center, surrounded by a shell of hydrophobic residues.

3.1.2 γC

The involvement of the IL-2Rγ subunit, or common γ chain, in forming heterodimeric IL-4 receptors was recognized by three groups in the early 90's (Kondo, et al., 1993, Leonard, et al., 1994, Russell, et al., 1993). The γC chain (CD132), which dimerizes with the IL-4Rα chain to form a functional type I IL-4 receptor, is a 60 kDa protein. The extracellular domain of γC possesses the tandem FN-III domains with four Cys residues and membrane-proximal WSXWS motif creating the classical CHR. Mouse γC chain was cloned in 1993 (Kumaki, et al., 1993) and human γC in 1992 (Takeshita, et al., 1992). Both human and mouse γC genes map to the X-chromosome in humans (Noguchi, et al., 1993) and mouse (Cao, et al., 1993). The γC subunit participates in the formation of many other cytokine receptor complexes including the IL-2, IL-7, IL-9, IL-15 , and IL-21 receptors. Thus, mutations that either diminish or eliminate γC expression or prevent association of the JAK3 kinase with γC impair activity of these cytokines important for the development and proliferation of many different cells of the immune system, resulting in X-linked severe combined immunodeficiency (XSCID) in humans (Leonard, et al., 1994). γC-deficient mice have no NK cells and severely diminished T- and B-cells, virtually absent lymph nodes and spontaneously develop inflammatory bowel lesions (Cao, et al., 1995).

3.1.3 IL-13 receptor α1 (IL-13Rα1)

The IL-13Rα1 chain (CD213a1) is a 65-70 kDa glycosylated protein, encoded on the X chromosome in mice and humans. The mouse IL-13Rα1 cDNA was cloned in 1996 (Hilton, et al., 1996), followed by characterization of the human gene (Aman, et al., 1996), revealing the characteristic WSXWS motif and four conserved Cys residues. IL-13Rα1 can act either as a ligand-binding chain for IL-13 or as a dimerization partner to the type II receptor's IL-4-IL-4Rα ternary complex (Zurawski, et al., 1993). The IL-13Rα1 chain is widely expressed on the surface of many hematopoietic and non-hematopoietic cells. It is through this Type II receptor complex that IL-4 and IL-13 mediate their effects on non-hematopoietic cells, which generally lack γC, and therefore Type I receptor expression. IL-13Rα1 surface expression is absent on resting mouse and human T-cells and on mouse B-cells (Ogata, et al., 1998, Umeshita-Suyama, et al., 2000), although recent studies suggested inducible expression on mouse and human CD4+ T-cells (Newcomb, et al., 2009, Newcomb, et al., 2011). Related evolutionarily to γC, IL-13Rα1 has acquired a third extra Ig-like domain, D1, allowing extra contacts with IL-13 in Type II receptor complexes (LaPorte, et al., 2008). This D1 domain is required for IL-13 binding and the formation of a functional Type II receptor, while it is not required for IL-4 binding or its activation of the Type II receptor (Ito, et al., 2009).

3.1.4 IL-13 receptor α2 (IL-13α2)

IL-13 binds to a second IL-13 receptor, IL-13Rα2 (CD213a2, IL13BP) that was cloned in humans (Caput, et al., 1996) and from mice (Donaldson, et al., 1998). The gene is also found on the X-chromosome. IL-13Rα2 (~65 kDa) is inducibly expressed on fibroblasts, keratinocytes, epithelial cells, macrophages, and certain tumor cells and requires STAT6 for its expression (David, et al., 2003). The soluble form can be generated by proteolytic cleavage of the membrane-bound form by matrix metalloproteinases (MMPS) (Matsumura, et al., 2007) or by alternative splicing (Tabata, et al., 2006). Interestingly, sIL-13Rα2 is detected in serum from mice but not humans (Chen, et al., 2009). Treatment of cells with IL-4 or IL-13 in combination with TNF-α upregulated IL-13Rα2 cell surface expression (Zheng, et al., 2003). In contrast to IL-13Rα1, IL-13Rα2 binds to IL-13 with very high affinity 10^{-11} M (Andrews, et al., 2002) one of the highest measured protein-protein interactions, possibly due to an interlocking IL-13-binding interface (Lupardus, et al., 2010). The IL-13Rα2 is proposed to act as a "decoy receptor" for IL-13 (Yoshikawa, et al., 2003) and, more recently, for IL-4 signaling (Rahaman, et al., 2002,). Consistent with this model, mice deficient in IL-13Rα2 have exaggerated IL-13 responses, such as severe liver fibrosis following *S. mansonii* infection (Chiaramonte, et al., 2003, Mentink-Kane, et al., 2004), reversible by soluble IL-13Rα2-Fc. A signaling role was hypothesized, however, in TNBS-induced colitis, tumor surveillance, and cancer (Strober, et al., 2009) and in monocytic cell lines through AP-1 (Fichtner-Feigl, et al., 2006).

3.2 Ligand binding properties

IL-4 binds to the IL-4 receptor α chain with high affinity with a *Kd* ranging between 20 - 300 pM (Lowenthal, et al., 1988), allowing ligand binding at low IL-4 concentrations, as would be present in the initiating phase of an allergic inflammatory response. There is species specificity for the IL-4:IL-4Rα interaction (Park, et al., 1987), yet dimerization of the binary IL-4:IL-4Rα complex with the γC chain is not species specific (Idzerda, et al., 1990). Dimerization with the γC chain forming Type I IL-4 receptors increases the affinity of IL-4 binding approximately three-fold (Russell, et al., 1993). The affinity of interaction of the binary IL-4:IL-4Rα complex with either of its dimerization partners, γC or IL-13Rα1, is low (559 nM for γC with IL-4:IL-4Rα (Andrews, et al., 2006, LaPorte, et al., 2008, Zhang, et al., 2002) and 487 nM for IL-13Rα1 (LaPorte, et al., 2008)). In contrast, IL-13 binding to IL-13Rα1 is a relatively low affinity interaction (Kd ~ 30 nM (Andrews, et al., 2002, LaPorte, et al., 2008)) that is not species-specific (Andrews, et al., 2001). Dimerization of IL-13:IL-13Rα1 with IL-4Rα to form the ternary Type II complex is a high affinity, species-specific interaction (Andrews, et al., 2001, LaPorte, et al., 2008).

The crystal structures of the three ternary complexes were solved in 2008 (LaPorte, et al., 2008) revealing that the IL-4/IL-13 receptor system was unique in that when forming a Type II receptor the "binder" (i.e. ligand-binding) and "trigger" (i.e. dimerizing partner) chains were switched depending on whether IL-4 or IL-13 is the ligand. Furthermore, there was a ~ 8° angle difference in the position of the IL-4Rα chain relative to the IL-13Rα1 chain between the two Type II structures. The impact of these subtle differences in initial binding affinities, order of chain assembly, and 3-dimensional structure of the extracellular domains of the ternary complexes on responsiveness to IL-4 and IL-13 is not clear. A recent study suggests that the relative abundance of the two receptor types and ratio of the ligand-binding chain to the trigger chain can fine-tune sensitivity to these cytokines (Junttila et al., 2008).

3.3 Signal transduction pathways activated by Type I and Type II receptor engagement

3.3.1 Janus kinases

Ligand-induced dimerization of the Type I or Type II IL-4 receptor activates receptor-associated kinases of the Janus kinase (JAK) family. JAK1 was activated by IL-4 and IL-13 (Welham, et al., 1995). IL-13 did not induce JAK3 activation, as the IL-13Rα1 does not recruit JAK3 (Keegan, et al., 1995, Welham, et al., 1995). JAK2 appeared to be constitutively associated with the IL-4Rα chain in human monocytes and stimulation of the Type II receptor complex with IL-13 enhanced the interaction (Roy, et al., 2002). IL-13 predominantly activates TYK2 (Murata & Puri, 1997), as well as JAK2 (Murata, et al., 1996). JAK1 is a substrate for other non-JAK kinases that can affect the activation of IL-4-induced signaling. PKCζ is required for full IL-4-induced JAK1 activation (Martin, et al., 2005). Mutational studies on cytoplasmic domain of IL-4Rα have revealed the presence of a membrane-proximal, proline-rich "box 1" motif (aa262 - 267 for hIL-4Rα and 263 - 271 for mIL-4Rα) to which JAK1 can bind (Fujiwara, et al., 1997, Russell, et al., 1994). The cytoplasmic domain of the γC also has a "box 1" motif :Pro-X-Pro and a preceding cluster of hydrophobic amino acids (aa286 - 294 that binds JAK3, Murakami, et al., 1991)).

The proline-rich region in the IL-13Rα1 (aa 373 - 378 in mouse and aa 376 - 381 in human) and the next six amino acids downstream mediate the interaction between IL-13Rα1 and the associated JAKs (TYK2, JAK1 in a transfected FDCP-1 cell line (Orchansky, et al., 1999)). The cytoplasmic domain of the IL-13Rα1 chain is shorter than that of the IL-4Rα or γC. It contains the box 1 motif and two tyrosines, Y402 and Y405, which act as STAT3 binding motifs (Orchansky, et al., 1999, Umeshita-Suyama, et al., 2000). Engagement of the receptor chain by IL-13 activates JAK1 and TYK2 and triggers a variety of signaling cascades which will be discussed below.

Tyrosine residues within the cytoplasmic domains of the Type I and Type II receptor subunits are targets for rapid phosphorylation by the JAKs (**Figure 2**). Both IL-4 and IL-13 induce tyrosine phosphorylation of IL-4Rα (Wang, et al., 1992). Tyrosine phosphorylation of IL-13Rα1 was not detected in immunoprecipitated lysates from IL-13-stimulated FD-5 cells transfected with the IL-13Rα1 subunit (Orchansky, et al., 1999) although mutational studies suggested that IL-13Rα1 tyrosines would indeed become phosphorylated (Umeshita-Suyama, et al., 2000). Studies using deletion, Y-to-F mutants, and chimeric forms of the IL-4Rα (Deutsch, et al., 1995, Keegan, et al., 1994, Koettnitz & Kalthoff, 1993, Seldin & Leder, 1994) have characterized distinct regions of the IL-4Rα cytoplasmic domain containing five essential tyrosine residues (Y1-Y5). These phosphotyrosines become docking sites for SH2- and PTB-containing proteins: Y1 (Y497) recruits IRS proteins, Y2-Y4 (Y575, Y603, Y631) recruit STAT6 and Y5 (Y713) is bound by the phosphatases, SHP-1, -2 and SHIP (Hanson, et al., 2003, Kashiwada, et al, 2001).

3.3.2 IRS proteins

IL-4 strongly induced the tyrosine phosphorylation of a ~170 kDa protein in the mouse IL-3-dependent hematopoietic cell line, FDCP-2 (Wang, et al., 1992), named IL-4-induced phosphotyrosine substrate (4PS) and it associated with PI3-K and PI3-K activity. This protein was identical to that tyrosine phosphorylated in response insulin and IGF-I in FDC cells (Wang, et al., 1993). 4PS was cloned from myeloid progenitor cells and renamed IRS-2 due to similarity to IRS-1 (Sun, et al., 1995). IRS-1 is also tyrosine phosphorylated in response to IL-4 stimulation and whether IRS-1 or IRS-2 or both are tyrosine phosphorylated after IL-4 stimulation depends on cellular expression of each protein and the surface expression of Type I or II receptors (Sun, et al., 1997). IRS-2 is predominantly found in hematopoietic cells and IRS-1 in non-hematopoietic cells: studies in 32D cells, which express neither IRS protein, revealed the role of both IRS-1 and IRS-2 in IL-4-induced cellular proliferation (Wang, et al., 1993).

The sequence of amino acids important for IRS binding to the IL-4 receptor was determined by truncation mutational analysis (between aa437 and 557). Within this interval, there is a homologous sequence that binds IRS proteins in the insulin and IGF-I receptor, known as the insulin and IL-4 receptor (I4R) motif, whose sequence is ^{488}PL-$(X)_4$-NPXYXSXSD^{502}. The central tyrosine when phosphorylated is critical for association of the PTB domain of IRS proteins with the I4R motif of the IL-4Rα (Keegan, et al., 1994, Zhou, et al., 1996).

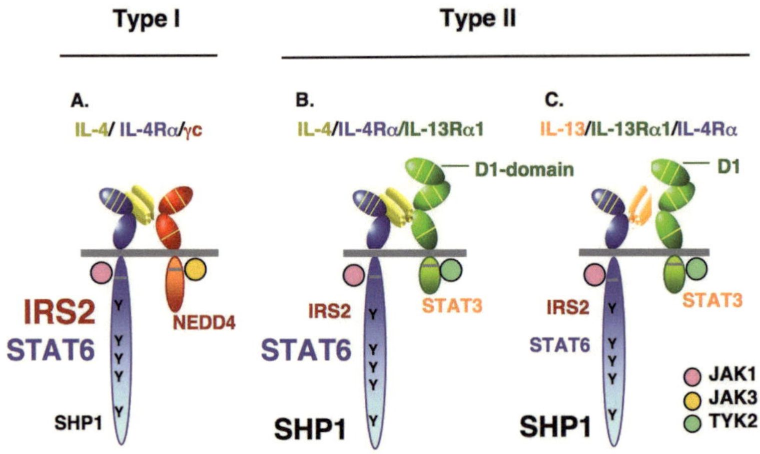

Fig. 2. **Signaling by the Type I and Type II receptors.** The signaling pathways activated by the Type I and Type II receptor complexes are shown in cartoon form. The *font size* is an indication of the *relative strength* of activation of IRS-2, STAT6, and SHP1 by the IL-4 or IL-13 receptor complexes. Differences in signaling by the receptor complexes are highlighted. A. Type I Receptor. IL-4 (yellow), IL-4Rα (blue) and γc (red). IL-4Rα binds JAK1 (pink) while γc binds JAK3 (rust). γc associates with Nedd4. B. Type II Receptor bound to IL-4. IL-4 (yellow), IL-4Rα (blue), and IL-13Rα1 (green). The D1 domain of IL-13Rα1 is shown. IL-13Rα1 binds to TYK2 (green). IL-13Rα1 recruits STAT3 (orange). C. Type II Receptor bound to IL-13. IL-13 (orange), IL-13Rα1 (green), IL-4Rα (blue). The relative ability of these receptor complexes to activate Shc or the MAP kinase pathways is unclear.

The IRS proteins are tyrosine phosphorylated in response to engagement of the IL-4 receptors. JAK1 is required for this to occur (Wang, et al., 1997). Once phosphorylated, tyrosines that are part of typical SH2-binding motifs (Sun, et al., 1991) provide docking sites for a variety of different SH2-domain-containing downstream molecules, such as the p85 subunit of PI3-K and Grb2 (Pruett, et al., 1995). There are three tyrosines, part of classical YXXM motifs, that act as p85 binding sites in IRS-1 and two in IRS-2 (White, 2002). Binding of p85 can activate PI3-K thus allowing IL-4 to initiate a large number of downstream signaling cascades. The IRS proteins can also bind SHP-2 following IL-4 stimulation and IRS-2 can recruit PLC-γ in response to IL-13 (Sozzani, et al., 1998). The IRS proteins also interact with the SOCS proteins that are negative regulators of IL-4 signaling and will be discussed in more detail in a later section.

The contribution of IRS-2 to allergy and asthma is not well understood. Transgenic overexpression of IRS-2 enhanced IgE production *in vivo*, and increased IL-5 secretion from *in vitro* differentiated CD4+ Th2 cells (Kelly-Welch, et al., 2004). Early studies of T-cells isolated from IRS2$^{-/-}$ mice found reduced T-cell proliferation and IL-5 production by Th2 cells compared to wildtype T-cells (Wurster, et al., 2002). Surprisingly, mice with a mutation in the IRS-2 docking site of the IL-4Rα (Y500F) demonstrated enhanced allergic inflammation, suggesting a significant contribution of this region of the IL-4Rα to inflammation control *in vivo* (Blaeser, et al., 2003). Activation of the IRS-2 pathway was abrogated but this Y500 region of the IL-4Rα also recruits a number of other signaling molecules including Shc, FRIP1, p62DOK, and p85β (Nelms, et al., 1998) that may negatively regulate the pathway (described below).

3.3.3 Activation of PI3-K

The p85 or regulatory subunit of PI3-K binds phosphotyrosines on the IRS protein via SH2-domains and the resulting conformational change releases inhibition of the enzymatic activity of the p110 (catalytic) subunit and allows it to translocate to the plasma membrane. Activation of PI3K activity in response to IL-4 was first demonstrated in hematopoietic FDCP cells inducing mitogenic signals (Wang, et al., 1992). The kinase transfers a phosphate group from ATP to phosphoinositol (PI) to rapidly form PIP3, activating a myriad of downstream pathways. PIP3 has the potential to activate protein kinase C (PKC) and protein kinase B (PKB)/Akt. Activation of Akt in response to IL-4 has been shown in human eosinophils (Coffer, et al., 1998), although we found no induction of phosphorylation on Akt^{Ser473} in mouse eosinophils by IL-4 or IL-13 (Heller et al, under review).

3.3.4 Signal Transducers and Activators of Transcription (STATs)

IL-4 receptor engagement can activate a number of members of the STAT family. STAT6 is the predominantly activated STAT but other members of the STAT family can also be activated to a lesser degree. The human STAT6 gene was cloned in 1994 and the same group determined that STAT6 (IL-4 Stat) directly interacted with the IL-4 receptor cytoplasmic domain, homodimerized via its SH2-domain and characterized the DNA binding motif recognized by STAT6 (Hou, et al., 1994). STAT6 docks via its highly conserved SH2-domain to the "gene regulation domain" (aa 557 - 657) encompassing three of the five conserved tyrosines of human IL-4Rα (Ryan, et al., 1996). STAT6 becomes tyrosine phosphorylated on Y641 and forms homodimers through pY641-SH2 interactions (Mikita et al., 1996). The C-terminus of STAT6 contains the transcriptional activation domain (Goenka, et al., 1999). In addition to tyrosine phosphorylation, the STAT6 protein can be post-translationally modified in other ways to affect its function: methylation (Chen, et al., 2003), serine phosphorylation (Pesu, et al., 2000) on S756 (Wang, et al., 2004) and S707 (Shirakawa, et al., 2011) and acetylation (Shankaranarayanan, et al., 2001).

Once in the nucleus, STAT6 homodimers bind to consensus DNA motifs in STAT6-responsive genes (reviewed in Goenka & Kaplan, 2011). The preferred DNA binding motif recognized by STAT6 is a dyad symmetric recognition element TTC-GAA separated by four nucleotides although STAT6 can also bind the dyad element separated by three nucleotides. STAT6 often co-operates with other transcription factors and co-activators to activate transcription including NK-κB, CEBPβ, CBP and p300 and p160 steroid receptor nuclear coactivator (NCoA-1).

STAT6 deficiency (Takeda, et al., 1996) is protective in many different *in vivo* models of allergy including allergic airway disease, food allergy, eosinophilic esophagitis and atopic dermatitis. In contrast, mice expressing constitutively active STAT6 are predisposed to an allergic phenotype (Sehra, et al., 2008, Sehra, et al., 2010). Hyperactive STAT6 can lead to cellular transformation and various cancers, due to dysregulated $p27^{Kip}$/cell cycle progression (Bruns, et al., 2003). Mice deficient in STAT6 have compromised expulsion of helminth parasites: they cannot produce Th2-cells, mount an effective IgE response, produce mucus or chemokines (Kaplan, et al., 1998).

While STAT6 is clearly the dominant STAT family member activated by IL-4 and IL-13, there are reports of activation of several other STATs to varying degrees. Some STAT1a activation was documented in the mouse T-helper cell line, HT-2, in response to IL-4 (Brunn, et al., 1995) and by IL-4 and IL-13 in five primary human cell types generally to a lesser degree than STAT6 (Wang, et al., 2004). Primary human monocytes respond to IL-13 with tyrosine phosphorylation of STAT1a (Roy, et al., 2002). Furthermore, STAT5 phosphorylation was detected in human B-cells in response to IL-4 and IL-13 (Rolling, et al., 1996) and in primary human monocytes by IL-13 (Roy, et al., 2002). The role of STAT1 and STAT5 in IL-4- or IL-13-induced responses is unknown.

The cytoplasmic domain of IL-13Rα1 contains two STAT3 binding motifs (Y402 andY405, (Orchansky, et al., 1999)). STAT3 activation by IL-4 and IL-13 is dependent upon expression of the IL-13Rα1 (Orchansky, et al., 1999) and occurs in response to IL-4 and IL-13 in human B-cells (Rolling, et al., 1996) and weakly in HMVEC-L and NHLF cells (Wang, et al., 2004). STAT3 phosphorylation was induced by IL-13 in primary human monocytes (Roy, et al., 2002) and by IL-4 in keratinocytes (Wery-Zennaro, et al., 1999). We have observed the relatively weak induction of STAT3 phosphorylation by IL-4 and IL-13 in murine bone-marrow-derived macrophages and the human lung adenocarcinoma cell line A549 (LaPorte, et al., 2008). The specific function of STAT3 in mediating responses to IL-4 and IL-13 is unclear. A recent report demonstrated that STAT3 played a role in Th2 differentiation, however the cytokines responsible for STAT3 activation in that setting were thought to be IL-6 or IL-21 (Stritesky, et al., 2011).

3.3.5 Other pathways activated by IL-4Rα (Ras/MAPK, Shc, Dok)

Activation of the Ras/MAPK pathway is not generally observed in response to IL-4 despite IRS activation leading to interaction with the adapter molecule, Grb2 (Pruett, et al., 1995, Wang, et al., 1995). Since Grb2 is constitutively associated with the guanine nucleotide exchange protein, SOS, that catalyzes exchange of GDP bound to Ras for GTP, it is often assumed that IL-4 will trigger the phosphorylation cascade of Raf/MEK/ERK-1/-2. However, IL-4 does not activate p21ras (Duronio, et al., 1992, Satoh, et al., 1991, Welham, et al., 1994), Raf1 or ERK1/2 (Welham, et al., 1992, Welham, et al., 1994). We too have been unable to detect ERK-1/2 activation in response to IL-4 or IL-13 in primary mouse bone marrow-derived macrophages (Heller, et al., 2008) or peripheral blood eosinophils. Activation of the Ras/MAPK pathway was demonstrated to enhance IL-4 signaling, possibly through MEK phosphorylation of JAK1 and STAT6 (Yamashita, et al., 1999).

Activation of Shc can be linked to Ras activation, via the Grb2 adapter-Sos interaction. There are three widely-expressed Shc proteins (~46, 52 and 66 kDa) containing a C-terminal SH2 domain, regions homologous to the a1 chain of collagen (Pelicci, et al., 1992) and an N-terminal PTB domain, similar in structure to IRS protein PTB domain (Zhou, et al., 1996). Shc moves to the plasma membrane and docks to the phosphorylated I4R motifs on activated IL-4 receptors via its SH2 and PTB domains (Wolf, et al., 1995). Phospho-Shc is then bound by the SH2/3 motifs of the Grb2 adaptor and bound Sos is activated. Shc activation in response to IL-4 appears to be dependent on cell type (Crowley, et al., 1996, Wery, et al., 1996, Welham, et al., 1994).

Two hematopoietically-expressed members of the Dok proteins play a role in IL-4R-induced responses. The N-terminal PH and PTB domains of the Dok proteins suggest that they could bind phosphotyrosines in membrane-localized receptors (Mashima, et al., 2009). Indeed, Dok-2 (also known as FRIP, Dok-R or p56^{dok}) has been shown to interact with the I4R motif of the IL-4Rα (Nelms, et al., 1998). T-cells from Dok-2-deficient mice (the *hairless* allele, *hr/hr*) have an increased proliferative response to IL-2 and IL-4 (Nelms, et al., 1998). Studies of Dok-1 (p62^{dok})-deficient cells suggest this protein plays a positive role in sustaining IL-4 signaling responses (IL-4-induced T-cell proliferation and CD23 expression and IgE class switching in B-cells (Inoue, et al., 2007)). The Dok proteins have multiple docking sites for SH2-containing proteins in their C-terminus and thus act as adaptor proteins. Because both Dok proteins bind RasGAP, which inactivates Ras by hydrolysis of GTP, it is thought that they might be negative regulators of the Ras/MAPK pathway. Recruitment of the Dok proteins to the IL-4Rα may explain the lack of Ras activation by IL-4 in some cell types.

3.4 Negative regulation of receptor signaling

3.4.1 SHP-1 and SHP-2

Protein tyrosine phosphatases (PTP) that remove phosphate groups from phosphotyrosine residues that are activating signals can downregulate the signaling cascades initiated by IL-4. SHP-1 and SHP-2 are PTP molecules containing two N-terminal SH2-domains, a single central phophatase domain and C-termini with two potential tyrosine phosphorylation sites that affect activity. The SH2-domain targets the phosphatase to a particular cellular location and binds to and inhibits the catalytic domain when the phosphatase is not bound to substrate. The expression of SHP-1 is restricted to hematopoietic cells (Yi, et al., 1992) and low expression is also found in epithelial cells. SHP-2, on the other hand, is widely expressed including in cells that express SHP-1.

SHP-1 may positively (White, et al., 2001) or negatively (Imani, et al., 1997) regulate IL-4 responses , depending upon the cell type (Huang, et al., 2005). Interestingly, SHP-1 constitutively associates with the IL-4Rα chain even in resting lymphocytes(Huang & Paul, 2000). Subsequent studies have indicated that SHP-1 also negatively regulates signaling responses to IL-13 by downregulating the phosphorylation of STAT6 (Haque, et al., 1998).

SHP SH2-domains bind to ITIM sequences [I/V/L]xY(p)xx[I/V/L] in activated receptors (Ravetch & Lanier, 2000). The cytoplasmic domain of the IL-4Rα possesses a putative ITIM surrounding the fifth tyrosine, Y713 (**Figure 2**) and a variety of studies have indicated this motif may interact with SHP-1, SHP-2, Shc and SHIP (Kashiwada, et al., 2001,Hershey, et al., 1997, Kruse, et al., 2002). Our group showed that Y^{713} in human IL-4Rα mediated recruitment of SHP-1 (Hanson, et al., 2003) and SHIP (Zamorano & Keegan, 1998) to the IL-4 receptor complex. Knock-in of a Y713F mutant of IL-4Rα in mice resulted in enhanced STAT6 phosphorylation, IgE production, and allergic lung inflammation (Tachdjian, et al., 2010). Loss of Y^{713} had a more dramatic effect on the magnitude of responses to IL-13 *vs.* IL-4. Taken together these results suggest that IL-4 and IL-13 signaling is modulated by SHP1 or other phosphatases capable of binding to Y^{713}, and that this modulation may be more profound for the Type II receptor complex (**Figure 2**).

While tyrosine phosphorylation of SHP-1 increases its phosphatase activity, tyrosine phosphorylation of SHP-2 has been proposed to allow this molecule to function as an adaptor protein by providing docking sites for other SH2-domain-containing proteins (Lorenz, 2009). Conflicting data describe that SHP-2 was (Kruse, et al., 2002, Wang, et al., 1999) or was not (Gadina, et al., 1999) tyrosine phosphorylated in response to IL-4 stimulation. IL-13 stimulation of PBMC also induced tyrosine phosphorylation of SHP-2 (Kruse, et al., 2002). SHP-2 interacts with IRS-1 (Xiao, et al., 2002), JAK1, JAK3 and coprecipitates with Grb-2 and p85 after cytokine stimulation (Gadina, et al., 1998, Kuhne, et al., 1993). Peptides derived from the IL-4Rα (aa 545–558) were able to pull down SHP-2 from lysates of IL-13-stimulated PBMC (Kruse, et al., 2002).

Hematopoietically-expressed SH2-domain-containing inositol 5'-phosphatase (SHIP) dephosphorylates PIP3, the product of the PI3-K enzyme, to form PIP2. IL-4 stimulation can induce tyrosine phosphorylation of SHIP, suggesting that SHIP can dock to multiple sites in the IL-4Rα (Zamorano & Keegan, 1998). SHIP-1-deficient mice spontaneously developed allergic lung inflammation, have increased mast cells that spontaneously released histamine indicating a potential homeostatic role for SHIP-1 in regulating Th2-responses *in vivo* (Oh, et al., 2007). Recent exciting data have defined a role for SHIP-1 in the skewing of macrophage phenotype (Rauh, et al., 2005).

3.4.2 Suppressors of Cytokine Signaling (SOCS)

The suppressor of cytokine signaling (SOCS) proteins are a family of cytokine-induced negative regulators of cytokine signaling (Starr, et al., 1997, Yoshimura, et al., 2003). The general structure of the SOCS protein includes a central SH2-domain, critical for binding to their tyrosine phosphorylated substrates, and a C-terminal SOCS box that mediates ubiquitin-dependent proteolysis. SOCS-1), -3 and CIS are induced by IL-4 and SOCS-1 and -3 were shown to inhibit IL-4 signaling transduction (Haque, et al., 2000, Losman, et al., 1999). SOCS-1 and SOCS-3, both of which are induced by IL-4, have an additional kinase inhibitory region that functions as a pseudosubstrate to inhibit JAK activity (Yasukawa, et al., 1999). Another mechanism of action is by SOCS interaction with the phosphorylated tyrosines within the cytoplasmic domains of the receptor. SOCS-3 directly interacted with IL-4α (O'Connor, et al., 2007). SOCS proteins can also target activated signaling intermediates to the proteasome. SOCS-1 is able to regulate the half-life of JAKs and insulin/IGF-I-induced IRS-2 (Rui, et al., 2001) in this manner.

4. Differential roles for IL-4 and IL-13 acting via the Type I or Type II receptors on features of allergic lung inflammation

Recent evidence suggests that even though IL-4 and IL-13 share receptor components and signaling proteins, and elicit overlapping responses *in vitro*, they can elicit different functional responses *in vivo*. IL-4 is primarily responsible for regulating Th2 development and inflammation while IL-13 is responsible for effector activities such as airway hypersensitivity, collagen production, and mucus hypersecretion (Gavett, et al., 1994, Pernis & Rothman, 2002, Wills-Karp, et al., 1998). The molecular basis for this variation is not understood clearly, since both IL-4 and IL-13 use the Type II receptor complex. It has been postulated that differences in the relative abundance of the Type I or Type II receptor subunits in different cell types may be responsible for the differences in responses elicited by IL-4 versus IL-13. Certainly the presence or absence of individual receptor subunits and appropriate Janus kinases in each cell determines whether a cell can respond to IL-4 or IL-13. However, many of the cell types involved in the effector activities express the Type II receptor that is activated by both IL-4 and IL-13.

4.1 Different receptor signaling pathways utilized by IL-4 and IL-13 via the Type I and Type II receptors

One reason proposed for differential functions of these cytokines is the observed differences in the amounts of IL-4 and IL-13 produced in tissues during Type II inflammation. Various reports have shown that IL-13 is secreted by large number of cell types and in much greater quantities than IL-4 during Th2 responses in both asthma patients (Huang, et al., 1995) as well as mouse models of this disease (Munitz, et al., 2008). However, analysis of the binding affinities of the Type I and Type II receptors with their respective ligands have shown that the relative amounts of each cytokine does not necessarily explain the functional differences between IL-4 and IL-13.

As discussed above, LaPorte and colleagues have shown that although IL-4 binding to the IL-4Rα chain occurs with high affinity, complex formation of IL-4: IL-4Rα with γC or IL-13Rα1 is quite unstable and inefficient (LaPorte, et al., 2008). On the other hand, IL-13 binds to IL-13Rα1 with low affinity, but the interaction of IL-13: IL-13Rα1 with IL-4Rα is more favorable and stable. As a result even at very low concentrations, IL-4 is able to mediate efficient and rapid STAT6 phosphorylation via Type I and Type II receptors, while cells have to be stimulated with much higher concentrations of IL-13 and for a longer time to obtain similar responses via the Type II receptor. Since the IL-4 bound complexes are less stable, LaPorte *et. al.* proposed that when expression of receptor chains in cells become limiting, IL-4 responses would be limited, while IL-13 responses would take over.

However, experiments using transgenic overexpression of large quantities of IL-4 or IL-13 still showed differences in the pathophysiology elicted by these two cytokines (Rankin, et al., 1996, Zhu, et al., 1999). These results suggest that there are real signaling differences between IL-4 and IL-13. To analyze potential signaling differences, we undertook a careful, side-by-side comparison of primary cells and cell lines that expressed either both Type I and II receptors or Type II receptors only. IL-4 stimulated tyrosine phosphorylation of STAT6 in the human airway epithelial cell line, A549, and the human B-cell line, Ramos, at significantly lower doses than IL-13. We demonstrated that IL-4 signaling through the Type I receptor induced robust tyrosine phosphorylation of the downstream adaptor protein IRS-2 and greater expression of the mRNAs for a subset of alternatively activated macrophage genes in primary mouse bone marrow-derived macrophages (BMM) (Heller, et al., 2008). This was in contrast to IL-4/IL-13 signaling through the Type II receptor which resulted in weaker tyrosine phosphorylation of IRS-2 and less mRNA for the AAM genes studied. This marked difference in IRS-2 phosphorylation and AAM gene expression induced by IL-4 was dependent upon expression of the γC subunit.

4.2 Differential functions of IL-4 and IL-13 in allergic lung inflammation

In both humans and mice, IL-4 and IL-13 signaling through the Type I and Type II receptors play a critical role in inducing asthma. The hallmark features of this disease include excessive pulmonary inflammation, periodic narrowing of airways, airway hyperesponsiveness (AHR) and enhanced mucus secretion. IL-4 and IL-13 have differential roles in asthma pathogenesis. Studies using IL-4Rα$^{-/-}$ and STAT6$^{-/-}$ mice in our lab and by other investigators have suggested that many of the asthma symptoms mentioned above are regulated by IL-4Rα and STAT6 (Cohn, et al., 1997, Corry, et al., 1998, Grunig, et al., 1998, Kelly-Welch, et al., 2004, Kuperman, et al., 1998, Mathew, et al., 2001, Wills-Karp, et al., 1998). However, since IL-4/IL-13 binding to either the Type I or Type II receptor activates STAT6, the contributions of these individual pathways in inducing the pathophysiology associated with this disease was unclear, until recently.

It is known that IL-4 is predominantly required for Th2 cell differentiation and proliferation (Kaplan, et al., 1996). Since most naive T cells lack the Type II receptor, they are unresponsive to IL-13. IL-4 signaling through the Type I IL-4R/STAT6 axis upregulates GATA3, the Th2 master transcription factor (reviewed in (Zhu & Paul, 2008)). STAT6-deficient T cells cannot differentiate into Th2 cells *in vitro* (Kaplan, et al., 1996). Recent studies have shown that STAT6 is not required for *in vivo* differentiation, although it is required for stabilization of Th2 cells and generating memory responses (reviewed in (Chapoval, et al., 2010)). Activated Th2 cells then secrete large quantities of IL-4, IL-5 and IL-13 which can act on many different cell types. IL-4 induces expression of MHC Class II in resting B cells and also causes antibody class switching from IgM to IgE and IgG1 (reviewed in Nelms, et al., 1999). Treatment with anti-IL-4 antibody blocks both primary and secondary IgE responses *in vivo,* when administered at the time of antigenic challenge (Finkelman, et al., 1988). IL-13 on the other hand is thought to be responsible for causing AHR, excessive mucus production and lung fibrosis. Neutralization of IL-13 was able to completely reverse allergen induced airway resistance and abolished mucus production by airway epithelial cells seen in control mice (Grunig, et al., 1998, Wills-Karp, et al., 1998).

Apart from its action on lymphocytes, IL-4 also activates mast cells. This cytokine enhances surface expression of FcεRI, the high affinity receptor for IgE (Toru, et al., 1996). Binding of IgE to FcεRI causes crosslinking of the cytoplasmic Fc domain of this receptor and triggers degranulation (release of mast cell granules). This process causes rapid release of many inflammatory mediators such as histamine, leukotrienes and prostaglandins (reviewed in (Weller, et al., 2011)). Histamine increases blood circulation and permeability of blood vessels, causing increased recruitment of inflammatory cells, including eosionophils, T cells, dendritic cells and monocytes. Leukotrienes and prostaglandins promote bronchoconstriction and stimulate epithelial cell induced mucus production. The importance of FcεRI in allergic responses has been demonstrated in studies using a soluble form of FcεRI and mice lacking the α chain of this receptor (Dombrowicz, et al., 1993, Ra, et al., 1993). In both cases IgE-mediated allergic responses were abrogated.

In addition to mast cells, eosinophils are closely associated with asthma pathogenesis. Increased numbers of eosinophils in the lung and other tissues in asthmatic patients usually correlate with disease severity and it is thought to be the central effector cell involved in airway inflammation (reviewed in (Hogan, et al., 2008)). IL-5 plays an important role in eosinophil development, proliferation and survival in the bone marrow. It is also required for migration of eosinophils into the blood and subsequently the lung. Recruitment of eosinophils to the peribronchial regions of the lung is thought to be mediated by secretion of various eotaxins (eotaxin 1, 2 and 3) by airway epithelial cells. Moreover, IL-5 and the eotaxins cooperate to induce tissue eosinophilia. Various eosinophilic granule components such as major basic protein (MBP) and eosinophilic cationic protein (ECP) have been implicated in initiating and propagating many features of asthma including pulmonary inflammation, airway hyperresponsiveness and bronchoconstriction. Eosinophils express both the Type I and Type II receptors. We have shown that IL-4, but not IL-13, can enhance chemotaxis of eosinophils to eotaxin 1 *in vitro* through the Type I receptor (Heller and Keegan, unpublished). Studies using IL-13Rα1$^{-/-}$ mice have shown that while eotaxin production and secretion by epithelial cells was completely dependent on IL-13 signaling through the Type II receptor, recruitment of eosinophils into the lungs was not (Munitz, et al., 2008, Ramalingam, et al., 2008). Therefore, it is possible that the Type I receptor is compensating for the absence of the Type II receptor. Alternatively, IL-5 may be playing a role in this response. Unlike hematopoietic cells, epithelial, endothelial and smooth muscle cells contain only the Type II receptor. Although both IL-4 and IL-13 can bind to this receptor complex, IL-13 is considered to be the main effector cytokine responsible for AHR, excessive mucus production and lung fibrosis.

The unique contributions of the Type II receptor in allergic lung inflammation have been studied using IL-13Rα1-/- mice. Mucus secretion, airway resistance, eotaxin production and induction of pro-fibrotic mediators such as TGFβ were completely dependent on the IL-13Rα1 chain, and thus the Type II receptor (Munitz, et al., 2008, Ramalingam, et al., 2008). However, the authors showed that Th2 cell differentiation, IgE secretion in response to T cell dependent antigens (such as ovalbumin) and recruitment of eosinophils and other inflammatory cells into the lungs could occur independently of IL-13Rα1 . In addition, DNA microarray analysis of cells isolated from allergen or IL-4 treated WT or IL-13Rα1-/- mice indicated that several AAM genes were differentially regulated. Munitz *et.al.* showed that allergen and IL-4 induced *Retnla* expression levels were similar in both WT and IL-13Rα1-/- mice, but induction of chitinase (*Chia*) was completely dependent on IL-13Rα1 (Munitz, et al., 2008). Interestingly enough, allergen induced arginase 1 expression required the Type II receptor, but IL-4 induced arginase 1 expression did not. Thus, it appears that IL-4 utilizes both the Type I and Type II receptors to stimulate AAM development in the lung.
Studies conducted by us as well as other groups have shown that IL-4 preferentially induces robust AAM gene expression, while IL-13 does so only weakly (Heller, et al., 2008, Munitz, et al., 2008, Ramalingam, et al., 2008). Intriguingly, mutation of the ITIM motif in the IL-4Rα chain resulted in increased sensitivity of macrophages to IL-13 mediated AAM activation. As demonstrated earlier, the Y709 (WT) BMMs treated with IL-4 led to significantly higher expression of AAM genes (*Arginase1, Chi3l3*) and also *Ccl11* in contrast to IL-13. Mutation of Y709 residue to F709 resulted in dramatic amplification of *Arginase1, Chi3l3* and *Ccl11* genes in response to IL-13, while leaving the IL-4 induced responses intact or slightly enhanced (Tachdjian, et al., 2010). IL-13 but not IL-4 induced similar responses in primary lung fibroblasts. These results suggest that there is a disproportionate increase in AAM activation induced by IL-13 signaling via the Type II receptor. The authors hinted that differential recruitment of SHP-1 by the Type I and Type II receptors may be the reason behind these observations (**Figure 2**). Although much progress has been made in understanding the mechanisms by which IL-4 and IL-13 may elicit different responses in different cell types and in the lung during allergic diseases and asthma, many more questions remain unanswered. Future research in this area will shed light on the molecular basis of the separation of functions of IL-4 and IL-13 and their consequences *in vivo*.

4.3 Single nucleotide polymorphisms leading to amino acid changes are commonly found in the IL-4Rα

Commonly occurring genetic polymorphisms leading to amino acid changes in the IL-4Rα have been linked to susceptibility to asthma and/or to asthma severity (Hershey, et al., 1997, Ober, et al., 2000, Risma, et al., 2002, Shirakawa, et al., 2000). The E400A, Q576R and the S503P polymorphisms reside in the cytoplasmic domain while the I50V resides in the extracellular domain of the IL-4Rα chain. Two of the polymorphisms located in the cytoplasmic domain, S503 to P and the Q576 to R, are frequently linked (Kruse, et al., 1999). This double mutation (S503P/Q576R) was associated with lower total IgE concentrations, similar to the single S503P polymorphism, and an increase in the phosphorylation of IRS2. E400A is especially prevalent in African-American populations and was associated with severe asthma exacerbations (Wenzel, et al., 2007). An I^{50} in the extracellular domain of the IL-4Rα chain was linked with enhanced signal transduction culminating in an increase in the production of IgE (Mitsuyasu, et al., 1998, Mitsuyasu, et al., 1999). On the other hand, several other studies reported no correlation of this polymorphism with enhanced IgE levels in patients (Khoo, et al., 2006, Noguchi, et al., 1999). Furthermore, the V^{50} polymorphism has been linked with enhanced CD23 expression, an increase in atopic asthma, and an increase in allergic bronchopulmonary aspergillosis (Knutsen, et al., 2006, Risma, et al., 2002). More recently the V^{50} polymorphism reduced the ability of IL-4 to suppress IL-17 production by human peripheral mononuclear cells (Wallis, et al., 2011). Because many of these polymorphisms are located in the cytoplasmic domain of the IL-4Rα, many investigators have hypothesized that they modulate signal transduction. However, experiments designed to analyze the direct effects of these polymorphisms on receptor signaling have lead to contradictory reports (Franjkovic, et al., 2005, Kruse, et al., 1999, Mitsuyasu, et al., 1998, Mitsuyasu, et al., 1999, Prots, et al., 2006, Risma, et al., 2002, Stephenson, et al., 2004).

We analyzed the impact of the Q576R, S503P, and I50V polymorphisms on signal transduction by the Type I receptor complex *in vitro*. While the R^{576} and P^{503} polymorphisms had no effect on STAT6 or IRS2 activation induced by IL-4 (Wang, et al., 1999), we found that the V^{50} polymorphism located in the extracellular domain of the IL-4Rα mediated a prolonged STAT6 signaling induced by IL-4 through the Type I receptor (Ford, et al., 2009). This was associated with a prolonged expression of the SOCS family member *Cis*. The effect of this polymorphism on signaling by the Type II receptor is unknown.

Using mouse knock-in strategies, the murine IL-4Rα-Q^{576} was replaced with IL-4Rα expressing the R^{576} polymorphism (Tachdjian, et al., 2009). This change was shown to enhance allergic asthma *in vivo*. The IL-4Rα-R^{576} enhanced Th2 differentiation and IgE production; both of these responses are Type I receptor dependent in the mouse model. Furthermore, it enhanced the production of CCL11 by BMM, fibroblasts, and tracheal epithelial cells (TEC) in response to IL-4 or IL-13. These results suggest the R^{576} polymorphism affects STAT6-dependent responses down stream of both the Type I and Type II receptors. However, there was no apparent effect of the R^{576} on the tyrosine phosphorylation of STAT6 (Tachdjian, et al., 2009), consistent with our study in cell lines (Wang, et al., 1999). Furthermore, there was no effect on the tyrosine phosphorylation of Shc. The effect of the R^{576} on IRS2 phosphorylation was not reported. Interestingly, the longevity of Erk1,2 phosphorylation in TEC was dramatically enhanced by R^{576}, however the mechanism by which R^{576} leads to Erk phosphorylation is still unclear. It will be important to understand the effects of the polymorphisms and their interactions on both IL-4 and IL-13 signaling since they are linked to different clinical phenotypes in human populations (Wenzel, et al., 2007).

5. Contribution of Type I and Type II receptor complexes to the control of regulatory mechanisms that act to modulate allergic inflammation

During Th2-driven allergic lung inflammation, a number of effector and regulatory mechanisms are orchestrated by IL-4 and IL-13 through Type I and Type II receptors. Several of these regulatory mechanisms allow for the amplification of Th2 differentiation and function, while others function as part of a negative feed-back loop to limit Th2-driven inflammation (**Figure 3**). Just as IL-4 and IL-13 are differentially involved in promoting various features of allergic lung disease, these cytokines utilize separate mechanisms to negatively regulate the signaling pathways activated by each other. These regulatory mechanisms will need to be considered in the design of inhibitors of the IL-4/IL-13 system.

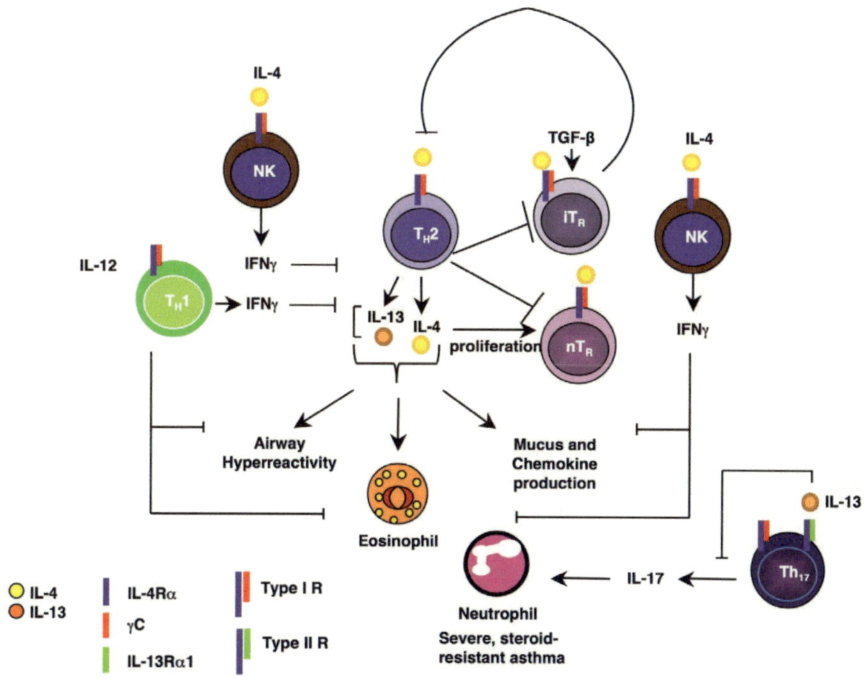

Fig. 3. **Differential control of regulatory mechanisms by the Type I and II Receptors.** IL-4 signaling through the Type I receptor on Th2 cell surfaces renders them resistant to control by T regulatory cells. Furthermore, IL-4 signaling STAT6 activation through the Type I receptor on naive CD4+ T-cells inhibits the differentiation of iTregs and Th1 cells. These responses lead to enhanced allergic inflammation. On the other hand, IL-4 signals through the Type I receptor on NK cell surfaces to induce IFNγ production. IFNγ in turn suppresses Th2 differentiation and inhibits signaling by both Type I and Type II receptors by inducing SOCS family members. IL-13 signals through the Type II receptor that is induced on the surface of Th17 cells and decreases IL-17 production. This suppression of IL-17 production by Th17 cells would limit the influx of neutrophils that are present in steroid resistant asthma.

5.1 Type I IL-4 receptor modulation of regulatory T-cells

Signaling through the Type I IL-4 receptor antagonizes the differentiation and function of regulatory T cells (Tregs). Tregs are a subset of T lymphocytes that regulate immune responses and prevent excessive immune system activation (Sakaguchi, et al., 2008, Shevach, 2009). The most studied Tregs are $CD4^+CD25^+FoxP3^+$, which have been found to play a role in allergic disease. FoxP3 is a transcription factor important for Treg development and function. Mice lacking FoxP3 expression (Scurfy mice) or humans with mutations in their *foxP3* gene (X-linked autoimmunity-allergic dysregulation syndrome) develop widespread autoimmune disease with a Th2-mediated allergic component (Khattri, et al., 2003). There are many mechanisms elicited by Tregs to suppress effector T cells, such as: (1) cell-mediated presentation of TGF-β or galectin-1 (Shevach, 2009), (2) secretion of the immunosuppressive cytokines IL-10 or TGF-β (Bettini & Vignali, 2009), or (3) consumption of IL-2, a limiting growth factor for T cells (Scheffold, et al., 2007). Th2 cells utilize several methods to inhibit immunosuppression by Tregs. Gata3 is the master transcriptional regulator of Th2 cells and is activated by signal transduction through the Type I IL-4 receptor. Using co-immunoprecipitation assays, Dardalhon and colleagues have shown physical interaction between Gata3 and FoxP3 in transiently transfected human embryo kidney 293 cells. The authors also observed IL-4 inhibition of FoxP3 induction in Ag-specific adaptive (inducible) Tregs, which was dependent on STAT6 expression (Dardalhon, et al., 2008). Our recent findings are in support of this antagonistic relationship between STAT6 and Tregs and IL-4-induced, STAT6-dependent inhibition of FoxP3. We have found that $STAT6^{-/-}$ mice have higher numbers of Tregs than wildtype mice (Chapoval, et al., 2011). This observation has also been confirmed by Takaki and colleagues who identified a STAT6-binding site in the silencer region in the FoxP3 mRNA transcript. STAT6 binding to this site reduced TGF-β1 induction of FoxP3 transcriptional activation (Takaki, et al., 2008).

Additionally, IL-4 was found to serve as a survival factor for $CD4^{+}CD25^{(-)}$ T helper (Th) cells and to aid in their protection from immunosuppression by $CD4^{+}CD25^{+}$ Tregs (Pace, et al., 2005). IL-13 failed to have this same effect. Therefore, this phenomenon was found to be dependent on Th cell surface expression of IL-4Rα chain and a functional Type I IL-4 receptor complex, as $IL\text{-}4R\alpha^{-/-}$ Th cells were not protected by IL-4 from Treg immunosuppression. IL-4 activation of the Type I IL-4 receptor, but not the Type II receptor, maintains anti-apoptotic and pro-proliferative processes in Th cells and protects them from Treg-induced perturbed cell growth and proliferation. Surprisingly, CSFE-labeled cocultures of $IL\text{-}4R\alpha^{-/-}$ Th cells and $IL\text{-}4R\alpha^{+/+}$ Tregs revealed that although IL-4 has on effect on Treg immunosuppression of $IL\text{-}4R\alpha^{-/-}$ Th cells, it promoted proliferation of Tregs *in-vitro* (Pace, et al., 2006). This could be a direct effect of IL-4 that would further complicate the role of this Th2 cytokine in modulating Treg immunosuppression.

5.2 Role of Type I receptors in control of Th1 responses that act to suppress allergic inflammation

Th1 cell programming antagonizes Th2 cell differentiation and could serve as a regulatory mechanism to suppress Th2-mediated allergic response. Gavett and colleagues showed that IL-12 can inhibit antigen induced-airway hyperreactivity and inflammation and to also reduce Th2 cytokine production (Gavett, et al., 1995). Th2 cells inhibit Th1 cell induction during the allergic response. Gata3 is activated downstream of STAT6 phosphorylation, which is induced by signaling through the Type I receptor (Kurata, et al., 1999, Nelms, et al., 1999). Not only does it serve as the master regulator transcription factor (TF) for Th2 cells, but Gata3 has also been shown to inhibit Th1 cell-specific factors. Gata3-deficient cell clones produced high levels of the Th1 cytokine, IFNγ, and had enhanced expression of T-bet (the Th1 cell master regulator TF) (Zhu, et al., 2006). Therefore, activation of the Type I IL-4 receptor could lead to activation of Gata3, which in turn inhibits Th1-inducing factors during the Th2-mediated allergic response. Th1 cells have also been shown to play a potentially stimulatory role in airway inflammation. Hansen et al. found that Th1 cells decreased airway eosinophilia, but failed to reduce airway hyperreactivity in ovalbumin-immunized Balb/c mice (Hansen, et al., 1999). But this may be a late phenomenon in airway inflammation during which additional non-Th2 inflammatory cells aid in amplifying chronic lung inflammation. This would be in direct contrast to the initiation of allergic airway inflammation which is characterized by strong Th2 immune responses and can be inhibited by non-Th2-promoting immune cells.

5.3 Modulation of NK cells

Although IL-4 and IFNγ are antagonistic towards each other during T cell differentiation, IL-4 can increase IL-2 and IL-12 induced IFNγ secretion by Natural Killer (NK) cells. Bream and co-authors also found that the increase in IFNγ production caused by IL-4 in conjunction with IL-2 was STAT6 dependent, while IL-4 synergy with IL-12 was independent of STAT6 activation (Bream, et al., 2003, Morris, et al., 2006). Further studies have shown that IL-13 was unable to cause a similar increase in NK cell derived IFNγ release (Morris, et al., 2006). This result is in agreement with the fact that IL-13 signals through the Type II receptor, and this receptor complex is absent in NK cells. IL-4 stimulated IFNγ production by NK cells has significant implications in the context for allergic lung inflammation. One group has shown that Sendai virus infection of mice suppressed NK cell derived IFNγ secretion. This led to enhanced Th2 responses and subsequent development of exacerbated allergic lung disease (Kaiko, et al., 2010). IFNγ production would suppress Th2 differentiation and inhibit signaling by both Type I and Type II receptors by inducing SOCS family members.
The role of NK cells in human allergic disease has been extensively examined; because of their ability to produce cytokines, NK cells have the potential to heavily influence the adaptive allergic immune response. Based on cytokine production, NK cells can be divided into 2 classes: (1) NK1 cells produce Th1 cytokines, such as IFNγ (Romagnani, 1992) and (2) NK2 cells produce Th2 cytokines IL-4, 5, and 13 (Hoshino, et al., 1999, Peritt, et al., 1998, Warren, et al., 1995). In a recent study analyzing NK cell populations in healthy and allergic patients, the authors found a predominance of NK2 cells in the peripheral blood of allergic patients. These NK2 cells produced high amounts of Th2 cytokines that could promote allergic inflammation (Timonen & Stenius-Aarniala, 1985, Wei, et al., 2005).

5.4 IL-13 inhibition of Th17 cells via the Type II receptor in severe asthma

It has long been thought that naïve T cells do not express the IL-13Rα1 chain of the Type II receptor complex and therefore cannot be regulated by IL-13. Due to restricted expression of IL-13Rα1 on non-hematopoetic cells, Type II receptor signaling has been limited to those cells and not seen in T cells. But this central dogma has been recently challenged by observations that Th17 cells are able to induce surface expression of IL-13Rα1 chain (Newcomb, et al., 2009, Newcomb, et al., 2011).
Th17 cells are a distinct population of CD4+ T cells, whose differentiation is induced by IL-6 or IL-21 and TGFβ (McGeachy, et al., 2007). Th17 cells produce IL-17, IL-6, and tumor necrosis factor. They have been shown to play a role in autoimmune diseases including the experimental autoimmune encephalitis (EAE) model of multiple sclerosis (Langrish, et al., 2005). Th17 cells also provide protection from some extracellular pathogens, such as *Klebsiella pneumoniae* infection of the lung (Happel, et al., 2005).
A statistically higher number of IL-17 + cells can be found in the sputum and BAL of asthmatic patients compared to controls and the greater expression of IL-17A in the lungs was associated with increased asthma severity. (Jatakanon, et al., 1999, Molet, et al., 2001). IL-17A induces neutrophil recruitment to the airway and augments the pathogenesis of steroid-resistant, severe asthma (McKinley, et al., 2008). Th17 cells alone cannot induce eosinophillic infiltration into the airway following immunization and challenge, but in the presence of Th2 cells, antigen-specific Th17 cells can enhance the eosinophil-activating properties of Th2 cells (Wakashin, et al., 2008).

Th17 polarized cells from mouse spleens were shown to have increased mRNA and protein levels of IL-13Rα1 after stimulation *in vitro*. When added to Th17 cell cultures, IL-13 reduced IL-17A production by Th17 cells and decreased the percentage of CD4+ Th17 cells. Additionally, IL-13 caused a reduction in the expression of RORγτ, the master regulator transcription factor for Th17 cells (Newcomb, et al., 2009). This phenomenon of IL-13 suppression of IL-17A production by Th17 cells was also observed *in vitro* using human CD4+ T cells (Newcomb, et al., 2011). Therefore, activated Th17 cells upregulate their surface expression of IL-13Rα1 chain and this allows for IL-13 to signal through a functional Type II receptor complex to decrease IL-17 production by Th17 cells. Thus, paradoxically, IL-13, a major effector cytokine of atopic asthma, inhibits the Th17 component of severe asthma. This concept could also explain the observation that IL-25-induced production of IL-13 inhibited Th17-mediated EAE disease progression (Kleinschek, et al., 2007). This is a unique mechanism whereby a Th2 immune-mediated illness is prevented from becoming more severe by IL-13, a Th2 cytokine. Consequently, efforts to suppress IL-13 function to treat allergic asthma may lead to Th17 induction and severe and persistent asthma in susceptible individuals.

6. Conclusion

The importance of the Type I IL-4 receptor in regulating T cells to become Th2 cells has been well documented. Furthermore, numerous studies have indicated the IL-4Rα expressed on lung epithelium is necessary for goblet cell differentiation and mucus hypersecretion. In addition, the IL-4Rα is expressed on many cell types that could contribute to the overall pathology and severity of asthma. The relative role of the Type I and Type II receptors on these cells has not yet been fully delineated. Using mice lacking one or the other complex (i.e. $\gamma C^{-/-}$ or IL-13Rα1$^{-/-}$) several groups have recently delineated interesting differences in their contributions to lung pathology. The Type I receptor is the major regulator of eosinophilic inflammation and the alternative activation of macrophages while the Type II receptor controls mucus hypersecretion and airway hyperresponsiveness. These receptors differentially regulate potential regulatory pathways including the control of T regulatory cells and the production of cytokines by NK cells; both of these responses are controlled by the Type I receptor complex. The Type II receptor complex can be induced on Th17 cells and allows IL-13 to down regulate Th17 differentiation. This could be of clinical importance for severe, steroid resistant forms of human asthma that may be mediated by Th17 cells. In this scenario, inhibiting IL-13 could be detrimental to the patient and illustrates the need to stratify patients prior to treatment.

As mentioned above, the intricate differences between the Type I and Type II receptor complexes could impact the therapeutic effectiveness of agents designed to target these receptors in asthma. Indeed initial trials to inhibit IL-4 using the soluble IL-4Rα in asthmatic patients were largely unsuccessful and possibly detrimental (Borish, et al., 2001, Wenzel, et al., 2007). The ability of IL-4 to suppress TNFα production, a highly pro-inflammatory cytokine, was suggested to be part of a negative regulatory mechanism that was unintentionally blocked by the therapy (Borish, 2010). Studies using soluble IL-13Rα2 to inhibit IL-13 signaling are ongoing. However, blocking one cytokine at a time may not prove beneficial. Since both cytokines can elicit effector functions, blocking only one could actually exacerbate disease because of the loss of a negative regulatory pathway. The most promising approach thus far has been to use a mutant IL-4 (Pitrakinra) that binds to the IL-4Rα, and blocks dimerization with either the γC or the IL-13Rα1 (Wenzel, et al., 2007). Thus, this single agent can prevent the formation of both the Type I and the Type II receptor complexes. Further understanding of the complex IL-4/IL-13 receptor system and its contribution to various features of allergic asthma will be essential to fine-tune therapeutic strategies for the treatment of asthma.

7. Acknowledgement

The authors acknowledge their financial support from the National Institutes of Health: RO1 AI038985 (ADK); T32HL06798 and K99/R00 HL096897 (NMH); Meyerhoff Graduate Research Fellowship, Minority Biomedical Research Support - Initiative for Maximizing Student Diversity, NIGMS, T32HL06798 and AI007540 (NJD): and R21AI076736 (SPC).

8. References

Akbari, O., Stock, P., Meyer, E., Kronenberg, M., Sidobre, S., Nakayama, T., Taniguchi, M., Grusby, M. J., DeKruyff, R. H., & Umetsu, D. T. (2003). Essential role of NKT cells producing IL-4 and IL-13 in the development of allergen-induced airway hyperreactivity. *Nature Medicine*, Vol. 9, No. 5, (May, 2003), pp. 582-588.

Aman, M. J., Tayebi, N., Obiri, N. I., Puri, R. K., Modi, W. S., & Leonard, W. J. (1996). cDNA cloning and characterization of the human interleukin 13 receptor alpha chain. *Journal of Biological Chemistry*, Vol. 271, No. 46, (Nov 15, 1996), pp. 29265-29270.

Andrews, A. L., Holloway, J. W., Holgate, S. T., & Davies, D. E. (2006). IL-4 receptor alpha is an important modulator of IL-4 and IL-13 receptor binding: implications for the development of therapeutic targets. *Journal of Immunology*, Vol. 176, No. 12, (Jun 15, 2006), pp. 7456-7461.

Andrews, A. L., Holloway, J. W., Puddicombe, S. M., Holgate, S. T., & Davies, D. E. (2002). Kinetic analysis of the interleukin-13 receptor complex. *Journal of Biological Chemistry*, Vol. 277, No. 48, (Nov 29, 2002), pp. 46073-46078.

Andrews, A. L., Nasir, T., Bucchieri, F., Holloway, J. W., Holgate, S. T., & Davies, D. E. (2006). IL-13 receptor alpha 2: a regulator of IL-13 and IL-4 signal transduction in primary human fibroblasts. *Journal of Allergy and Clinical Immunology*, Vol. 118, No. 4, (Oct, 2006), pp. 858-865.

Andrews, R., Rosa, L., Daines, M., & Khurana Hershey, G. (2001). Reconstitution of a functional human type II IL-4/IL-13 receptor in mouse B cells: demonstration of species specificity. *Journal of Immunology*, Vol. 166, No. 3, (Feb 1, 2001), pp. 1716-1722.

Bahadori, K., Doyle-Waters, M. M., Marra, C., Lynd, L., Alasaly, K., Swiston, J., & FitzGerald, J. M. (2009). Economic burden of asthma: a systematic review. *BMC Pulm Med*, Vol. 9, No., (2009), pp. 24, 1471-2466.

Ben-Sasson, S. Z., Le Gros, G., Conrad, D. H., Finkelman, F. D., & Paul, W. E. (1990). Cross-linking Fc receptors stimulate splenic non-B, non-T cells to secrete interleukin 4 and other lymphokines. *Proceedings of the National Academy of Sciences of the United States of America*, Vol. 87, No. 4, (Feb, 1990), pp. 1421-1425.

Bettini, M., & Vignali, D. A. (2009). Regulatory T cells and inhibitory cytokines in autoimmunity. *Current Opinion in Immunology*, Vol. 21, No. 6, (Dec, 2009), pp. 612-618.

Blaeser, F., Bryce, P. J., Ho, N., Raman, V., Dedeoglu, F., Donaldson, D. D., Geha, R. S., Oettgen, H. C., & Chatila, T. A. (2003). Targeted inactivation of the IL-4 receptor alpha chain I4R motif promotes allergic airway inflammation. *Journal of Experimental Medicine*, Vol. 198, No. 8, (Oct 20, 2003), pp. 1189-1200.

Borish, L. (2010). IL-4 and IL-13 dual antagonism: a promising approach to the dilemma of generating effective asthma biotherapeutics. *American Journal of Respiratory and Critical Care Medicine*, Vol. 181, No. 8, (Apr 15, 2010), pp. 769-770.

Borish, L. C., Nelson, H. S., Corren, J., Bensch, G., Busse, W. W., Whitmore, J. B., & Agosti, J. M. (2001). Efficacy of soluble IL-4 receptor for the treatment of adults with asthma. *Journal of Allergy and Clinical Immunology*, Vol. 107, No. 6, (Jun, 2001), pp. 963-970.

Bream, J. H., Curiel, R. E., Yu, C. R., Egwuagu, C. E., Grusby, M. J., Aune, T. M., & Young, H. A. (2003). IL-4 synergistically enhances both IL-2- and IL-12-induced IFN-gamma expression in murine NK cells. *Blood*, Vol. 102, No. 1, (Jul 1, 2003), pp. 207-214.

Brown, M. A., Pierce, J. H., Watson, C. J., Falco, J., Ihle, J. N., & Paul, W. E. (1987). B cell stimulatory factor-1/interleukin-4 mRNA is expressed by normal and transformed mast cells. *Cell*, Vol. 50, No. 5, (Aug 28, 1987), pp. 809-818.

Bruns, H. A., Schindler, U., & Kaplan, M. H. (2003). Expression of a constitutively active Stat6 in vivo alters lymphocyte homeostasis with distinct effects in T and B cells. *Journal of Immunology*, Vol. 170, No. 7, (Apr 1, 2003), pp. 3478-3487.

Burd, P. R., Thompson, W. C., Max, E. E., & Mills, F. C. (1995). Activated mast cells produce interleukin 13. *Journal of Experimental Medicine*, Vol. 181, No. 4, (Apr 1, 1995), pp. 1373-1380.

Cao, X., Kozak, C. A., Liu, Y. J., Noguchi, M., O'Connell, E., & Leonard, W. J. (1993). Characterization of cDNAs encoding the murine interleukin 2 receptor (IL-2R) gamma chain: chromosomal mapping and tissue specificity of IL-2R gamma chain expression. *Proceedings of the National Academy of Sciences of the United States of America*, Vol. 90, No. 18, (Sep 15, 1993), pp. 8464-8468.

Cao, X., Shores, E. W., Hu-Li, J., Anver, M. R., Kelsall, B. L., Russell, S. M., Drago, J., Noguchi, M., Grinberg, A., Bloom, E. T., & et al. (1995). Defective lymphoid development in mice lacking expression of the common cytokine receptor gamma chain. *Immunity*, Vol. 2, No. 3, (Mar, 1995), pp. 223-238.

Caput, D., Laurent, P., Kaghad, M., Lelias, J. M., Lefort, S., Vita, N., & Ferrara, P. (1996). Cloning and characterization of a specific interleukin (IL)-13 binding protein structurally related to the IL-5 receptor alpha chain. *Journal of Biological Chemistry*, Vol. 271, No. 28, (Jul 12, 1996), pp. 16921-16926.

Chapoval, S., Dasgupta, P., Dorsey, N. J., & Keegan, A. D. (2010). Regulation of the T helper cell type 2 (Th2)/T regulatory cell (Treg) balance by IL-4 and STAT6. *Journal of Leukocyte Biology*, Vol. 87, No. 6, (Jun, 2010), pp. 1011-1018.

Chapoval, S. P., Dasgupta, P., Smith, E. P., DeTolla, L. J., Lipsky, M. M., Kelly-Welch, A. E., & Keegan, A. D. (2011). STAT6 expression in multiple cell types mediates the cooperative development of allergic airway disease. *Journal of Immunology*, Vol. 186, No. 4, (Feb 15, 2011), pp. 2571-2583.

Chen, W., Daines, M. O., & Khurana Hershey, G. K. (2003). Arginine 27, a conserved methylation site in Stat6, is essential for IL-4-induced tyrosine phosphorylation, DNA binding activity, and nuclear translocation of Stat6. *Journal of Allergy and Clinical Immunology*, Vol. 111, No. 2, (2003), pp. S855.

Chen, W., Sivaprasad, U., Tabata, Y., Gibson, A. M., Stier, M. T., Finkelman, F. D., & Hershey, G. K. (2009). IL-13R alpha 2 membrane and soluble isoforms differ in humans and mice. *Journal of Immunology*, Vol. 183, No. 12, (Dec 15, 2009), pp. 7870-7876.

Chiaramonte, M. G., Mentink-Kane, M., Jacobson, B. A., Cheever, A. W., Whitters, M. J., Goad, M. E., Wong, A., Collins, M., Donaldson, D. D., Grusby, M. J., & Wynn, T. A. (2003). Regulation and function of the interleukin 13 receptor alpha 2 during a T helper cell type 2-dominant immune response. *Journal of Experimental Medicine*, Vol. 197, No. 6, (Mar 17, 2003), pp. 687-701.

Chomarat, P., & Banchereau, J. (1998). Interleukin-4 and interleukin-13: their similarities and discrepancies. *International Reviews of Immunology*, Vol. 17, No. 1-4, (1998), pp. 1-52, 0883-0185.

Coffer, P. J., Schweizer, R. C., Dubois, G. R., Maikoe, T., Lammers, J. W., & Koenderman, L. (1998). Analysis of signal transduction pathways in human eosinophils activated by chemoattractants and the T-helper 2-derived cytokines interleukin-4 and interleukin-5. *Blood*, Vol. 91, No. 7, (Apr 1, 1998), pp. 2547-2557.

Cohn, L., Homer, R. J., Marinov, A., Rankin, J., & Bottomly, K. (1997). Induction of airway mucus production By T helper 2 (Th2) cells: a critical role for interleukin 4 in cell recruitment but not mucus production. *Journal of Experimental Medicine*, Vol. 186, No. 10, (Nov 17, 1997), pp. 1737-1747.

Corry, D. B., Grunig, G., Hadeiba, H., Kurup, V. P., Warnock, M. L., Sheppard, D., Rennick, D. M., & Locksley, R. M. (1998). Requirements for allergen-induced airway hyperreactivity in T and B cell-deficient mice. *Molecular Medicine*, Vol. 4, No. 5, (May, 1998), pp. 344-355.

Crowley, M. T., Harmer, S. L., & DeFranco, A. L. (1996). Activation-induced association of a 145-kDa tyrosine-phosphorylated protein with Shc and Syk in B lymphocytes and macrophages. *Journal of Biological Chemistry*, Vol. 271, No. 2, (Jan 12, 1996), pp. 1145-115.

Dardalhon, V., Awasthi, A., Kwon, H., Galileos, G., Gao, W., Sobel, R. A., Mitsdoerffer, M., Strom, T. B., Elyaman, W., Ho, I. C., Khoury, S., Oukka, M., & Kuchroo, V. K. (2008). IL-4 inhibits TGF-beta-induced Foxp3+ T cells and, together with TGF-beta, generates IL-9+ IL-10+ Foxp3(-) effector T cells. *Nature Immunology*, Vol. 9, No. 12, (Dec, 2008), pp. 1347-1355.

Das, J., Eynott, P., Jupp, R., Bothwell, A., Van Kaer, L., Shi, Y., & Das, G. (2006). Natural killer T cells and CD8+ T cells are dispensable for T cell-dependent allergic airway inflammation. *Nature Medicine*, Vol. 12, No. 12, (Dec, 2006), pp. 1345-1346; author reply 1347.

David, M. D., Bertoglio, J., & Pierre, J. (2003). Functional characterization of IL-13 receptor alpha2 gene promoter: a critical role of the transcription factor STAT6 for regulated expression. *Oncogene*, Vol. 22, No. 22, (2003), pp. 3386-3394.

Deutsch, H. H., Koettnitz, K., Chung, J., & Kalthoff, F. S. (1995). Distinct sequence motifs within the cytoplasmic domain of the human IL-4 receptor differentially regulate apoptosis inhibition and cell growth. *Journal of Immunology*, Vol. 154, No. 8, (Apr 15, 1995), pp. 3696-3703.

Devouassoux, G., Saxon, A., Metcalfe, D. D., Prussin, C., Colomb, M. G., Brambilla, C., & Diaz-Sanchez, D. (2002). Chemical constituents of diesel exhaust particles induce IL-4 production and histamine release by human basophils. *Journal of Allergy and Clinical Immunology*, Vol. 109, No. 5, (May, 2002), pp. 847-853.

Dombrowicz, D., Flamand, V., Brigman, K. K., Koller, B. H., & Kinet, J. P. (1993). Abolition of anaphylaxis by targeted disruption of the high affinity immunoglobulin E receptor alpha chain gene. *Cell*, Vol. 75, No. 5, (Dec 3, 1993), pp. 969-976.

Donaldson, D. D., Whitters, M. J., Fitz, L. J., Neben, T. Y., Finnerty, H., Henderson, S. L., O'Hara, R. M., Jr., Beier, D. R., Turner, K. J., Wood, C. R., & Collins, M. (1998). The murine IL-13 receptor alpha 2: molecular cloning, characterization, and comparison with murine IL-13 receptor alpha 1. *Journal of Immunology*, Vol. 161, No. 5, (Sep 1, 1998), pp. 2317-2324.

Duronio, V., Welham, M. J., Abraham, S., Dryden, P., & Schrader, J. W. (1992). p21ras activation via hemopoietin receptors and c-kit requires tyrosine kinase activity but not tyrosine phosphorylation of p21ras GTPase-activating protein. *Proceedings of the National Academy of Sciences of the United States of America*, Vol. 89, No. 5, (Mar 1, 1992), pp. 1587-1591.

Ferrick, D. A., Schrenzel, M. D., Mulvania, T., Hsieh, B., Ferlin, W. G., & Lepper, H. (1995). Differential production of interferon-gamma and interleukin-4 in response to Th1- and Th2-stimulating pathogens by gamma delta T cells in vivo. *Nature*, Vol. 373, No. 6511, (Jan 19, 1995), pp. 255-257.

Fichtner-Feigl, S., Strober, W., Kawakami, K., Puri, R. K., & Kitani, A. (2006). IL-13 signaling through the IL-13alpha2 receptor is involved in induction of TGF-beta1 production and fibrosis. *Nature Medicine*, Vol. 12, No. 1, (Jan, 2006), pp. 99-106.

Finkelman, F. D., Katona, I. M., Urban, J. F., Jr., Holmes, J., Ohara, J., Tung, A. S., Sample, J. V., & Paul, W. E. (1988). IL-4 is required to generate and sustain in vivo IgE responses. *Journal of Immunology*, Vol. 141, No. 7, (Oct 1, 1988), pp. 2335-2341

Ford, A. Q., Heller, N. M., Stephenson, L., Boothby, M. R., & Keegan, A. D. (2009). An Atopy-Associated Polymorphism in the Ectodomain of the IL-4R{alpha} Chain (V50) Regulates the Persistence of STAT6 Phosphorylation. *Journal of Immunology*, Vol. 183, No. 3, (August 1, 2009, 2009), pp. 1607-1616.

Franjkovic, I., Gessner, A., Konig, I., Kissel, K., Bohnert, A., Hartung, A., Ohly, A., Ziegler, A., Hackstein, H., & Bein, G. (2005). Effects of common atopy-associated amino acid substitutions in the IL-4 receptor alpha chain on IL-4 induced phenotypes. *Immunogenetics*, Vol. 56, No. 11, (Feb, 2005), pp. 808-817.

Fujiwara, H., Hanissian, S. H., Tsytsykova, A., & Geha, R. S. (1997). Homodimerization of the human interleukin 4 receptor alpha chain induces Cepsilon germline transcripts in B cells in the absence of the interleukin 2 receptor gamma chain. *Proceedings of the National Academy of Sciences of the United States of America*, Vol. 94, No. 11, (May 27, 1997), pp. 5866-5871.

Gadina, M., Stancato, L. M., Bacon, C. M., Larner, A. C., & O'Shea, J. J. (1998). Involvement of SHP-2 in multiple aspects of IL-2 signaling: evidence for a positive regulatory role. *Journal of Immunology*, Vol. 160, No. 10, (May 15, 1998), pp. 4657-4661.

Gadina, M., Sudarshan, C., & O'Shea, J. J. (1999). IL-2, but not IL-4 and other cytokines, induces phosphorylation of a 98-kDa protein associated with SHP-2, phosphatidylinositol 3'-kinase, and Grb2. *Journal of Immunology*, Vol. 162, No. 4, (Feb 15, 1999), pp. 2081-2086.

Galizzi, J. P., Zuber, C. E., Harada, N., Gorman, D. M., Djossou, O., Kastelein, R., Banchereau, J., Howard, M., & Miyajima, A. (1990). Molecular cloning of a cDNA encoding the human interleukin 4 receptor. *International Immunology*, Vol. 2, No. 7, (1990), pp. 669-675.

Gavett, S. H., Chen, X., Finkelman, F., & Wills-Karp, M. (1994). Depletion of murine CD4+ T lymphocytes prevents antigen-induced airway hyperreactivity and pulmonary eosinophilia. *American Journal of Respiratory Cell and Molecular Biology*, Vol. 10, No. 6, (Jun, 1994), pp. 587-593.

Gavett, S. H., O'Hearn, D. J., Li, X., Huang, S. K., Finkelman, F. D., & Wills-Karp, M. (1995). Interleukin 12 inhibits antigen-induced airway hyperresponsiveness, inflammation, and Th2 cytokine expression in mice. *The Journal of experimental medicine*, Vol. 182, No. 5, (Nov 1, 1995), pp. 1527-1536

Goenka, S., & Kaplan, M. H. (2011). Transcriptional regulation by STAT6. *Immunologic Research*, Vol. 50, No. 1, (May, 2011), pp. 87-96.

Goenka, S., Youn, J., Dzurek, L. M., Schindler, U., Yu-Lee, L. Y., & Boothby, M. (1999). Paired Stat6 C-terminal transcription activation domains required both for inhibition of an IFN-responsive promoter and trans-activation. *Journal of Immunology*, Vol. 163, No. 9, (Nov 1, 1999), pp. 4663-4672.

Grunig, G., Warnock, M., Wakil, A. E., Venkayya, R., Brombacher, F., Rennick, D. M., Sheppard, D., Mohrs, M., Donaldson, D. D., Locksley, R. M., & Corry, D. B. (1998). Requirement for IL-13 independently of IL-4 in experimental asthma. *Science*, Vol. 282, No. 5397, (Dec 18, 1998), pp. 2261-2263.

Haan, C., Rolvering, C., Raulf, F., Kapp, M., Druckes, P., Thoma, G., Behrmann, I., & Zerwes, H. G. (2011). Jak1 has a dominant role over Jak3 in signal transduction through gammac-containing cytokine receptors. *Chemistry and Biology*, Vol. 18, No. 3, (Mar 25, 2011), pp. 314-323.

Hage, T., Sebald, W., & Reinemer, P. (1999). Crystal structure of the IL-4/IL-4 receptor alpha chain complex reveals a mosaic binding interface. *Cell*, Vol. 97, No. 2, (April 16, 1999), pp 271-281.

Hansen, G., Berry, G., DeKruyff, R. H., & Umetsu, D. T. (1999). Allergen-specific Th1 cells fail to counterbalance Th2 cell-induced airway hyperreactivity but cause severe airway inflammation. *The Journal of Clinical Investigation*, Vol. 103, No. 2, (Jan, 1999), pp. 175-183.

Hanson, E. M., Dickensheets, H., Qu, C. K., Donnelly, R. P., & Keegan, A. D. (2003). Regulation of the dephosphorylation of Stat6. Participation of Tyr-713 in the interleukin-4 receptor alpha, the tyrosine phosphatase SHP-1, and the proteasome. *Journal of Biological Chemistry*, Vol. 278, No. 6, (2003), pp. 3903-3911.

Happel, K. I., Dubin, P. J., Zheng, M., Ghilardi, N., Lockhart, C., Quinton, L. J., Odden, A. R., Shellito, J. E., Bagby, G. J., Nelson, S., & Kolls, J. K. (2005). Divergent roles of IL-23 and IL-12 in host defense against Klebsiella pneumoniae. *The Journal of experimental medicine*, Vol. 202, No. 6, (Sep 19, 2005), pp. 761-769.

Haque, S. J., Harbor, P., Tabrizi, M., Yi, T., & Williams, B. R. (1998). Protein-tyrosine phosphatase Shp-1 is a negative regulator of IL-4- and IL-13-dependent signal transduction. *Journal of Biological Chemistry*, Vol. 273, No. 51, (1998), pp. 33893-33896.

Haque, S. J., Harbor, P. C., & Williams, B. R. (2000). Identification of critical residues required for suppressor of cytokine signaling-specific regulation of interleukin-4 signaling. *Journal of Biological Chemistry*, Vol. 275, No. 34, (2000), pp. 26500-26506.

Heller, N. M., Qi, X., Junttila, I. S., Shirey, K. A., Vogel, S. N., Paul, W. E., & Keegan, A. D. (2008). Type I IL-4Rs selectively activate IRS-2 to induce target gene expression in macrophages. *Sci Signal*, Vol. 1, No. 51, (2008), pp. ra17.

Hershey, G. K., Friedrich, M. F., Esswein, L. A., Thomas, M. L., & Chatila, T. A. (1997). The association of atopy with a gain-of-function mutation in the alpha subunit of the interleukin-4 receptor. *New England Journal of Medicine*, Vol. 337, No. 24, (Dec 11, 1997), pp. 1720-1725.

Hilton, D. J., Zhang, J. G., Metcalf, D., Alexander, W. S., Nicola, N. A., & Willson, T. A. (1996). Cloning and characterization of a binding subunit of the interleukin 13 receptor that is also a component of the interleukin 4 receptor. *Proceedings of the National Academy of Sciences of the United States of America*, Vol. 93, No. 1, (Jan 9, 1996), pp. 497-501.

Hogan, S. P., Rosenberg, H. F., Moqbel, R., Phipps, S., Foster, P. S., Lacy, P., Kay, A. B., & Rothenberg, M. E. (2008). Eosinophils: biological properties and role in health and disease. *Clinical and Experimental Allergy*, Vol. 38, No. 5, (May, 2008), pp. 709-750.

Hoshino, T., Winkler-Pickett, R. T., Mason, A. T., Ortaldo, J. R., & Young, H. A. (1999). IL-13 production by NK cells: IL-13-producing NK and T cells are present in vivo in the absence of IFN-gamma. *Journal of immunology (Baltimore, Md: 1950)*, Vol. 162, No. 1, (Jan 1, 1999), pp. 51-59, 0022-1767; 0022-1767.

Hou, J., Schindler, U., Henzel, W. J., Ho, T. C., Brasseur, M., & McKnight, S. L. (1994). An interleukin-4-induced transcription factor: IL-4 Stat. *Science*, Vol. 265, No. 5179, (1994), pp. 1701-1706.

Huang, H., & Paul, W. E. (2000). Protein tyrosine phosphatase activity is required for IL-4 induction of IL-4 receptor alpha-chain. *Journal of Immunology*, Vol. 164, No. 3, (Feb 1, 2000), pp. 1211-1215.

Huang, S. K., Xiao, H. Q., Kleine-Tebbe, J., Paciotti, G., Marsh, D. G., Lichtenstein, L. M., & Liu, M. C. (1995). IL-13 expression at the sites of allergen challenge in patients with asthma. *Journal of Immunology*, Vol. 155, No. 5, (Sep 1, 1995), pp. 2688-2694.

Huang, Z., Coleman, J. M., Su, Y., Mann, M., Ryan, J., Shultz, L. D., & Huang, H. (2005). SHP-1 regulates STAT6 phosphorylation and IL-4-mediated function in a cell type-specific manner. *Cytokine*, Vol. 29, No. 3, (Feb 7, 2005), pp. 118-124.

Idzerda, R. L., March, C. J., Mosley, B., Lyman, S. D., Vanden Bos, T., Gimpel, S. D., Din, W. S., Grabstein, K. H., Widmer, M. B., Park, L. S., & et al. (1990). Human interleukin 4 receptor confers biological responsiveness and defines a novel receptor superfamily. *Journal of Experimental Medicine*, Vol. 171, No. 3, (Mar 1, 1990), pp. 861-873.

Imani, F., Rager, K. J., Catipovic, B., & Marsh, D. G. (1997). Interleukin-4 (IL-4) induces phosphatidylinositol 3-kinase (p85) dephosphorylation. Implications for the role of SHP-1 in the IL-4-induced signals in human B cells. *Journal of Biological Chemistry*, Vol. 272, No. 12, (Mar 21, 1997), pp. 7927-7931.

Inoue, A., Yasuda, T., Yamamoto, T., & Yamanashi, Y. (2007). Dok-1 is a positive regulator of IL-4 signalling and IgE response. *J Biochem*, Vol. 142, No. 2, (Aug, 2007), pp. 257-263.

Ito, T., Suzuki, S., Kanaji, S., Shiraishi, H., Ohta, S., Arima, K., Tanaka, G., Tamada, T., Honjo, E., Garcia, K. C., Kuroki, R., & Izuhara, K. (2009). Distinct structural requirements for interleukin-4 (IL-4) and IL-13 binding to the shared IL-13 receptor facilitate cellular tuning of cytokine responsiveness. *Journal of Biological Chemistry*, Vol. 284, No. 36, (Sep 4, 2009), pp. 24289-24296.

Izuhara, K., & Harada, N. (1993). Interleukin-4 (IL-4) induces protein tyrosine phosphorylation of the IL-4 receptor and association of phosphatidylinositol 3-kinase to the IL-4 receptor in a mouse T cell line, HT2. *Journal of Biological Chemistry*, Vol. 268, No. 18, (Jun 25, 1993), pp. 13097-13102.

Jatakanon, A., Uasuf, C., Maziak, W., Lim, S., Chung, K. F., & Barnes, P. J. (1999). Neutrophilic inflammation in severe persistent asthma. *American Journal of Respiratory and Critical Care Medicine*, Vol. 160, No. 5 Pt 1, (Nov, 1999), pp. 1532-1539.

Junttila, I. S., Mizukami, K., Dickensheets, H., Meier-Schellersheim, M., Yamane, H., Donnelly, R. P., Paul, W. E. (2008). Tuning sensitivity to IL-4 and IL-13: Differential expression of IL-4Rα, IL-13Rα1 and γc regulates relative cytokine sensitivity. *Journal of Experimental Medicine*, Vol., No., (2008), pp.

Kaiko, G. E., Phipps, S., Angkasekwinai, P., Dong, C., & Foster, P. S. (2010). NK cell deficiency predisposes to viral-induced Th2-type allergic inflammation via epithelial-derived IL-25. *Journal of Immunology*, Vol. 185, No. 8, (Oct 15, 2010), pp. 4681-4690.

Kang, C. M., Jang, A. S., Ahn, M. H., Shin, J. A., Kim, J. H., Choi, Y. S., Rhim, T. Y., & Park, C. S. (2005). Interleukin-25 and interleukin-13 production by alveolar macrophages in response to particles. *American Journal of Respiratory Cell and Molecular Biology*, Vol. 33, No. 3, (Sep, 2005), pp. 290-296.

Kaplan, M. H., Schindler, U., Smiley, S. T., & Grusby, M. J. (1996). Stat6 is required for mediating responses to IL-4 and for development of Th2 cells. *Immunity*, Vol. 4, No. 3, (1996), pp. 313-319.

Kaplan, M. H., Whitfield, J. R., Boros, D. L., & Grusby, M. J. (1998). Th2 cells are required for the Schistosoma mansoni egg-induced granulomatous response. *Journal of Immunology*, Vol. 160, No. 4, (Feb 15, 1998), pp. 1850-1856.

Kashiwada, M., Giallourakis, C. C., Pan, P. Y., & Rothman, P. B. (2001). Immunoreceptor tyrosine-based inhibitory motif of the IL-4 receptor associates with SH2-containing phosphatases and regulates IL-4-induced proliferation. *Journal of Immunology*, Vol. 167, No. 11, (Dec 1, 2001), pp. 6382-6387.

Keegan, A. D., Johnston, J. A., Tortolani, P. J., McReynolds, L. J., Kinzer, C., O'Shea, J. J., & Paul, W. E. (1995). Similarities and differences in signal transduction by interleukin 4 and interleukin 13: analysis of Janus kinase activation. *Proceedings of the National Academy of Sciences of the United States of America*, Vol. 92, No. 17, (Aug 15, 1995), pp. 7681-7685.

Keegan, A. D., Nelms, K., White, M., Wang, L. M., Pierce, J. H., & Paul, W. E. (1994). An IL-4 receptor region containing an insulin receptor motif is important for IL-4-mediated IRS-1 phosphorylation and cell growth. *Cell*, Vol. 76, No. 5, (Mar 11, 1994), pp. 811-820.

Kelly-Welch, A. E., Melo, M. E., Smith, E., Ford, A. Q., Haudenschild, C., Noben-Trauth, N., & Keegan, A. D. (2004). Complex role of the IL-4 receptor alpha in a murine model of airway inflammation: expression of the IL-4 receptor alpha on nonlymphoid cells of bone marrow origin contributes to severity of inflammation. *Journal of Immunology*, Vol. 172, No. 7, (Apr 1, 2004), pp. 4545-4555.

Kelly-Welch, A. E., Wang, H. Y., Wang, L. M., Pierce, J. H., Jay, G., Finkelman, F., & Keegan, A. D. (2004). Transgenic expression of insulin receptor substrate 2 in murine B cells alters the cell density-dependence of IgE production in vitro and enhances IgE production in vivo. *Journal of Immunology*, Vol. 172, No. 5, (Mar 1, 2004), pp. 2803-2810.

Khattri, R., Cox, T., Yasayko, S. A., & Ramsdell, F. (2003). An essential role for Scurfin in CD4+CD25+ T regulatory cells. *Nature Immunology*, Vol. 4, No. 4, (Apr, 2003), pp. 337-342.

Khoo, S. K., Zhang, G., Backer, V., Porsbjerg, C., Nepper-Christensen, S., Creegan, R., Baynam, G., de Klerk, N., Rossi, G. A., Hagel, I., Di Prisco, M. C., Lynch, N., Britton, J., Hall, I., Musk, A. W., Goldblatt, J., & Le Souef, P. N. (2006). Associations of a novel IL4RA polymorphism, Ala57Thr, in Greenlander Inuit. *Journal of Allergy and Clinical Immunology*, Vol. 118, No. 3, (Sep, 2006), pp. 627-634.

Kleinschek, M. A., Owyang, A. M., Joyce-Shaikh, B., Langrish, C. L., Chen, Y., Gorman, D. M., Blumenschein, W. M., McClanahan, T., Brombacher, F., Hurst, S. D., Kastelein, R. A., & Cua, D. J. (2007). IL-25 regulates Th17 function in autoimmune inflammation. *The Journal of experimental medicine*, Vol. 204, No. 1, (Jan 22, 2007), pp. 161-170.

Knutsen, A. P., Kariuki, B., Consolino, J. D., & Warrier, M. R. (2006). IL-4 alpha chain receptor (IL-4Ralpha) polymorphisms in allergic bronchopulmonary sspergillosis. *Clin Mol Allergy*, Vol. 4, No., (2006), pp. 3.

Koettnitz, K., & Kalthoff, F. S. (1993). Human interleukin-4 receptor signaling requires sequences contained within two cytoplasmic regions. *European Journal of Immunology*, Vol. 23, No. 4, (Apr, 1993), pp. 988-991.

Kondo, M., Takeshita, T., Ishii, N., Nakamura, M., Watanabe, S., Arai, K., & Sugamura, K. (1993). Sharing of the interleukin-2 (IL-2) receptor gamma chain between receptors for IL-2 and IL-4. *Science*, Vol. 262, No. 5141, (Dec 17, 1993), pp. 1874-1877.

Kopf, M., Brombacher, F., Hodgkin, P. D., Ramsay, A. J., Milbourne, E. A., Dai, W. J., Ovington, K. S., Behm, C. A., Kohler, G., Young, I. G., & Matthaei, K. I. (1996). IL-5-deficient mice have a developmental defect in CD5+ B-1 cells and lack eosinophilia but have normal antibody and cytotoxic T cell responses. *Immunity*, Vol. 4, No. 1, (Jan, 1996), pp. 15-24.

Kruse, S., Braun, S., & Deichmann, K. A. (2002). Distinct signal transduction processes by IL-4 and IL-13 and influences from the Q551R variant of the human IL-4 receptor alpha chain. *Respir Res*, Vol. 3, No., (2002), pp. 24.

Kruse, S., Japha, T., Tedner, M., Sparholt, S. H., Forster, J., Kuehr, J., & Deichmann, K. A. (1999). The polymorphisms S503P and Q576R in the interleukin-4 receptor alpha gene are associated with atopy and influence the signal transduction. *Immunology*, Vol. 96, No. 3, (Mar, 1999), pp. 365-371.

Kuhne, M. R., Pawson, T., Lienhard, G. E., & Feng, G. S. (1993). The insulin receptor substrate 1 associates with the SH2-containing phosphotyrosine phosphatase Syp. *Journal of Biological Chemistry*, Vol. 268, No. 16, (Jun 5, 1993), pp. 11479-11481.

Kumaki, S., Kondo, M., Takeshita, T., Asao, H., Nakamura, M., & Sugamura, K. (1993). Cloning of the mouse interleukin 2 receptor gamma chain: demonstration of functional differences between the mouse and human receptors. *Biochemical and Biophysical Research Communications*, Vol. 193, No. 1, (May 28, 1993), pp. 356-363.

Kuperman, D., Schofield, B., Wills-Karp, M., & Grusby, M. J. (1998). Signal transducer and activator of transcription factor 6 (Stat6)- deficient mice are protected from antigen-induced airway hyperresponsiveness and mucus production. *Journal of Experimental Medicine*, Vol. 187, No. 6, (1998), pp. 939-948.

Kurata, H., Lee, H. J., O'Garra, A., & Arai, N. (1999). Ectopic expression of activated Stat6 induces the expression of Th2-specific cytokines and transcription factors in developing Th1 cells. *Immunity*, Vol. 11, No. 6, (Dec, 1999), pp. 677-688.

Langrish, C. L., Chen, Y., Blumenschein, W. M., Mattson, J., Basham, B., Sedgwick, J. D., McClanahan, T., Kastelein, R. A., & Cua, D. J. (2005). IL-23 drives a pathogenic T cell population that induces autoimmune inflammation. *The Journal of experimental medicine*, Vol. 201, No. 2, (Jan 17, 2005), pp. 233-240.

LaPorte, S. L., Juo, Z. S., Vaclavikova, J., Colf, L. A., Qi, X., Heller, N. M., Keegan, A. D., & Garcia, K. C. (2008). Molecular and structural basis of cytokine receptor pleiotropy in the interleukin-4/13 system. *Cell*, Vol. 132, No. 2, (Jan 25, 2008), pp. 259-272.

Leonard, W. J., Noguchi, M., & Russell, S. M. (1994). Sharing of a common gamma chain, gamma c, by the IL-2, IL-4, and IL-7 receptors: implications for X-linked severe combined immunodeficiency (XSCID). *Advances in Experimental Medicine and Biology*, Vol. 365, No., (1994), pp. 225-232.

Lorenz, U. (2009). SHP-1 and SHP-2 in T cells: two phosphatases functioning at many levels. *Immunological Reviews*, Vol. 228, No. 1, (Mar, 2009), pp. 342-359.

Losman, J., Chen, X. P., Jiang, H., Pan, P. Y., Kashiwada, M., Giallourakis, C., Cowan, S., Foltenyi, K., & Rothman, P. (1999). IL-4 signaling is regulated through the recruitment of phosphatases, kinases, and SOCS proteins to the receptor complex. *Cold Spring Harbor Symposia on Quantitative Biology*, Vol. 64, No., (1999), pp. 405-416.

Lowenthal, J. W., Castle, B. E., Christiansen, J., Schreurs, J., Rennick, D., Arai, N., Hoy, P., Takebe, Y., & Howard, M. (1988). Expression of high affinity receptors for murine interleukin 4 (BSF-1) on hemopoietic and nonhemopoietic cells. *Journal of Immunology*, Vol. 140, No. 2, (Jan 15, 1988), pp. 456-464.

Lupardus, P. J., Birnbaum, M. E., & Garcia, K. C. (2010). Molecular basis for shared cytokine recognition revealed in the structure of an unusually high affinity complex between IL-13 and IL-13Ralpha2. *Structure*, Vol. 18, No. 3, (Mar 10, 2010), pp. 332-342.

Martin, P., Villares, R., Rodriguez-Mascarenhas, S., Zaballos, A., Leitges, M., Kovac, J., Sizing, I., Rennert, P., Marquez, G., Martinez, A. C., Diaz-Meco, M. T., & Moscat, J. (2005). Control of T helper 2 cell function and allergic airway inflammation by PKCzeta. *Proceedings of the National Academy of Sciences of the United States of America*, Vol. 102, No. 28, (Jul 12, 2005), pp. 9866-9871.

Mashima, R., Hishida, Y., Tezuka, T., & Yamanashi, Y. (2009). The roles of Dok family adapters in immunoreceptor signaling. *Immunological Reviews*, Vol. 232, No. 1, (Nov, 2009), pp. 273-285.

Mathew, A., MacLean, J. A., DeHaan, E., Tager, A. M., Green, F. H., & Luster, A. D. (2001). Signal transducer and activator of transcription 6 controls chemokine production and T helper cell type 2 cell trafficking in allergic pulmonary inflammation. *Journal of Experimental Medicine*, Vol. 193, No. 9, (2001), pp. 1087-1096.

Matsumura, M., Inoue, H., Matsumoto, T., Nakano, T., Fukuyama, S., Matsumoto, K., Takayama, K., Saito, M., Kawakami, K., & Nakanishi, Y. (2007). Endogenous metalloprotease solubilizes IL-13 receptor alpha2 in airway epithelial cells. *Biochemical and Biophysical Research Communications*, Vol. 360, No. 2, (Aug 24, 2007), pp. 464-469.

McGeachy, M. J., Bak-Jensen, K. S., Chen, Y., Tato, C. M., Blumenschein, W., McClanahan, T., & Cua, D. J. (2007). TGF-beta and IL-6 drive the production of IL-17 and IL-10 by T cells and restrain T(H)-17 cell-mediated pathology. *Nature Immunology*, Vol. 8, No. 12, (Dec, 2007), pp. 1390-1397.

McKinley, L., Alcorn, J. F., Peterson, A., Dupont, R. B., Kapadia, S., Logar, A., Henry, A., Irvin, C. G., Piganelli, J. D., Ray, A., & Kolls, J. K. (2008). TH17 cells mediate steroid-resistant airway inflammation and airway hyperresponsiveness in mice. *Journal of immunology (Baltimore, Md: 1950)*, Vol. 181, No. 6, (Sep 15, 2008), pp. 4089-4097.

Mentink-Kane, M. M., Cheever, A. W., Thompson, R. W., Hari, D. M., Kabatereine, N. B., Vennervald, B. J., Ouma, J. H., Mwatha, J. K., Jones, F. M., Donaldson, D. D.,

Grusby, M. J., Dunne, D. W., & Wynn, T. A. (2004). IL-13 receptor alpha 2 down-modulates granulomatous inflammation and prolongs host survival in schistosomiasis. *Proceedings of the National Academy of Sciences of the United States of America*, Vol. 101, No. 2, (Jan 13, 2004), pp. 586-590.

Mikita, T., Campbell, D., Wu, P., Williamson, K., & Schindler, U. (1996). Requirements for interleukin-4-induced gene expression and functional characterization of Stat6. *Molecular and Cellular Biology*, Vol. 16, No. 10, (1996), pp. 5811-5820.

Min, B., & Paul, W. E. (2008). Basophils and type 2 immunity. *Current Opinion in Hematology*, Vol. 15, No. 1, (Jan, 2008), pp. 59-63.

Mitsuyasu, H., Izuhara, K., Mao, X. Q., Gao, P. S., Arinobu, Y., Enomoto, T., Kawai, M., Sasaki, S., Dake, Y., Hamasaki, N., Shirakawa, T., & Hopkin, J. M. (1998). Ile50Val variant of IL4R alpha upregulates IgE synthesis and associates with atopic asthma. *Nature Genetics*, Vol. 19, No. 2, (Jun, 1998), pp. 119-120.

Mitsuyasu, H., Yanagihara, Y., Mao, X. Q., Gao, P. S., Arinobu, Y., Ihara, K., Takabayashi, A., Hara, T., Enomoto, T., Sasaki, S., Kawai, M., Hamasaki, N., Shirakawa, T., Hopkin, J. M., & Izuhara, K. (1999). Cutting edge: dominant effect of Ile50Val variant of the human IL-4 receptor alpha-chain in IgE synthesis. *Journal of Immunology*, Vol. 162, No. 3, (Feb 1, 1999), pp. 1227-1231.

Molet, S., Hamid, Q., Davoine, F., Nutku, E., Taha, R., Page, N., Olivenstein, R., Elias, J., & Chakir, J. (2001). IL-17 is increased in asthmatic airways and induces human bronchial fibroblasts to produce cytokines. *The Journal of Allergy and Clinical Immunology*, Vol. 108, No. 3, (Sep, 2001), pp. 430-438.

Morris, S. C., Orekhova, T., Meadows, M. J., Heidorn, S. M., Yang, J., & Finkelman, F. D. (2006). IL-4 induces in vivo production of IFN-gamma by NK and NKT cells. *Journal of Immunology*, Vol. 176, No. 9, (May 1, 2006), pp. 5299-5305.

Mosley, B., Beckmann, M. P., March, C. J., Idzerda, R. L., Gimpel, S. D., VandenBos, T., Friend, D., Alpert, A., Anderson, D., Jackson, J., & et al. (1989). The murine interleukin-4 receptor: molecular cloning and characterization of secreted and membrane bound forms. *Cell*, Vol. 59, No. 2, (Oct 20, 1989), pp. 335-348.

Munitz, A., Brandt, E. B., Mingler, M., Finkelman, F. D., & Rothenberg, M. E. (2008). Distinct roles for IL-13 and IL-4 via IL-13 receptor alpha1 and the type II IL-4 receptor in asthma pathogenesis. *Proceedings of the National Academy of Sciences of the United States of America*, Vol. 105, No. 20, (May 20, 2008), pp. 7240-7245.

Murakami, M., Narazaki, M., Hibi, M., Yawata, H., Yasukawa, K., Hamaguchi, M., Taga, T., & Kishimoto, T. (1991). Critical cytoplasmic region of the interleukin 6 signal transducer gp130 is conserved in the cytokine receptor family. *Proceedings of the National Academy of Sciences of the United States of America*, Vol. 88, No. 24, (Dec 15, 1991), pp. 11349-11353.

Murata, T., Noguchi, P. D., & Puri, R. K. (1996). IL-13 induces phosphorylation and activation of JAK2 Janus kinase in human colon carcinoma cell lines: similarities between IL-4 and IL-13 signaling. *Journal of Immunology*, Vol. 156, No. 8, (Apr 15, 1996), pp. 2972-2978.

Murata, T., & Puri, R. K. (1997). Comparison of IL-13- and IL-4-induced signaling in EBV-immortalized human B cells. *Cellular Immunology*, Vol. 175, No. 1, (Jan 10, 1997), pp. 33-40.

Nelms, K., Keegan, A. D., Zamorano, J., Ryan, J. J., & Paul, W. E. (1999). The IL-4 receptor: signaling mechanisms and biologic functions. *Annual Review of Immunology*, Vol. 17, No., (1999), pp. 701-738.

Nelms, K., Snow, A. L., Hu-Li, J., & Paul, W. E. (1998). FRIP, a hematopoietic cell-specific rasGAP-interacting protein phosphorylated in response to cytokine stimulation. *Immunity*, Vol. 9, No. 1, (Jul, 1998), pp. 13-24.

Nelson, B. H., Lord, J. D., & Greenberg, P. D. (1996). A membrane-proximal region of the interleukin-2 receptor gamma c chain sufficient for Jak kinase activation and induction of proliferation in T cells. *Molecular and Cellular Biology*, Vol. 16, No. 1, (Jan, 1996), pp. 309-317.

Newcomb, D. C., Boswell, M. G., Zhou, W., Huckabee, M. M., Goleniewska, K., Sevin, C. M., Hershey, G. K., Kolls, J. K., & Peebles, R. S., Jr. (2011). Human TH17 cells express a functional IL-13 receptor and IL-13 attenuates IL-17A production. *Journal of Allergy and Clinical Immunology*, Vol. 127, No. 4, (Apr, 2011), pp. 1006-1013.

Newcomb, D. C., Zhou, W., Moore, M. L., Goleniewska, K., Hershey, G. K., Kolls, J. K., & Peebles, R. S., Jr. (2009). A functional IL-13 receptor is expressed on polarized murine CD4+ Th17 cells and IL-13 signaling attenuates Th17 cytokine production. *Journal of Immunology*, Vol. 182, No. 9, (May 1, 2009), pp. 5317-5321.

Noguchi, E., Shibasaki, M., Arinami, T., Takeda, K., Yokouchi, Y., Kobayashi, K., Imoto, N., Nakahara, S., Matsui, A., & Hamaguchi, H. (1999). No association between atopy/asthma and the ILe50Val polymorphism of IL-4 receptor. *American Journal of Respiratory and Critical Care Medicine*, Vol. 160, No. 1, (Jul, 1999), pp. 342-345.

Noguchi, M., Adelstein, S., Cao, X., & Leonard, W. J. (1993). Characterization of the human interleukin-2 receptor gamma chain gene. *Journal of Biological Chemistry*, Vol. 268, No. 18, (Jun 25, 1993), pp. 13601-13608.

Noguchi, M., Yi, H., Rosenblatt, H. M., Filipovich, A. H., Adelstein, S., Modi, W. S., McBride, O. W., & Leonard, W. J. (1993). Interleukin-2 receptor gamma chain mutation results in X-linked severe combined immunodeficiency in humans. *Cell*, Vol. 73, No. 1, (Apr 9, 1993), pp. 147-157.

O'Connor, J. C., Sherry, C. L., Guest, C. B., & Freund, G. G. (2007). Type 2 diabetes impairs insulin receptor substrate-2-mediated phosphatidylinositol 3-kinase activity in primary macrophages to induce a state of cytokine resistance to IL-4 in association with overexpression of suppressor of cytokine signaling-3. *Journal of Immunology*, Vol. 178, No. 11, (Jun 1, 2007), pp. 6886-6893.

Ober, C., Leavitt, S. A., Tsalenko, A., Howard, T. D., Hoki, D. M., Daniel, R., Newman, D. L., Wu, X., Parry, R., Lester, L. A., Solway, J., Blumenthal, M., King, R. A., Xu, J., Meyers, D. A., Bleecker, E. R., & Cox, N. J. (2000). Variation in the interleukin 4-receptor alpha gene confers susceptibility to asthma and atopy in ethnically diverse populations. *American Journal of Human Genetics*, Vol. 66, No. 2, (Feb, 2000), pp. 517-526.

Ogata, H., Ford, D., Kouttab, N., King, T. C., Vita, N., Minty, A., Stoeckler, J., Morgan, D., Girasole, C., Morgan, J. W., & Maizel, A. L. (1998). Regulation of interleukin-13 receptor constituents on mature human B lymphocytes. *Journal of Biological Chemistry*, Vol. 273, No. 16, (Apr 17, 1998), pp. 9864-9871.

Oh, S. Y., Zheng, T., Bailey, M. L., Barber, D. L., Schroeder, J. T., Kim, Y. K., & Zhu, Z. (2007). Src homology 2 domain-containing inositol 5-phosphatase 1 deficiency leads to a spontaneous allergic inflammation in the murine lung. *Journal of Allergy and Clinical Immunology*, Vol. 119, No. 1, (Jan, 2007), pp. 123-131.

Orchansky, P. L., Kwan, R., Lee, F., & Schrader, J. W. (1999). Characterization of the cytoplasmic domain of interleukin-13 receptor-alpha. *Journal of Biological Chemistry*, Vol. 274, No. 30, (Jul 23, 1999), pp. 20818-20825.

Pace, L., Pioli, C., & Doria, G. (2005). IL-4 modulation of CD4+CD25+ T regulatory cell-mediated suppression. *Journal of Immunology*, Vol. 174, No. 12, (Jun 15, 2005), pp. 7645-7653.

Pace, L., Rizzo, S., Palombi, C., Brombacher, F., & Doria, G. (2006). Cutting edge: IL-4-induced protection of CD4+CD25- Th cells from CD4+CD25+ regulatory T cell-mediated suppression. *Journal of Immunology)*, Vol. 176, No. 7, (Apr 1, 2006), pp. 3900-3904.

Paliard, X., de Waal Malefijt, R., Yssel, H., Blanchard, D., Chretien, I., Abrams, J., de Vries, J., & Spits, H. (1988). Simultaneous production of IL-2, IL-4, and IFN-gamma by activated human CD4+ and CD8+ T cell clones. *Journal of Immunology*, Vol. 141, No. 3, (Aug 1, 1988), pp. 849-855.

Park, L. S., Friend, D., Grabstein, K., & Urdal, D. L. (1987). Characterization of the high-affinity cell-surface receptor for murine B-cell-stimulating factor 1. *Proceedings of the National Academy of Sciences of the United States of America*, Vol. 84, No. 6, (Mar, 1987), pp. 1669-1673.

Park, L. S., Friend, D., Sassenfeld, H. M., & Urdal, D. L. (1987). Characterization of the human B cell stimulatory factor 1 receptor. *Journal of Experimental Medicine*, Vol. 166, No. 2, (Aug 1, 1987), pp. 476-488.

Pelicci, G., Lanfrancone, L., Grignani, F., McGlade, J., Cavallo, F., Forni, G., Nicoletti, I., Pawson, T., & Pelicci, P. G. (1992). A novel transforming protein (SHC) with an SH2 domain is implicated in mitogenic signal transduction. *Cell*, Vol. 70, No. 1, (Jul 10, 1992), pp. 93-104.

Peritt, D., Robertson, S., Gri, G., Showe, L., Aste-Amezaga, M., & Trinchieri, G. (1998). Differentiation of human NK cells into NK1 and NK2 subsets. *Journal of Immunology* Vol. 161, No. 11, (Dec 1, 1998), pp. 5821-5824.

Pesu, M., Takaluoma, K., Aittomaki, S., Lagerstedt, A., Saksela, K., Kovanen, P. E., & Silvennoinen, O. (2000). Interleukin-4-induced transcriptional activation by stat6 involves multiple serine/threonine kinase pathways and serine phosphorylation of stat6. *Blood*, Vol. 95, No. 2, (Jan 15, 2000), pp. 494-502.

Piccinni, M. P., Macchia, D., Parronchi, P., Giudizi, M. G., Bani, D., Alterini, R., Grossi, A., Ricci, M., Maggi, E., & Romagnani, S. (1991). Human bone marrow non-B, non-T cells produce interleukin 4 in response to cross-linkage of Fc epsilon and Fc gamma receptors. *Proceedings of the National Academy of Sciences of the United States of America*, Vol. 88, No. 19, (Oct 1, 1991), pp. 8656-8660.

Plaut, M., Pierce, J. H., Watson, C. J., Hanley-Hyde, J., Nordan, R. P., & Paul, W. E. (1989). Mast cell lines produce lymphokines in response to cross-linkage of Fc epsilon RI or to calcium ionophores. *Nature*, Vol. 339, No. 6219, (May 4, 1989), pp. 64-67.

Pouliot, P., Turmel, V., Gelinas, E., Laviolette, M., & Bissonnette, E. Y. (2005). Interleukin-4 production by human alveolar macrophages. *Clinical and Experimental Allergy*, Vol. 35, No. 6, (Jun, 2005), pp. 804-810.

Prots, I., Skapenko, A., Wendler, J., Mattyasovszky, S., Yone, C. L., Spriewald, B., Burkhardt, H., Rau, R., Kalden, J. R., Lipsky, P. E., & Schulze-Koops, H. (2006). Association of the IL4R single-nucleotide polymorphism I50V with rapidly erosive rheumatoid arthritis. *Arthritis and Rheumatism*, Vol. 54, No. 5, (May, 2006), pp. 1491-1500.

Pruett, W., Yuan, Y., Rose, E., Batzer, A. G., Harada, N., & Skolnik, E. Y. (1995). Association between GRB2/Sos and insulin receptor substrate 1 is not sufficient for activation of extracellular signal-regulated kinases by interleukin-4: implications for Ras activation by insulin. *Molecular and Cellular Biology*, Vol. 15, No. 3, (Mar, 1995), pp. 1778-1785.

Ra, C., Kuromitsu, S., Hirose, T., Yasuda, S., Furuichi, K., & Okumura, K. (1993). Soluble human high-affinity receptor for IgE abrogates the IgE-mediated allergic reaction. *International Immunology*, Vol. 5, No. 1, (Jan, 1993), pp. 47-54.

Rahaman, S. O., Sharma, P., Harbor, P. C., Aman, M. J., Vogelbaum, M. A., & Haque, S. J. (2002). IL-13R(alpha)2, a decoy receptor for IL-13 acts as an inhibitor of IL-4-dependent signal transduction in glioblastoma cells. *Cancer Research*, Vol. 62, No. 4, (Feb 15, 2002), pp. 1103-1109.

Ramalingam, T. R., Pesce, J. T., Sheikh, F., Cheever, A. W., Mentink-Kane, M. M., Wilson, M. S., Stevens, S., Valenzuela, D. M., Murphy, A. J., Yancopoulos, G. D., Urban, J. F., Jr., Donnelly, R. P., & Wynn, T. A. (2008). Unique functions of the type II interleukin 4 receptor identified in mice lacking the interleukin 13 receptor alpha1 chain. *Nat Immunol*, Vol. 9, No. 1, (Jan, 2008), pp. 25-33.

Rankin, J. A., Picarella, D. E., Geba, G. P., Temann, U. A., Prasad, B., DiCosmo, B., Tarallo, A., Stripp, B., Whitsett, J., & Flavell, R. A. (1996). Phenotypic and physiologic characterization of transgenic mice expressing interleukin 4 in the lung: lymphocytic and eosinophilic inflammation without airway hyperreactivity. *Proceedings of the National Academy of Sciences of the United States of America*, Vol. 93, No. 15, (Jul 23, 1996), pp. 7821-7825.

Rauh, M. J., Ho, V., Pereira, C., Sham, A., Sly, L. M., Lam, V., Huxham, L., Minchinton, A. I., Mui, A., & Krystal, G. (2005). SHIP represses the generation of alternatively activated macrophages. *Immunity*, Vol. 23, No. 4, (Oct, 2005), pp. 361-374.

Ravetch, J. V., & Lanier, L. L. (2000). Immune inhibitory receptors. *Science*, Vol. 290, No. 5489, (Oct 6, 2000), pp. 84-89.

Reichel, M., Nelson, B. H., Greenberg, P. D., & Rothman, P. B. (1997). The IL-4 receptor alpha-chain cytoplasmic domain is sufficient for activation of JAK-1 and STAT6 and the induction of IL-4-specific gene expression. *Journal of Immunology*, Vol. 158, No. 12, (Jun 15, 1997), pp. 5860-5867.

Risma, K. A., Wang, N., Andrews, R. P., Cunningham, C. M., Ericksen, M. B., Bernstein, J. A., Chakraborty, R., & Hershey, G. K. (2002). V75R576 IL-4 receptor alpha is associated with allergic asthma and enhanced IL-4 receptor function. *Journal of Immunology*, Vol. 169, No. 3, (Aug 1, 2002), pp. 1604-1610.

Rolling, C., Treton, D., Pellegrini, S., Galanaud, P., & Richard, Y. (1996). IL4 and IL13 receptors share the gamma c chain and activate STAT6, STAT3 and STAT5 proteins in normal human B cells. *FEBS Letters*, Vol. 393, No. 1, (1996), pp. 53-56.

Romagnani, S. (1992). Induction of TH1 and TH2 responses: a key role for the 'natural' immune response? *Immunology Today*, Vol. 13, No. 10, (Oct, 1992), pp. 379-381.

Roy, B., Bhattacharjee, A., Xu, B., Ford, D., Maizel, A. L., & Cathcart, M. K. (2002). IL-13 signal transduction in human monocytes: phosphorylation of receptor components, association with Jaks, and phosphorylation/activation of Stats. *Journal of Leukocyte Biology*, Vol. 72, No. 3, (Sep, 2002), pp. 580-589.

Rui, L., Fisher, T. L., Thomas, J., & White, M. F. (2001). Regulation of insulin/insulin-like growth factor-1 signaling by proteasome-mediated degradation of insulin receptor substrate-2. *Journal of Biological Chemistry*, Vol. 276, No. 43, (Oct 26, 2001), pp. 40362-40367.

Russell, S. M., Johnston, J. A., Noguchi, M., Kawamura, M., Bacon, C. M., Friedmann, M., Berg, M., McVicar, D. W., Witthuhn, B. A., Silvennoinen, O., & et al. (1994). Interaction of IL-2R beta and gamma c chains with Jak1 and Jak3: implications for XSCID and XCID. *Science*, Vol. 266, No. 5187, (Nov 11, 1994), pp. 1042-1045.

Russell, S. M., Keegan, A. D., Harada, N., Nakamura, Y., Noguchi, M., Leland, P., Friedmann, M. C., Miyajima, A., Puri, R. K., Paul, W. E., & et al. (1993). Interleukin-2 receptor gamma chain: a functional component of the interleukin-4 receptor. *Science*, Vol. 262, No. 5141, (Dec 17, 1993), pp. 1880-1883.

Ryan, J. J., McReynolds, L. J., Keegan, A., Wang, L. H., Garfein, E., Rothman, P., Nelms, K., & Paul, W. E. (1996). Growth and gene expression are predominantly controlled by distinct regions of the human IL-4 receptor. *Immunity*, Vol. 4, No. 2, (Feb, 1996), pp. 123-132.

Sabin, E. A., Kopf, M. A., & Pearce, E. J. (1996). Schistosoma mansoni egg-induced early IL-4 production is dependent upon IL-5 and eosinophils. *Journal of Experimental Medicine*, Vol. 184, No. 5, (Nov 1, 1996), pp. 1871-1878.

Sakaguchi, S., Yamaguchi, T., Nomura, T., & Ono, M. (2008). Regulatory T cells and immune tolerance. *Cell*, Vol. 133, No. 5, (May 30, 2008), pp. 775-787.

Satoh, T., Nakafuku, M., Miyajima, A., & Kaziro, Y. (1991). Involvement of ras p21 protein in signal-transduction pathways from interleukin 2, interleukin 3, and granulocyte/macrophage colony-stimulating factor, but not from interleukin 4. *Proceedings of the National Academy of Sciences of the United States of America*, Vol. 88, No. 8, (Apr 15, 1991), pp. 3314-3318.

Scheffold, A., Murphy, K. M., & Hofer, T. (2007). Competition for cytokines: T(reg) cells take all. *Nature Immunology*, Vol. 8, No. 12, (Dec, 2007), pp. 1285-1287.

Schroeder, J. T., Kagey-Sobotka, A., & Lichtenstein, L. M. (1995). The role of the basophil in allergic inflammation. *Allergy*, Vol. 50, No. 6, (Jun, 1995), pp. 463-472.

Seder, R. A., Boulay, J. L., Finkelman, F., Barbier, S., Ben-Sasson, S. Z., Le Gros, G., & Paul, W. E. (1992). CD8+ T cells can be primed in vitro to produce IL-4. *Journal of Immunology*, Vol. 148, No. 6, (Mar 15, 1992), pp. 1652-1656.

Sehra, S., Bruns, H. A., Ahyi, A. N., Nguyen, E. T., Schmidt, N. W., Michels, E. G., von Bulow, G. U., & Kaplan, M. H. (2008). IL-4 is a critical determinant in the generation of allergic inflammation initiated by a constitutively active Stat6. *Journal of Immunology*, Vol. 180, No. 5, (Mar 1, 2008), pp. 3551-3559.

Sehra, S., Yao, Y., Howell, M. D., Nguyen, E. T., Kansas, G. S., Leung, D. Y., Travers, J. B., & Kaplan, M. H. (2010). IL-4 regulates skin homeostasis and the predisposition toward allergic skin inflammation. *Journal of Immunology*, Vol. 184, No. 6, (Mar 15, 2010), pp. 3186-3190.

Seldin, D. C., & Leder, P. (1994). Mutational analysis of a critical signaling domain of the human interleukin 4 receptor. *Proceedings of the National Academy of Sciences of the United States of America*, Vol. 91, No. 6, (Mar 15, 1994), pp. 2140-2144.

Shankaranarayanan, P., Chaitidis, P., Kuhn, H., & Nigam, S. (2001). Acetylation by histone acetyltransferase CREB-binding protein/p300 of STAT6 is required for transcriptional activation of the 15-lipoxygenase- 1 gene. *Journal of Biological Chemistry*, Vol. 276, No. 46, (2001), pp. 42753-42760.

Shevach, E. M. (2009). Mechanisms of foxp3+ T regulatory cell-mediated suppression. *Immunity*, Vol. 30, No. 5, (May, 2009), pp. 636-645.

Shirakawa, I., Deichmann, K. A., Izuhara, I., Mao, I., Adra, C. N., & Hopkin, J. M. (2000). Atopy and asthma: genetic variants of IL-4 and IL-13 signalling. *Immunology Today*, Vol. 21, No. 2, (Feb, 2000), pp. 60-64.

Shirakawa, T., Kawazoe, Y., Tsujikawa, T., Jung, D., Sato, S., & Uesugi, M. (2011). Deactivation of STAT6 through serine 707 phosphorylation by JNK. *Journal of Biological Chemistry*, Vol. 286, No. 5, (Feb 4, 2011), pp. 4003-4010.

Shirey, K., Cole, L. E., Keegan, A. D., Elkins, K. E., Vogel, S. N. (2008). *Francisella tularensis* LVS induces Macrophage Alternative Activation as a Survival Mechanism. *Journal of Immunology*, Vol., No., (2008), pp.

Shirey, K. A., Pletneva, L. M., Puche, A. C., Keegan, A. D., Prince, G. A., Blanco, J. C., & Vogel, S. N. (2010). Control of RSV-induced lung injury by alternatively activated macrophages is IL-4R alpha-, TLR4-, and IFN-beta-dependent. *Mucosal Immunol*, Vol. 3, No. 3, (May, 2010), pp. 291-300.

Sozzani, P., Hasan, L., Seguelas, M. H., Caput, D., Ferrara, P., Pipy, B., & Cambon, C. (1998). IL-13 induces tyrosine phosphorylation of phospholipase C gamma-1 following IRS-2 association in human monocytes: relationship with the inhibitory effect of IL-13 on ROI production. *Biochemical and Biophysical Research Communications*, Vol. 244, No. 3, (Mar 27, 1998), pp. 665-670.

Starr, R., Willson, T. A., Viney, E. M., Murray, L. J., Rayner, J. R., Jenkins, B. J., Gonda, T. J., Alexander, W. S., Metcalf, D., Nicola, N. A., & Hilton, D. J. (1997). A family of cytokine-inducible inhibitors of signalling. *Nature*, Vol. 387, No. 6636, (Jun 26, 1997), pp. 917-921.

Stephenson, L., Johns, M. H., Woodward, E., Mora, A. L., & Boothby, M. (2004). An IL-4R alpha allelic variant, I50, acts as a gain-of-function variant relative to V50 for Stat6, but not Th2 differentiation. *Journal of Immunology*, Vol. 173, No. 7, (Oct 1, 2004), pp. 4523-4528.

Stritesky, G. L., Muthukrishnan, R., Sehra, S., Goswami, R., Pham, D., Travers, J., Nguyen, E. T., Levy, D. E., & Kaplan, M. H. (2011). The transcription factor STAT3 is required for T helper 2 cell development. *Immunity*, Vol. 34, No. 1, (Jan 28, 2011), pp. 39-49.

Strober, W., Kitani, A., Fichtner-Feigl, S., & Fuss, I. J. (2009). The signaling function of the IL-13Ralpha2 receptor in the development of gastrointestinal fibrosis and cancer surveillance. *Curr Mol Med*, Vol. 9, No. 6, (Aug, 2009), pp. 740-750.

Sun, X. J., Pons, S., Wang, L. M., Zhang, Y., Yenush, L., Burks, D., Myers, M. G., Jr., Glasheen, E., Copeland, N. G., Jenkins, N. A., Pierce, J. H., & White, M. F. (1997). The IRS-2 gene on murine chromosome 8 encodes a unique signaling adapter for insulin and cytokine action. *Molecular Endocrinology*, Vol. 11, No. 2, (Feb, 1997), pp. 251-262.

Sun, X. J., Rothenberg, P., Kahn, C. R., Backer, J. M., Araki, E., Wilden, P. A., Cahill, D. A., Goldstein, B. J., & White, M. F. (1991). Structure of the insulin receptor substrate IRS-1 defines a unique signal transduction protein. *Nature,* Vol. 352, No. 6330, (Jul 4, 1991), pp. 73-77.

Sun, X. J., Wang, L. M., Zhang, Y., Yenush, L., Myers, M. G., Jr., Glasheen, E., Lane, W. S., Pierce, J. H., & White, M. F. (1995). Role of IRS-2 in insulin and cytokine signalling. *Nature,* Vol. 377, No. 6545, (Sep 14, 1995), pp. 173-177.

Suzuki, K., Nakajima, H., Kagami, S., Suto, A., Ikeda, K., Hirose, K., Hiwasa, T., Takeda, K., Saito, Y., Akira, S., & Iwamoto, I. (2002). Proteolytic processing of Stat6 signaling in mast cells as a negative regulatory mechanism. *Journal of Experimental Medicine*, Vol. 196, No. 1, (Jul 1, 2002), pp. 27-38.

Tabata, Y., Chen, W., Warrier, M. R., Gibson, A. M., Daines, M. O., & Hershey, G. K. (2006). Allergy-driven alternative splicing of IL-13 receptor alpha2 yields distinct membrane and soluble forms. *Journal of Immunology*, Vol. 177, No. 11, (Dec 1, 2006), pp. 7905-7912.

Tachdjian, R., Al Khatib, S., Schwinglshackl, A., Kim, H. S., Chen, A., Blasioli, J., Mathias, C., Kim, H. Y., Umetsu, D. T., Oettgen, H. C., & Chatila, T. A. (2010). In vivo regulation of the allergic response by the IL-4 receptor alpha chain immunoreceptor tyrosine-based inhibitory motif. *Journal of Allergy and Clinical Immunology*, Vol. 125, No. 5, (May, 2010), pp. 1128-1136.

Tachdjian, R., Mathias, C., Al Khatib, S., Bryce, P. J., Kim, H. S., Blaeser, F., O'Connor, B. D., Rzymkiewicz, D., Chen, A., Holtzman, M. J., Hershey, G. K., Garn, H., Harb, H., Renz, H., Oettgen, H. C., & Chatila, T. A. (2009). Pathogenicity of a disease-associated human IL-4 receptor allele in experimental asthma. *Journal of Experimental Medicine*, Vol. 206, No. 10, (Sep 28, 2009), pp. 2191-2204.

Takaki, H., Ichiyama, K., Koga, K., Chinen, T., Takaesu, G., Sugiyama, Y., Kato, S., Yoshimura, A., & Kobayashi, T. (2008). STAT6 Inhibits TGF-beta1-mediated Foxp3 induction through direct binding to the Foxp3 promoter, which is reverted by retinoic acid receptor. *The Journal of biological chemistry*, Vol. 283, No. 22, (May 30, 2008), pp. 14955-14962.

Takeda, K., Tanaka, T., Shi, W., Matsumoto, M., Minami, M., Kashiwamura, S., Nakanishi, K., Yoshida, N., Kishimoto, T., & Akira, S. (1996). Essential role of Stat6 in IL-4 signalling. *Nature,* Vol. 380, No. 6575, (Apr 18, 1996), pp. 627-630.

Takeshita, T., Asao, H., Ohtani, K., Ishii, N., Kumaki, S., Tanaka, N., Munakata, H., Nakamura, M., & Sugamura, K. (1992). Cloning of the gamma chain of the human IL-2 receptor. *Science,* Vol. 257, No. 5068, (Jul 17, 1992), pp. 379-382.

Timonen, T., & Stenius-Aarniala, B. (1985). Natural killer cell activity in asthma. *Clinical and Experimental Immunology*, Vol. 59, No. 1, (Jan, 1985), pp. 85-90.

Toru, H., Pawankar, R., Ra, C., Yata, J., & Nakahata, T. (1998). Human mast cells produce IL-13 by high-affinity IgE receptor cross-linking: enhanced IL-13 production by IL-4-primed human mast cells. *Journal of Allergy and Clinical Immunology*, Vol. 102, No. 3, (Sep, 1998), pp. 491-502.

Toru, H., Ra, C., Nonoyama, S., Suzuki, K., Yata, J., & Nakahata, T. (1996). Induction of the high-affinity IgE receptor (Fc epsilon RI) on human mast cells by IL-4. *International Immunology*, Vol. 8, No. 9, (Sep, 1996), pp. 1367-1373.

Umeshita-Suyama, R., Sugimoto, R., Akaiwa, M., Arima, K., Yu, B., Wada, M., Kuwano, M., Nakajima, K., Hamasaki, N., & Izuhara, K. (2000). Characterization of IL-4 and IL-13 signals dependent on the human IL-13 receptor alpha chain 1: redundancy of requirement of tyrosine residue for STAT3 activation. *International Immunology*, Vol. 12, No. 11, (Nov, 2000), pp. 1499-1509.

van Panhuys, N., Prout, M., Forbes, E., Min, B., Paul, W. E., & Le Gros, G. (2011). Basophils are the major producers of IL-4 during primary helminth infection. *Journal of Immunology*, Vol. 186, No. 5, (Mar 1, 2011), pp. 2719-2728.

Voehringer, D., Shinkai, K., & Locksley, R. M. (2004). Type 2 immunity reflects orchestrated recruitment of cells committed to IL-4 production. *Immunity*, Vol. 20, No. 3, (Mar, 2004), pp. 267-277.

Wakashin, H., Hirose, K., Maezawa, Y., Kagami, S., Suto, A., Watanabe, N., Saito, Y., Hatano, M., Tokuhisa, T., Iwakura, Y., Puccetti, P., Iwamoto, I., & Nakajima, H. (2008). IL-23 and Th17 cells enhance Th2-cell-mediated eosinophilic airway inflammation in mice. *American Journal of Respiratory and Critical Care Medicine*, Vol. 178, No. 10, (Nov 15, 2008), pp. 1023-1032.

Wallis, S. K., Cooney, L. A., Endres, J. L., Lee, M. J., Ryu, J., Somers, E. C., & Fox, D. A. (2011). A polymorphism in the interleukin-4 receptor affects the ability of interleukin-4 to regulate Th17 cells: a possible immunoregulatory mechanism for genetic control of the severity of rheumatoid arthritis. *Arthritis Res Ther*, Vol. 13, No. 1, (Feb 4, 2011), pp. R15.

Wang, H. Y., Shelburne, C. P., Zamorano, J., Kelly, A. E., Ryan, J. J., & Keegan, A. D. (1999). Cutting edge: effects of an allergy-associated mutation in the human IL-4R alpha (Q576R) on human IL-4-induced signal transduction. *Journal of Immunology*, Vol. 162, No. 8, (Apr 15, 1999), pp. 4385-4389.

Wang, H. Y., Zamorano, J., & Keegan, A. D. (1998). A role for the insulin-interleukin (IL)-4 receptor motif of the IL-4 receptor alpha-chain in regulating activation of the insulin receptor substrate 2 and signal transducer and activator of transcription 6 pathways. Analysis by mutagenesis. *Journal of Biological Chemistry*, Vol. 273, No. 16, (Apr 17, 1998), pp. 9898-9905.

Wang, H. Y., Zamorano, J., Yoerkie, J. L., Paul, W. E., & Keegan, A. D. (1997). The IL-4-induced tyrosine phosphorylation of the insulin receptor substrate is dependent on JAK1 expression in human fibrosarcoma cells. *Journal of Immunology*, Vol. 158, No. 3, (Feb 1, 1997), pp. 1037-1040.

Wang, I. M., Lin, H., Goldman, S. J., & Kobayashi, M. (2004). STAT-1 is activated by IL-4 and IL-13 in multiple cell types. *Molecular Immunology*, Vol. 41, No. 9, (Jul, 2004), pp. 873-884.

Wang, L. M., Keegan, A. D., Li, W., Lienhard, G. E., Pacini, S., Gutkind, J. S., Myers, M. G., Jr., Sun, X. J., White, M. F., Aaronson, S. A., & et al. (1993). Common elements in interleukin 4 and insulin signaling pathways in factor-dependent hematopoietic cells. *Proceedings of the National Academy of Sciences of the United States of America*, Vol. 90, No. 9, (May 1, 1993), pp. 4032-4036.

Wang, L. M., Keegan, A. D., Paul, W. E., Heidaran, M. A., Gutkind, J. S., & Pierce, J. H. (1992). IL-4 activates a distinct signal transduction cascade from IL-3 in factor-dependent myeloid cells. *EMBO Journal*, Vol. 11, No. 13, (Dec, 1992), pp. 4899-4908.

Wang, L. M., Michieli, P., Lie, W. R., Liu, F., Lee, C. C., Minty, A., Sun, X. J., Levine, A., White, M. F., & Pierce, J. H. (1995). The insulin receptor substrate-1-related 4PS substrate but not the interleukin-2R gamma chain is involved in interleukin-13-mediated signal transduction. *Blood*, Vol. 86, No. 11, (Dec 1, 1995), pp. 4218-4227.

Wang, L. M., Myers, M. G., Jr., Sun, X. J., Aaronson, S. A., White, M., & Pierce, J. H. (1993). IRS-1: essential for insulin- and IL-4-stimulated mitogenesis in hematopoietic cells. *Science*, Vol. 261, No. 5128, (Sep 17, 1993), pp. 1591-1594.

Wang, X. Y., Gelfanov, V., Sun, H. B., Tsai, S., & Yang, Y. C. (1999). Distinct actions of interleukin-9 and interleukin-4 on a hematopoietic stem cell line, EMLC1. *Experimental Hematology*, Vol. 27, No. 1, (Jan, 1999), pp. 139-146.

Wang, Y., Malabarba, M. G., Nagy, Z. S., & Kirken, R. A. (2004). Interleukin 4 regulates phosphorylation of serine 756 in the transactivation domain of Stat6. Roles for multiple phosphorylation sites and Stat6 function. *Journal of Biological Chemistry*, Vol. 279, No. 24, (Jun 11, 2004), pp. 25196-25203.

Warren, H. S., Kinnear, B. F., Phillips, J. H., & Lanier, L. L. (1995). Production of IL-5 by human NK cells and regulation of IL-5 secretion by IL-4, IL-10, and IL-12. *Journal of Immunology*, Vol. 154, No. 10, (May 15, 1995), pp. 5144-5152.

Wei, H., Zhang, J., Xiao, W., Feng, J., Sun, R., & Tian, Z. (2005). Involvement of human natural killer cells in asthma pathogenesis: natural killer 2 cells in type 2 cytokine predominance. *The Journal ofAllergy and Clinical Immunology*, Vol. 115, No. 4, (Apr, 2005), pp. 841-847.

Welham, M. J., Duronio, V., Leslie, K. B., Bowtell, D., & Schrader, J. W. (1994). Multiple hemopoietins, with the exception of interleukin-4, induce modification of Shc and mSos1, but not their translocation. *Journal of Biological Chemistry*, Vol. 269, No. 33, (Aug 19, 1994), pp. 21165-21176.

Welham, M. J., Duronio, V., Sanghera, J. S., Pelech, S. L., & Schrader, J. W. (1992). Multiple hemopoietic growth factors stimulate activation of mitogen-activated protein kinase family members. *Journal of Immunology*, Vol. 149, No. 5, (Sep 1, 1992), pp. 1683-1693.

Welham, M. J., Duronio, V., & Schrader, J. W. (1994). Interleukin-4-dependent proliferation dissociates p44erk-1, p42erk-2, and p21ras activation from cell growth. *Journal of Biological Chemistry*, Vol. 269, No. 8, (Feb 25, 1994), pp. 5865-5873.

Welham, M. J., Learmonth, L., Bone, H., & Schrader, J. W. (1995). Interleukin-13 signal transduction in lymphohemopoietic cells. Similarities and differences in signal transduction with interleukin-4 and insulin. *Journal of Biological Chemistry*, Vol. 270, No. 20, (May 19, 1995), pp. 12286-12296.

Weller, C. L., Collington, S. J., Williams, T., & Lamb, J. R. (2011). Mast cells in health and disease. *Clin Sci (Lond)*, Vol. 120, No. 11, (Jun, 2011), pp. 473-484.

Wen, L., Barber, D. F., Pao, W., Wong, F. S., Owen, M. J., & Hayday, A. (1998). Primary gamma delta cell clones can be defined phenotypically and functionally as Th1/Th2 cells and illustrate the association of CD4 with Th2 differentiation. *Journal of Immunology*, Vol. 160, No. 4, (Feb 15, 1998), pp. 1965-1974.

Wenzel, S., Wilbraham, D., Fuller, R., Getz, E. B., & Longphre, M. (2007). Effect of an interleukin-4 variant on late phase asthmatic response to allergen challenge in asthmatic patients: results of two phase 2a studies. *Lancet*, Vol. 370, No. 9596, (Oct 20, 2007), pp. 1422-1431.

Wenzel, S. E., Balzar, S., Ampleford, E., Hawkins, G. A., Busse, W. W., Calhoun, W. J., Castro, M., Chung, K. F., Erzurum, S., Gaston, B., Israel, E., Teague, W. G., Curran-Everett, D., Meyers, D. A., & Bleecker, E. R. (2007). IL4R alpha mutations are associated with asthma exacerbations and mast cell/IgE expression. *American Journal of Respiratory and Critical Care Medicine*, Vol. 175, No. 6, (Mar 15, 2007), pp. 570-576.

Wery-Zennaro, S., Letourneur, M., David, M., Bertoglio, J., & Pierre, J. (1999). Binding of IL-4 to the IL-13Ralpha(1)/IL-4Ralpha receptor complex leads to STAT3 phosphorylation but not to its nuclear translocation. *FEBS Letters*, Vol. 464, No. 1-2, (Dec 24, 1999), pp. 91-96.

Wery, S., Letourneur, M., Bertoglio, J., & Pierre, J. (1996). Interleukin-4 induces activation of mitogen-activated protein kinase and phosphorylation of shc in human keratinocytes. *Journal of Biological Chemistry*, Vol. 271, No. 15, (Apr 12, 1996), pp. 8529-8532.

Wesch, D., Glatzel, A., & Kabelitz, D. (2001). Differentiation of resting human peripheral blood gamma delta T cells toward Th1- or Th2-phenotype. *Cellular Immunology*, Vol. 212, No. 2, (Sep 15, 2001), pp. 110-117.

White, E. D., Andrews, R. P., & Hershey, G. K. (2001). Sulfhydryl-2 domain-containing protein tyrosine phosphatase-1 is not a negative regulator of interleukin-4 signaling in murine mast cells. *Journal of Leukocyte Biology*, Vol. 69, No. 5, (2001), pp. 825-830.

White, M. F. (2002). IRS proteins and the common path to diabetes. *Am J Physiol Endocrinol Metab*, Vol. 283, No. 3, (Sep, 2002), pp. E413-422.

Wills-Karp, M., Luyimbazi, J., Xu, X., Schofield, B., Neben, T. Y., Karp, C. L., & Donaldson, D. D. (1998). Interleukin-13: central mediator of allergic asthma. *Science*, Vol. 282, No. 5397, (Dec 18, 1998), pp. 2258-2261.

Witthuhn, B. A., Silvennoinen, O., Miura, O., Lai, K. S., Cwik, C., Liu, E. T., & Ihle, J. N. (1994). Involvement of the Jak-3 Janus kinase in signalling by interleukins 2 and 4 in lymphoid and myeloid cells. *Nature*, Vol. 370, No. 6485, (Jul 14, 1994), pp. 153-157.

Wolf, G., Trub, T., Ottinger, E., Groninga, L., Lynch, A., White, M. F., Miyazaki, M., Lee, J., & Shoelson, S. E. (1995). PTB domains of IRS-1 and Shc have distinct but overlapping binding specificities. *Journal of Biological Chemistry*, Vol. 270, No. 46, (Nov 17, 1995), pp. 27407-27410.

Wu, L., Bijian, K., & Shen, S. H. (2009). CD45 recruits adapter protein DOK-1 and negatively regulates JAK-STAT signaling in hematopoietic cells. *Molecular Immunology*, Vol. 46, No. 11-12, (Jul, 2009), pp. 2167-2177.

Wurster, A. L., Rodgers, V. L., White, M. F., Rothstein, T. L., & Grusby, M. J. (2002). Interleukin-4-mediated protection of primary B cells from apoptosis through Stat6-dependent up-regulation of Bcl-xL. *Journal of Biological Chemistry*, Vol. 277, No. 30, (Jul 26, 2002), pp. 27169-27175.

Wymann, M. P., & Pirola, L. (1998). Structure and function of phosphoinositide 3-kinases. *Biochimica et Biophysica Acta*, Vol. 1436, No. 1-2, (Dec 8, 1998), pp. 127-150.

Yamashita, M., Kimura, M., Kubo, M., Shimizu, C., Tada, T., Perlmutter, R. M., & Nakayama, T. (1999). T cell antigen receptor-mediated activation of the Ras/mitogen-activated protein kinase pathway controls interleukin 4 receptor function and type-2 helper T cell differentiation. *Proceedings of the National Academy of Sciences of the United States of America*, Vol. 96, No. 3, (Feb 2, 1999), pp. 1024-1029.

Yi, T. L., Cleveland, J. L., & Ihle, J. N. (1992). Protein tyrosine phosphatase containing SH2 domains: characterization, preferential expression in hematopoietic cells, and localization to human chromosome 12p12-p13. *Molecular and Cellular Biology*, Vol. 12, No. 2, (Feb, 1992), pp. 836-846.

Yoshikawa, M., Nakajima, T., Tsukidate, T., Matsumoto, K., Iida, M., Otori, N., Haruna, S., Moriyama, H., & Saito, H. (2003). TNF-alpha and IL-4 regulate expression of IL-13 receptor alpha2 on human fibroblasts. *Biochemical and Biophysical Research Communications*, Vol. 312, No. 4, (Dec 26, 2003), pp. 1248-1255.

Yoshimura, A., Mori, H., Ohishi, M., Aki, D., & Hanada, T. (2003). Negative regulation of cytokine signaling influences inflammation. *Current Opinion in Immunology*, Vol. 15, No. 6, (Dec, 2003), pp. 704-708.

Zamorano, J., & Keegan, A. D. (1998). Regulation of apoptosis by tyrosine-containing domains of IL-4R alpha: Y497 and Y713, but not the STAT6-docking tyrosines, signal protection from apoptosis. *Journal of Immunology*, Vol. 161, No. 2, (Jul 15, 1998), pp. 859-867.

Zhang, J. L., Buehner, M., & Sebald, W. (2002). Functional epitope of common gamma chain for interleukin-4 binding. *European Journal of Biochemistry*, Vol. 269, No. 5, (Mar, 2002), pp. 1490-1499.

Zheng, T., Liu, W., Oh, S. Y., Zhu, Z., Hu, B., Homer, R. J., Cohn, L., Grusby, M. J., & Elias, J. A. (2008). IL-13 receptor alpha2 selectively inhibits IL-13-induced responses in the murine lung. *Journal of Immunology*, Vol. 180, No. 1, (Jan 1, 2008), pp. 522-529.

Zheng, T., Zhu, Z., Liu, W., Lee, C. G., Chen, Q., Homer, R. J., & Elias, J. A. (2003). Cytokine regulation of IL-13Ralpha2 and IL-13Ralpha1 in vivo and in vitro. *Journal of Allergy and Clinical Immunology*, Vol. 111, No. 4, (Apr, 2003), pp. 720-728.

Zhou, M. M., Huang, B., Olejniczak, E. T., Meadows, R. P., Shuker, S. B., Miyazaki, M., Trub, T., Shoelson, S. E., & Fesik, S. W. (1996). Structural basis for IL-4 receptor phosphopeptide recognition by the IRS-1 PTB domain. *Nature Structural Biology*, Vol. 3, No. 4, (Apr, 1996), pp. 388-393.

Zhu, J., & Paul, W. E. (2008). CD4 T cells: fates, functions, and faults. *Blood*, Vol. 112, No. 5, (Sep 1, 2008), pp. 1557-1569.

Zhu, J., Yamane, H., Cote-Sierra, J., Guo, L., & Paul, W. E. (2006). GATA-3 promotes Th2 responses through three different mechanisms: induction of Th2 cytokine production, selective growth of Th2 cells and inhibition of Th1 cell-specific factors. *Cell Research*, Vol. 16, No. 1, (Jan, 2006), pp. 3-10.

Zhu, Z., Homer, R. J., Wang, Z., Chen, Q., Geba, G. P., Wang, J., Zhang, Y., & Elias, J. A. (1999). Pulmonary expression of interleukin-13 causes inflammation, mucus hypersecretion, subepithelial fibrosis, physiologic abnormalities, and eotaxin production. *Journal of Clinical Investigation*, Vol. 103, No. 6, (Mar, 1999), pp. 779-788.

Zurawski, S. M., Vega, F., Jr., Huyghe, B., & Zurawski, G. (1993). Receptors for interleukin-13 and interleukin-4 are complex and share a novel component that functions in signal transduction. *EMBO Journal*, Vol. 12, No. 7, (Jul, 1993), pp. 2663-2670.

4

Enzymatic and Chemical Modifications of Food Allergens

Dragana Stanić-Vučinić and Tanja Ćirković Veličković
Faculty of Chemistry, University of Belgrade, Serbia

1. Introduction

Food allergy is defined as an abnormal immunological reaction to food proteins, which causes an adverse clinical reaction. Today 4-6% of children and 1-3% of adults are affected with food allergy in Europe (Mills et al., 2007), while in the USA 6- 8% of children and 4% of adults are affected (Gupta et al., 2008). The incidence of food allergy has been increasing over the years, and to date, no effective treatment of food allergies is available. Therapies involving drugs (antihistamines, decongestants, or steroids) only combat the symptoms of an allergic reaction and do not prevent allergenic reactions due to future exposures to the allergen. Specific immunotherapy (SIT) is the only prophylactic desensitizing therapy for allergy (Bousquet et al., 1998; Durham et al., 1999). However, for food allergies immunotherapy safety-profile is extremely poor because allergic reactions are associated with a significant risk of anaphylactic side-effects (Nelson et al., 1997; Skripak et al., 2008), even with fatal outcome. Therefore, allergen modification resulting in almost complete reduction of IgE-binding, while retaining its immunogenicity, could improve formulations for immunotherapy of food allergies.

The best way to prevent unintended exposure to a food allergen is the strict avoidance of foodstuffs containing allergens. Such avoidance may not always be possible, and in certain instances impossible. Furthermore, complete elimination of foodstuffs causing allergy also has negative impact on healthy diet as about 90 % of allergens are present in food of high nutrition value (milk, eggs, fish, shellfish, tree nuts, peanuts, wheat, and soybeans) (Thompson et al., 2006). Therefore production of hypoallergenic food become increasingly indispensable part of food industry with growing demand for methods aimed to reduce allergenic potential of food products. There is increasing number of publications describing successful attempts to reduce allergenicity of food allergens. A number of studies of food processing on allergen reactivity are largely focused on thermal treatments. Although thermal treatments can be used on many products to alter food allergen reactivity, thermal processing has also been known to modify organoleptic properties, including flavor, color, and nutrient content (Holdsworth, 1985). Therefore, novel non-thermal food processing techniques are being explored in order to create hypoallergenic products (Shriver & Yang, 2011). Variable success of methods for allergenicity reduction, due to limited knowledge of allergen and epitope structures and the factors governing their stability, imposes need for an empirical approach (Soler-Rivas & Wichers, 2001). Chemical or enzymatic modification of allergen molecule may alter its structure or physically obstruct binding of IgE antibodies to conformational or linear epitopes. The objective of this review is to thoroughly explore chemical and enzymatic processing techniques utilized to modify food allergens, highlighting the efficacy of these methods in their ability to alter food allergen reactivity. As there are comprehensive reviews on food allergen treatment with digestive enzymes and the effects of fermentation on food reactivity, this review is focused on chemical and enzymatic modification of food allergen in the narrow sense.

2. Methods for assessing allergenicity of food products

The efficacy of chemical and enzymatic methods used to alter food allergen reactivity must be verified by analyzing the treated allergen's (or treated allergenic food) ability to trigger an immune response. As the reactivity of an allergen is often described by its ability to bind IgE antibodies, reduced IgE activity may indicate a modification or removal of food allergen(s). A variety of rapid assay methods are in use as analytical tools in research of molecular structure, integrity and biological activity of food allergens and their epitopes. Allergen reactivity can be determined by *in vitro, ex vivo* and *in vivo* testing. *In vitro* tests are often inexpensive, quick and without a threat to human or animal subjects. On the other hand *in vivo* assays provide a more accurate representation of the research. *Ex vivo* tests are advantageous because they are measuring allergenic response on effector cell level, using human subject blood without exposing them to risk. Animal models may also be used, though these models are not always analogous to the human. However, animal models may be a useful tool for predicting sensitizing potential of proteins introduced into diet by genetic manipulation or modified allergens which may carry higher allergenic risk.

In vivo **tests**. In vivo detection includes skin prick tests (SPT) and oral food challenges (OFC). SPT is simple and inexpensive, but the wheal sizes can vary by allergen and subject (Sampson, 1999), subjective results can differ between evaluators (Poulsen, 2001) and patients with atopic dermatitis may develop false-positive wheals (Fleischer et al., 2010). OFC is considered the "gold standard" in diagnosing food allergy as it can provide more accurate information regarding food allergy. However, these tests are complex, expensive and time consuming. As subject may experience severe adverse reactions patients who are susceptible to anaphylaxis should not be included in this type of study (Fleischer et al., 2010). However, final proof of improved safety of potentially less allergenic foods must be provided through human test studies, via double-blind placebo-controlled food challenge (DBPCFC)-tests.

Animal models. Rodent animal models are the most often exploited animal models of food allergy. Though the dosage of the allergen, route of exposure and duration of the build-in phase of allergy may differ depending on the allergen used and animal strain, many food allergy models have been described in the literature providing generation of IgE in the serum upon immunization and/or anaphylaxis reaction upon challenge with allergen. Animal models are useful in elucidation of mechanisms involved in reduction of allerenicity, especially on B cell and T cell level (Hattori et al., 2000; Kobayashi et al., 2001; Kobayashi et al., 2003).

Ex vivo tests. Ex vivo tests include histamine release or up regulation of surface molecules CD63 or CD203c on basophile granulocytes, known as the basophile activation test, BAT. By measuring specific IgE we only measure one interaction, between IgE and an allergen, whilst an allergic response requires two simultaneous interactions of allergen with IgE on the same effector cell. This is simulated in the *ex vivo* tests based on basophile granulocytes.

In vitro tests. *In vitro* studies for determining allergen reactivity include the measurement of serum IgE using radio-allergosorbent tests (RAST), enzyme-allergosorbent tests (EAST), enzyme linked immunosorbent assay (ELISA), ImmunoCAP assays (Phadia, Uppsala, Sweden); and immunobloting. By RAST, EAST and ELISA (competitive inhibition and indirect) multiple samples can be tested at once. However, due to differences with solid phase and sample preparation among analysts standardization is the main problem. Furthermore, IgG antibodies can compete with IgE antibodies for similar epitopes. Although expensive, an ImmunoCAP tests have increased sensitivity compared to RAST, EAST and ELISA with minimized nonspecific binding by non-IgE binding antibodies. Immunoblotting includes Western blot and dot blot allergen analysis. In Western blotting proteins are most often tested in their linear conformation so that conformational epitopes may not be represented and new IgE binding epitopes, in native conformation hidden within the protein, may be uncovered. Immunobloting is frequently used since protein bands can be individually analyzed to determine the changes in a specific allergen. In dot blot conformational epitopes may be preserved due to non-denaturing conditions, but in the case of protein mixture immunogenicity of the entire sample is analyzed.

Digestibility assays for food protein allergenicity assessment. The observation that many food allergens exhibit proteolytic stability led to allergy assessment strategy that use of digestion stability as a criterion for protein allergenicity assessment (Becker, 1997; Besler er al., 2001; Taylor & Lehrer, 1996). Although the relationship between the stability of proteins in simulated gastric fluid (SGF) and allergenicity has been inconsistent among studies, many recent reports proved increased incidence of food allergies in relation to impaired gastric digestion in human and animal studies. (Untersmayr & Jensen-Jarolim, 2008). Thomas et al. (Thomas et al., 2008) demonstrated that common protocol for evaluating the *in vitro* digestibility of proteins is reproducible and yields consistent results when performed using the same proteins at different laboratories. However, digestibility assays of pure proteins may not be always relevant in assessing allergenicity potential as they do not account for the effects of food matrices (Ofori-Anti et al., 2008). Therefore, *in vitro* gastrointestinal digestion protocols should be preferably combined with immunological assays in order to elucidate the role of large digestion-resistant fragments and the influence of the food matrix (Moreno, 2007). For a comprehensive review on digestibility of food allergens refer to Cirkovic Velickovic et al. (Cirkovic Velickovic et al., 2009). Anyway, comparison of unmodified and modified food allergen in digestibility studies can give valuable information about allergic potential of modified food protein and efficiency of modifying method used. As enzymatic and chemical methods change allergen structure digestibility of modified allergen can be increased or decreased thus directly influencing allergen availability to gut immune system.

3. Chemical modifications

The aim of chemical modifications of proteins used for nutritional purposes, in addition to reduction of allergenic properties, is obtaining of proteins with required techno-functional properties (solubility, emulsification, foaming, gelling, etc.) and preserved nutritional value. Chemical modifications of food proteins can lead to a change in the charge and hydrophobicity of proteins, which in turn can diminish or eliminate allergenicity of food allergens. However, regardless the application of non-toxic reagents, chemical modifications are not so often applied in the food industry regarding complex procedures of removing remaining chemical agents.

3.1 Covalent modifications

Acylation. Acylation of allergens by treatment with anhydrides, such as acetic or succinic, blocks positively charged amino groups on the protein molecule and the remaining free carboxyl groups of aspartic and glutamic acid residues make the net charge of the modified protein more negative. Szymkiewicz & Jędrychowski (Szymkiewicz & Jedrychowski, 2009) modified pea proteins with acetic or succinic anhydride. Immunoreactivity of albumins and legumin, as estimated by ELISA with rabbit polyclonal antibodies, was reduced by 91-99% and 78-97% after succinylation and acetylation, respectively, while immunoreactivity of vicilin fraction was reduced down to 12% and 17%, respectively. In their other study (Szymkiewicz & Jędrychowski, 2008) the authors combined enzymatic hydrolysis by Alcalase with chemical modification by acylation of pea proteins. The enzyme hydrolysis of acylation-modified pea proteins caused significant reduction in the immunoreactivity of pea proteins, especially vicilin, whose epitopes were the most resistant to the modifications, both chemical (Szymkiewicz & Jedrychowski, 2009) and enzymatic one (Szymkiewicz & Jędrychowski, 2005), applied separately. The application of Alcalase lowered the immunoreactivity of vicilin to 2-2.5%, while immunoreactivity of legumin and albumin decreased by nearly 100%. Thus, combining various methods of protein modification is more efficient and can be a promising approach for preparing products with reduced allergenicity. However, in ELISA tests with individual sera of patients allergic to leguminous seeds, IgE binging of pea proteins were reduced only by 40-75%, indicating that considerable decrease in the antigenicity of proteins not always guarantees their lower allergenicity and also shows differences in individual patients.

Carbamoylation. Mistrello et al. (Mistrello et al., 1996) chemically modified ovalbumin by reaction with potassium cyanate (KCNO), which transforms the ε-amino group of the lysine of proteinaceous allergens into ureido groups. KCNO-modified (carbamylated) allergens have low allergenic potency, as demonstrated in *vitro* (RAST inhibition) and in vivo (passive cutaneous anaphylaxis). When used to immunize rabbits, carbamylated allergens still induce IgG antibodies able to cross-react with native allergens (immunoblotting experiments). Although potentially useful for immunotherapy formulations preparation this method is not suitable for hypoallergic food preparation.

Nitration. In study of Untersmayr et al. (Untersmayr et al., 2010) BALB/c mice were immunized intragastrically by feeding untreated ovalbumin (OA) and nitrated ovalbumin (nOA) with or without acid-suppression. While oral immunizations of nOA under anti-acid treatment did not result in IgG and IgE formation, intraperitoneal immunization induced high levels of OA specific IgE, which were significantly increased in the group that received nOA by injection. Furthermore, nOA triggered significantly enhanced mediator release of effector cells of sensitized allergic animals. In gastric digestion experiments nOA was degraded within few minutes, whereas OA remained stable up to 120 min. Additionally, one tyrosine residue being very efficiently nitrated is part of an ovalbumin epitope recognized exclusively after oral sensitization. These data indicated that despite the enhanced triggering capacity in existing allergy, nitration of OVA may be associated with a reduced *de novo* sensitizing capability via the oral route due to enhanced protein digestibility and/or changes in antibody epitopes. Although the authors considered effects of endogenously nitrated allergen, these results imply that nitration of food allergen as method have no potential for reducing its allergenic potential.

Conjugation with synthetic copolymer. Conjugates of ovalbumin (OA) and the copolymer of N-vinyl pyrrolidone and maleic anhydride (VMA) modified with epsilon-aminocaproic acid (Acp) were prepared by Babakhin et al. (Babakhin et al., 1995). Of all conjugates injected intraperitoneally into mice only the conjugate containing 20%OA (OA-Acp-VMA) did induce anti-OA IgG antibodies without significant quantities of anti-OA IgE. In passive cutaneous anaphylaxis, RAST inhibition and leukocyte histamine release, OA-Acp-VMA have shown significant reduction of allergenicity and stimulated activation of the OA-specific T-cell comparable to that of unconjugated OA. During experimental allergen-specific hyposensitization with OA-Acp-VMA, suppression of anti-OA IgE response and elevation of anti-OA IgG responses were noted. By using the carrier Acp-VMA to reduce allergenicity there is selective blockage of B-cell epitopes of allergen without affecting T-cell epitopes, thereby preserving immunogenicity, which enable creation of preparations for allergen-specific immunotherapy.

Polymerization by glutaraldehyde. By treatment with glutaraldehyde aldehyde groups of glutaraldehyde react with the amino groups of protein resulting in cross-linked allergen proteins with altered immunological characteristics (Patterson et al., 1979). Recently the ability of glutaraldehyde-treated allergens to stimulate T-cells has been disputed (Wurtzen et al., 2007). XiYang et al. (Yang et al., 1993) demonstrated that whereas *in vivo* administration of ovalbumin (OA) induces cytokine synthesis that is neither Thl nor Th2 dominated, administration of glutaraldehyde polymerized, high relative molecular weight OA (OA-POL) leads to 20-fold increase in the ratio of interferon γ (IFN-γ)/IL-4 and IFN-γ/IL-10 synthesis observed after short-term, antigen-mediated restimulation directly *ex vivo*. In contrast, concurrent in vivo administration of anti-IFN-γ/mAb and OA or OA-POL results in marked increases in IL-4 and IL-10, and decreased IFN-γ production, reflecting a polarization of the response towards a Th2-1ike pattern of cytokine synthesis. This is approach that allows selective activation of strongly Thl-dominated immune responses to protein antigens and it may be useful in clinical settings where the ability to actively select specific patterns of cytokine gene expression would be advantageous. Koppelman et al. (Koppelman et al., 2010) demonstrated that modification of peanut conglutin with glutaraldehyde (GA) does not result nor in a change of secondary structure nether in substantial decrease of IgE binding (only 2-3 fold). Reduction/alkylation treatment (RA) change secondary structures, whereas RA treatment followed by GA modification (RA-GA) results in a tertiary structure that differs from that of conglutin treated only with RA, due to modification of Cys and Lys residues. As demonstrated by IgE-ELISA and IgE blot treatment with RA-GA decreases IgE-binding up to a hundred fold and also induce a strong T cell response in T cell proliferation tests. These data demonstrate that all three modifications lead to a reduction in IgE binding, with the strongest reduction observed after both reduction/alkylation and glutaraldehyde treatment.

3.1.1 Covalent hydrophilisation - conjugation with polysaccharides

The shielding of epitopes by materials having low-antigenicity and immunogenicity may be efficient way of reducing allergenicity of the protein, especially with the use of a high molecular weight modifier to achieve effective shielding of epitopes.

Carboxymethyldextran. Hattori et al. (Hattori et al., 2000) prepared BLG-carboxymethyl dextran conjugates (BLG-CMD), by using a water-soluble carbodiimide. The anti-BLG antibody response was markedly reduced after immunization with the BLG-CMD conjugates in mice. Linear epitope profiles of the BLG-CMD conjugates were similar to those of BLG, while the antibody response for each epitope was dramatically reduced. Reduction of immunogenicity of BLG depend on CMD content indicating that masking of epitopes by

CMD is responsible for the decreased immunogenicity of the BLG conjugates due to effective shielding by CMD. Similar result were obtained by Kobayashi et al. (Kobayashi et al., 2001) who prepared BLG-CMD with different molar ratios. Results of both studies show that conjugation with CMD of higher molecular weight is effective in reducing the immunogenicity of BLG by masking of B cell epitopes by CMD. In their further study Kobayashi et al. (Kobayashi et al., 2003), investigated changes in the T cell response to BLG after conjugation with CMDs. When lymph node cells from mice immunized with BLG or the conjugates were stimulated with BLG, T cells from the conjugate-immunized mice showed a lower proliferative response comparing to BLG-immunized mice (Fig.1). T cell epitope profiles of the conjugates were similar to those of BLG, whereas the proliferative response to each epitope was reduced, indicating that the lower *in vivo* T cell response with the conjugates was not due to induction of conjugate-specific T cells, but due to a decrease in the number of BLG-specific T cells. In addition, conjugation with CMD enhanced the resistance of BLG to cathepsin B and cathepsin D, suggesting that conjugation with CMD inhibited the degradation of BLG by proteases in antigen presenting cells (APC) and led to suppression of the generation of antigenic peptides including T cell epitopes from BLG. Therefore, the authors considered that the suppressive effect on the generation of T cell epitopes reduced the antigen presentation of the conjugates and this reduction led to a decrease in the number of BLG-specific T cells *in vivo*. As a result, the decreased help to B cells by T cells would have reduced the antibody response to BLG leading to conclusion that suppression of the generation of T cell epitopes by conjugation with CMD is important to the mechanism for the reduced immunogenicity of BLG.

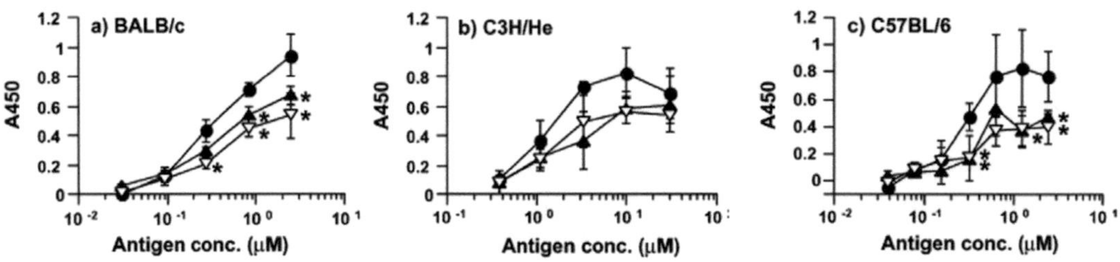

Fig. 1. Proliferative response to BLG of lymph node cells from mice immunized with BLG (circles) or the BLG-CMD conjugates (triangles) and stimulated with BLG at various concentrations. The magnitude of the *in vivo* T cell response was evaluated as the *ex vivo* proliferative response by BrdU ELISA. Each value is expressed as the mean absorbance at 450 nm and standard deviation of triplicate cultures after subtracting the background values (stimulated with PBS). Significant differences ($p < 0.05$) between BLG and each conjugate were determined by Student's t-test and are indicated by asterisks. Reprinted with permission from (Kobayashi et al., 2003). Copyright (2003) American Chemical Society.

Acidic polysaccharides. Hattori et al. (Hattori et al., 2004) conjugated BLG with the acidic oligosaccharides, alginic acid oligosaccharide (ALGO) and phosphoryl oligosaccharides (Pos), by the Maillard reaction. Fluorescence studies indicated surface of each conjugate was covered with a saccharide chain. The anti-BLG antibody response was markedly reduced after immunization with both conjugates in mice. Linear epitope profiles of the conjugates were found to be similar to those of BLG, whereas the antibody response to each epitope was dramatically reduced. In particular, effective reduction of the antibody response was observed in the vicinity of the carbohydrate-binding sites. Obtained conjugates are edible, have higher thermal stability and improved emulsifying properties than those of native BLG, thus being very useful for food application. Yoshida et al. (Yoshida et al., 2005) demonstrate that the T cell response was reduced when mice were immunized with BLG-ALGO conjugates and that novel epitopes were not generated by conjugation. The authors clarified that the BLG-ALGO conjugate modulated the immune response to Th1 dominance and considered that this property of the BLG-ALGO conjugate would be effective for preventing food allergy as well as by its reduced immunogenicity. Therefore, conjugation with acidic oligosaccharides could be applied to various food allergens to achieve reduced allergenicity with multiple improvements in their properties.

Galactomannan. Babiker et al. (Babiker et al., 1998) prepared soy protein-galactomannan conjugate by the Maillard reaction. Conjugation removed the allergenicity of the 34 kDa protein which is frequently recognized by the IgE antibody in the sera of soybean-sensitive patients as a major allergen. Monitoring of polyclonal antibody titers by an indirect enzyme-linked immunosorbent assay and immunoblotting of rabbit sera, monoclonal antibody, and human allergic sera showed that soy protein-galactomannan conjugation was more effective in reducing the allergenicity of the soy protein than transglutaminase treatments and/or chymotrypsin. Additionally, heat stability, solubility and emulsifying properties were greatly improved by conjugation with galactomannan.

Chitosan. Aoki et al. (Aoki et al., 2006) conjugated BLG with chitosan (CHS) by means of a water-soluble carbodiimide to reduce its immunogenicity. The antigenicity of the BLG-CHS conjugates was similar to that of BLG in C3H/He mice, while immunogemicity of BLG was reduced by conjugation. The linear epitope profiles of the conjugates were found to be similar to those of BLG, while the antibody response to each epitope was dramatically reduced. The researchers suggested masking of B cell epitopes as one of the mechanisms in reduction of immunogenicity.

Dextran-glycylglycine and amylose-glycylglycine. Nodake et al. (Nodake et al., 2010) conjugated BLG with the N-hydroxysuccinimide ester of the dextran-glycylglycine adduct (DG-ONSu) to reduce the immunogenicity of BLG. Conjugation with DG-ONSu greatly decreased the reactivity of BLG with anti-BLG antibodies and suppressed their production *in vivo* due to its shielding action for epitope(s) on the protein's molecular surface. Beside, DG-BLG was resistant to proteolytic enzymes. In the other study (Nodake et al., 2011) these authors demonstrated that conjugation BLG with the *N*-hydroxysuccinimide ester of the amylose-glycylglycine adduct (AG-ONSu) also greatly decreased the reactivity of BLG. The authors proposed usage of DG-ONSu and AG-ONSu to suppress the hypersensitivity mediated by IgE antibodies in milk allergy.

3.1.2 Covalent lipophilization

Stearic acid. In the study of Akita and Nakai (Akita & Nakai, 1990) BLG was chemically modified by covalent attachment of different levels of stearic acid. A decreased *in vitro* digestibility was observed with extent of stearic acid incorporation (lipophilization). At low lipophilization increased ability to elicit IgE antibodies, determined by heterologous passive cutaneous anaphylaxis, was observed. Medium level of lipophilization decreased this ability, while high lipophilization almost destroyed the ability to elicit IgE antibodies. The researchers also found that low- and medium-lipophilization increased while high lipophilization decreased the IgG binding ability, measured by ELISA.

3.2 Noncovalent modifications

Components of food matrix can interact noncovalentlly with food allergens resulting insoluble complexes thus lowering the level of soluble allergens and reducing their allergenic properties. Also they can reduce digestibility of food allergens and consequently their allergenicity by hindering access of digestive enzymes. Phenolic compounds and phytic acid are known to form soluble and insoluble complexes with proteins. For instance, it was shown that multivalent hydrophobic interactions cause compaction of cow's milk caseins with the polyphenol epigallocatechin in way that individual casein molecules "wrap around" polyphenol (Jobstl et al., 2006).

Phytic acid. Chung et al. (Chung & Champagne, 2007) treated peanut extract with phytic acid and demonstrated that phytic acid formed complexes with the major peanut allergens (Ara h 1 and Ara h 2), reducing their solubility in acidic and neutral conditions. Also, 6-fold reduction in IgE binding of the extract was observed after treatment with phytic acid, observed by competitive inhibition ELISA using a pooled serum from peanut-allergic individuals. Similar result obtained with peanut butter slurry led to the suggestion that phytic acid treatment might reduce the allergenicity of peanut-based products due to reducing their solubility (Fig 2). In another study by the same group of authors, a facilitated IgE binding in vitro was observed was peanut allergens and phytic acid. Apparently, phytic acid was able to stabilize allergen-antibody interactions (Chung & Champagne, 2006) However, usage of phytic acid might be limited considering its anti-nutritive properties due to ability to chelate iron.

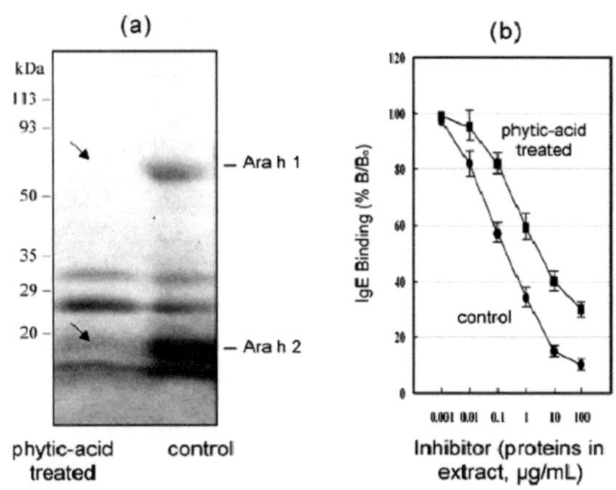

Fig. 2. a) SDS-PAGE and b) competitive inhibition ELISA of natural peanut butter slurry treated and centrifugated with and without phytic acid. Values are means ± SD (n=3). Values of the treated samples at 0.01–100 μg/mL are significantly different from those of the control ($P < 0.05$, n=3). Reprinted with permission from (Chung & Champagne, 2007). Copyright (2003) American Chemical Society.

Phenolic compounds: Adding of phenolics such as caffeic, chlorogenic and ferulic acids to peanut extracts, liquid peanut butter and peanut butter slurries, precipitated most of the major peanut allergens, Ara h 1 and Ara h 2, and complexation was irreversible (Chung & Champagne, 2008; Chung & Champagne, 2009). Of the three phenolics, caffeic acid formed the most precipitates with peanut extracts. IgE binding was reduced approximately 10- to 16-fold as determined by inhibition ELISA (Fig. 3). Assuming that the insoluble complexes are not absorbed by the body the researchers concluded that reducing IgE binding by phenolics is feasible and have a great potential in development of less allergenic liquid peanut-based products.

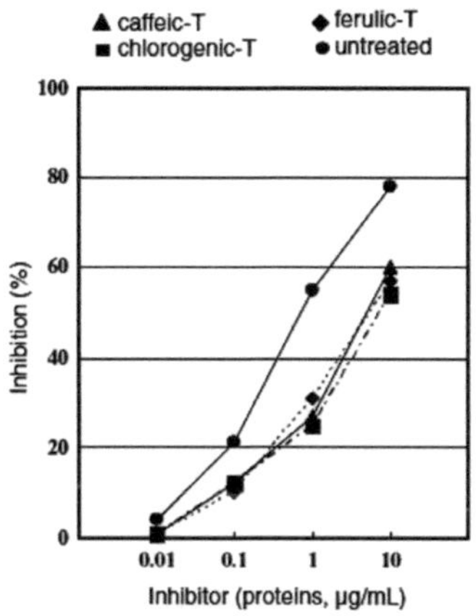

Fig. 3. IgE binding of phenolic-treated and untreated peanut extracts in competitive inhibition ELISA using pooled human plasma from peanut-allergic individuals. Values (on semi-log scale) are mean of three determinations. Values between treatments (caffeic, chlorogenic, and ferulic) are not significantly different from each other but from the untreated ($P < 0.05$). Reprinted from (Chung & Champagne, 2009), Copyright (2009), with permission from Elsevier.

Polysaccharides. Mouecoucou et al. (Mouecoucou et al., 2004) examined the influence of polysaccharides, i.e., gum arabic, low methylated pectin (LMP) and xylan, on the in vitro hydrolysis of peanut protein isolate (PPI) and the in vitro allergenicity of the digestion products. PPI was hydrolyzed in vitro by pepsin, followed by a trypsin/ chymotrypsin (T/C) mixture in dialysis bags. Hydrolysis by all of the digestive enzymes showed retention of some proteins in the dialysis bags in the presence of gum arabic and xylan. The retentates were recognized by IgG and IgE, but IgE binding of retentate containing xylan was reduced. The immunoreactivity of hydrolysis products in dialysates was considerably reduced by polysaccharides. Polovic et al. (Polovic et al., 2007) demonstrated that addition of apple fruit pectin (1.5% and 3%) to the purified kiwi allergen Act c 2 was able to protect it from pepsin digestion *in vitro. In vivo* experiments on healthy non-atopic volunteers have shown that 1 h after ingestion of kiwi fruit in gastric content intact Act c 2 was still present. In their further work Polovic et al. (Polovic et al., 2010) discovered that after *in vivo* digestion of Act c 2 with pure pectin in rats both gastric acidity, as well as specific and total pepsin activity declined and thus protected 23% of the ingested allergen from digestion for 90 minutes. These results show that although presence of polysaccharides can be effective in masking of IgE epitopes, thus reducing allergenicity, it also reduces allergen digestibility, enabling higher dosages of the allergen to reach the immune system.

Oxidized lipids. In study of Doke et al. (Doke et al., 1989) though oxidized soybean oil did not show any allergenicity, the IgE titer of sera from soybean-sensitive patients (in ELISA) was greatly increased when oxidized soybean oil was incubated with soybean 2S-globulin. The IgE titer became higher when greater amounts of oxidized soybean oil were used, but little difference was noted when soybean 2S-globulin was replaced by other food proteins. A similar tendency was noted when soybean oil was replaced by other vegetable oils or fatty acids. The authors speculated that proteins interacted with oxidized lipid are allergenic to soybean-sensitive patients probably due to creation of new epitopes.

3.3 Modifications by oxidation/reduction

Oxidation. Heavy metal ions (Cu2+, Fe 2+, etc.) with hydrogen peroxide can cross-link proteins through oxidation of their tyrosine residues and forming dityrosine and isodityrosine, as well as by oxidation of sulfhydriles resulting in disulfides. In study of Chung et al. (Chung, 2005) extracts from raw and roasted peanuts were treated with Cu^{2+}/H_2O_2 and only roasted peanuts were affected by Cu^{2+}/H_2O_2 . In this case cross-links were formed and levels of Ara h 1 and Ara h 2 were reduced as shown in competitive inhibition ELISA with pooled serum of peanut-allergic individuals. IgE binding, overall, was lower despite some binding of IgE to cross-links leading to conclusion that Cu^{2+}/H_2O_2 reduced peanut allergenicity by inducing the decrease and cross-linking of peanut allergens.
Reduction. The proteins are allergenically active and less digestible in the oxidized (S--S) state. When reduced (SH state), they lose their allergenicity and/or become more digestible. Allergen reduction can be performed by using a reducing agent such as 2-mercaptoethanol, dithiothreitol, cysteine, glutathione, etc., or by using proteins glutaredoxin or thioredoxin. In study of Buchanan et al. (Buchanan et al., 1997) thioredoxin mitigated the allergenicity of whey flour proteins, gliadins and glutenins, as determined by skin tests with a canine model for food allergy, but gave less consistent results with albumins and globulins. In the study of de Val et al. (del Val et al., 1999) after reduction of one or both of its disulfide bonds by thioredoxin, BLG became strikingly sensitive to pepsin in simulated gastric fluid and lost its allergenicity as determined by skin test responses and gastrointestinal symptoms in inbred colony of high IgE–producing dogs sensitized to milk. Koppelman et al. (Koppelnan et al., 2007) modified 2S albumins by reduction by thioredoxin, resulting in breakage of disulfide bonds, followed by alkylation for prevention of reformation of disulfide bonds. Oral administration of native 2S albumin resulted in the development of Th-1 mediated IgG1- and Th-2 mediated IgG2a and IgE responses in the rat, as determined by ELISA. Oral exposure to RA-2S albumin did not result in the development of specific IgE against RA-2S, but IgGl and IgG2a antibodies against RA-2S albumin were formed in a lower level compared to native 2S albumin. Dosing of the animals with the low dose RA-2S albumin (0.1 mg protein/rat/day) did not result in an antibody response at all in the rats whereas the same dose of native 2S albumin induced specific IgGI, IgG2a and IgE responses, again indicating a lesser immunogenicity. Taken together, these data show that reduction of the disulphide bonds of 2S albumin results in loss of allergenicity and an increased sensitivity to digestion. All these results provide evidence that thioredoxin can be applied to enhance digestibility and lower allergenicity of food proteins. However, thioredoxins represent a novel family of cross-reactive allergens involved in the pathogenesis of atopic eczema and asthma. Also, cross-reactivity to human thioredoxin can contribute to the exacerbation of severe atopic diseases by involvement of IgE-mediated autoreactivity (Glaser et al., 2008). Considering these facts usage of thioredoxin in food allergen modification might be limited.

4. Enzymatic modifications

Beside proteolytic enzymes, enzymes able to cross-link proteins have shown to be promising tools for reduction of allergenicity of food proteins. Enzymatic cross-linking of proteins, by transglutaminases, peroxisases and phenol oxidases (such as tyrosinases and laccases), is currently exploited in the food processing industry (Buchert et al., 2007).

4.1 Transglutaminases

Transglutaminases (TG) catalyze formation of a covalent bond between a primary amines (including ε-amino group of lysine residues) and the γ-carboxamid group of protein-bound glutamine leading to protein cross-linking.

Villas-Boas et al. (Villas-Boas et al., 2010) polymerized heat treated BLG and TG (BLG-TG) and untreated BLG in the presence of cysteine and TG (BLG-Cys-TG). BALB/c mice sensitized with BLG-Cys-TG showed lower levels of IgG1 and IgE than those immunized with native BLG or BLG-TG, suggesting that polymerization in the presence of Cys modified or hid epitopes, reducing the potential antigenicity of BLG. Clare et al. (Clare et al., 2007) cross-linked peanut flour dispersions with transglutaminase in the presence and absence of the dithiothreitol. Transglutaminase treatment did not diminish IgE binding responses in ELISA implying only that transglutaminase cross-linking do not enhance potential for allergic responses. In their further study Clare et al. (Clare et al., 2008) cross-linked light roasted peanut flour (PF) with transglutaminase with casein (CN) as co-substrate. In immunoblotting, in some patient sera IgE binding to TGase-treated PF-CN fractions appeared less compared to equivalent polymeric PF dispersions lacking supplemental CN and non-cross-linked PF-CN samples. The researchers assumed that covalent modification masked IgE peanut protein binding epitopes, at least to some degree, on an individual patient basis.

In study of Wroblewska et al. (Wroblewska et al., 2008) whey protein concentrate (WPC) was modified by two enzymes: proteinase Alcalase and transglutaminase. The new products were characterized by 2D electrophoresis, immunoblotting, and ELISA methods. The WPC hydrolysate obtained with Alcalase contained proteins and peptides showing strong immunoreactive properties, as revealed by immunoblotting with α-la and β-lg polyclonal rabbit antibodies. However, the immunoblot analysis demonstrated that WPC showed a stronger reactivity towards IgE of allergic patients then WPC treated with transglutaminase. ELISA assay with human sera showed that two-step modification with Alcalase followed by TG significantly reduced the immunoreactive properties of whey proteins. Patients with wheat-dependent, exercise-induced anaphylaxis (WDEIA) experience recurrent anaphylactic reactions when exercising after ingestion of wheat products.

Palosuo et al. (Palosuo et al., 2003) digested purified ω-5 gliadin, major allergen in WDEIA, with pepsin or with pepsin/trypsin and treated with tissue transglutaminase (tTG). The IgE-binding ability of ω-5 gliadin was retained after pepsin and pepsin-trypsin digestion, as shown in IgE ELISA test. tTG treatment of the whole peptic digest resulted in cross-linked aggregates which bound IgE antibodies in immunoblotting more intensely than untreated, pepsin-digested, or pepsin-trypsin–digested ω-5 gliadin. In the 20 WDEIA patients the mean skin prick test wheal elicited by tTG treated peptic fraction was 77% larger than that elicited by the untreated peptic fraction and 56% larger than that elicited by intact ω-5 gliadin. These results suggest that activation of tTG during exercise in the intestinal mucosa of patients with WDEIA could lead to the formation of large allergen complexes capable of eliciting anaphylactic reactions. Leszczynska et al. (Leszczynska et al., 2006) modified wheat flour by the treatment with transglutaminase and demonstrated, in indirect non-competitive ELISA with human sera, reduction of glutenin immunoreactivity to below 30%.

Watanabe et al. (Watanabe, 2004) have made hypoallergenic flour by flour treatment with actinase, collagenase, and transglutaminase and that TG is the least effective of tested enzymes in reducing flour allergenicity. Soy protein-galactomannan conjugation was more effective in reducing the allergenicity of the soy protein than transglutaminase treatments (Babiker et al., 1998) (Fig. 4). In the study of Monogioudi et al. (Monogioudi et al., 2011) β-casein was cross-linked of by transglutaminase and demonstrated that enzymatically cross-linked β-casein was stable under acidic conditions and was more resistant to pepsin digestion when compared to non cross-linked β-casein. In the study of Stanic et al (Stanic et al., 2010) TG-treated casein showed no mitigated IgE binding reactivity compared with the untreated CN in BAT.

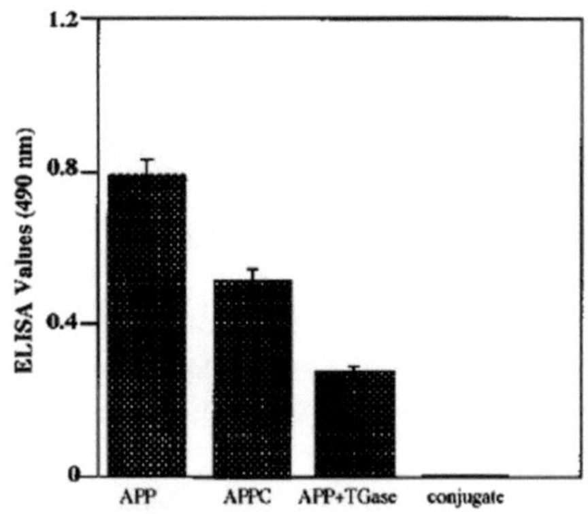

Fig. 4. Determination of antibody titers by indirect ELISA of acid precipitated soy protein (APP), chymotrypsin digest (APPC), transglutaminase treated APP and galactomannan conjugate dry heated for 7 days. Error bars indicate the standard deviations (n=6). Reprinted with permission from (Babiker et al., 1998). Copyright (1998) American Chemical Society.

As a microbial TG is included in many food technological processes, safety of the TG itself, as well as safety of the deamidated/cross-linked proteins generated by this enzyme should be checked (Malandain, 2005). In their study, Pedersen et al. (Pedersen et al., 2004) investigated the allergenicity of TG from *Streptoverticillium mobaraens* by evaluation of amino acid sequence similarity to known allergens, pepsin resistance, and detection of protein binding to specific serum immunoglobulin E (IgE) (RAST) evaluated as recommended by 2001 FAO/WHO Decision Tree, recommended for evaluation of proteins from genetically modified organisms (GMOs). All tests demonstrated that there is no safety concerns with regard to the allergenic potential of tested TG.

4.2 Peroxidases

Peroxidases (POD) are a heme-containing enzymes catalyzing the oxidation of a variety of organic compounds by hydrogen peroxide or hydroperoxides. Acting on phenolic compounds POD generate o-quinones, which further react with other phenolics, amino, or sulfhydryl compounds in proteins to form cross-linked products.

In their study Chung et al. (Chung et al., 2004) have treated protein extracts from raw and roasted defatted peanut meals with POD in the presence of hydrogen. While POD treatment had no effect on raw peanuts, a significant cross-linking and decrease in the levels of the major allergens, Ara h 1 and Ara h 2, in roasted peanuts (Fig.7) was observed in imunoblots and IgE ELISA. The authors suppose that POD induced the cross-linking of mainly Ara h 1 and Ara h 2 from roasted peanuts and that, due to POD treatment, IgE binding was reduced.

Garcia et al. (Garcia et al., 2007) investigated effect of peroxidase and antioxidant diethyldithiocarbamic acid (DIECA) on IgE-binding by Mal d 1, the major apple allergen. In competitive ELISA IgE-binding by Mal d 1 decreased by adding peroxidase with more pronounced effect in presence of catechin. DIECA protected the IgE-binding by the allergen, protection being less strong in the presence of exogenous peroxidase (Fig 5).

Weangsripanaval et al. (Weangsripanaval et al., 2003) purified and characterized new allergenic protein from the tomato identified as suberization-associated anionic peroxidase 1. Furthermore, SanchezMonge et al. (SanchezMonge et al., 1997) purified and characterized allergenic protein from wheat flour identified as seed-specific peroxidase. These facts imply that peroxidases themselves can be allergens and safety for use them must be assessed.

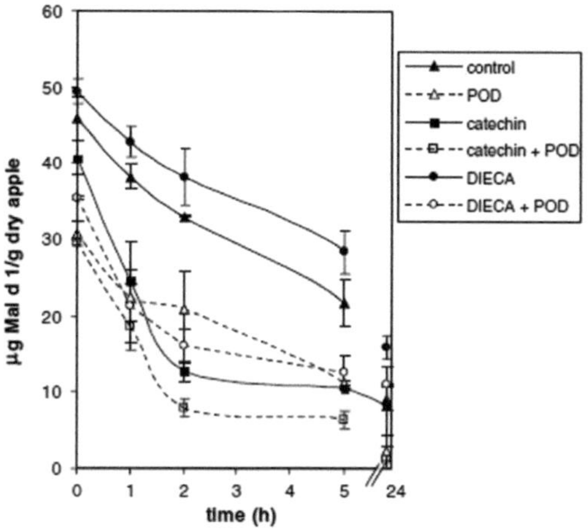

Fig. 5. Influence of the treatments performed on apple peel samples on Mal d 1 concentration determined by competitive ELISA using a pool of sera. The treatments consisted of: additional peroxidase (POD), additional substarte catechin, additional catechin combined with POD, additional diethyldithiocarbamic acid (DIECA) and additional DIECA combined with POD.T he incubation times were 0, 1, 2, 5, and 24 h at room temperature. Reprinted from (Garcia et al., 2007), Copyright (2007), with permission from Elsevier.

4.3 Phenol oxidases

4.3.1 Polyphenoloxidases (tyrosinases)

Polyphenol oxidases (PPO) or tyrosinases are bifunctional enzymes catalyzing o-hydroxylation of monophenols (including protein-bound tyrosine residues) to o-diphenols and subsequent oxidation of o-diphenols to o-quinones (Lerch, 1983). Reactive o-quinones can further undergo non-enzymatic polymerization or can react with amino acid residues in proteins.

In the study of Gruber et al. (Gruber et al., 2004) incubation of recombinant Pru av 1, major cherry allergen, with phenol compounds in the presence of tyrosinase led to decrease in IgE-binding activity of the protein as revealed by EAST and inhibition assays. Caffeic acid and epicatechin showed to be the most efficient in decreasing of rPru av 1 IgE-binding activity, followed by catechin and gallic acid, while quercetin and rutin were the least efficient. However, PPO without the addition of a phenolic compound did not display a reduction in IgE binding. The researchers speculated that, reactive intermediates formed during enzymatic polyphenol oxidation are responsible for modifying nucleophilic amino acid side chains of proteins, thus inducing an irreversible change in the tertiary structure of the protein and resulting in a loss of conformational epitopes of the allergen. In study of Chung et al. (Chung et al., 2005) peanut extracts were treated with and without PPO, PPO/caffeic and caffeic acid. All treatments resulted in cross-linking and decreased the levels and IgE binding (competitive inhibition ELISA) of two peanut major allergens, Ara h 1 and Ara h 2, with PPO/caffeic as the most effective (Fig.6).

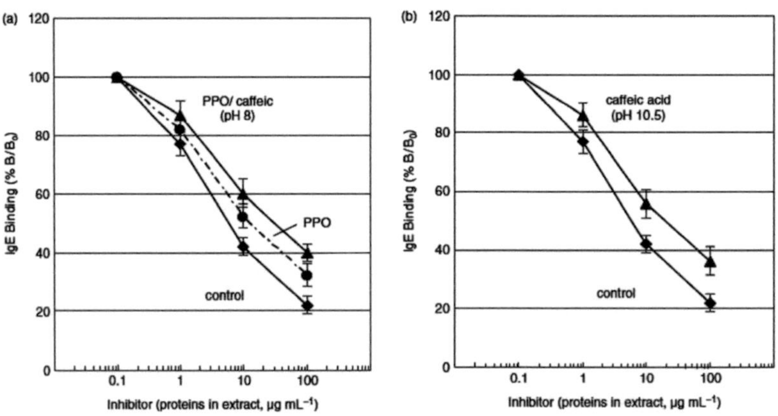

Fig. 6. Inhibition of IgE antibodies in a competitive inhibition ELISA by (a) PPO- and PPO/caffeic-treated extracts, pH 8, and (b) caffeic-treated extract, pH 10.5. Extracts, diluted at the concentration indicated, were each mixed with a pooled serum from peanut allergic individuals, and then added to an allergen-coated microtiter plate. Values are means ± SD (n = 3). Values of the treated samples at 1–100 µg mL^{-1} are significantly different from those of the control ($P < 0.05$, $n = 3$).Reprinted from (Chung et al., 2005), Copyright (2005), with permission from John Wiley and Sons.

In their further study Chung et al. (Chung & Champagne, 2008) treated peanut butter slurries with phenolic compounds/PPO and obtained reduction in IgE-binding, despite the formation of soluble allergen complexes or cross-links, for which authors assume that are less allergenic. Novotna et al. (Novotna et al., 2011) investigated effects of celery juice by oxidation by utilising its natural polyphenol oxidase (PPO) content on the reduction of the content of the Api g1, the main celery allergen. Oxidation failed to eliminate the allergenicity of pure celery juice, but oxidation in apple-celery juices reduced the allergenicity of the mixture. However, the basophil activation test showed no reduction in the allergic response to the oxidised juice mixture. Skin testing showed that the prolonged oxidation of juice mixture showed significantly lower reaction, while apple juice stabilised with ascorbic acid did not have effect. Due to the contradictory results in different tests, the method cannot be declared successful or safe, even for mixtures of apple-celery juices. In competitive ELISA Garcia et al. (Garcia et al., 2007) demonstrated decreased IgE binding of Mal d 1 after enrichment of apple extract with PPO, with the strongest effect in presence of catechin. Antioxidant DIECA protected the IgE-binding by the allergen, protection being less strong in the presence of exogenous PPO. Schmitz et al. (Schmitz-Eiberger & Matthes, 2011) evaluated relationship between Mal d 1, the main apple allergen, content and PPO, total phenol content and antioxidative capacity in different apple varietie. Whereas higher PPO activities and polyphenols contents result in less extractable Mal d 1, higher antioxidative activity can inhibit the interaction between oxidised phenols and Mal d 1, resulting in higher allergenicity (extractable Mal d 1). In the study of Monogioudi et al. (Monogioudi et al., 2011) β-casein was cross-linked of by tyrosinase and demonstrated that enzymatically cross-linked b-casein was stable under acidic conditions and was more resistant to pepsin digestion when compared to non cross-linked b-casein. In the study of Stanic et al. (Stanic et al., 2010) tyrosinase treated casein showed mitigated IgE binding reactivity, compared with the untreated CN, only in the presence of caffeic acid as mediator in BAT.

4.3.2 Laccases

Laccases catalyse oxidation of various phenolic compounds with one electron mechanism generating free radical species. Reactive free radicals can further undergo non-enzymatic polymerization or can react with high redox potential substrate targets, such as amino acid residues in proteins (Canfora et al., 2008).

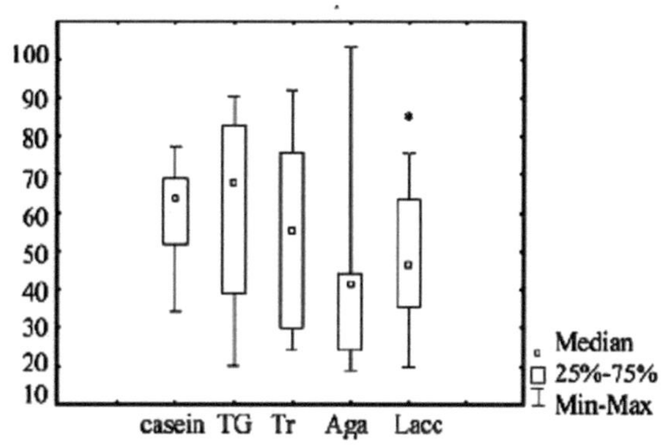

Fig. 7. Basophil activation to casein and crosslinked caseins in seven patients with CMA. $p<0.05$ was statistically significant difference in a Wilcoxon-maitched pairs test. Reprinted from (Stanic et al., 2009), Copyright (2009), with permission from John Wiley and Sons.

Tantoush et al. (Tantoush et al., 2011) cross-linked BLG by laccase in the presence of an sour cherry phenolics. In a BAT assay, the allergenicity of the cross-linked protein was shown to decrease in all nine cow's milk-allergic patients, while digestibility of the remaining monomeric BLG in simulated conditions of the gastrointestinal tract increased. In the further study of Tantoush et al. (Tantoush et al., 2011) cross-linking BLG by laccase in the presence of apple phenolics (APE) rendered the protein insoluble in the reaction mixture consisting of cross-linked BLG, with a fraction of the BLG remaining monomeric. Enzymatic processing of BLG decrease the bi-phasal pepsin–pancreatin digestibility of the monomeric and cross-linked protein, thus decreasing its nutritional value. Stanic et al. (Stanic et al., 2010) crosslinked β-casein (CN) by laccase and caffeic acid and demonstrated that crosslinking was not very efficient, leaving mostly monomeric CN modified by caffeic acid. Regardless to that ability of crosslinked CNs to activate basophils was significantly reduced in seven

patients and reduced inhibition potential is possibly due to hindering of epitopes by monomer modification. Also, digestion of crosslinked CN by pepsin was hampered.
As enzyme preparations used in food technology are food grade, but often not of the highest purity, they can contain contaminating enzyme activities. These so-called ''side activities'' even if present only in trace quantities, can have unpredictable influence on functional properties, nutritional quality and safety of food implying that effects of contaminating enzymes in used enzyme preparations should be carefully monitored. Stanic et al. (Stanic et al., 2009) found out that in the presence of high purity commercial laccase and tyrosinase preparations, both variants of BLG (A and B) underwent removal of a peptide from the N-terminus. The truncated forms were more susceptible to digestion by pepsin and thus with lower allergenic potential.

5. Conclusion

In development of new methods for food allergen modification there are two main applications. First one, and the most frequent, is creation of hypoallergic food and food additives, and the second one is preparation of formulations for safe immunotherapy of food allergies. In addition to the main aim, reduction of allergenicity, there are several other requirements that must be satisfied for certain application. For both applications safety is obligatory, implicating usage of minimal toxic and nonalleregnic agents, including the main and auxiliary one. Preferred reagents used for allergen modification are those acceptable for the production of foodstuffs or pharmaceuticals. In that sense, recent researches are more focused on usage of enzymes as modification agents, as well as compounds naturally occurring in food. Also, all products of modification reaction, not only modified allergen, must be safe or successfully eliminated/degraded in further processing and expenses of method have to be reasonable. For food industry desirable physico-chemical properties of modified proteins are important as they determine technological properties such as solubility, pH stability, gelling, foaming, emulsifying properties etc., as well as nutritional value and impact on taste and flavor. Allergen modifications, although efficient in reducing allergenicity, do not bare potential for application in food industry if mentioned properties are significantly disturbed, as for food industry the most important is consumer`s acceptance of certain food (texture, taste, stability, natural origin, etc.). Typical example are extensive protein hydrolysates, although highly hypoallergenic, having bitter taste, which is difficult to mask, and high osmolarity. For immunotherapy preparations, in addition to reduced/eliminated allergenicity and preserved immunogenicity, immunomodulatory properties are highly desirable for increasing immunotherapy efficiency. Also, physico-chemical properties of modified proteins define their stability, such as susceptibility for proteolysis and heat denaturation.
There is numerous studies focusing on modification of food protein as new properties enable design of more different food products and exploitation of cheap high nutritional food sources. Many of methods for reducing food protein allergenicity emerged from these studies, as evidenced by in parallel investigation of techno-functional properties and allergenicity testing in some publications. Reducing of allergenic properties by chemical or enzymatic methods was demonstrated on full extract, raw or pretreated, or on isolated allergens from peanut, wheat, whey, soy, pea and cherry. The most frequently modified food allergens are BLG and ovalbumin. BLG was interesting due to its high nutritional value, important functional properties and its availability as by-product cheese industry.

Ovalbumin was the most frequently used as a model allergen in studies using animal models.

As reducing of alleregenicity can be achieved by removal of epitopes, destruction of epitopes, and by their masking, knowledge of the structural aspects of allergenicity and of the factors that determine epitope integrity will lead to novel and more specific approaches to decrease allergenicity. By treatment with chemical or enzyme agent only few amino acid residues of allergen react, such as residues of lysine, arginine, cystein, tyrosine. Therefore, epitope containing these residues are expected to be changed/masked in significant extent and knowing the epitope structure can help in prediction which method would be the most successful. In addition to B cell epitope changes, changes in T cell eptopes can significantly contribute reduction of allergic response as well. T cells provide help to B cells, by direct interaction and secretion of cytokines, and promote their proliferation and differentiation into antibody producing cells (Kaminogava, 1996). Therefore, during allergen modification formation of bonds non-hydrolisabile by processing machinery in APC, can change T cell epitope profiles of allergens and have influence on direction of immune response, potentiating allergy or tolerance.

It seems that the most effective approach for allergen modification is combination of two or more methods acting by different mechanisms, such as combination of acylation and proteolysis (Szymkiewicz & Jedrychowski, 2008), reduction, alkylation and cross-linking (Koppelman et al., 2010), cross-linking and reduction (Villas-Boas et al., 2010), proteolysis and cross-linking (Wroblewska et al., 2008). Covalent modification of allergens by edible high molecular mass polysaccharides is effective and acceptable way for designing hypoallergic food formulatios offering also improved techno-functional properties. However, low immugenicity of modifications limits this method for creation of effective immunotherapy preparations.

Of all applied cross-linking enzymes it seems that transglutaminase is the least efficient in reducing protein allergenicity, and only when it is combined with allergen reduction or in the presence of co-substrate or with proteolysis. Although for the efficiency of peroxidase there are only sparse data, food allergen cross-linking with phenol oxidases (tyrosinases, laccases) with assistance of small phenolic compounds have great potential. It looks like that protein cross-linking itself is not enough for significant masking IgE epitopes and that phenolic mediators contribute by modification of the nucleophilic surface residues in the protein and the hindering of the epitopes by their covalent attachment in a highly aggregated product, as well as to monomer allergen. Also, it seems that cross-linked allergens are more resistant to digestion then their monomeric form. It is well known that proteins resistant to both gastric and intestinal digestion are not allergenic. The data from animal models show that both gastric and intestinal-resistant allergens do not carry strong food-allergy risk or induce oral tolerance, simply because both food-allergy and oral-tolerance are MHC class II-dependent processes and require antigen presentation to the immune system i.e. readily available peptides in intestinal fluids (Bowman & Selgrade, 2008).

For the most methods mentioned in this review exhaustive studies on human subjects, including DBPCFC tests, are needed in order to design food with label hypoallergenic. As substantial part of the population reacts to very low amounts of allergens, residual unmodified allergen that remain after modification can still bind IgE and elicit symptoms in highly sensitive patients (Wensing et al., 2002). Also some modifications may be clinically relevant for some allergic individuals but not for others. The method for allergen modification applied to food source, such as wheat, peanut, soy flour or WPI, may change different allergens to a different extent. Therefore, methods enabling a reduction of allergenicity of all proteins should be used or different types of modification should be applied simultaneously.

In the future further and more fundamental researches in this multidisciplinary field is necessary in order to develop novel hypoallergenic foods and food additives on one hand, and to obtain suitable preparations enabling safe and efficient food allergen-specific immunotherapy in clinical practice on the other hand.

6. Acknowledgment

This study was supported by the grant No. 172024 obtained from the Ministry of Education and Science of the Republic of Serbia and FP7 project FCUB ERA, GA No. 256716.

7. References

Akita, E. M. & Nakai, S. (1990). Lipophilization of β-lactoglobulin: effect on allergenicity and digestibility. *Journal of Food Science,* Vol. 55 No. 3, (May 1990), pp. 718-723, ISSN 1750-3841

Aoki, T., Iskandar, S., Yoshida, T., Takahashi, K., & Hattori, M. (2006). Reduced immunogenicity of beta-lactoglobulin by conjugating with chitosan. *Bioscience, biotechnology and biochemistry,*Vol.70, No.10, (October 2006), pp 2349-2356, ISSN 0916-8451 (Print), 0916-8451 (Linking)

Babakhin, A. A., DuBuske, L. M., Wheeler, A. W., Stockinger, B., Nolte, H., Andreev, S. M., et al. (1995). Immunological properties of allergen chemically modified with synthetic copolymer of N-vinylpyrrolidone and maleic anhydride. *Allergy Proccedings,* Vol. 16, No. 5, (September 1995), pp 261-268, ISSN 1046-9354 (Print), 1046-9354 (Linking)

Babiker, E. E., Hiroyuki, A., Matsudomi, N., Iwata, H., Ogawa, T., Bando, N., et al. (1998). Effect of polysaccharide conjugation or transglutaminase treatment on the allergenicity and functional properties of soy protein. *Journal of Agricultural and Food Chemistry,* Vol. 46, No. 3, (March 1998), pp 866-871, ISSN 0021-8561

Becker, W. M. (1997). Characterization of Ara h 1 by two-dimensional electrophoresis immunoblot and recombinant techniques: new digestion experiments with peanuts imitating the gastrointestinal tract. *International Archives of Allergy and Immunology,* Vol. 113, No. 1-3, (May 1997), pp 118-121, ISSN 1018-2438 (Print), 1018-2438 (Linking)

Besler, M., Steinhart, H., & Paschke, A. (2001). Stability of food allergens and allergenicity of processed foods. *Journal of Chromatography B: Biomedical Sciences and Applications,* Vol. 756, No. 1-2, (May 2001), pp 207-228, ISSN 1387-2273

Bousquet, J., Lockey, R., & Malling, H. J. (1998). Allergen immunotherapy: therapeutic vaccines for allergic diseases. A WHO position paper. *Journal of Allergy and Clinical Immunology,* Vol. 102, No. 4 Pt 1, (October 1998), pp 558-562, ISSN

Bowman, C.C., Selgrade, M.J.K. 2008. (2008). Failure to induce oral tolerance in mice is predictive of dietary allergenic potency among foods with sensitizing capacity *Toxicological Sciences,* Vol. 106, No.2, (December 2008), pp 435, ISSN 1096-6080

Buchanan, B. B., Adamidi, C., Lozano, R. M., Yee, B. C., Momma, M., Kobrehel, K., et al. (1997). Thioredoxin-linked mitigation of allergic responses to wheat. *Proceedings of the National Academy of Sciences of the United States of America,* Vol. 94, No. 10, (May 1997), pp 5372-5377, ISSN 0027-8424 (Print), 0027-8424 (Linking)

Buchert, J., Selinheimo, E., Kruus, K., Mattinen, M.L., Lantto, R. & Autio, K. (2007). Using crosslinking enzymes to improve textural and other properties of food, In: Novel enzyme technology for food applications, Rastall, R. (Ed.), pp 101 - 139, Woodhead Publishing Limited, ISBN 1 84569 132 6, Cambridge, UK

Canfora, L., Iamarino, G., Rao, M. A., & Gianfreda, L. (2008). Oxidative transformation of natural and synthetic phenolic mixtures by Trametes versicolor laccase. *Journal of Agricultural and Food Chemistry, Vol.* 56, No.4, (February 2008), pp 1398-1407, ISSN 0021-8561 (Print), 0021-8561 (Linking)

Chung, S., & Champagne, E. T. (2006). Effect of phytic acid on IgE binding to peanut allergens. *Journal of Allergy and Clinical Immunology,* Vol. 117, No. 2, (February 2006), pp S38-S38, ISSN 0091-6749

Chung, S.Y., Kato, Y. & Champagne, E.T. (2007). Reducing the allergenic properties of peanut allergens by copper/hydrogen peroxide, In: Recent progress in medicinal plants, Vol.15, V.K.Singh, J.N.Govil, Khalil Ahmad, Rajeev Kr.Sharma, (Ed.), pp 443-453, Studium Press (India) Pvt. Ltd. , ISBN 9780976184973, India

Chung, S., & Champagne, E. T. (2008). Using phenolic compounds to reduce the allergenic properties of peanut extracts and peanut butter slurries. *Journal of Allergy and Clinical Immunology,* Vol. 121, No. 2, (February 2008), pp S249-S249, ISSN 0091-6749

Chung, S. Y., & Champagne, E. T. (2007). Effects of Phytic acid on peanut allergens and allergenic properties of extracts. *Journal of Agricultural and Food Chemistry,* Vol. 55, No. 22, (October 2007), pp 9054-9058, ISSN 0021-8561

Chung, S. Y., & Champagne, E. T. (2009). Reducing the allergenic capacity of peanut extracts and liquid peanut butter by phenolic compounds. *Food Chemistry,* Vol. 115, No. 4, (August 2009), pp 1345-1349, ISSN 0308-8146

Chung, S. Y., Kato, Y., & Champagne, E. T. (2005). Polyphenol oxidase/caffeic acid may reduce the allergenic properties of peanut allergens. *Journal of the Science of Food and Agriculture,* Vol. 85, No. 15, (December 2005), pp 2631-2637, ISSN 0022-5142

Chung, S. Y., Maleki, S. J., & Champagne, E. T. (2004). Allergenic properties of roasted peanut allergens may be reduced by peroxidase. *Journal of Agricultural and Food Chemistry,* Vol. 52, No. 14, (July 2004), pp 4541-4545, ISSN 0021-8561

Cirkovic Velickovic, T., Radosavljevic, J., & Stanic, D. (2009). Digestibility of food allergens. *CAB Reviews: Perspectives in Agriculture, Veterinary Science, Nutrition and Natural Resources,* Vol. 4, No. 034, pp 1–17, ISSN 1749-8848 (Linking), Available form: http://www.cababstractsplus.org/cabreviews

Clare, D. A., Gharst, G., Maleki, S. J., & Sanders, T. H. (2008). Effects of transglutaminase catalysis on the functional and immunoglobulin binding properties of peanut flour dispersions containing casein. *Journal of Agricultural and Food Chemistry,* Vol. 56, No. 22, (November 2008), pp 10913-10921, ISSN 1520-5118 (Electronic), 0021-8561 (Linking)

Clare, D. A., Gharst, G., & Sanders, T. H. (2007). Transglutaminase polymerization of peanut proteins. *Journal of Agricultural and Food Chemistry,* Vol. 55, No. 2, (January 2007), pp 432-438, ISSN 0021-8561 (Print), 0021-8561 (Linking)

del Val, G., Yee, B. C., Lozano, R. M., Buchanan, B. B., Ermel, R. W., Lee, Y. M., et al. (1999). Thioredoxin treatment increases digestibility and lowers allergenicity of milk. *Journal of Allergy and Clinical Immunology,* Vol. 103, No. 4, (April 1999), pp 690-697, ISSN 0091-6749

Doke, S., Nakamura, R. & Torii S. (1989). Allergenicity of Food Proteins Interacted with Oxidized Lipids in Soybean-Sensitive Individuals. *Agricultural and Biological Chemistry,* Vol. 53, No. 5, (May 1989), pp 1231-1235, ISSN 0002-1369

Durham, S. R., Walker, S. M., Varga, E. M., Jacobson, M. R., O'Brien, F., Noble, W., et al. (1999). Long-term clinical efficacy of grass-pollen immunotherapy. *New England Journal of Medicine,* Vol. *341,* No. 7, (August 1999), pp 468-475, ISSN 0028-4793

Fleischer, D. M., Byrne, A. M., Malka-Rais, J., & Burks, A. W. (2010). How do we know when peanut and tree nut allergy have resolved, and how do we keep it resolved? *Clinical and Experimental Allergy,* Vol. 40, No. 9, (September 2010), pp 1303-1311, ISSN 0954-7894

Garcia, A., Wichers, J. H., & Wichers, H. J. (2007). Decrease of the IgE-binding by Mal d 1, the major apple allergen, by means of polyphenol oxidase and peroxidase treatments. *Food Chemistry,* Vol. 103, No. 1, (October 2006), pp 94-100, ISSN 0308-8146

Glaser, A. G., Menz, G., Kirsch, A. I., Zeller, S., Crameri, R., & Rhyner, C. (2008). Auto- and cross-reactivity to thioredoxin allergens in allergic bronchopulmonary aspergillosis. *Allergy,* Vol. 63, No. 12, (December 2008), pp 1617-1623, ISSN 0105-4538

Gruber, P., Vieths, S., Wangorsch, A., Nerkamp, J., & Hofmann, T. (2004). Maillard reaction and enzymatic browning affect the allergenicity of Pru av 1, the major allergen from cherry (Prunus avium). *Journal of Agricultural and Food Chemistry,* Vol. *52,* No. 12, (June 2004), pp 4002-4007, ISSN 0021-8561

Gupta, R. S., Kim, J. S., Barnathan, J. A., Amsden, L. B., Tummala, L. S., & Holl, J. L. (2008). Food allergy knowledge, attitudes and beliefs: focus groups of parents, physicians and the general public. *BMC Pediatrics,* Vol. 8, No. 1, (September 2008), pp 36-46, ISSN 1471-2431 (Electronic), 1471-2431 (Linking)

Hattori, M., Miyakawa, S., Ohama, Y., Kawamura, H., Yoshida, T., To-o, K., et al. (2004). Reduced immunogenicity of beta-lactoglobulin by conjugation with acidic oligosaccharides. *Journal of Agricultural and Food Chemistry,* Vol. 52, No. 14, (July 2004), pp 4546-4553, ISSN 0021-8561 (Print), 0021-8561 (Linking)

Hattori, M., Nagasawa, K., Ohgata, K., Sone, N., Fukuda, A., Matsuda, H., et al. (2000). Reduced immunogenicity of beta-lactoglobulin by conjugation with carboxymethyl dextran. *Bioconjugate Chemistry,* Vol. *11,* No. 1, (January 2000), pp 84-93, ISSN 1043-1802 (Print), 1043-1802 (Linking)

Holdsworth, S. (1985). Optimisation of thermal processing—a review. *Journal of Food Engeenering,* Vol. 4, No. 2, (September 1985), pp 89–116, ISSN 0260-8774

Jobstl, E., Howse, J. R., Fairclough, J. P. A., & Williamson, M. P. (2006). Noncovalent cross-linking of casein by epigallocatechin gallate characterized by single molecule force microscopy. *Journal of Agricultural and Food Chemistry,* Vol. 54, No. 12, (Jun 2006), pp 4077-4081, ISSN 0021-8561

Kaminogawa, S. (1996). Food allergy, oral tolerance and immunomodulation--their molecular and cellular mechanisms. *Bioscience, Biotechnology and Biochemistry,* Vol.

60, No. 11, (November 1996), pp 1749-1756, ISSN 0916-8451 (Print), 0916-8451 (Linking)

Kobayashi, K., Hirano, A., Ohta, A., Yoshida, T., Takahashi, K., & Hattori, M. (2001). Reduced immunogenicity of beta-lactoglobulin by conjugation with carboxymethyl dextran differing in molecular weight. *Journal of Agricultural and Food Chemistry,* Vol. 49, No. 2, (February 2001), pp 823-83, ISSN 0021-8561 (Print), 0021-8561 (Linking)

Kobayashi, K., Yoshida, T., Takahashi, K., & Hattori, M. (2003). Modulation of the T cell response to beta-lactoglobulin by conjugation with carboxymethyl dextran. *Bioconjugate Chemistry,* Vol. 14, No. 1, (January 2003), pp 168-176, ISSN 1043-1802 (Print), 1043-1802 (Linking)

Koppelman, S. J. (2007). Immunotherapy for food allergy by reduced and alkylated food allergens, 2007, Patent Number US20070190069

Koppelman, S. J., Van Den, H. R. H. J. A., Sleijster-selis, H. E. & Luijkx, D. M. A. M. (2010). Modification of allergens, 2010, Patent Number US20100086568

Lerch, K. (1983). Neurospora tyrosinase: structural, spectroscopic and catalytic properties. *Molecular and Cellular Biochemistry,* Vol. 52, No. 2, (January 1983), pp 125-138, ISSN 0300-8177 (Print), 0300-8177 (Linking)

Leszczynska, J., Lacka, A., & Bryszewska, M. (2006). The use of transglutaminase in the reduction of immunoreactivity of wheat flour. *Food and Agricultural Immunology,* Vol. 17, No. 2, (February 2006), pp 105-113, ISSN 0954-0105

Malandain, H. (2005). Transglutaminases: a meeting point for wheat allergy, celiac disease, and food safety. *European annals of allergy and clinical immunology,* Vol. 37, No. 10, (December 2005), pp 397-403, ISSN 1764-1489 (Print),1764-1489 (Linking)

Mills, E. N., Mackie, A. R., Burney, P., Beyer, K., Frewer, L., Madsen, C., et al. (2007). The prevalence, cost and basis of food allergy across Europe. *Allergy,* Vol. *62,* No. 7, (July 2007), pp (717-722), ISSN 0105-4538 (Print), 0105-4538 (Linking)

Mistrello, G., Brenna, O., Roncarolo, D., Zanoni, D., Gentili, M., & Falagiani, P. (1996). Monomeric chemically modified allergens: immunologic and physicochemical characterization. *Allergy,* Vol. *51,* No. 1, (January 2006), pp (8-15), ISSN 0105-4538 (Print), 0105-4538 (Linking)

Monogioudi, E., Faccio, G., Lille, M., Poutanen, K., Buchert, J., & Mattinen, M. L. (2011). Effect of enzymatic cross-linking of beta-casein on proteolysis by pepsin. *Food Hydrocolloids,* Vol. 25, No.1, (January 2011), pp 71-81, ISSN 0268-005X

Moreno, F. J. (2007). Gastrointestinal digestion of food allergens: effect on their allergenicity. *Biomedicine and Pharmacotherapy,* Vol. 61, No. 1, (January 2007), pp 50-60, ISSN 0753-3322 (Print)

Mouecoucou, J., Fremont, S., Sanchez, C., Villaume, C., & Mejean, L. (2004). In vitro allergenicity of peanut after hydrolysis in the presence of polysaccharides. *Clinical and Experimental Allergy,* Vol. 34, No.9, (September 2004), pp 1429-1437, ISSN 0954-7894 (Print), 0954-7894 (Linking)

Nelson, H. S., Lahr, J., Rule, R., Bock, A., & Leung, D. (1997). Treatment of anaphylactic sensitivity to peanuts by immunotherapy with injections of aqueous peanut extract. *J Allergy Clin Immunol,* Vol. 99, No. 6 Pt 1, (Jun 1997), pp 744-751, ISSN 0091-6749 (Print), 0091-6749 (Linking)

Nodake, Y., Fukumoto, S., Fukasawa, M., Sakakibara, R., & Yamasaki, N. (2010). Reduction of the immunogenicity of beta-lactoglobulin from cow's milk by conjugation with a dextran derivative. *Bioscience, biotechnology and biochemistry,* Vol. 74, No. 4, (April 2010), pp 721-726, ISSN 1347-6947 (Electronic), 0916-8451 (Linking)

Nodake, Y., Fukumoto, S., Fukasawa, M., Yamasaki, N., & Sakakibara, R. (2011). Preparation and immunological characterization of beta-lactoglobulin-amylose conjugate. *Bioscience, biotechnology and biochemistry,* Vol. 75, No. 1, (January 2011), pp (165-167), ISSN 1347-6947 (Electronic), 0916-8451 (Linking)

Novotna, P., Setinova, I., Heroldova, M., Kminkova, M., Pruchova, J., Strohalm, J., et al. (2011). Deallergisation Trials of Pure Celery Juice and Apple-Celery Juice Mixture by Oxidation. *Czech Journal of Food Sciences,* Vol. 29, No. 2, (February 2011), pp 190-200, ISSN 1212-1800

Ofori-Anti, A. O., Ariyarathna, H., Chen, L., Lee, H. L., Pramod, S. N., & Goodman, R. E. (2008). Establishing objective detection limits for the pepsin digestion assay used in the assessment of genetically modified foods. *Regulatory toxicology and pharmacology,* Vol. 52, No. 2, (November 2008), pp (94-103), ISSN 1096-0295 (Electronic)

Palosuo, K., Varjonen, E., Nurkkala, J., Kalkkinen, N., Harvima, R., Reunala, T., et al. (2003). Transglutaminase-mediated cross-linking of a peptic fraction of omega-5 gliadin enhances IgE reactivity in wheat-dependent, exercise-induced anaphylaxis. *Journal of Allergy and Clinical Immunology,* Vol. 111, No. 6, (Jun 2003), pp 1386-1392, ISSN 0091-6749

Patterson, R., Suszko, I. M., Bacal, E., Zeiss, C. R., Kelly, J. F., & Pruzansky, J. J. (1979). Reduced allergenicity of high molecular weight ragweed polymers. *The Journal of Allergy and Clinical Immunology,* Vol. 63, No. 1, (January 1979), pp 47-50, ISSN 0091-6749 (Print), 0091-6749 (Linking)

Pedersen, M. H., Hansen, T. K., Sten, E., Seguro, K., Ohtsuka, T., Morita, A., et al. (2004). Evaluation of the potential allergenicity of the enzyme microbial transglutaminase using the 2001 FAO/WHO Decision Tree. *Molecular Nutrition and Food Research,* Vol. 48, No. 6, (November 2004), pp 434-440, ISSN 1613-4125

Polovic, N., Blanusa, M., Gavrovic-Jankulovic, M., Atanaskovic-Markovic, M., Burazer, L., Jankov, R., et al. (2007). A matrix effect in pectin-rich fruits hampers digestion of allergen by pepsin in vivo and in vitro. *Clinical and Experimental Allergy,* Vol. 37, No. 5, (May 2007), pp 764-771, ISSN 0954-7894 (Print), 0954-7894 (Linking)

Polovic, N., Obradovic, A., Spasic, M., Plecas-Solarovic, B., Gavrovic-Jankulovic, M. & Cirkovic Velickovic, T. (2010). In Vivo Digestion of a Thaumatin-Like Kiwifruit Protein in Rats. *Food digestion,* Vol. 1, No. 1-2, (February 2010), pp 5-13, ISSN 1869-1986

Poulsen, L. K. (2001). In vivo and in vitro techniques to determine the biological activity of food allergens. *Journal of Chromatography B,* Vol. 756, No. 1-2, (May 2001), pp 41-55, ISSN 0378-4347

Sampson, H. A. (1999). Food allergy. Part 2: Diagnosis and management. *Journal of Allergy and Clinical Immunology,* Vol. *103,* No. 6, (January 1999), pp 981-989, ISSN 0091-6749

SanchezMonge, R., GarciaCasado, G., LopezOtin, C., Armentia, A., & Salcedo, G. (1997). Wheat flour peroxidase is a prominent allergen associated with baker's asthma.

Clinical and Experimental Allergy, Vol. 27, No. 10, (October 1997), pp 1130-1137, ISSN 0954-7894

Schmitz-Eiberger, M., & Matthes, A. (2011). Effect of harvest maturity, duration of storage and shelf life of apples on the allergen Mal d 1, polyphenoloxidase activity and polyphenol content. *Food Chemistry,* Vol. 127, No. 4, (August 2011), pp 1459-1464, ISSN 0308-8146

Shriver, S. K., & Yang, W. W. (2011). Thermal and Nonthermal Methods for Food Allergen Control. *Food Engineering Reviews,* Vol. 3, No. 1, (March 2011), pp 26-43, ISSN 1866-7910

Skripak, J. M., Nash, S. D., Brereton, N. H., Rowley, H., Oh, S., Hamilton, R. G., et al. (2008). A randomized, double-blind, placebo-controlled (DBPC) study of milk oral immunotherapy (MOIT) for cow's milk allergy (CMA). *Journal of Allergy and Clinical Immunology,* Vol. 121, No. 2, (February 2008), pp S137-S137, ISSN 0091-6749

Soler-Rivas, C., & Wichers, H. J. (2001). Impact of (bio)chemical and physical procedures on food allergen stability. *Allergy,* Vol. 56, No. Suppl 67, (April 2001), pp 52-55, ISBN 0105-4538 (Print), 0105-4538 (Linking)

Stanic, D., Radosavljevic, J., Polovic, N., Jadranin, M., Popovic, M., Vuckovic, O., Burazer, L., Jankov, R. and Cirkovic Velickovic, T. (2009). Removal of N-terminal peptides from beta-lactoglobulin by proteolytic contaminants in a commercial phenol oxidase preparation. *International Dairy Journal,* Vol. 19, No. 12, (December 2009), pp 746-752, ISSN 0958-6946

Stanic, D., Monogioudi, E., Dilek, E., Radosavljevic, J., Atanaskovic-Markovic, M., Vuckovic, O., Lannto, R., Mattinen, M., Buchert, J. and Cirkovic Velickovic, T. (2010). Digestibility and allergenicity assessment of enzymatically crosslinked beta-casein. *Molecular Nutrition and Food Research,* Vol. 54, No. 9, (September 2010), pp 1273-1284, ISSN 1613-4125

Szymkiewicz, A. & Jędrychowski L. (2005). Reduction of immunoreactive properties of pea globulins as the result of enzymatic modification. *Acta Alimentaria,* Vol. 34, No.3, (March 2005), pp 295–306, ISSN 0139-3006

Szymkiewicz, A. & Jędrychowski L. (2008). Effect of acylation and enzymatic modification on pea proteins allergenicity. *Polish Journal of Food and Nutrition Sciences,* Vol. 58, No. 3, pp. 345-350, ISSN 1230-0322.

Szymkiewicz, A., & Jedrychowski, L. (2009). Immunoreactivity of Acetylated and Succinylated Pea Proteins. *Acta Alimentaria,* Vol. 38, No. 3, (September 2009), pp 329-339, ISSN 0139-3006

Tantoush, Z., Stanic, D., Stojadinovic, M., Ognjenovic, J., Mihajlovic, L., Atanaskovic-Markovic, M., et al. (2011). Digestibility and allergenicity of beta-lactoglobulin following laccase-mediated cross-linking in the presence of sour cherry phenolics. *Food Chemistry,* Vol. 125, No. 1, pp 84-91, ISSN 0308-8146

Tantoush, Z., Mihajlovic, L., Kravic, B., Ognjenovic, J., Jankov, R. M., Cirkovic Velickovic, T. & Stanic-Vucinic, D. (2011). Digestibility of β-lactoglobulin following cross-linking by *Trametes versicolor* laccase and apple polyphenols . *Journal of Serbian Chemical Society,* Vol. 76, No. 6, (June 2011), pp 847–855, ISSN 0352-5139

Taylor, S. L., & Lehrer, S. B. (1996). Principles and characteristics of food allergens. *Critical Reviews in Food Science and Nutrition,* Vol. 36 Suppl, pp S91-118, ISSN 1040-8398 (Print), 1040-8398 (Linking)

Thomas, K., Herouet-Guicheney, C., Ladics, G., McClain, S., MacIntosh, S., Privalle, L., et al. (2008). Current and future methods for evaluating the allergenic potential of proteins: international workshop report 23-25 October 2007. *Food Chemistry and Toxicology,* Vol. 46, No. 9, (September 2008), pp 3219-3225, ISSN 0278-6915 (Print)

Thompson, T., Kane, R. R., & Hager, M. H. (2006). Food Allergen Labeling and Consumer Protection Act of 2004 in effect. *Journal of the American Dietetic Association,* Vol. 106, No. 11, (November 2006), pp 1742-1744, ISSN 0002-8223 (Print), 0002-8223 (Linking)

Untersmayr, E., Diesner, S. C., Oostingh, G. J., Selzle, K., Pfaller, T., Schultz, C., et al. (2010). Nitration of the egg-allergen ovalbumin enhances protein allergenicity but reduces the risk for oral sensitization in a murine model of food allergy. *PLoS One,* Vol. 5, No. 12, (December 2010), pp e14210, ISSN 1932-6203 (Electronic), 1932-6203 (Linking)

Untersmayr, E., & Jensen-Jarolim, E. (2008). The role of protein digestibility and antacids on food allergy outcomes. *The Journal of Allergy and Clinical Immunology,* Vol. 121, No. 6, (Jun 2008), pp 1301-1308, ISSN 1097-6825 (Electronic), 0091-6749 (Linking)

Villas-Boas, M. B., Vieira, K. P., Trevizan, G., Zollner, R. D., & Netto, F. M. (2010). The effect of transglutaminase-induced polymerization in the presence of cysteine on beta-lactoglobulin antigenicity. *International Dairy Journal,* Vol. 20, No.6, (Jun 2010), pp 386-392, ISSN 0958-6946

Weangsripanaval, T., Nomura, N., Moriyama, T., Ohta, N., & Ogawa, T. (2003). Identification of suberization-associated anionic peroxidase as a possible allergenic protein from tomato. *Bioscience Biotechnology and Biochemistry,* Vol. 67, No. 6, (Jun 2003), pp 1299-1304, ISSN 0916-8451

Wensing, M., Penninks, A. H., Hefle, S. L., Koppelman, S. J., Bruijnzeel-Koomen, C. A., & Knulst, A. C. (2002). The distribution of individual threshold doses eliciting allergic reactions in a population with peanut allergy. *The Journal of Allergy and Clinical Immunology,* Vol. 110, No. 6, (December 2002), pp 915-920, ISSN 0091-6749 (Print), 0091-6749 (Linking)

Wroblewska, B., Jedrychowski, L., Hajos, G., & Szabo, E. (2008). Influence of Alcalase and transglutaminase on immunoreactivity of cow milk whey proteins. *Czech Journal of Food Sciences,* Vol. 26, No. 1, (January 2008), pp 15-23, ISSN 1212-1800

Wurtzen, P. A., Lund, L., Lund, G., Holm, J., Millner, A., & Henmar, H. (2007). Chemical modification of birch allergen extract leads to a reduction in allergenicity as well as immunogenicity. *International Archives of Allergy and Immunology,* Vol. 144, No. 4, (February 2007), pp 287-295, ISSN 0091-6749

Yang, X., Gieni, R. S., Mosmann, T. R., & HayGlass, K. T. (1993). Chemically modified antigen preferentially elicits induction of Th1-like cytokine synthesis patterns in vivo. *Journal of Experimental Medicine,* Vol. 178, No. 1, (July 2007), pp (349-353), ISSN 0022-1007 (Print), 0022-1007 (Linking)

Yoshida, T., Sasahara, Y., Miyakawa, S., & Hattori, M. (2005). Reduced T cell response to beta-lactoglobulin by conjugation with acidic oligosaccharides. *Journal of Agricultural and Food Chemistry,* Vol. 53, No. 17, (August 2005), pp 6851-6857, ISSN 0021-8561

5

Characterization of Seafood Proteins Causing Allergic Diseases

Anas M. Abdel Rahman[1], Robert J. Helleur[2],
Mohamed F. Jeebhay[3] and Andreas L. Lopata[4]
[1]*Samuel Lunenfeld Research Institute, Mount Sinai Hospital, Toronto, ON,*
[2]*Department of Chemistry, Memorial University of Newfoundland, St. John's, NL*
[3]*Centre for Occupational and Environmental Health Research, University of Cape Town*
[4]*School of Pharmacy and Molecular Science, James Cook University*
[1,2]*Canada*
[3]*South Africa*
[4]*Australia*

1. Introduction

Food allergy is increasing at a faster rate than any other allergic disorder (Gupta et al., 2007). In the last few decades, a large movement toward healthier eating makes seafood one of the major foods consumed worldwide (Wild & Lehrer, 2005). Consequently, the international trade of seafood has been growing rapidly, which reflects the popularity and frequency of consumption worldwide. The United States has become the third largest consumer of seafood in the world, with 1.86 billion kg of crustaceans in 2007 (6.04 kg/capita/year)(Food and Agriculture Organisation, 2007). Since seafood ingestion can cause severe acute hypersensitivity reactions and is recognized as one of the most common food allergies, the increased production and consumption of seafood has resulted in more frequent health problems (Lopata & Lehrer, 2009; Lopata et al., 2010). Exposure to seafood can cause a variety of health problems, including gastrointestinal disorders, urticaria, immunoglobulin E (IgE)-mediated asthma and anaphylaxis (Bang et al., 2005; Lopata & Lehrer, 2009; Malo & Cartier, 1993; Sicherer et al., 2004; Wild & Lehrer, 2005).

A true allergy is known as type-one hypersensitivity that activates the human mast cells, a type of white blood cells, producing an IgE response as seen in Fig. 1. This activation releases histamine and other inflammatory mediators such as cytokines. These immunological activities result in different allergenic symptoms such as itchiness, dyspnea, and anaphylaxis. High-molecular mass proteins seem to be the cause of chronic dermatitis (Greenberg et al., 2003).

Allergic reactions are directed to two major groups: fish and shellfish. Shellfish includes crustaceans and mollusks. Fish is subdivided into bony fish and cartilaginous fish (sharks and rays), whereas most edible species belong to bony fish such as cod and carp (see Table1) (Lopata & Lehrer, 2009).

Phylum	Class	Family species (common name)
Arthropoda	Gastropoda	Crabs, lobsters, prawns, shrimp, scampi, shrimpmeal
Mollusca	Gastropoda	Ablone
	Bivalvia	Clams, oysters, mussels, scallops
	Cephalopoda	Cuttlefish (and bone), octopus, squid
Pisces (sub-phylum Chordata)	Osteichthyes (bony fish)	Salmon, plaice, tuna, hake, cod, herring, pilchard, anchovy, trout, swordfish, sole, pomfret, yellowfin, fishmeal (flour)
	Chondrichthyes (Cartilaginous fish)	shark (cartilage)
Other non-seafood associated biological agents		Hoya (sea-squirt), Anisakis, Red soft coral, Daphnia, Marine sponge, Algae

Table 1. Seafood species causing occupational allergy and asthma [Reproduced with permission from (Jeebhay et al., 2001)].

1.1 Shellfish allergens

In shellfish, crustaceans and mollusks, the protein tropomyosin (TM) seems to be the major allergen responsible for ingestion-related allergic reactions (Table1). Tropomyosin belongs to the family of actin filament-binding proteins with different isoforms that can be expressed in muscle, and non-muscle tissues. A complex of TM and troponin regulates the calcium sensitive interaction of actin and myosin. Tropomyosin in crustaceans was first identified in shrimp in 1981 by Hoffman *et al* (Hoffman et al., 1981). Shanti *et al.* reported an 86% amino acid sequence homology between the *Penaeus indicus* shrimp allergen Pen i 1 and fruit fly (*Drosophila melanogaster*) TM (Shanti et al., 1993). The open reading frame of the cloned TM in invertebrates was reported to be 281-amino acids with a monomeric molecular weight ranging from 38-41 kDa. The highly conserved amino acid sequence of TM is responsible for its identification as a panallergen for cross-reactivity between crustaceans, insects, arachnids, and different classes of mollusks (Rodriguez et al., 1997; Wild & Lehrer, 2005). In addition, the allergenicity of TM was confirmed in six species of crustaceans: black tiger prawn, kuruma prawn, pink shrimp, king crab, snow crab, and horsehair crab by immunoblotting and the overall sequence identity showed more than 90% homology (Motoyama et al., 2007).

Many other allergens have been identified in crustaceans. Yu's group identified arginine kinase (AK) (40 kDa) as a novel shrimp allergen (Yu et al., 2003). The amino acid sequence of

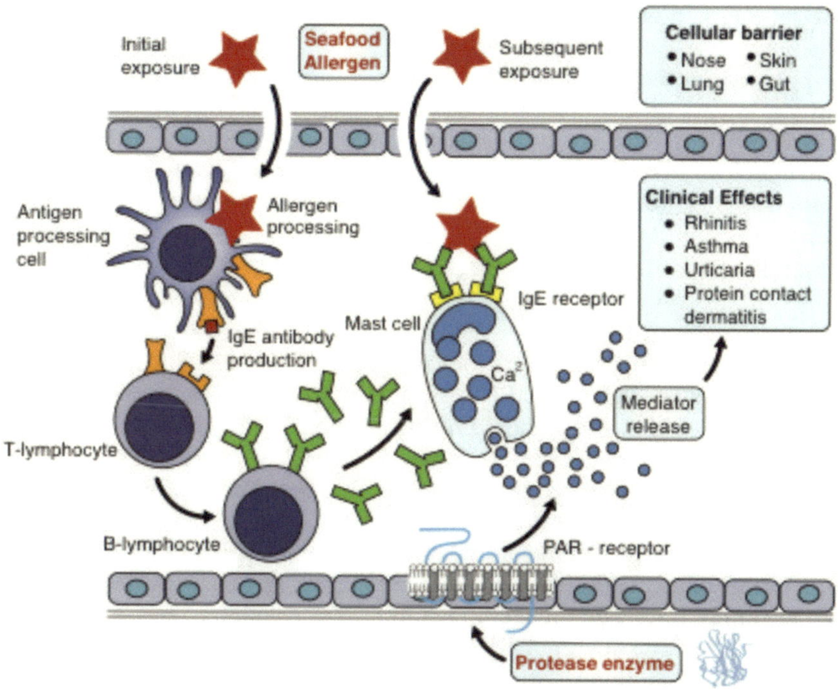

Fig. 1. Mechanisms of allergic and non-allergic inflammation in seafood exposed individuals (Modified and adapted from (Lehrer et al., 1996).

this protein showed 60% similarity to AK of the crustacean, kuruma prawn (*Penaeus japonicas*) (Yu et al., 2003). AK was recently reported as an allergen in different crustacean species which was identified in white shrimp (*Litopenaeus vannamei*) (García-Orozco et al., 2007), gulf shrimp (*Penaeus aztecus*) (France et al., 1997), chinese shrimp (*Fenneropenaeus chinensis*) (Yao et al., 2005), black tiger prawn (*Penaeus monodon*) and other shrimp species using a proteomics approach (Abdel Rahman et al., 2010a; Yu et al., 2003). Moreover, AK has been identified in other crab species: mud crab (*Scylla serrata*) (Shen et al., 2011), and by our group in snow crab (*Chionoecetes opilio*) (Abdel Rahman et al., 2011), where 49% of the participant patient's sera have a reactivity with AK. Arginine kinase also has been reported is allergen in some other invertebrates, such as the house dust mite (*Dermatophagoides farinae*) (Bi & Chew, 2004), Indian-meal moth (*Plodia interpunctella*) (Binder et al., 2001), and silkworm larvae (*Bombyx mori*) (Liu et al., 2009).

Recent studies have reported other novel crustacean allergens. In 2008, Shiomi *et al*. identified the immunoreactive band (20 kDa) as sarcoplasmic reticulum Ca-binding protein, which was consequently extracted from black tiger shrimp (*Penaeus monodon*) (Shiomi et al., 2008). Recently, this allergen was also identified in white shrimp (*Litopenaeus vannamei*) (Ayuso et al., 2009), and in snow crab (*Chionoecetes opilio*) (Abdel Rahman et al., 2011). Sarcoplasmic calcium binding protein (SCP) is an invertebrate EF-hand calcium buffering protein that fulfills a similar function in muscle relaxation as vertebrate major allergen parvalbumin (White et al., 2011).

In 2008, myosin light chain was identified as an allergen in white shrimp (*Litopenaeus vannamei*) (Ayuso et al., 2008; 2010), and our group also identified in black tiger prawn (*Penaeus monodon*) (Abdel Rahman et al., 2010a). Since TM is a common allergen in both crustaceans and mollusks (Ishikawa et al., 1998a;b; Lopata et al., 1997; Miyazawa et al., 1996; Suma et al., 2007), other potent allergens such as myosin heavy chain (Martins et al., 2004), troponin, actine, hemocyanin (Juji et al., 1990; Koshte et al., 1989; Maeda et al., 1991), and amylase (Azofra & Lombardero, 2003) are reported also in molluscan shellfish. These allergens were identified and characterized in different species such as mussel, oyster, and could exist alone in crustaceans (Table 2) (Taylor, 2008). Some of these allergenic proteins are rapidly degraded within a short period of digestion time, while TM seems to be relatively resistant to acidic digestion (Huang et al., 2010; Liu et al., 2010; 2011).

1.2 Fish allergens

The Atlantic cod was the first model for studying fish allergens, Gad c 1(12 kDa) (Aas & Elsayed, 1969; Aas & Lundkvist, 1973; Elsayed & Aas, 1970). This glycoprotein is identified later as parvalbumin, which buffers calcium during muscle relaxation. Parvalbumin has a higher natural abundance in the lower invertebrates than the fast twitch muscles of higher vertebrates (Lehky et al., 1974). Parvalbumin represents the major clinical cross-reactive fish allergen with sequence homology ranging from 60-80%. This feature was comprehensively applied to exploit the closeness between fish allergens and their human homologs (Jenkins et al., 2007). Parvalbumin, with allergen molecular mass ranges from 10-13 kDa, contains heat-resistant linear epitopes that are stabilized by the interaction of metal-binding domains (Lopata & Lehrer, 2009). The allergenicity of the parvalbumin was studied in purified forms from different types of fish along with two other high molecular weight allergens: 29 and 54 kDa (Beale et al., 2009; Lim et al., 2008; Rehbein & Lopata, 2011). The polymeric form of the parvalbumin is also reported as a high molecular weight allergen (Besler et al., 2000; Rosmilah et al., 2005). In addition, other fish allergens are characterized such as collagen and gelatin isolated from skin (Sakaguchi et al., 2000) and muscle tissues (Taylor et al., 2004), fish hormones like vitellogenin in caviar (Escudero et al., 2007; Perez-Gordo et al., 2008), and many other allergens reviewed in detail by Lopata and Lehrer 2009. The literature reports that there is no cross-reactivity between fish allergens and shellfish (Lopata & Lehrer, 2009).

2. Allergen discovery platforms

Raw and cooked seafood extracts are used to diagnose allergic sensitization in individuals by skin prick test (Jeebhay et al., 2008). These in-vivo assays lack the molecular information needed for component resolved diagnostics and initiated the development of various biomolecular and chemical approaches.

The seafood allergens discovery platform is reviewed as described in Fig. 2, which starts with the allergenic protein separation, western blotting, and amino acid sequencing. This developed strategy for allergen identification has expedited the discovery of the seafood allergens in two dimensions: among the same species (different allergens) and between other species (cross-reactivity). The cross-reactivity between the novel allergen and the equivalent protein in other species can be investigated by applying the same strategy that is used for the investigation but using the same antibody. The idea for this strategy is based mainly on the high level of homology between the same functional proteins, which makes the extensive characterization using molecular biology techniques more feasible. The most common seafood allergens and the used method(s) for the characterization and quantification are summarized in Table 2.

Species			Allergen/code	Techniques		Reference
				Characterization	Quantification	
Shellfish	Crustaceans	Shrimp	Tropomyosin Cra c1, Lit v1, Met e1, Pan b1, Pen a1, Pen i1, Pen m1	RAST, MG, MS	ELISA, MS	(Abdel Rahman et al., 2010a; Leung et al., 1994; Motoyama et al., 2008; 2007)
			Arginine kinase/ Cra c2, Lit v2, Pen m2, Met e 2, Met j 2	MG, MS	MS	(Abdel Rahman et al., 2010a; García-Orozco et al., 2007; Yoon et al., 2004; Yu et al., 2003)
			Sarcoplasmic calcium-binding protein/ Cra c4, Pen e4, Pen m4, Lit v4	ELISA, Edman, WB, LC-MSMS, MG	N/A	(Ayuso et al., 2009; Shiomi et al., 2008)
			Myosin, light chain /Art fr 5, Cra c5, Lit v3, Pen m3	MS, Edmand, MG, WB, Peptide microarray	N/A	Submitted (JUN-2007) to the EMBL/GenBank/ DDBJ databases), (Ayuso et al., 2008; 2010)
			Troponin C/ Pen m6, Cra c6	MG	N/A	WHO-IUIS Allergen DB
			Triosephosphate isomerase/Cra c8	MG	N/A	WHO-IUIS Allergen DB

Table 2. The most common known seafood allergens and the method of their characterization and quantification. [MG: Molecular genetics, WB: western blotting, MS: Mass spectrometry, ELISA: Enzyme-linked immunosorbent assay]

Species			Allergen/code	Techniques		Reference
				Characterization	Quantification	
Shellfish	Crustaceans	Crab	Tropomyosin/Cha f 1, Chi o1, Can p 1, Eri i 1, Par c 1, Por s 1, Por tr 1, Ran ra 1, Scy o 1, Scy pa 1, Scy s 1	MG, ELISA, RAST, WB, MS	ELISA, LCMSMS, RAST	(Abdel Rahman et al., 2010b;c; Huang et al., 2010; Kunimoto et al., 2009; Leung & Chu, 1998; Liang et al., 2008; Motoyama et al., 2007; Shibahara et al., 2009; Werner et al., 2007; Yu et al., 2010)
			Argine kinase/Chi o2, Scy s 2, Lim p 2	MG, WB, RAST, MS	MG, WB, RAST, MS	(Abdel Rahman et al., 2011; Bobolea et al., 2010; Werr et al., 2009; Yu et al., 2003)
			Troponin / Chi o 6	MS	N/A	(Shiomi et al., 2008); (Abdel Rahman et al., 2011)
			Sarcoplasmic calcium-binding protein/ Chi o 4	MG, MS	N/A	(Abdel Rahman et al., 2011; Shiomi et al., 2008)
		Lobster	Tropomyosin/Hom a1, Hom g 1, Jas la 1, Met ja 1, Nep n 1, Pan h 1, Pan j 1, Pan s 1	MG, WB, RAST, MS	ELISA	(DeWitt et al., 2004; Leung et al., 1996; Leung & Chu, 1998; Motoyama et al., 2007; Mykles et al., 1998; Shibahara et al., 2009; Werr et al., 2009)
			Arginine kinase/ Hom g 2	WB, MS, MG, ELISA	N/A	(Werr et al., 2009; Yu et al., 2003)
			Myosin light chain 2/ Hom a3	MG	N/A	(Towle & Smith, 2006)

Table 2. The most common known seafood allergens ..... continued from previous page

Species			Allergen/code	Techniques		Reference
				Characterization	Quantification	
Shellfish	Crustaceans	Lobster	Troponin C/ Hom a6	MG	N/A	(Garone et al., 1991)
			Sarcoplasmic calcium-binding/ Hom a 4	MG	N/A	(Shiomi et al., 2008)
		Crayfish	Tropomyosin/ Pro cl 1	WB, MG	LCMSMS	(Faeste et al., 2011)
			Sarcoplasmic calcium-binding protein/ Pon I4	MS	N/A	(Jauregui-Adell et al., 1989)
			Ast f	WB	ELISA	(Lopata & Jeebhay, 2007)
			Troponin I/Pon I7	Edman	LCMSMS	(Faeste et al., 2011; Kobayashi et al., 1989)
		Krill	Tropomyosin/ Eup p1, Eup s 1	MG, WB	N/A	(Motoyama et al., 2008; Nakano et al., 2007)
	Mollusks		Tropomyosin/ Hel as 1, Hal a 1, Tod p 1	MG, WB, ELISA	N/A	(Asturias et al., 2000; Suma et al., 2007; Suzuki et al., 2010)
			Hemocyanin / Meg c	Microarray	N/A	(Oyelaran & Gildersleeve, 2010)

Table 2. The most common known seafood allergens ..... continued from previous page

Species		Allergen/code	Techniques		Reference
			Characterization	Quantification	
Shellfish	Mollusks	Paramyosin/ Hal di, Myt g, Oct v, Tur c	MG, WB, ELISA	N/A	(Suzuki et al., 2010)
		Hal r 49kD	RAST, ELISA	N/A	(Lopata et al., 1997)
Fish		Che ag	RAST	N/A	(Koyama et al., 2006)
		Lop pi	Clinically	N/A	(Gimenez-Arnau et al., 2008)
		Gelatin/ Ore a	ELISA	N/A	(Weber et al., 2010)
		Parvalbumin/Seb m, Ore a 1, Seb m 1, Sar sa 1.0101	MG, WB, MS, Edman	ELISA	(Beale et al., 2009; Chen et al., 2006; Faeste & Plassen, 2008; Gajewski & Hsieh, 2009; Jeebhay et al., 2005; Kuehn et al., 2010; Van der Ventel et al., 2010; Weber et al., 2009)
		Albumin/ Onc ma	WB	ELISA, MS	(Nakamura et al., 2009)
		glyceraldehyde-3-phosphate dehydrogenase	WB	N/A	(Beale et al., 2009)

Table 2. The most common known seafood allergens ..... continued from previous page

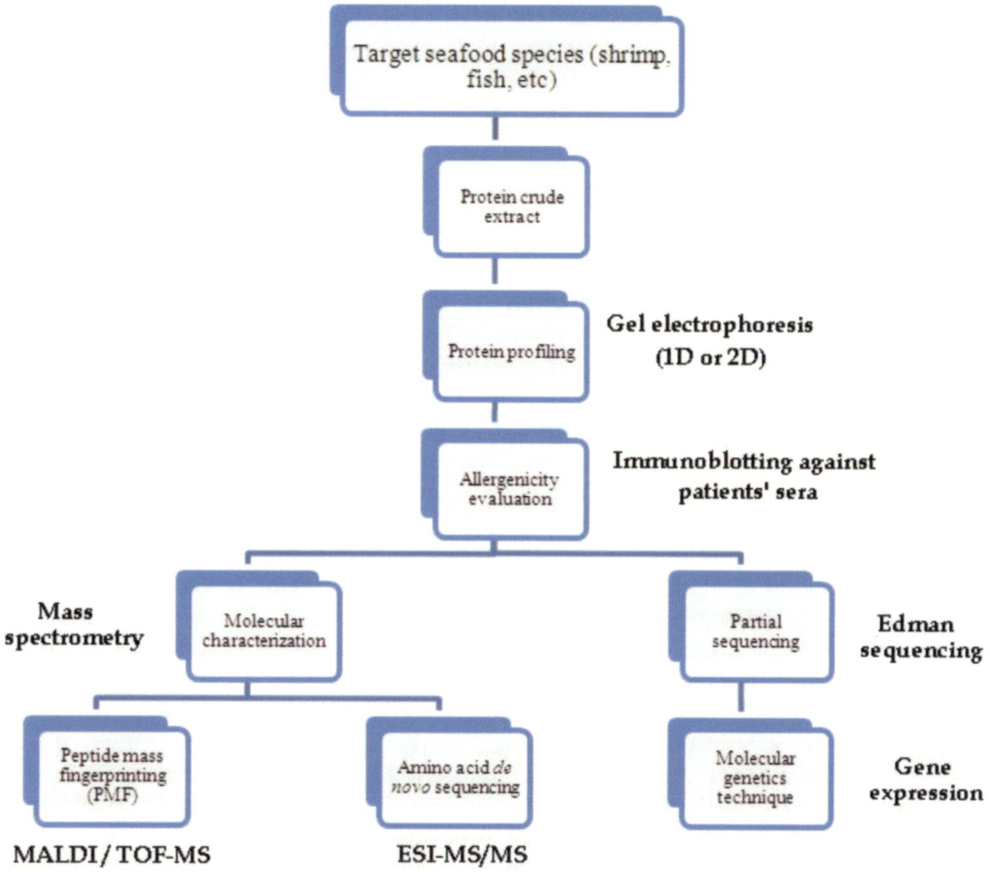

Fig. 2. The allergen discovery platform: starting from the seafood meat and ending by the characterization and quantification approaches

2.1 protein profiling and the allergenicity evaluation

2.1.1 Protein separation using gel electrophoresis

To characterize seafood allergens, it is necessary to profile the complex crude extracts by separating the protein content by gel electrophoresis. This technique plays a central role in seafood allergen research, wherein it provides a powerful separation and semi-quantification information. The principle of separation by gel electrophoretic techniques is mainly based on the ability of molecules to move through the pores of the gel media under the influence of an electric field. In this experiment, proteins carry charges from either a uniform coating by sodium dodecyl sulphate (SDS) or its natural net charge state isoelectric point (pI). The rate of protein mobility is based on the protein size and pI in both sodium dodecyl sulfate polyacrylamide gel electrophoresis (SDS-PAGE) and isoelectric focusing (IEF), respectively, where the larger difference in mobility gives better resolutions (Kinter & Sherman, 2000). Combining both electrophoresis separation behaviors, SDS-PAGE and IEF, gives better resolution and sensitive detection of allergen profile. In two dimensional gel electrophoresis (2-DE), the first dimension separates proteins based on their pI and consequently, the IPGstrip of isoelectric focusing gel is saturated in SDS buffer and then applied to the SDS-PAGE, as the second dimension. The resulting gel profile shows pI values on the abscissa and the molecular weight along the ordinate. These two sources of information are very important in identifying proteins and comparing different profiles originating from different species. In addition, the 2-DE profile gives a relative amount of the allergens in each single spot (Rabilloud, 2000).

2.1.2 Western blotting

After separating the complex of proteins that might contain allergens by gel electrophoresis, the separation profile should be applied to the immunoblotting experiment using allergic patients' sera. Immunoblotting is a powerful, selective, and sensitive technique, used to detect a small amount of protein or to study antibody-antigen reactivity. The protein profile in gel electrophoresis is electrophoretically transferred to a membrane which is usually nitrocellulose or polyvinylidene fluoride (PVDF). The membranes are soaked with a blocking reagent, either bovine serum albumin or skim milk in tris-buffered saline (TBS), to prevent any non-specific binding of the primary antibody on the membrane (Habsah et al., 2000). Consequently, the blot is incubated with sera collected from individuals who have tested positive in the skin test (Abdel Rahman et al., 2011; 2010b). After that, the peroxidase-conjugated antihuman IgE secondary antibody is added for the purpose of visualization (Towbin et al., 1979). Then the color development substrate is added in solution to visualize the immuno-reacted bands. Once the allergen is identified, the antibody against this protein can be produced in animals such as rats, rabbits, or goats.These allergen specific antibodies can subsequently be used for cross-reactivity studies and for developing quantitative approaches that will be discussed later.

This basic profile is very important to determine the target allergenic protein, which can subsequently be further analyzed with different techniques for further molecular characterization using molecular cloning or MS techniques. The allergen bands could be cut and introduced to Edman sequencing to identify the amino acid sequence of the N-terminal protein region. This information is very important to develop the primers that will be used for producing a recombinant protein from the related gene. The Edman sequencing can be omitted if the allergen is identified as being related to other known allergens.

2.2 Edman sequencing

Edman sequencing was in the past the only technique to identify the amino acid sequence of the N-terminus of seafood allergens, which is necessary to design the appropriate primers for isolating the relevant gene and deoxyribonucleic acid (DNA) sequencing (Ayuso et al., 2008; Hamada et al., 2004; Ma et al., 2008). The Edman reaction is performed on the protein N-terminus, where the amine side of the N-terminal amino acid reacts with phenylisothiocyanate (PITC) to form a phenylthiocarbamyl (PTC) protein. Consequently, trifluoroacetic acid is used to cleave the PTC, which then gives phenylthiohydantoin (PTH) amino acid derivatives as final products. These final products have different chemical structures, depending on the side chain of the N-terminal amino acid, and can subsequently be separated by high-performance liquid chromatography (HPLC) and compared to a standard to identify the N-terminal amino acid. Through this reaction, the N-terminal amino acid is removed from the protein, and produces a cleaved derivative of that amino acid along with a protein that is shortened by one amino acid and has a new N-terminus. This shortened protein is re-exposed to the same procedure for removing the next amino acid (Findlay et al., 1989).

Edman degradation is a part of modern protein analysis because of its ability to sequence a protein in its intact form as well as the proteolytic peptides. Furthermore, Edman sequencing has many other advantages, making it the main technique used worldwide in the last few decades before the use of mass spectrometry (MS) took over this kind of analysis. Advantages include its sensitivity, which is sufficient for analyzing proteins detected by Coomassie staining, the ease of operation, and the clarity of the data. However, this technique has a number of serious drawbacks compared to tandem MS, which will be discussed later, to be used in a proteomics platform. The time required to accomplish each cycle is very long (45 min/amino acid) and it cannot be used with proteins having blocked N-termini (Kinter & Sherman, 2000). However, Edman sequencing was the only technique to identify the amino acid sequence of the N-terminus of seafood allergens, which are necessary to design the proper primer for isolating the relevant gene and DNA sequencing.

2.3 Sequencing of proteins by cDNA analysis

After collecting the N-terminus amino acid sequence of the target protein, specific DNA primers are designed for amplifying the equivalent gene using polymerase chain reaction (PCR). The complete amino acid sequence of the target allergen is deduced from the DNA sequence of its equivalent gene(s) for the isolated genome. A recombinant protein from the target gene can be produced inside bacteria. After the gene amplification, a restriction enzyme is used to produce staggered cuts on the specific sequence of one of the gene strands. The same enzyme is also used to have a complementary cut on the bacteria plasmid. The gene is incorporated in the plasmid sequence by insertion, where the cohesive ends are bound and form a full plasmid. While the bacteria are cultured, the gene is transcripted, translated, and then produces the target protein. The recombinant allergen is isolated from the bacteria-media complex using some affinity techniques such as affinity chromatography or immuno-precipitation (Reese et al., 1997; Swoboda et al., 2002). This protein should have the same allergenicity and identity as seen in the native protein that was extracted from the seafood meat.

2.4 Characterization of seafood allergen using molecular genetics approach

The molecular genetics based-method is followed by the allergen discovery, which is based on the charcterization of its primary structure. The first shellfish allergen characterized was from the shrimp (Hoffman et al., 1981), where the target allergen was applied to a crossed immunoelectrophoresis technique against rabbit and pig antisera. In that time, the identity of the allergen was limited to its reactivity with the patient sera, native and reduction size, the molecular contents, such as carbohydrates and amino acids, and the isoelectric point (Hoffman et al., 1981). Using the same molecular information, cross-reactivity studies between shrimp extracts with other species were commenced with homology ranging from 60-80% among the sequenced peptides (Halmepuro et al., 1987; Lehrer et al., 1985; Lin et al., 1993). The 36-kDa allergen was identified as TM by comparing the molecular characterization of Pen a 1 with the fruit fly (*Drosophila melanogaster*) (Daul et al., 1994). This study gave a remarkable movement in allergen characterization by comparing experimentally the known allergen's structural features with other species' known proteins (Table 2). Among different fish species, another cross-reactivity study was commenced with more molecular identification (Van der Ventel et al., 2010). The Atlantic cod major allergen Gad m 1 (Aas & Elsayed, 1969) was identified as parvalbumin, by profiling the protein in isolectric focusing, SDS-PAGE, immunoblotting, and later identified using a recombinant form in Atlantic salmon (Do et al., 1999; ONeil et al., 1993; Pascual et al., 1992). The primary structure of the major shrimp allergen Met e 1, was also identified for the first time by a cloning technique, nucleotide sequencing, and translation to the amino acid sequence (Leung et al., 1994). Allergenicity of the recombinant protein was subsequently examined using the same protocol that has been used for the fish allergen discovery. After applying this informative strategy, the seafood allergen characterization, a new era in the field of seafood allergy research has begun. Other research groups started to focus on other novel allergens from mollusks, such as 49 kDa which is known as Hal m 1 (Lopata et al., 1997), and to study the cross-reactivity among different species: lobster (Zhang et al., 2006), crab (Leung & Chu, 1998) and among shellfish; crustaceans and mollusks, such as squid (Miyazawa et al., 1996). Motoyama *et al.*, used the gene cloning technique to identify the reactive TM protein in six species of crustaceans using immunoblotting against sensitized patient sera and also a specific monoclonal antibody (Mabe et al., 2009; Motoyama et al., 2007).

2.5 Protein mass spectrometry

Mass spectrometry is a technique used to characterize the gas-phase chemical structure of compounds after having them ionized. Based on the ion source, the ions in mass spectrometer can be formed in either of five different mechanisms: protonation, deprotonation, electron capturing, electron ejection, and adduct formation. The molecular ions, positive or negative, are electrically attracted and focused to get them in the mass analyzer, where the ions are separated based on their mass-to-charge ratio (m/z). This experiment usually gives the molecular weight of the target compound. For further structural analysis, tandem MS is performed by separating the target ions in the first mass analyzer, and then exposed to the collision cell. The produced fragment ions are separated in the second mass analyzer based on their mass-to-charge ratio to give a chemical structure.

Analyzing large molecules using tandem MS was only possible for the energetic stable molecules, such as polymers. Proteins were analyzed by MS after the invention of the matrix-based laser desorption techniques, like fast atom bombardment (FAB) and matrix assisted laser desorption ionization (MALDI), where the laser energy transferred indirectly and softely to the protein via the matrices. Although, MALDI and time-of-flight (TOF) is a good combination between an ion source and mass analyzer for protein MW determination, generating a fragmentation pattern for the protein's ion is a challenge. This dilemma is limited to the fact that the MALDI mainly forms mono-charged ions, which requires higher energy in acceleration voltage for the effective fragmentation process, as well as the difficulties of coupling a TOF MS to another analyzer for tandem process. The electrospray ionization (ESI) invention offered a historical shift for protein characterization using MS, where this ion source produces the multiply charged ions with lower demand on fragmentation energy. The primary structure of the allergenic proteins can now be identified using MS, where it helps to understand the other proteins' structural features and functional activity. In addition, the amino acid sequence directly corresponds to the DNA sequence of the corresponding gene (s), which helps to study the activity of proteins by detecting the common mutations at the molecular level.

Amino acid sequencing is performed by determining the structure and the position of each amino acid residue within the protein. This target demands a method sensitive and specific enough to analyze native proteins in highly throughput manner. In addition, it must provide reliable information with sufficient mass accuracy (Kinter & Sherman, 2000). The ESI generates multiply-charged ions, which are easily accelerated and fragmented in tandem

MS experiments. Allergen analysis can be performed in MS by peptide mass fingerprinting (PMF) as an identification technique or by tandem MS for *de novo* sequencing.

2.5.1 Peptide mass fingerprinting.

Mass spectrometry has become a major analytical tool for protein structural analyses. Generating the gas phase ions of protein molecule was a challenge before MALDI and ESI along with accurate mass analyzers, which offered a valuable tool for protein identification. Following the completion of the early genome sequencing projects, several search engines (i.e. Mascot and Sequest) were developed for the genome databases with MS interface. The enzymatic digested protein generates a highly unique peptide profile which is further analyzed by MS. These peptides are introduced to a mass spectrometer to give fingerprint profiles. The so called PMF technique is important for protein identification that already has genetic information in the databases. There are several factors that control the precision of the database search such as the resolving power of the MS, type of protease, availability of the gene data in data bank, and the purity of the target proteins (Aebersold & Mann, 2003).

2.5.2 Tandem mass spectrometry

Selected gas-phase ions of peptides and proteins are fragmented in the tandem MS mode, which gives a series of ions related to the amino acid sequence. This development in protein MS was extended to give high throughput protein identification, *de novo* sequencing, and identification of post-translational modifications (Aebersold & Mann, 2003). Protein tandem MS-based techniques are mainly divided into two major types; bottom-up or top-down. These terminologies are assigned for the point of sample handling before MS analysis and from the data processing and sequencing manipulation (Kinter & Sherman, 2000).

2.5.2.1 Bottom-up approach

In the bottom-up approach, the enzymatically-digested proteins are subjected to LC-MS/MS analyses. The precursor ions of the peptides are separated in the first mass event, and then fragmented to produce a series of informative product ions. These ions are separated and analyzed in the second mass event.

A distinctive series of product ions are directly related to the amino acid sequence, which then compared with 'in-silico' ions that are generated theoretically from the DNA databases by computers. The sequence will be assigned when both series of ions, experimental and theoretical, are matched perfectly as shown in peptide number 3 in Fig.3. This technique usually provides useful information about the post-translational modifications (i.e. phosphorylated, acetylated). Some of these post-translational modified residues are difficult to be identified due to poor chromatographic resolution or detector sensitivity (Chait, 2004; Scherperel & Reid, 2007), as seen for the two peptides number 2 and 5 in Fig. 3. On the other hand, introducing the whole protein to the mass spectrometer without any digestion, top-down (discussed below), is a very useful technique to identify most of the labile post translation modification groups with high amino acid sequencing coverage (Siuti & Kelleher, 2007).

Enzymatic digestion of the intact protein followed by purification and electrophoretic separation prior to MS analyses is routine but tedious work for bottom-up approach. The enzymatic peptides are normally separated by reversed phase chromatography and subjected ESI or MALDI with analysis by tandem MS. The sequence of each peptide is deduced from the product ion spectra after gas phase collision induced dissociation (CID) (Kinter & Sherman, 2000).

Generating a good sequencing coverage for the intact protein requires producing peptides that are readily soluble for chromatography. The chromatographic separation of peptides prior to MS ionization is very important. Generating ion of highly energetic gas-phase ions inside the field free region is required for facile fragmentation or dissociation. Sequencing the intact protein using a regular tandem mass spectrometer is limited to the energy of the dissociation and the resolving power of the mass analyzer, which leads to erroneously manipulation from the algorithms of the database. The labile post-translational and environmental modifications of proteins are difficult to be identified using energetic dissociation bottom-up method. As well the modified peptides are more sensitive to be detected by MS than the large hydrophobic proteins (Eidhammer et al., 2007). The bottom-up approach can usually deal with most types of proteins regardless of their size or function. This approach is still the most common, but the sequence coverage is limited (Eidhammer et al., 2007).

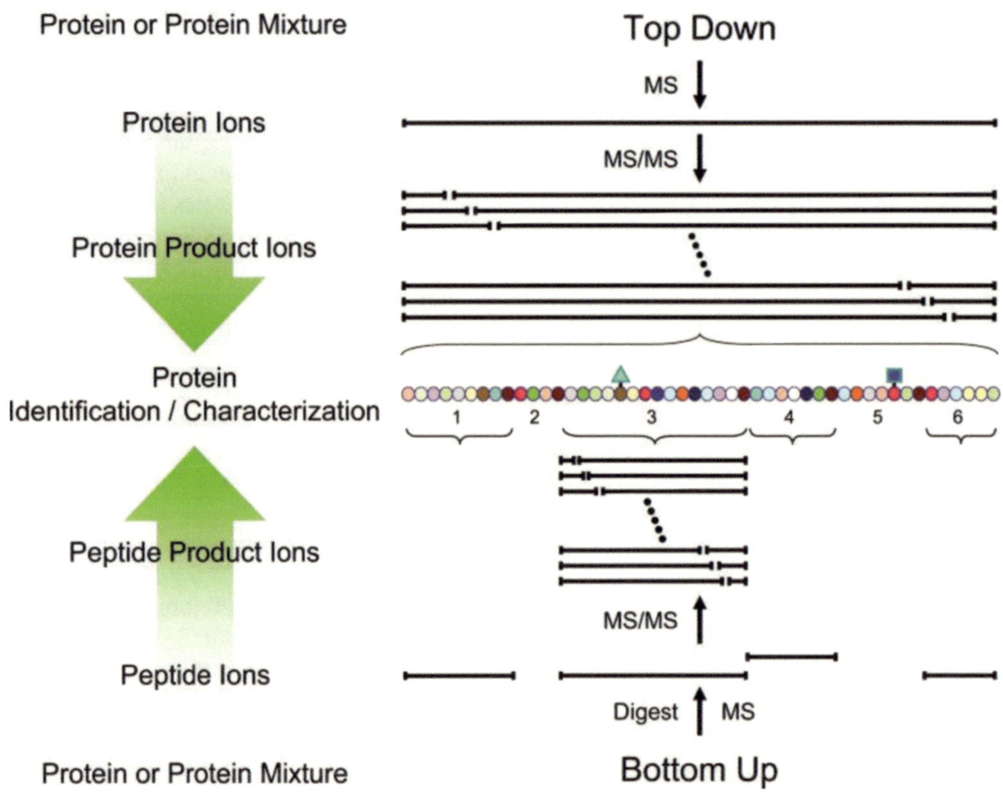

Fig. 3. Schematic overview of bottom-up and top-down approaches employed for tandem MS-based protein identification and characterization. The shaded circles represent the amino acids of a protein, while the shaded triangle and rectangle represents post-translational modifications. (Reproduced by permission of The Royal Society of Chemistry; (Scherperel & Reid, 2007)

2.5.2.2 Top-down approach

Manipulating the bottom-up approach data requires data availability in the gene bank. Thus, the top-down approach was found to improve protein identification even in case of the lack of genetic information in the databases. Understanding the chemical composition, molecular weight, and stability/solubility of the target protein(s) is paramount for achieving proper ionization and gas phase dissociation in the mass spectrometer. Kelleher and group introduced the top-down approach by analyzing an intact protein using an ESI ion source (Kelleher et al., 1999). This type of analysis requires high resolution mass analyzers as well as a high energy collision cell. The amino acid sequence, and post-translation modification structures were determined in this approach using in-time tandem MS experiments. The mass difference between the generated precursor ions and their equivalent predicted ions in the DNA databases were considered for amino acid sequencing of the intact protein (Reid & McLuckey, 2002).

The top-down approach was further developed for the analysis of a mixture of proteins without classical separation (chromatography or electrophoresis). The precursor ion of the target protein is selected and isolated in the first mass analysis event for amino acid sequencing (Reid & McLuckey, 2002). This approach still offers a comprehensive post-translation modification mapping. Several bioinformatic tools can be implemented to map the post-translation modification information in protein, which are mainly defined by the mass differences between the experimental and theoretical spectral data (Kelleher et al., 1999). The MS resolution is high enough to identify a disulfide bond, which increases the molecular weight of the protein by 2 Da after reduction. The top-down method has clearly been shown to identity even the labile post-translation modification groups (Scherperel & Reid, 2007). Two-dimensional correlation between MS/MS and MS/MS/MS was also developed to confirm the amino acid sequence in Fourier-transform ion cyclotron resonance (FTICR) instruments (Zhang & McElvain, 2000).

The top-down approach affords another valuable and powerful tool for proteomic analyses. Post-translation modification mapping can become a reliable tool for determining chemistry, location, and quantity of these modifications along with the primary structure of a protein. Using this method as the sequencing approach for an intact protein can provide close to 100% coverage. Moreover proteins can be part of a mixture, or have unusually large molecular weight. Analysis of these types of samples will still give the same accuracy and with less complexity compared to the bottom-up approach. Simple algorithm databases with more sophisticated data processing are readily available for top-down approaches. Including powerful and advanced MS instruments such as FTICR allowing for maximum mass accuracy and resolution reinforces the strength behind this approach

2.6 Characterization of seafood allergen using mass spectrometry

Mass spectrometry serves as a characterization technique of seafood allergens by determining the molecular weight, the primary structure, and the quantity of the intact allergenic protein. Unfortunately, a number of seafood allergen research articles that used MS is quite low compared with other protein-based food allergen research. The shortage of genomic data for many of the seafood species in GenBank and lack of expertise in facilitating the MS techniques in this research area are also the main reasons for this literature shortage. Officially, MS was recommended as a replacement technique for allergen detection in inspection labs back in 2005 (Hungerford, 2006; Hungerford & Trucksess, 2005).

Allergen analysis by MS started by determining the molecular weight of small allergens such as parvalbumin (12 kDa) in fish (Bugajska-Schretter et al., 2000; Cai et al., 2010; Swoboda et al., 2002). After completing the genome sequence and developing the MS-interface databases, some studies use the PMF approach to identify the seafood allergens evaluated by immunoblotting (Ayuso et al., 2009; García-Orozco et al., 2007; Mazzeo et al., 2008; Shen et al., 2011; Yamasaki et al., 2010; Yu et al., 2003). The best example of this kind of research was in 2003, when Pen m 2 shrimp allergen was identified using PMF, where the recognized spot proteins by a pool of patients' sera were tryptic digested and analyzed by MALDI-ToF (Yu et al., 2003). Consequently, the purified AK of white shrimp that was partially sequenced using the shot-gun MS method (García-Orozco et al., 2007) was also identified by comparing the MS data with the sequence of Pen m 2 in the MASCOT search engine. Instrumentally, most of this unambiguous characteristic information was generated by coupling MALDI ion source to the TOF mass analyzer, which can give the molecular weight of the purified intact protein with a margin of error of 0.1% (DeHoffmann & Stroobant, 2007) and perform the PMF experiments. The precision of MALDI-TOF is poorer with larger proteins, which provoked to use more advanced ion sources like ESI coupled with FTICR (Ma et al., 2008). The high resolution of MS analyzers are used to study seafood authentication by measuring the exact molecular weight of a marker protein (Mazzeo et al., 2008).

The seafood allergenic proteins can be also sequenced using tandem MS (Abdel Rahman et al., 2010a; 2011; 2010b; Misnan et al., 2010). This method was used in the seafood allergen studies as a confirmatory technique to study some biochemical and biophysical properties by collecting the amino acid sequence of a few peptides (Perez-Gordo et al., 2011). Ma *et al.* (2008) validated the using of high resolution MS profiles to evaluate the cross-reactivity of the allergens based on their structural similarities. The cross-reactivity between both the natural and recombinant forms of cod and carp parvalbumin was evaluated using patients' sera and the structure was also evaluated using both circular dichroism (CD) and nuclear magnetic resonance (NMR) (Ma et al., 2008).

In Helleur's group, the tandem MS technique was the method for *de novo* sequencing of seafood allergens. Tropomyosin, the major snow crab and black tiger prawn allergens, was used as a reference protein to develop a tandem MS strategy for the protein sequencing (Abdel Rahman et al., 2010a;b). Since the amino acid sequences of both allergens are available in the databases, it was an advantage to optimize the full sequence strategy. The multi-enzymatic digestions, multi-ion sources, and multi-derivatization reactions were used for obtaining the full amino acid coverage. This strategy was later applied for other allergens characterization (Abdel Rahman et al., 2011; Carrera et al., 2010; Liu et al., 2011). The high resolution tandem MS is also capable to study the heterogeneity of allergen isoforms in micro scale. Permyakov *et al.* studied the microheterogeneity of Pike α-parvalbumin, where precisely the MS output shows the presence of both amino acid sequences for $\alpha 1$ and $\alpha 2$ isoforms (Permyakov et al., 2009). Extensively, 25 new parvalbumin isoforms were identified and *de novo* sequenced from different 11 species using some bioinformtic tools (e.g. PEAK). The high mass accuracy of the FTICR (0.05-4.47 ppm) allowed for the amino acid sequence of the species which their genomes remain unsequenced (Carrera et al., 2010).

3. Allergen quantification

3.1 Immunological-based techniques

There are several techniques that can be used for the quantification of potential allergens. These techniques target either the allergenic protein itself or biomarker that indicates its presence. However, the allergen detection itself is a challenge, as their chemical properties are not be well characterized. In addition, many allergenic seafood species contain multiple allergenic proteins that can vary in their concentration. Once the allergenic protein is characterized and a specific antibody produced, this allergen can be routinely detected in one of the immunochemical detection protocols such as radio-allergosorbent test (RAST), enzyme allergosorbent test (Dearnaley et al., 2010), rocket Immuno-electrophoresis (RIE), immunoblotting, and enzyme-linked immunosorbent assay (ELISA). Whereas, RIE is only used for qualitative or semi-quantitative the same as immunoblotting, however, RAST, EAST, and ELISA are absolute quantitative methods. The choice of method depends on the availability of the antibody, the target of the analysis, and the method characteristic merits such as detection limit and precision.

3.1.1 Radio-allergosorbent inhibition

Radio-allergosorbent is a technique that can be used for the determination of allergen-specific IgE antibodies generated by the sensitized individuals, which is commonly used in the clinical diagnosis of most allergies. In addition, this technique has been used for the qualitative detection and determination of allergenicity of different seafood species. Basically, the target allergen in the RAST test is bound to a solid polymer. The specific IgE in the patient sera binds to the allergen. After removing non-specific IgE, antigens in a sample solution inhibit IgE binding to the antigen immobilized on the solid phase. Radio-labeled anti-human IgE antibody is added to form a complex, and then the unbound secondary antibody is washed away after incubation. The amount of radioactivity, detected in gamma counter, is proportional to the amount of the bound IgE (Malo et al., 1997). These methods have several drawbacks to be the major technique for allergen quantification, one of them is its reliance on human sera from allergic individual (Nordlee & S.L.Taylor, 1995)

3.1.2 Enzyme-linked immunosorbent assay.

Currently, ELISA is the main immunological reaction-based technique used for determination levels of allergens in different matrices. In principle, a calibration curve of a serial dilution from the allergen extracts is developed and the antigen/antibody reaction is optimized. There are two main approaches for allergen quantification using ELISA: competitive and sandwich. The sandwich ELISA is more specific and precise than the competitive, where the primary antibody is bound to the solid phase like the microtiter plate. The specific protein is captured and the non-bound species will be removed. The captured protein is detected by the enzyme-labeled secondary antibody. The complex is visualized by a reaction between a particular substrate with the conjugated enzyme on the secondary antibody and developing a colored product. The analyte concentration is proportional directly with the measured absorption. The relatively small proteins are preferably measured by the competitive ELISA. The patients' sera and the allergen extracts are pre-incubated, and then this mixture is added to the microtiter wells that have an antigen bound to the solid phase. The maximum binding between the solid phase-bound antigen and the enzyme-labeled antibody is performed when there is no antigen presence in the inhibitor sample. Antigens in the sample inhibit the binding of enzyme-labeled antibody to the immobilized antigen, where the concentration of the allergen is inversely proportional to the color absorption.

3.1.3 Detection and quantification of selected allergens in seafood

The RAST technique was used as a diagnosis method, where the positive skin test patient sera were evaluated using a crude extract of the potential allergenic seafood, such as in crustaceans, prawn, shrimp, crawfish, and lobster (Daul et al., 1988; Halmepuro et al., 1987; Nagano et al., 1984). This technique was used to study the cross-reactivity between the oyster and crustacean (Lehrer & McCants, 1987) and caddis fly with arthropoda and mollusca (Koshte et al., 1989),

which indicated to the non-specificity of RAST to be a diagnostic assay. However, the RAST inhibition technique was used to evaluate the species-specific shrimp allergen (Morgan et al., 1989). Shrimp allergy is estimated to be about 2% of the general population (Besler et al., 2001; Lopata et al., 2010). The threshold doses for shrimp allergic individual were evaluated to be 16g (Daul et al., 1988) and for fish ranging from 5-600 mg (Taylor et al., 2002) using the double-blind placebo controlled food challenges (DBPCFC). Cod fish allergen, the first reported allergen, was also evaluated by RAST to study the physico-chemical properties and the cross-reactivity with other fish species (Aas & Elsayed, 1975; Aas & Lundkvist, 1973; Aukrust et al., 1978).
The absolute quantification for the seafood allergen was initiated in 1997 by Lehrer's group (Jeoung et al., 1997). A sandwich ELISA method was developed using TM extracted and purified from brown shrimp. The detection limit was 4 ng/ml and the assay detected the TM-like allergen in different crustacean species such as crab and lobster. Recently, the method was optimized to evaluate the level of crustacean major allergen, TM, in processed food (Motoyama et al., 2008; Seiki et al., 2007) with a limit of detection of about 2.5 mg/kg (Rejeb et al., 2002). This assay demonstrated cross-reactivity between other crustaceans like crab and lobster. Although the TM sequence homology between the shrimp and pork or chicken was around 55%, this study showed no cross-reactivity between them (Reese et al., 1997). The fish major allergen, parvalbumin, was quantified for the first time by Lopata et al (2005) in its aerosolized form (Lopata et al., 2005). Recently, this method was applied for the evaluation of fish allergen levels in foodstuff (Faeste & Plassen, 2008), and for comparing the parvalbumin levels in different species (Kuehn et al., 2010). Commercially, there is only one ELISA kit available for detection of crustacean' allergens in foodstuff: however there is none available for the fish allergens.

3.2 Allergen quantification using mass spectrometry

Studying the large variety of proteins belonging to a certain biological system is known as proteomics. In recent decades, high throughput MS-based proteomics techniques have been developed for protein analysis and identification. The tandem MS tools have been very influential in the field of protein science as the genome sequence projects were being completed. The discovery and development of ESI and MALDI sources has given protein MS a huge push to become one of the dominating fields in proteomics. At its inception, MS proteomics research was mainly a qualitative discipline, where the outputs were limited to a list of identified proteins without any further information about abundances, distributions, or stoichiometry (Schulze & Usadel, 2010). In contrast, quantitative strategies were developed by analyzing the gene expression by microarray technology, real-time PCR, or evaluating the enzymes' activity that directly represent theirae quantity. Several MS-based tools are being developed for proteomics quantification, which help in characterizing the proteome complexities. For example, quantitative data can assist in the study the true protein interactions (interactoms) of a given bait protein over the background. These proteomics strategies are used to differentiate between stressed and normal samples or between knock-out and wild types for certain biological systems.

3.2.1 Proteomics quantification

Quantitative proteomics approaches are used as part of the larger framework of the available techniques for studying regulatory processes in the living cell. Choosing the quantification method is less important than the method's practical aspects which include good technical

reproducibility. By the same token, the biological system variations must be considered in the experimental design, along with financial costs. Since there is no amplification step at the protein level, the sample size is the most important limiting factor affecting the strategy of quantitative differential proteomics. Accordingly, enrichments and purification of protein are carried out to meet the sensitivity of the quantification technique. In this way, the sample size will influence the choice of analytical method (Schulze & Usadel, 2010).
The differences in the physical and chemical properties of different peptides, directly affect the proton affinity and the MS signal intensity. These peptide variables are their charge state, peptide length, amino acid composition, and any post-translational modification. These structural variations contribute to the peptides' ion intensities even if they belong to the same protein. Because of this, many MS-based quantitative methods produce only relatively quantitative data, which is based mainly on the MS response in contest with its sample matrix. Accordingly, careful experimental design and suitable data analysis are needed to obtain the desired analytical information.

3.2.2 Relative quantification MS-based techniques

The relative quantification MS-based techniques are categorized into two major groups: stable-isotope-labeling and the label-free approach. The relative standard deviation for most stable-isotope-labeling techniques is below 10% and the accuracy is approximately 30%, based on peak intensities or extracted ion chromatograms. However, the precision obtainable from label-free approaches, based on spectral counting or derived indices, is as high as 50% RSD (Schulze & Usadel, 2010).
The label-free quantification methods are based mainly on precursor signal intensity, which requires a high precision mass spectrometer. The label-free approaches are inexpensive (no labeled material to purchase) and can be applied to any biological material. The proteome coverage for quantified proteins can be very high, because any protein with one or more identified peptides can be quantified. Thus the sample complexity does not normally increase by mixing different proteomes together. Hence the protein expression can be quantified between different biological samples from different treatments. These samples can be analyzed by the free-label MS approach due to its analytical power and flexible dynamic range (Old et al., 2005). There are two main label-free approaches; protein-based methods (spectral count or derived indices) and peptide-based methods (ion intensities and protein correlation profile). The protein-based method looks to the protein expression levels among proteins of the same sample and compares them with another sample. In contrast, the peptide-based method utilizes the averaged and normalized ion intensities of the identified peptides (of specific proteins) for quantification.
The isotopic-labeling methods are classified with respect to the labeling strategy; metabolic labeling and isobaric mass tags. The metabolic labeling approach introduces the whole cell or organism to a labeled culture media (e.g. stable-isotope labeling by amino acid (SILAC) in cultured cells). On the other hand, chemical labeling (isobaric mass tags) can be attached to the protein or proteolytic peptides by a chemical reaction. Equivalent quantities of the labeled and unlabeled samples are mixed and treated in the same manner prior to the MS analysis. The differences between the labeled peptides' intensities and those of unlabeled represent the levels of that specific protein in the original sample. The drawback in this method is interference by co-eluting isobaric compounds when tandem MS is not used.
The isobaric mass tags method can overcome any co-eluting interferences by developing reagents that co-elute with the target peptide ion, then they will have a significant resolution

after fragmentation in the product ion spectra. Each product ion spectrum is the result of a different chemical tag with its intensity equivalent to the level of protein expression in the original sample. These fragments (tags) are in the low mass range, which make interferences from other peptides' fragments difficult. There are some commercial isobaric reagents that offer this type of quantification strategy such as the isobaric tag for relative and absolute quantification (iTRAQ) and the tandem mass tag (TMT).

3.2.3 Absolute quantification and isotopic dilution mass spectrometric techniques

A technique called absolute quantification (AQUA) using the stable-isotopic-labeled technique was reported for the first time by Desiderio and Kai (1983) (Desiderio & Kai, 1983). By using selected reaction monitoring (SRM) in triple quadruple tandem mass spectrometer, the AQUA became a standard protocol in protein quantification. The informatics combination between the retention time, peptide precursor ion, and the fragmentation profile gives this method high specificity toward the particular target peptide. The signal-to-noise ratio in SRM is very high, which gives an extended linear dynamic range up to 5 orders of magnitude. By spiking a protein sample with a known amount of the stable-isotopic-labeled peptide, the concentration of the native protein can be calculated. However, this may not cover all levels of the expressed protein in the tissue, because sample preparation steps may lead to loss or enrichment of the target peptide that are not addressed by the AQUA method. The absolute quantification of large proteins (MW>15kDa) by MS can be performed using the bottom-up approach. The intact protein is digested and the signature peptide is selected to represent the target protein. The stable-isotopic-labeled and natural (light) forms of the signature peptide are chemically synthesized, where the heavy form is used as an internal standard. Before MS analysis, the heavy form of the signature peptide is added to the sample in a deliberate manner; hence the method is called 'isotope dilution' MS. Small proteins (<15kDa) can also be quantified using the top-down approach, whereby the internal standard is prepared as a metabolic labeling strategy using labeled culture media (Brun et al., 2009).

3.2.4 Validation of bioanalytical methods

Once the AQUA method for the target protein is developed, the validity of the method is studied and evaluated to meet successfully the minimum standards of the Food and Drug Administration (Marko-Varga et al., 2005) guidelines for accuracy, precision, selectivity, sensitivity, reproducibility, and stability (Food and Drug Administration, 2001). This guideline was specifically developed for studying the bioanalytical method validation of small molecules or drugs, however, Helleur's group has modified this protocol to be developed for studying the AQUA method for allergen quantification using multiple reaction monitoring (MRM) tandem MS (Abdel Rahman et al., 2010c).

3.2.5 Insight of using mass spectrometry for seafood allergen quantification

The seafood allergen discovery platform, starting from the seafood species and ending by allergens absolute quantification, can be expedited efficiently by applying the allergenomics approach as discriped in Fig 4. Allergenomics is one of the functional proteomics strategies that focus on potential allergen discovery of such species. Whereas the primary structure and the relative and absolute quantification of the target allergen are determined. This strategy gives a reliable tool for monitoring the immuno-reactivity proteins in various conditions such as heating or adding food additives. Helleur's group commenced this strategy in seafood allergen, where the snow crab and black tiger prawn were the species of choice

(Abdel Rahman et al., 2010a;b). The real seafood allergen quantification by MS was performed for measuring the level of aerosolized snow crab major allergens in the workplaces. The TM and AK were simultaneously measured using MRM-MS/MS in air samples collected from crab processing plants (Abdel Rahman et al., 2012; 2010c) and from fishing vessels as joint project between SafteyNet and Rural Center at Memorial University of Newfound land and Dalhousie University, respectively (in preparation).

For developing allergenomics quantification method for any species, the crude extract samples should be profiled in 2D-gel electrophoresis (Fig. 4). The allergenicity of the protein profile is evaluated by immunoblotting the 2D-gels with a pool of patients' sera. The reactive proteins would then be cut, tryptic digested, and characterized using MS. The relative abundances of the discovered allergens can be evaluated using either the label-free or the isobaric mass tags methods such as iTRAQ. It is highly recommended to have an allergenomics profile and absolute multi-allergens quantification method. Therefore, proteomics quantification methods such as iTRAQ or TMT can be used to give a relative quantification profile for all detected allergens in a very specific and sensitive manner. All candidate allergens that have been shown up in the iTRAQ profile will be considered for developing an absolute quantification method. An artificial polypeptide is designed to produce all the signature peptides of all target allergens as soon as digested by trypsin. The heavy form standard of this polypeptide is added to the target sample (e.g. food or air filters), as an internal standard right before the extraction and digestion. Stoichiometrically, this process will control completeness of the digestion and sample loss as well as give an absolute quantification for each single allergen in the sample in a single run. This approach can be performed in air samples as well as for monitoring the levels of allergens in food as a quality control test (food grades) for the sake of reporting the nutritional facts.

4. Occupational/inhalant allergy and asthma associated with seafood

The increasing growth of the seafood market in the past two decades has led to an increasing number of workers engaged in various harvesting and aquaculture activities. Aside from increased consumption worldwide, more than 45 million workers are also involved in seafood production and are therefore exposed to seafood allergens in various contexts (Food and Agriculture Organisation, 2010). Adverse reactions have increasingly been reported in individuals consuming, handling or processing seafood in various settings. Aside from the ingestion route, seafood proteins can also enter the body through inhalation of aerosols or vapours containing allergens.

In domestic settings, a Spanish study reported 11% of children from a group of 197 children with fish allergy/hypersensitivity, placed on a strict fish avoidance diet, who experienced repeated allergic reactions upon incidental inhalation of fish odors or vapors. In most cases, these episodes occurred at home when other people were eating fish (James & Crespo, 2007). A similar observation in a South African study of 105 individuals with self-reported seafood allergy, reported 30% of individuals with allergic symptoms after handling or inhaling seafood in the domestic home environment (Lopata & Jeebhay, 2001).

In the workplace setting, occupational asthma was first reported in 1937 by De Besche in a fisherman who developed allergic symptoms when handling codfish. Since then various other seafood has been reported to cause occupational allergy and asthma including crustaceans as summarized in Table 1 (shrimp and shrimpmeal, prawn, lobsters), mollusc's (mussels, octopus, scallops, abalone) and other bony fish (trout, salmon, pilchard, anchovy, plaice, hake, tuna, haddock, cod, pollack). These incidents have been reported on board

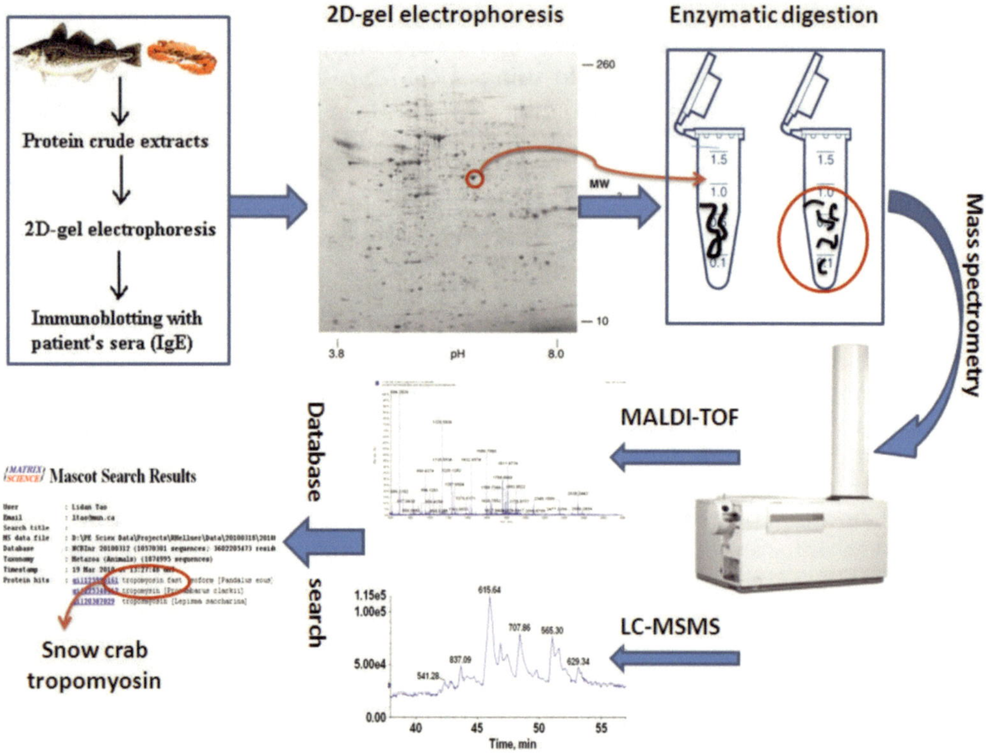

Fig. 4. The allergenomics strategy for allergen discovery, which uses the seafood crude extracts and the proteomics-MS based approach for characterization

fishing vessels and among workers involved with land-based seafood processing factories. Various epidemiological studies among seafood processors indicate that the prevalence of occupational asthma is between 2% and 36%. These differences in prevalence are partly due to varying definitions of occupational asthma used by investigators; the allergenic potential of the seafood proteins involved; and the type of work process resulting in excessive exposure such as steam, organic dust, air blowing and water jets. What is notable, however, is that these studies show that occupational asthma is more commonly associated with shellfish (4-36%) than with bony fish (2-8%) (Jeebhay & Cartier, 2010; Jeebhay et al., 2001).

Various studies show that the common work processes causing bioaerosol production include butchering or grinding; degilling, 'cracking' and boiling of crabs; cleaning and brushing of crab; 'tailing' of lobster; 'blowing' of prawn meat through shells; washing or scrubbing of shellfish; degutting, heading, and cooking/boiling of fish; mincing of seafood; and cleaning of the processing line or storage tanks with high pressured water hoses (Jeebhay et al., 2001). Processes that generate dry aerosol particulates such as prawn blowing operations using compressed air and fishmeal loading/bagging appear to generate higher levels of particulate than wet processes (prawn blowing with water jets). It is these aerosolized wet or dry particulates produced from seafood during processing operations that are inhaled by workers in the occupational setting. In domestic environments, it is highly probable that similar conditions prevail, although on a much smaller scale, resulting in allergic symptoms in highly exposed or allergic individuals.

Experimental studies in crab processing plants demonstrate that the aerosols generated in these factories contain mainly crab exoskeleton containing chitin, meat primarily muscle protein, gills and kanimiso/internal organs (Jeebhay et al., 2001). Fish juice produced in fish filleting and canning plants has various biogenic amines, degradation compounds associated with postmortem changes, digestive enzymes, skin slime/mucin, collagen and fish muscle proteins.

4.1 Aeroallergen quantification in seafood workplaces

There are several quantification approaches utilized to measure the levels of aeroallergens in workplace environments. These techniques are based mainly on the immunoreactivity of allergenic proteins with the specific IgE of sensitized patients' sera. Inhibition RIA, RAST, and ELISA are the most common techniques that have been used historically. Taylor et al. measured the level of raw fish aeroallergens in open-air fish markets using the inhibition RIA (Taylor et al., 2000). In 1997 Malo *et al.* applied the RAST test for the first time to measure seafood aeroallergens, where the air samples were collected from snow crab processing plants (Malo et al., 1997). In this study, total allergen extracts were prepared as a standard and the activity of these extracts was evaluated by skin test in patients known to have occupational asthma. The amount of the allergenic protein was estimated by percent inhibition of the RAST profile. A comprehensive study with four snow crab plants was accomplished in Newfoundland and Labrador, where air samples were analyzed using a similar process (Howse et al., 2006).

Inhibition ELISA techniques have also been used to study seafood aeroallergens. The water or meat protein extract and a pool of patients' sera were used as standard and primary antibody, respectively. Weytjens *et al.* measured the levels of snow crab allergen in workplaces and studied the gradient profile of the aeroallergens inside a processing plant using the ELISA technique with an ^{125}I-radiolabel (Weytjens et al., 1999). Using the same approach, Beaudet's group studied aerosolized crab levels aboard crab processing vessels in Alaska, where the concentration of crab allergen was reported to be similar across all job categories (Beaudet et al., 2002). ELISA techniques with a colorimetric detection system were developed for measuring the fish aeroallergen in processing plants (Lopata et al., 2005). In 2005, Jeebhay et al. quantified the level of aeroallergens to study the correlation between the levels of the aerosolized allergens and other major determinants of variability in an attempt to establish dose-response relationships for asthma due to fish antigen exposure (Jeebhay et al., 2008; 2005). Another comprehensive study was performed for examining the levels of bioaerosols in the seafood industry using the ELISA reader for quantification purposes (Bang et al., 2005). Recently, the aeroallergen levels of snow crab and northern shrimp in harvesting vessels and processing plants were measured directly using tandem MS techniques. The TM and the AK were detected in their aerosolized form in the processing plants; however, TM was the only allergen detected aboard the vessels holds and decks (Abdel Rahman et al., 2012; 2011; 2010c). Table 3 summarizes the results of the various exposure characterization studies conducted and demonstrates the wide range of total inhalable airborne particulate (0.001-11.293 mg/m^3), protein (0.001-6.4 mg/m^3) and allergen (0.001-75.748 mg/m^3) levels (Jeebhay & Cartier, 2010). Particulate and allergen levels reach very high levels in the processing operations aboard vessels at sea in the case of crab processing and during fishmeal operations.

In conclusion, the development of novel methods to characterize airborne seafood allergens have the potential to introduce accurate, sensitive, and specific advanced monitoring approaches that will contribute towards strategies to minimize allergen exposures among

Seafood Category		Particle fraction measured	Particulate conc. (mg/m³) Range	Protein conc. (mg/m³) Range	Allergen (µg/m³) Range
Crustaceans	crabs (snow, Tanner, common, King)	total inhalable	0.001-0.680	0.001-6.400	0.001-5.061
	crabs (snow)*	total inhalable	ND	ND	0.001-5.061
	crabs (snow, Tanner, common, King)	total inhalable	ND	ND	0.079-21.093
	prawns	total inhalable	0.100-3.300	ND	ND
	shrimp	total inhalable	ND	ND	1.500-6.260
	rock lobster	thoracic	LOD-0.661	LOD-0.002	ND
	scampi	total inhalable	ND	ND	0.047-1.042
Finfish	salmon	respirable	0.040-3.570	ND	0.100-1.00
	pollock	total inhalable	0.004	ND	ND
	whiff megrim/hake	total inhalable	ND	ND	0.002-0.025
	pilchard	thoracic	LOD-2.954	LOD-0.006	0.010-0.898
	cod	total inhalable	ND	ND	3.800-5.100
	salmon	total inhalable	ND	ND	LOD-1.600
	herring	total inhalable	ND	ND	0.300-1.900
	fishmeal (anchovy)	thoracic	LOD-11.293	LOD-0.004	0.069-75.748
	shark cartilage**	Respirable total inhalable	0.920 - 5.140 26.400 - 44.700	ND ND	ND ND

ND: Not done, LOD: Limit of detection,
* processing aboard vessels; and
** non-food-handling environment

Table 3. Exposure assessment studies of seafood processing workers on land and aboard vessels (Reproduced with permission from (Jeebhay & Cartier, 2010)

seafood processing workers in the seafood industry(Lopata & Jeebhay, 2007). Monitoring workplaces will contribute therefore towards engineering controls aimed at improving the ventilation and machine designs, which ultimately will decrease the incidence of asthma associated with seafood exposures.

5. References

Aas, K. & Elsayed, S. (1969). Characterization of a major allergen (cod): Effect of enzymic hydrolysis on the allergenic activity, *Journal of Allergy* 44(6): 333–343.

Aas, K. & Elsayed, S. (1975). Physico-chemical properties and specific activity of a purified allergen (codfish), *Developments in biological standardization* 29: 90–98.

Aas, K. & Lundkvist, U. (1973). The radioallergosorbent test with a purified allergen from codfish, *Clinical & Experimental Allergy* 3(3): 255–261.

Abdel Rahman, A., Gagne, S. & Helleur, R. (2012). Simultaneous determination of two major snow crab aeroallergens in processing plants by use of isotopic dilution tandem mass spectrometry, *Anal. Bioanal. Chem* (In press)DOI: *http://dx.doi.org/10.1007/s00216-012-5873-2*

Abdel Rahman, A., Kamath, S., Lopata, A. & Helleur, R. (2010a). Analysis of the allergenic proteins in black tiger prawn (penaeus monodon) and characterization of the major allergen tropomyosin using mass spectrometry, *Rapid communications in mass spectrometry* 24(16): 2462–2470.

Abdel Rahman, A., Kamath, S., Lopata, A., Robinson, J. & Helleur, R. (2011). Biomolecular characterization of allergenic proteins in snow crab (chionoecetes opilio) and de novo sequencing of the second allergen arginine kinase using tandem mass spectrometry, *Journal of proteomics* 74(2): 231–241.

Abdel Rahman, A., Lopata, A., O'Hehir, R., Robinson, J., Banoub, J. & Helleur, R. (2010b). Characterization and de novo sequencing of snow crab tropomyosin enzymatic peptides by both electrospary ionization and matrix-assisted laser desorption ionization qqtof tandem mass spectrometry, *Journal of Mass Spectrometry* 45(4): 372–381.

Abdel Rahman, A., Lopata, A., Randell, E. & Helleur, R. (2010c). Absolute quantification method and validation of airborne snow crab allergen tropomyosin using tandem mass spectrometry, *Analytica chimica acta* 681(1-2): 49–55.

Aebersold, R. & Mann, M. (2003). Mass spectrometry-based proteomics, *Nature* 422(6928): 198–207.

Asturias, J., Eraso, E., Arilla, M., Gómez-Bayón, N., Inácio, F. & Martínez, A. (2000). Cloning, isolation, and ige-binding properties of helix aspersa (brown garden snail) tropomyosin, *International archives of allergy and immunology* 128(2): 90–96.

Aukrust, L., Grimmer, O. & Aas, K. (1978). Demonstration of distinct allergens by means of immunological methods, *International Archives of Allergy and Immunology* 57(2): 183–192.

Ayuso, R., Grishina, G., Bardina, L., Carrillo, T., Blanco, C., Ibáñez, M., Sampson, H. & Beyer, K. (2008). Myosin light chain is a novel shrimp allergen, lit v 3, *Journal of Allergy and Clinical Immunology* 122(4): 795–802.

Ayuso, R., Grishina, G., Ibáñez, M., Blanco, C., Carrillo, T., Bencharitiwong, R., Sánchez, S., Nowak-Wegrzyn, A. & Sampson, H. (2009). Sarcoplasmic calcium-binding protein is an ef-hand-type protein identified as a new shrimp allergen, *Journal of Allergy and Clinical Immunology* 124(1): 114–120.

Ayuso, R., Sánchez-Garcia, S., Lin, J., Fu, Z., Ibáñez, M., Carrillo, T., Blanco, C., Goldis, M., Bardina, L., Sastre, J. et al. (2010). Greater epitope recognition of shrimp allergens by children than by adults suggests that shrimp sensitization decreases with age, *Journal of Allergy and Clinical Immunology* 125(6): 1286–1293.

Azofra, J. & Lombardero, M. (2003). Limpet anaphylaxis: cross-reactivity between limpet and house-dust mite dermatophagoides pteronyssinus, *Allergy* 58(2): 146–149.

Bang, B., Aasmoe, L., Aamodt, B., Aardal, L., Andorsen, G., Bolle, R., Bøe, R., Van, T., Evans, R., Florvåg, E. et al. (2005). Exposure and airway effects of seafood industry workers in northern norway, *Journal of occupational and environmental medicine* 47(5): 482.

Beale, J., Jeebhay, M. & Lopata, A. (2009). Characterisation of purified parvalbumin from five fish species and nucleotide sequencing of this major allergen from pacific pilchard, sardinops sagax, *Molecular immunology* 46(15): 2985–2993.

Beaudet, N., Brodkin, C., Stover, B., Daroowalla, F., Flack, J. & Doherty, D. (2002). Crab allergen exposures aboard five crab-processing vessels, *Aiha Journal* 63(5): 605–609.

Besler, M., Eigenmann, P. & Schwartz, R. (2000). Allergen data collection: Cow's milk (bos domesticus), *Internet Symposium on Food Allergens*, Publisher, conference location, pp. 9–74.

Besler, M., Steinhart, H. & Paschke, A. (2001). Stability of food allergens and allergenicity of processed foods, *Journal of Chromatography B: Biomedical Sciences and Applications* 756(1-2): 207–228.

Bi, X. & Chew, F. (2004). Molecular, proteomic and immunological characterization of isoforms of arginine kinase, a cross-reactive invertebrate pan-allergen, from the house dust mite, dermatophagoides farinae, *Journal of Allergy and Clinical Immunology* 113(2): S226–S226.

Binder, M., Mahler, V., Hayek, B., Sperr, W., Schöller, M., Prozell, S., Wiedermann, G., Valent, P., Valenta, R. & Duchêne, M. (2001). Molecular and immunological characterization of arginine kinase from the indianmeal moth, plodia interpunctella, a novel cross-reactive invertebrate pan-allergen, *The Journal of Immunology* 167(9): 5470.

Bobolea, I., Barranco, P., Pastor-Vargas, C., Iraola, V., Vivanco, F. & Quirce, S. (2010). Arginine kinase from the cellar spider (holocnemus pluchei): A new asthma-causing allergen, *International Archives of Allergy and Immunology* 155(2): 180–186.

Brun, V., Masselon, C., Garin, J. & Dupuis, A. (2009). Isotope dilution strategies for absolute quantitative proteomics, *Journal of proteomics* 72(5): 740–749.

Bugajska-Schretter, A., Grote, M., Vangelista, L., Valent, P., Sperr, W., Rumpold, H., Pastore, A., Reichelt, R., Valenta, R. & Spitzauer, S. (2000). Purification, biochemical, and immunological characterisation of a major food allergen: different immunoglobulin e recognition of the apo-and calcium-bound forms of carp parvalbumin, *Gut* 46(5): 661.

Cai, Q., Liu, G., Li, T., Hara, K., Wang, X., Su, W. & Cao, M. (2010). Purification and characterization of parvalbumins, the major allergens in red stingray (dasyatis akajei), *Journal of agricultural and food chemistry* 58(24): 12964–12969.

Carrera, M., Canas, B., Vazquez, J. & Gallardo, J. (2010). Extensive de novo sequencing of new parvalbumin isoforms using a novel combination of bottom-up proteomics, accurate molecular mass measurement by fticr-ms and selected ms/ms ion monitoring, *Journal of Proteome Research* 9(9): 4393–4406.

Chait, B. (2004). Chemistry: Mass spectrometry: Bottom-up or top-down?, *Neuroscience* 123: 931.

Chen, L., Hefle, S., Taylor, S., Swoboda, I. & Goodman, R. (2006). Detecting fish parvalbumin with commercial mouse monoclonal anti-frog parvalbumin igg, *Journal of agricultural and food chemistry* 54(15): 5577–5582.

Daul, C., Morgan, J., Hughes, J. & Lehrer, S. (1988). Provocation-challenge studies in shrimp-sensitive individuals, *Journal of allergy and clinical immunology* 81(6): 1180–1186.

Daul, C., Slattery, M., Reese, G. & Lehrer, S. (1994). Identification of the major brown shrimp (penaeus aztecus) allergen as the muscle protein tropomyosin, *International archives of allergy and immunology* 105(1): 49–55.

Dearnaley, D., Kote-Jarai, Z. & Eeles, R. (2010). Dietary fat and early-onset prostate cancer risk, *British Journal of Nutrition* 103(9): 1375–1380.

DeHoffmann, E. & Stroobant, V. (2007). *Mass spectrometry: principles and applications*, Wiley-Interscience.

Desiderio, D. & Kai, M. (1983). Preparation of stable isotope-incorporated peptide internal standards for field desorption mass spectrometry quantification of peptides in biologic tissue, *Biological Mass Spectrometry* 10(8): 471–479.

DeWitt, Å., Mattsson, L., Lauer, I., Reese, G. & Lidholm, J. (2004). Recombinant tropomyosin from penaeus aztecus (rpen a 1) for measurement of specific immuno-globulin e antibodies relevant in food allergy to crustaceans and other invertebrates, *Molecular nutrition & food research* 48(5): 370–379.

Do, T. V., Hordvik, I., Endresen, C. & Elsayed, S. (1999). Expression and analysis of recombinant salmon parvalbumin, the major allergen in atlantic salmon (salmo salar), *Scandinavian Journal of Immunology* 50(6): 619–625.

Eidhammer, I., Flikka, K., Martens, L. & Mikalsen, S. (2007). *Computational methods for mass spectrometry proteomics*, Wiley Online Library.

Elsayed, S. & Aas, K. (1970). Characterization of a major allergen (cod). chemical composition and immunological properties, *International Archives of Allergy and Immunology* 38(5): 536–548.

Escudero, R., Gamboa, P., Anton, J. & Sanz, M. (2007). Food allergy due to trout roe., *Journal of investigational allergology & clinical immunology: official organ of the International Association of Asthmology (INTERASMA) and Sociedad Latinoamericana de Alergia e Inmunología* 17(5): 346.

Faeste, C. & Plassen, C. (2008). Quantitative sandwich elisa for the determination of fish in foods, *Journal of immunological methods* 329(1-2): 45–55.

Faeste, C., Ronning, H., Christians, U. & Granum, P. (2011). Liquid chromatography and mass spectrometry in food allergen detection, *Journal of Food Protection* 74(2): 316–345.

Food and Drug Administration, U. (2001). Guidance for industry: bioanalytical method validation, *Rockville, MD: CDER* .

Findlay, J., Geisow & Michael, J. (1989). *Protein Sequencing, Practical Approach Series*, Oxford University Press.

Food and Agriculture Organisation (FAO) (2007). The state of world fisheries and aquaculture. URL: *http://www.fao.org/docrep/013/i1820e/i1820e00.htm, accessed on 30 March 2011*

Food and Agriculture Organisation (FAO) (2010). The state of world fisheries and aquaculture. URL: *http://www.fao.org/docrep/013/i1820e/i1820e00.htm, accessed on 30 March 2011*

France, R., Sellers, D. & Grossman, S. (1997). Purification, characterization, and hydrodynamic properties of arginine kinase from gulf shrimp (penaeus aztecus)* 1, *Archives of biochemistry and biophysics* 345(1): 73–78.

Gajewski, K. & Hsieh, Y. (2009). Monoclonal antibody specific to a major fish allergen: parvalbumin, *Journal of Food Protection* 72(4): 818–825.

García-Orozco, K., Aispuro-Hernández, E., Yepiz-Plascencia, G., Calderón-de-la Barca, A. & Sotelo-Mundo, R. (2007). Molecular characterization of arginine kinase, an allergen from the shrimp(litopenaeus vannamei), *International archives of allergy and immunology* 144(1): 23–28.

Garone, L., Theibert, J., Miegel, A., Maeda, Y., Murphy, C. & Collins, J. (1991). Lobster troponin c: amino acid sequences of three isoforms, *Archives of biochemistry and biophysics* 291(1): 89–91.

Gimenez-Arnau, A., Maurer, M., De La Cuadra, J. & Maibach, H. (2008). Immediate contact skin reactions, an update of contact urticaria, contact urticaria syndrome and protein contact dermatitis–"a never ending story", *European Journal of Dermatology* 1(1).

Greenberg, M. I., Hamilton, R. J. andPhillips, S. D. & McCluskey, G. J. (2003). *Occupational, industrial, and environmental toxocology*, Mosby.

Gupta, R., Sheikh, A., Strachan, D. & Anderson, H. (2007). Time trends in allergic disorders in the uk, *Thorax* 62(1): 91–96.

Habsah, M., Amran, M., Mackeen, M., Lajis, N., Kikuzaki, H., Nakatani, N., Rahman, A. et al. (2000). Screening of zingiberaceae extracts for antimicrobial and antioxidant activities, *Journal of ethnopharmacology* 72(3): 403–410.

Halmepuro, L., Salvaggio, J. & Lehrer, S. (1987). Crawfish and lobster allergens: identification and structural similarities with other crustacea, *International Archives of Allergy and Immunology* 84(2): 165–172.

Hamada, Y., Nagashima, Y. & Shiomi, K. (2004). Reactivity of serum immunoglobulin e to bullfrog rana catesbeiana parvalbumins in fish-allergic patients, *Fisheries Science* 70(6): 1137–1143.

Hoffman, D., Day Jr, E. & Miller, J. (1981). The major heat stable allergen of shrimp., *Annals of allergy* 47(1): 17.

Howse, D., Gautrin, D., Neis, B., Cartier, A., Horth-Susin, L., Jong, M. & Swanson, M. (2006). Gender and snow crab occupational asthma in newfoundland and labrador, canada, *Environmental research* 101(2): 163–174.

Huang, Y., Liu, G., Cai, Q., Weng, W., Maleki, S., Su, W. & Cao, M. (2010). Stability of major allergen tropomyosin and other food proteins of mud crab (scylla serrata) by in vitro gastrointestinal digestion, *Food and Chemical Toxicology* 48(5): 1196–1201.

Hungerford, J. (2006). Committee on natural toxins and food allergens: Marine and freshwater toxins, *Journal of AOAC International* 89(1): 248–269.

Hungerford, J. & Trucksess, M. (2005). Committee on natural toxins and food allergens: Marine and freshwater toxins: Mycotoxins, *Journal of AOAC International* 88(1): 299–324.

Ishikawa, M., Ishida, M., Shimakura, K., Nagashima, Y. & Shiomi, K. (1998a). Purification and ige-binding epitopes of a major allergen in the gastropod turbo cornutus, *Bioscience, biotechnology, and biochemistry* 62(7): 1337–1343.

Ishikawa, M., Ishida, M., Shimakura, K., Nagashima, Y. & Shiomi, K. (1998b). Tropomyosin, the major oyster crassostrea gigas allergen and its ige-binding epitopes, *Journal of food science* 63(1): 44–47.

James, J. & Crespo, J. (2007). Allergic reactions to foods by inhalation, *Current allergy and asthma reports* 7(3): 167–174.

Jauregui-Adell, J., Wnuk, W. & Cox, J. (1989). Complete amino acid sequence of the sarcoplasmic calcium-binding protein (scp-i) from crayfish (astacus leptodactilus), *FEBS letters* 243(2): 209–212.

Jeebhay, M. & Cartier, A. (2010). Seafood workers and respiratory disease: an update, *Current opinion in allergy and clinical immunology* 10(2): 104–113.

Jeebhay, M., Robins, T., Lehrer, S. & Lopata, A. (2001). Occupational seafood allergy: a review, *Occupational and environmental medicine* 58(9): 553–562.

Jeebhay, M., Robins, T., Miller, M., Bateman, E., Smuts, M., Baatjies, R. & Lopata, A. (2008). Occupational allergy and asthma among salt water fish processing workers, *American journal of industrial medicine* 51(12): 899–910.

Jeebhay, M., Robins, T., Seixas, N., Baatjies, R., George, D., Rusford, E., Lehrer, S. & Lopata, A. (2005). Environmental exposure characterization of fish processing workers, *Annals of Occupational Hygiene* 49(5): 423–437.

Jenkins, J., Breiteneder, H. & Mills, E. (2007). Evolutionary distance from human homologs reflects allergenicity of animal food proteins, *Journal of Allergy and Clinical Immunology* 120(6): 1399–1405.

Jeoung, B., Reese, G., Hauck, P., Oliver, J., Daul, C. B. & Lehrer, S. (1997). Quantification of the major brown shrimp allergen pen a 1 (tropomyosin) by a monoclonal antibody-based sandwich elisa, *Journal of allergy and clinical immunology* 100(2): 229–234.

Juji, F., Takashima, H., Suko, M., Doi, M., Takaishi, T., Okudaira, H., Ito, K. & Miyamoto, T. (1990). A case of food-dependent-exercise induced anaphylaxis possibly induced by shellfish (sulculus supertexta and turbo cornutus), *Arerugī=[Allergy]* 39(11): 1515–1522.

Kelleher, N., Lin, H., Valaskovic, G., Aaserud, D., Fridriksson, E. & McLafferty, F. (1999). Top down versus bottom up protein characterization by tandem high-resolution mass spectrometry, *Journal of the American Chemical Society* 121(4): 806–812.

Kinter, M. & Sherman, N. (2000). *Protein sequencing and identification using tandem mass spectrometry*, LibreDigital.

Kobayashi, T., Takagi, T., Konishi, K. & Cox, J. (1989). Amino acid sequence of crayfish troponin i, *Journal of Biological Chemistry* 264(3): 1551–1557.

Koshte, V., Kagen, S. & Aalberse, R. (1989). Cross-reactivity of ige antibodies to caddis fly with arthropoda and mollusca, *Journal of Allergy and Clinical Immunology* 84(2): 174–183.

Koyama, H., Kakami, M., Kawamura, M., Tokuda, R., Kondo, Y., Tsuge, I., Yamada, K., Yasuda, T. & Urisu, A. (2006). Grades of 43 fish species in japan based on ige-binding activity, *Allergology International* 55: 311–316.

Kuehn, A., Scheuermann, T., Hilger, C. & Hentges, F. (2010). Important variations in parvalbumin content in common fish species: A factor possibly contributing to variable allergenicity, *International archives of allergy and immunology* 153(4): 359–366.

Kunimoto, A., Sisino, T., Sakai, K., Matsumoto, T., Takahashi, K., Yamashita, H., Hiemori, M., Tsuji, H. & Kimoto, M. (2009). Molecular cloning and allergenicity of pen j 1, a major allergen of kuruma prawn, penaeus japonicus, *Bioscience, biotechnology, and biochemistry* 73(4): 840–848.

Lehky, P., Blum, H., Stein, E. & Fischer, E. (1974). Isolation and characterization of parvalbumins from the skeletal muscle of higher vertebrates, *Journal of Biological Chemistry* 249(13): 4332–4334.

Lehrer, S., Horner, W., Reese, G. & Taylor, S. (1996). Why are some proteins allergenic? implications for biotechnology, *Critical reviews in food science and nutrition* 36(6): 553–564.

Lehrer, S. & McCants, M. (1987). Reactivity of ige antibodies with crustacea and oyster allergens: evidence for common antigenic structures, *The Journal of allergy and clinical immunology* 80(2): 133–139.

Lehrer, S., McCants, M. & Salvaggio, J. (1985). Identification of crustacea allergens by crossed radioimmunoelectrophoresis, *International Archives of Allergy and Immunology* 77(1-2): 192–194.

Leung, P., Chow, W., Duffey, S., Kwan, H., Gershwin, M. & Chu, K. (1996). Ige reactivity against a cross-reactive allergen in crustacea and mollusca: evidence for tropomyosin as the common allergen, *Journal of allergy and clinical immunology* 98(5): 954–961.

Leung, P. & Chu, K. (1998). Molecular and immunological characterization of shellfish allergens, *Front Biosci* 3: 306–312.

Leung, P., Chu, K., Chow, W. & andC.I. Bandea, A. A. (1994). Cloning, expression, and primary structure of metapenaeus ensis tropomyosin, the major heat-stable shrimp allergen, *Journal of allergy and clinical immunology* 94(5): 882–890.

Liang, Y., Cao, M., Su, W., Zhang, L., Huang, Y. & Liu, G. (2008). Identification and characterisation of the major allergen of chinese mitten crab (eriocheir sinensis), *Food Chemistry* 111(4): 998–1003.

Lim, D., Neo, K., Yi, F., Chua, K., Goh, D., Shek, L., Giam, Y., Bever, H. V. & Lee, B. (2008). Parvalbumin–the major tropical fish allergen, *Pediatric Allergy and Immunology* 19(5): 399–407.

Lin, R., Shen, H. & Han, S. (1993). Identification and characterization of a 30 kd major allergen from parapenaeus fissurus, *Journal of allergy and clinical immunology* 92(6): 837–845.

Liu, G., Cao, M., Huang, Y., Cai, Q., Weng, W. & Su, W. (2010). Comparative study of in vitro digestibility of major allergen tropomyosin and other food proteins of chinese mitten crab (eriocheir sinensis), *Journal of the Science of Food and Agriculture* 90(10): 1614–1620.

Liu, G., Huang, Y., Cai, Q., Weng, W., Su, W. & Cao, M. (2011). Comparative study of in vitro digestibility of major allergen, tropomyosin and other proteins between grass prawn (penaeus monodon) and pacific white shrimp (litopenaeus vannamei), *Journal of the Science of Food and Agriculture* 91(1): 163–170.

Liu, Z., Xia, L., Wu, Y., Xia, Q., Chen, J. & Roux, K. (2009). Identification and characterization of an arginine kinase as a major allergen from silkworm (bombyx mori) larvae, *International archives of allergy and immunology* 150(1): 8–14.

Lopata, A. & Jeebhay, M. (2001). Seafood allergy in south africa studies in the domestic and occupational setting, *Allergy and Clinical Immunology International* 13(5): 204–209.

Lopata, A. & Jeebhay, M. (2007). Allergy and asthma to indigenous seafood species in south africa, *Current Allergy & Clinical Immunology* 20(4): 197–200.

Lopata, A., Jeebhay, M., Reese, G., Fernandes, J., Swoboda, I., Robins, T. & Lehrer, S. (2005). Detection of fish antigens aerosolized during fish processing using newly developed immunoassays, *International archives of allergy and immunology* 138(1): 21–28.

Lopata, A. & Lehrer, S. (2009). New insights into seafood allergy, *Current opinion in allergy and clinical immunology* 9(3): 270–277.

Lopata, A., O'Hehir, R. & Lehrer, S. (2010). Shellfish allergy, *Clinical & Experimental Allergy* 40(6): 850–858.

Lopata, A., Zinn, C. & Potter, P. (1997). Characteristics of hypersensitivity reactions and identification of a unique 49 kd ige-binding protein (hal-m-1) in abalone (haliotis midae), *Journal of allergy and clinical immunology* 100(5): 642–648.

Ma, Y., Griesmeier, U., Susani, M., Radauer, C., Briza, P., Erler, A., Bublin, M., Alessandri, S., Himly, M., Vázquez-Cortés, S. et al. (2008). Comparison of natural and recombinant forms of the major fish allergen parvalbumin from cod and carp, *Allergenic and physico-chemical properties of parvalbumins* 52(Suppl 2): S196–207.

Mabe, D., Singh, T., Bello, B., Jeebhay, M., Lopata, A. & Wadee, A. (2009). Allergenicity of latex rubber products used in south african dental schools, *SAMJ: South African Medical Journal* 99(9): 672–674.

Maeda, S., Morikawa, A., Kato, M., Motegi, Y., Shigeta, M., Tokuyama, K., Kuroume, T., Naritomi, Y., Suehiro, K. & Kusaba, K. (1991). 11 cases of anaphylaxis caused by grand keyhole limpet (abalone like shellfish), *Arerugī=[Allergy]* 40(11): 1415.

Malo, J. & Cartier, A. (1993). Occupational reactions in the seafood industry, *Clinical Reviews in Allergy and Immunology* 11(2): 223–240.

Malo, J., Chretien, P., McCants, M. & Lehrer, S. (1997). Detection of snow-crab antigens by air sampling of a snow-crab production plant, *Clinical & Experimental Allergy* 27(1): 75–78.

Marko-Varga, G., Lindberg, H., Löfdahl, C., Jönsson, P., Hansson, L., Dahlbäck, M., Lindquist, E., Johansson, L., Foster, M. & Fehniger, T. (2005). Discovery of biomarker candidates within disease by protein profiling: principles and concepts, *Journal of proteome research* 4(4): 1200–1212.

Martins, L., Peltre, G., da Costa Faro, C., Vieira Pires, E. & da Cruz Inácio, F. (2004). The helix aspersa (brown garden snail) allergen repertoire, *International archives of allergy and immunology* 136(1): 7–15.

Mazzeo, M., Giulio, B., Guerriero, G., Ciarcia, G., Malorni, A., Russo, G. & Siciliano, R. (2008). Fish authentication by maldi-tof mass spectrometry, *Journal of agricultural and food chemistry* 56(23): 11071–11076.

Misnan, R., Murad, S., Jones, M., Taylor, G., Rahman, D., Arip, M., Abdullah, N. & Mohamed, J. (2010). Identification of the major allergens of indian scad (decapterus russelli), *Asian Pacific Journal of Allergy and Immunology* 26(4): 191–198.

Miyazawa, H., Fukamachi, H., Inagaki, Y., Reese, G., Daul, C., Lehrer, S., Inouye, S. & Sakaguchi, M. (1996). Identification of the first major allergen of a squid (todarodes pacificus), *Journal of allergy and clinical immunology* 98(5): 948–953.

Morgan, J., O'Neil, C., Daul, C. & Lehrer, S. (1989). Species-specific shrimp allergens: Rast and rast-inhibition studies, *Journal of allergy and clinical immunology* 83(6): 1112–1117.

Motoyama, K., Suma, Y., Ishizaki, S., Nagashima, Y., Lu, Y., Ushio, H. & Shiomi, K. (2008). Identification of tropomyosins as major allergens in antarctic krill and mantis shrimp and their amino acid sequence characteristics, *Marine Biotechnology* 10(6): 709–718.

Motoyama, K., Suma, Y., Ishizaki, S., Nagashima, Y. & Shiomi, K. (2007). Molecular cloning of tropomyosins identified as allergens in six species of crustaceans, *Journal of agricultural and food chemistry* 55(3): 985–991.

Mykles, D., Cotton, J., Taniguchi, H., Sano, K. & Maeda, Y. (1998). Cloning of tropomyosins from lobster (homarus americanus) striated muscles: fast and slow isoforms may be generated from the same transcript, *Journal of muscle research and cell motility* 19(2): 105–115.

Nagano, T., Kanao, K. & Sugai, T. (1984). Allergic contact urticaria caused by raw prawns and shrimps: three cases, *Journal of allergy and clinical immunology* 74(4): 489–493.

Nakamura, R., Satoh, R., Nakajima, Y., Kawasaki, N., Yamaguchi, T., Sawada, J., Nagoya, H. & Teshima, R. (2009). Comparative study of gh-transgenic and non-transgenic amago salmon (oncorhynchus masou ishikawae) allergenicity and proteomic analysis of amago salmon allergens, *Regulatory Toxicology and Pharmacology* 55(3): 300–308.

Nakano, S., Yoshinuma, T. & Yamada, T. (2007). Reactivity of shrimp allergy-related ige antibodies to krill tropomyosin, *International archives of allergy and immunology* 145(3): 175–181.

Nordlee, J. & S.L.Taylor (1995). Immunological analysis of food allergens and other food proteins, *Food technology (USA)* .

Old, W., Meyer-Arendt, K., Aveline-Wolf, L., Pierce, K., Mendoza, A., Sevinsky, J., Resing, K. & Ahn, N. (2005). Comparison of label-free methods for quantifying human proteins by shotgun proteomics, *Molecular & Cellular Proteomics* 4(10): 1487.

ONeil, C., Helbling, A. & Lehrer, S. (1993). Allergic reactions to fish, *Clinical Reviews in Allergy and Immunology* 11(2): 183–200.

Oyelaran, O. & Gildersleeve, J. (2010). Evaluation of human antibody responses to keyhole limpet hemocyanin on a carbohydrate microarray, *PROTEOMICS–Clinical Applications* 4(3): 285–294.

Pascual, C., Esteban, M. & Crespo, J. (1992). Fish allergy: evaluation of the importance of cross-reactivity, *The Journal of pediatrics* 121(5): S29–S34.

Perez-Gordo, M., Cuesta-Herranz, J., Maroto, A., Cases, B., Ibáñez, M., Vivanco, F. & Pastor-Vargas, C. (2011). Identification of sole parvalbumin as a major allergen: study of cross-reactivity between parvalbumins in a spanish fish-allergic population, *Clinical & Experimental Allergy* 41(5): 750–758.

Perez-Gordo, M., Sanchez-Garcia, S., Cases, B., Pastor, C., Vivanco, F. & Cuesta-Herranz, J. (2008). Identification of vitellogenin as an allergen in beluga caviar allergy, *Allergy* 63(4): 479–480.

Permyakov, S., Karnoup, A., Bakunts, A. & Permyakov, E. (2009). Sequence microheterogeneity of parvalbumin pi 5.0 of pike: A mass spectrometric study, *Biochimica et Biophysica Acta (BBA)-Proteins & Proteomics* 1794(1): 129–136.

Rabilloud, T. (2000). *Proteome research: two-dimensional gel electrophoresis and identification methods*, Springer verlag.

Reese, G., Jeoung, B., Daul, C. & Lehrer, S. (1997). Characterization of recombinant shrimp allergen pen a 1 (tropomyosin), *International archives of allergy and immunology* 113(1-3): 240–242.

Rehbein, H. & Lopata, A. (2011). Presence of parvalbumin in different tissues of three sturgeon species (acipenser baeri, a. gueldenstaedtii, a. ruthenus), *Journal of Applied Ichthyology* 27(2): 219–225.

Reid, G. & McLuckey, S. (2002). 'top-down' protein characterization via tandem mass spectrometry, *Journal of mass spectrometry* 37(7): 663–675.

Rejeb, S. B., Davies, D., Cleroux, C., Langlois, D. & Delahaut, P. (2002). Enzyme immunoassay for the detection of crustacean proteins in foods, Publisher, conference location, p. 102.

Rodriguez, J., Reano, M., Vives, R., Canto, G., Daroca, P., Crespo, J., Vila, C., Villarreal, O. & Bensabat, Z. (1997). Occupational asthma caused by fish inhalation, *Allergy* 52(8): 866–869.

Rosmilah, M., Shahnaz, M., Masita, A., Noormalin, A. & Jamaludin, M. (2005). Identification of major allergens of two species of local snappers: Lutjanus argentimaculatus (merah/red snapper) and lutjanus johnii (jenahak/golden snapper), *Trop Biomed* 22(2): 171–177.

Sakaguchi, M., Toda, M., Ebihara, T., Irie, S., Hori, H., Imai, A., Yanagida, M., Miyazawa, H., Ohsuna, H., Ikezawa, Z. et al. (2000). Ige antibody to fish gelatin (type i collagen) in patients with fish allergy, *Journal of allergy and clinical immunology* 106(3): 579–584.

Scherperel, G. & Reid, G. (2007). Emerging methods in proteomics: top-down protein characterization by multistage tandem mass spectrometry, *Analyst* 132(6): 500–506.

Schulze, W. & Usadel, B. (2010). Quantitation in mass-spectrometry-based proteomics, *Annual review of plant biology* 61: 491–516.

Seiki, K., Oda, H., Yoshioka, H., Sakai, S., Urisu, A., Akiyama, H. & Ohno, Y. (2007). A reliable and sensitive immunoassay for the determination of crustacean protein in processed foods, *Journal of agricultural and food chemistry* 55(23): 9345–9350.

Shanti, K., Martin, B., Nagpal, S., Metcalfe, D. & Rao, P. (1993). Identification of tropomyosin as the major shrimp allergen and characterization of its ige-binding epitopes, *The Journal of Immunology* 151(10): 5354.

Shen, Y., Cao, M., Cai, Q., Su, W., Yu, H., Ruan, W. & Liu, G. (2011). Purification, cloning, expression and immunological analysis of scylla serrata arginine kinase, the crab allergen, *Journal of the Science of Food and Agriculture* 91(7): 1326–1335.

Shibahara, Y., Yamada, I., Uesaka, Y., Uneo, N., Abe, A., Ohashi, E. & Shiomi, K. (2009). Extraction method suitable for detection of unheated crustaceans including cephalothorax by elisa., *Shokuhin Eiseigaku Zasshi= Journal of the Food Hygienic Society of Japan* 50(4): 153–159.

Shiomi, K., Sato, Y., Hamamoto, S., Mita, H. & Shimakura, K. (2008). Sarcoplasmic calcium-binding protein: Identification as a new allergen of the black tiger shrimp (penaeus monodon), *International archives of allergy and immunology* 146(2): 91–98.

Sicherer, S., Muñoz-Furlong, A. & Sampson, H. (2004). Prevalence of seafood allergy in the united states determined by a random telephone survey, *Journal of allergy and clinical immunology* 114(1): 159–165.

Siuti, N. & Kelleher, N. (2007). Decoding protein modifications using top-down mass spectrometry, *Nature methods* 4(10): 817–821.

Suma, Y., Ishizaki, S., Nagashima, Y., Lu, Y., Ushio, H. & Shiomi, K. (2007). Comparative analysis of barnacle tropomyosin: divergence from decapod tropomyosins and role as a potential allergen, *Comparative Biochemistry and Physiology Part B: Biochemistry and Molecular Biology* 147(2): 230–236.

Suzuki, M., Kobayashi, Y., Hiraki, Y., Nakata, H. & Shiomi, K. (2010). Paramyosin of the disk abalone haliotis discus discus: identification as a new allergen and cross-reactivity with tropomyosin, *Food Chemistry* 124(3): 921–926.

Swoboda, I., Bugajska-Schretter, A., Verdino, P., Keller, W., Sperr, W., Valent, P., Valenta, R. & Spitzauer, S. (2002). Recombinant carp parvalbumin, the major cross-reactive fish allergen: a tool for diagnosis and therapy of fish allergy, *The Journal of Immunology* 168(9): 4576–4584.

Taylor, A., Swanson, M., Jones, R., Vives, R., Rodriguez, J., Yunginger, J. & Crespo, J. (2000). Detection and quantitation of raw fish aeroallergens from an open-air fish market, *Journal of allergy and clinical immunology* 105(1): 166–169.

Taylor, S. (2008). Molluscan shellfish allergy, *Advances in Food and Nutrition Research* 54: 139–177.

Taylor, S., Hefle, S., Bindslev-Jensen, C., Bock, S., Jr, A. B., Christie, L., Hill, D., Host, A., Hourihane, J., Lack, G. et al. (2002). Factors affecting the determination of threshold doses for allergenic foods: How much is too much?, *Journal of Allergy and Clinical Immunology* 109(1): 24–30.

Taylor, S., Kabourek, J. & Hefle, S. (2004). Fish allergy: fish and products thereof, *Journal of food science* 69(8): R175–R180.

Towbin, H., Staehelin, T. & Gordon, J. (1979). Electrophoretic transfer of proteins from polyacrylamide gels to nitrocellulose sheets: procedure and some applications, *Proceedings of the National Academy of Sciences* 76(9): 4350–4354.

Towle, D. & Smith, C. (2006). Gene discovery in carcinus maenas and homarus americanus via expressed sequence tags, *Integrative and Comparative Biology* 46(6): 912–918.

Van der Ventel, M., Nieuwenhuizen, N., Kirstein, F., Hikuam, C., Jeebhay, M., Swoboda, I., Brombacher, F. & Lopata, A. (2010). Differential responses to natural and recombinant allergens in a murine model of fish allergy, *Molecular Immunology* 48(4): 637–646.

Weber, P., Steinhart, H. & Paschke, A. (2009). Competitive indirect elisa for the determination of parvalbumins from various fish species in food grade fish gelatins and isinglass with parv-19 anti-parvalbumin antibodies, *Journal of agricultural and food chemistry* 57(23): 11328–11334.

Weber, P., Steinhart, H. & Paschke, A. (2010). Characterization, antigenicity and detection of fish gelatine and isinglass used as processing aids in wines, *Food Additives & Contaminants: Part A* 27(3): 273–282.

Werner, M., Fæste, C. & Egaas, E. (2007). Quantitative sandwich elisa for the determination of tropomyosin from crustaceans in foods, *Journal of agricultural and food chemistry* 55(20): 8025–8032.

Werr, M., Cramer, J. & Ilg, T. (2009). Identification and characterization of two arginine kinases from the parasitic insect ctenocephalides felis, *Insect biochemistry and molecular biology* 39(9): 634–645.

Weytjens, K., Cartier, A., Malo, J., Chretien, P., Essiembre, F., Lehrer, S. & Swanson, M. (1999). Aerosolized snow-crab allergens in a processing facility, *Allergy* 54(8): 892–893.

White, A., Northcutt, M., Rohrback, S., Carpenter, R., Niehaus-Sauter, M., Gao, Y., Wheatly, M. & Gillen, C. (2011). Characterization of sarcoplasmic calcium binding protein (scp) variants from freshwater crayfish procambarus clarkii, *Comparative Biochemistry and Physiology Part B: Biochemistry and Molecular Biology* . in press.

Wild, L. & Lehrer, S. (2005). Fish and shellfish allergy, *Current Allergy and Asthma Reports* 5(1): 74–79.

Yamasaki, A., Higaki, H., Nakashima, K., Yamamoto, O., Hein, K., Takahashi, H., Chinuki, Y. & Morita, E. (2010). Identification of a major yolk protein as an allergen in sea urchin roe, *Acta dermato-venereologica* 90(3): 235–238.

Yao, C., Wu, C., Xiang, J. & Dong, B. (2005). Molecular cloning and response to laminarin stimulation of arginine kinase in haemolymph in chinese shrimp, fenneropenaeus chinensis, *Fish & shellfish immunology* 19(4): 317–329.

Yoon, S., Kim, H., Kim, H., Choi, J., Suh, C., Nahm, D., Kim, Y., Min, K. & Park, H. (2004). Identification of the major allergen in the shrimp (metapenaeus joyneri): Effects of heating and digestive enzymes, *Korean Journal of Asthma, Allergy and Clinical Immunology* 24(2): 211–216.

Yu, C., Lin, Y., Chiang, B. & Chow, L. (2003). Proteomics and immunological analysis of a novel shrimp allergen, pen m 2, *The Journal of Immunology* 170(1): 445–453.

Yu, H., Cao, M., Cai, Q., Weng, W., Su, W. & Liu, G. (2010). Effects of different processing methods on digestibility of scylla paramamosain allergen (tropomyosin), *Food and Chemical Toxicology* 49(4): 791–798.

Zhang, Y., Matsuo, H. & Morita, E. (2006). Cross-reactivity among shrimp, crab and scallops in a patient with a seafood allergy, *The Journal of dermatology* 33(3): 174–177.

Zhang, Z. & McElvain, J. (2000). De novo peptide sequencing by two-dimensional fragment correlation mass spectrometry, *Analytical chemistry* 72(11): 2337–2350.

6

Birch Pollen-Related Food Allergy: An Excellent Disease Model to Understand the Relevance of Immunological Cross-Reactivity for Allergy

Brinda Subbarayal, Marija Geroldinger-Simic and Barbara Bohle
Department of Pathophysiology and Allergy Research, Christian Doppler Laboratory for Immunomodulation, Medical University of Vienna, Vienna, Austria

1. Introduction

According to the position paper from the European Academy for Allergy and Clinical Immunology (EAACI) "food allergy" summarizes immune-mediated, non-toxic adverse reactions to foods (Figure 1)(Bruijnzeel-Koomen et al., 1995). The most common form of food allergy is mediated by immunoglobulin (Ig)E antibodies and reflects an immediate-type ("Type 1 hypersensitivity") reaction, i.e. acute onset of symptoms after ingestion or inhalation of foods. IgE-mediated food allergy is further classified into primary (class 1) and secondary (class 2) food allergy. This distinction is based on clinical appearance, the predominantly affected group of patients (children or adults), disease-eliciting food allergens and the underlying immune mechanisms. Primary (class 1) or "true" food allergy starts in early life and often represents the first manifestation of the atopic syndrome. The most common foods involved are cow´s milk, hen´s egg, legumes (peanuts and soybean), fish, shellfish and wheat. Of note, allergens contained in these foods do not only elicit allergic reactions in the gastrointestinal tract but often cause or influence urticaria, atopic dermatitis as well as bronchial obstruction. With a few exceptions (peanut and fish) most children outgrow class 1 food allergy within the first 3 to 6 years of life.

Secondary (class 2) food allergy describes allergic reactions to foods in mainly adolescent and adult individuals with established respiratory allergy, for example to pollen of birch, mugwort or ragweed. This form of food allergy is believed to be a consequence of immunological cross-reactivity between respiratory allergens and structurally related proteins in the respective foods. In principle, the recognition of homologous proteins in foods by IgE-antibodies specific for respiratory allergens can induce clinical symptoms. Foods inducing allergic reactions in the different groups of patients vary according to the manifested respiratory allergy. Different syndromes have been defined, such as the birch-fruit-hazelnut-vegetable syndrome, the mugwort-celery-spice syndrome or the latex-shrimp syndrome.

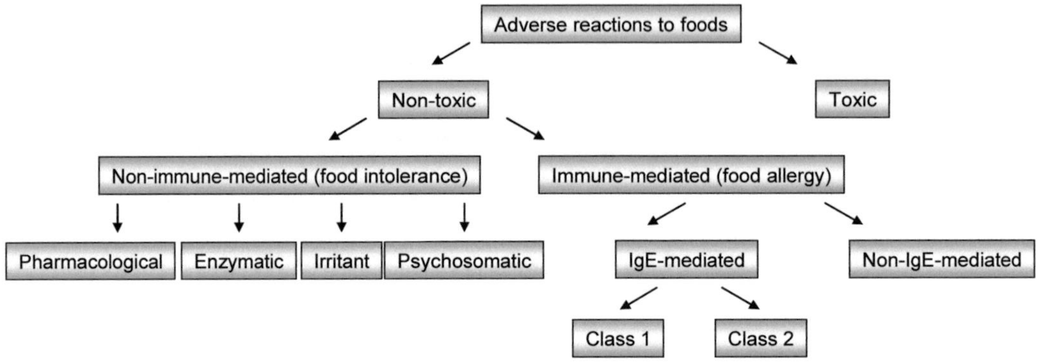

Fig. 1. Classification of adverse reactions to foods according to the pathophysiology (Bruijnzeel-Koomen et al., 1995). Adverse reactions to foods comprise toxic and non-toxic reactions. The latter reactions are either non-immune-mediated or immune-mediated. IgE-mediated reactions constitute type I hypersensitivity while non-IgE-mediated reactions are suspected to be mediated by IgG or IgM immune complex reactions (type III hypersensitivity) or cell-mediated delayed-type reactions (type IV hypersensitivity).

2. Immune mechanisms underlying IgE-mediated allergy

IgE-mediated allergy develops upon contact with an allergenic protein leading to sensitisation. The allergen is absorbed through the mucosal membrane of the respiratory or the gastrointestinal tract or the skin and can enter tissues through disrupted epithelium and gain access to antigen-presenting cells (APC), most importantly dendritic cells, which takes up allergen and migrate to lymph nodes. There they present small peptide fragments resulting from allergen processing bound to major histocompatibility complex (MHC) class II molecules to naïve $CD4^+$ Th lymphocytes. Depending on key cytokines present during the initial interaction with APC naïve $CD4^+$ cells differentiate into five different (and maybe more) "classical" effector cell subsets, Th2, Th1, Th17, Th22 cells and induced regulatory T (Treg) cells (Figure 2). The presence of interleukin (IL)-4 promotes T cell differentiation towards allergen-specific Th2 cells that produce high amounts of the signature cytokines IL-4, IL-5, IL-9 and IL-13 but little or no interferon-γ (IFN-γ). IL-4 is the major switch factor for IgE synthesis in B cells. The presence of IL-12 and IL-27 during T cell priming fosters the differentiation of Th1 cells that produce high amounts of the signature cytokine IFN-γ, which is a potent antagonist of IL-4 and inhibits the differentiation of Th2 cells. Human Th17 cells differentiate in the presence of IL-1β and IL-23. This subset synthesizes the signature cytokines IL-17a, IL-17f, IL-22 and IL-21. Th17 cells are important for the defence against extracellular bacteria and fungi and play a role in inflamed skin in atopic dermatitis. Moreover, Th17 cells have been shown to be involved in initiation and augmentation of inflammation in the airways and in the gut mucosa. Th22 cells produce IL-22 but not IL-17 and differentiate in the presence of IL-6 and TNF-α (Duhen et al., 2009). IL-22 is a growth factor for keratinocytes and Th22 cells have been considered to have a role in protective and regenerative epithelial cell responses (Eyerich et al., 2009). Induced Treg cells suppress the differentiation and effector phases of other T cell subsets either by cell-cell contact and/or by IL-10 and/or TGF-β. Different subsets of Treg cells have been described. So-called Th3 cells producing high amounts of TGF-β have been implicated as mediators of oral tolerance.

The term "Tr1 cells" was proposed for all IL-10-producing regulatory T cell populations that are induced by IL-10. Additional subsets of Treg cells may exist as well as additional subsets of effector cells, e.g. the more recently described Th9 (Veldhoen et al., 2008, Wong et al., 2010). In addition, evidence accumulates that there is a significant degree of overlap and plasticity between the different subsets of CD4+ T effector and regulatory lymphocytes.

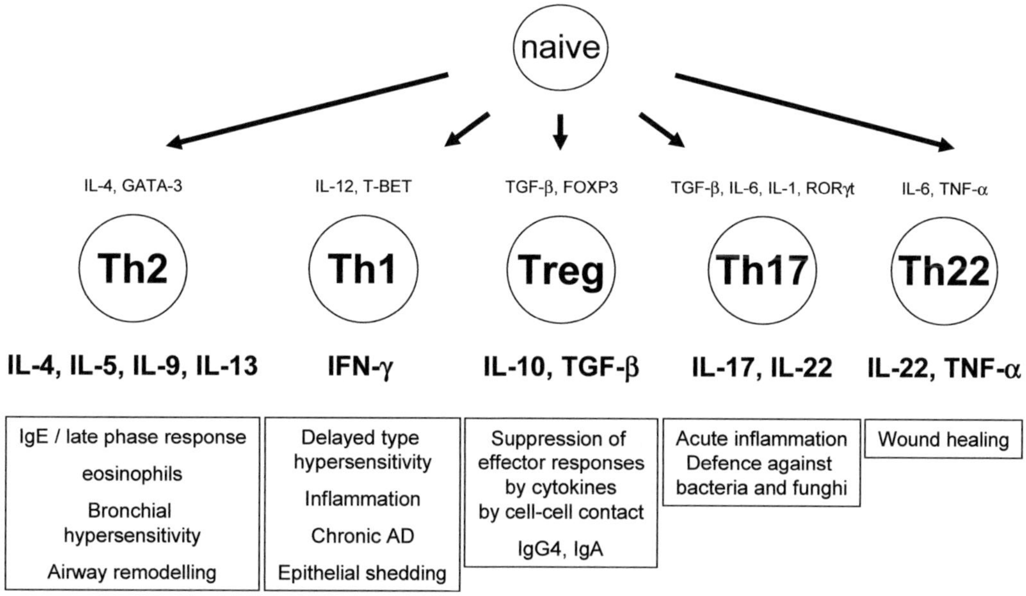

Fig. 2. Classical CD4+ T cell subsets and their role in IgE-mediated allergy. Naïve CD4+ T lymphocytes differentiate into different subsets directed by cytokines in the microenvironment during their activation *via* the T cell receptor. The presence of high concentrations of IL-4 promotes the induction of Th2 cells, IL-12 of Th1 cells, TGF-β Treg cells, TGF-β and IL-6 and/or IL-1 Th17 cells and IL-6 and TNF-α Th22 cells. The different subsets are characterized by the expression of different transcription factors (GATA-3, T-bet, Foxp3, RORγt). The transcription factor of Th22 cells has not yet been identified. Upon activation the different subsets of CD4+ effector cells produce different signature cytokines and thereby exert different effector functions.

IgE-mediated disorders result from an aberrant Th2-dominated response to allergens due to ineffective counter-regulation by allergen-specific Th1 and Treg cells. The overshooting allergen-specific Th2 response promotes the production of allergen-specific IgE antibodies which subsequently are bound to the high affinity receptor (FcεRI) on the surface of effector cells such as mast cells and basophils (Figure 3). Cross-linking of IgE by allergen induces effector cell activation and the release of preformed mediators, most importantly histamine, which cause immediate allergic symptoms. After 6-48 hours late phase reactions occur which are mediated by eosinophils and allergen-specific T cells that have migrated to the site of inflammation. Allergen-IgE-complexes bind to low affinity IgE receptors (FcεRII, CD23) expressed on lymphocytes, monocytes, macrophages and platelets. Receptor-mediated endocytosis of allergens *via* FcεRII is an important way of allergen uptake by B lymphocytes which is thought to increase allergic responses by promoting Th2 responses.

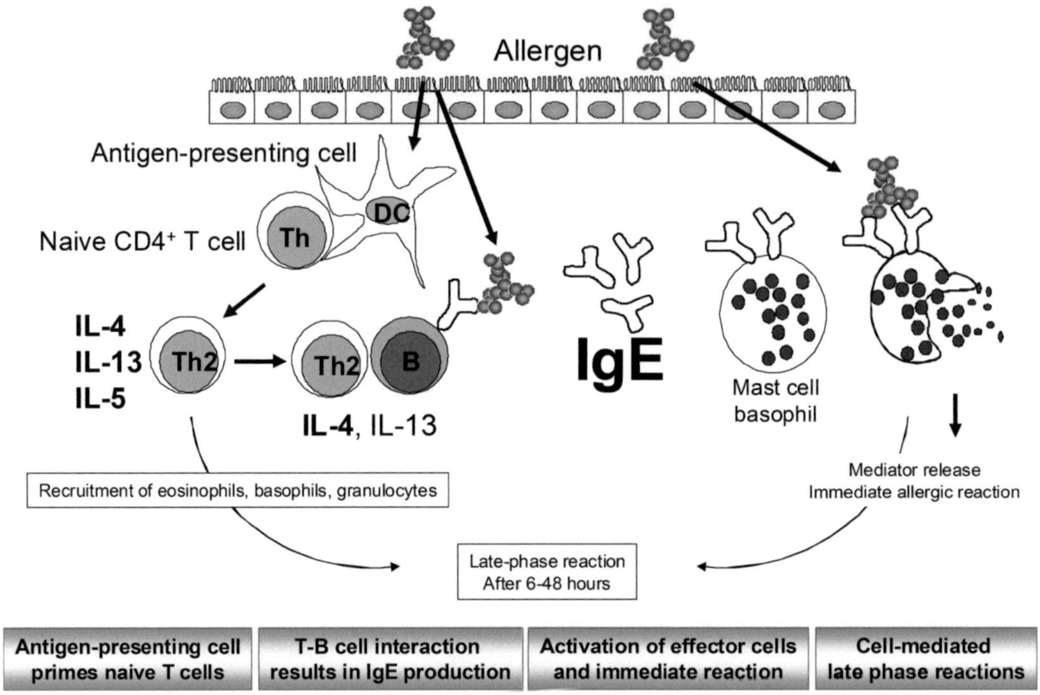

Fig. 3. The pathophysiology of IgE-mediated allergy. Allergens enter the human body through mucosal sites, e.g. in the respiratory or gastrointestinal tract, or via the skin. Antigen-presenting cells, most importantly dendritic cells (DC), take up allergens and migrate to lymph nodes where they present allergens to naïve CD4+ T helper (Th) cells. In atopic individuals, the majority of allergen-specific T cells differentiate into Th2 cells producing high amounts of the signature cytokine IL-4. Interaction of Th2 cells and B cells leads to the production of IgE antibodies which are bound on the surface of effector cells. Upon repeated allergen encounter, these effector cells are activated and release preformed mediators, most importantly histamine, causing immediate allergic symptoms. After 6-48 hours cell-mediated late phase reactions in target organs can occur because different types of granulocytes and allergen-specific T cells have migrated to inflammatory sites.

3. Birch pollen-related food allergy: Clinical appearance

Birch pollen is one of the most common causes of rhinoconjunctivitis and allergic asthma in Northern and Central Europe and North America (Lin et al., 2002, Stevens et al., 2003). Already in 1948 it has been recognized that birch pollen-allergic patients tend to develop allergic reactions to fruits and vegetables in addition to seasonal respiratory symptoms (Juhlin-Dannfelt, 1948). An association between birch pollinosis and allergic reactions to diverse foods was first demonstrated in the late seventies (Hannuksela and Lahti, 1977). In this report, more than 380 Finish patients with various atopic disorders were tested for allergic reactivity to common fruits and vegetables. Of the patients with hypersensitivity to birch pollen, 36% showed immediate positive responses to fresh fruits and vegetables whereas such reactions were rare among patients without allergy to birch pollen. One year later a correlation between birch pollen allergy and allergic symptoms to nuts, apple, peach, cherry, pear, plum, carrot and new potato was reported in 1120 adult Swedish patients (Eriksson, 1978). A subsequent interrogation of 600 patients with pollen allergy again confirmed that hypersensitivity to various nuts, fruits and roots was reported more often by patients with (70%) than by patients without birch pollen allergy (19%) and that grass pollen allergy negatively correlated with food hypersensitivity (Eriksson et al., 1982).

Approximately, 100 million people suffer from birch pollen allergy worldwide and approximately 70% of these individuals develop birch pollen-related food allergy. Therefore, this secondary food allergy has to be regarded as one of the most common plant food allergies in adolescent and adult individuals today. Interestingly, birch pollen-related food allergy is perennial in more than 80% of the affected individuals, i.e. affecting the patients also outside of the birch pollen season (Geroldinger-Simic et al., 2011). Around 40% of the patients suffer from more severe symptoms during the pollen season as compared to the pollen-free time period. The most frequent triggers of birch pollen-related food allergy are stone-fruits (apple, peach) and hazelnuts. In addition, particular vegetables (celery, carrot), peanuts and soy products can also induce allergic reactions in birch pollen-allergic patients (Asero et al., 1996, Eriksson et al., 1982, Geroldinger-Simic et al., 2011, Ghunaim et al., 2005, Osterballe et al., 2005). In the majority of patients allergic reactions to these foods manifest as contact urticaria of the oral mucosa (oral allergy syndrome, OAS). Typical symptoms comprise itching of the lips, tongue and throat, sometimes accompanied by oedema of the lips and tongue and occur within minutes after contact with the food (Ortolani et al., 1988). Many patients also describe itching in their ears. Usually, these reactions disappear within 20-30 minutes. In addition to OAS which is confined to the site of allergen exposure, systemic and more severe IgE-mediated reactions such as urticaria, asthma or anaphylactic shock may occur occasionally. In particular, the consumption of soy-containing food products which contain the Bet v 1-homologous protein Gly m 4 have been described to trigger anaphylactic reactions such as swollen tongue, angioedema, urticaria, rhino-conjunctivitis and/or hypotension within 15-30 min after consumption (Kleine-Tebbe et al., 2002, van Zuuren et al., 2010). However, several patients experiencing severe systemic reactions to soy-products were found to show IgE-reactivity to seed storage proteins in soy which are primary food allergens and also likely candidates to cause the observed severe soy allergy (van Zuuren et al., 2010).

4. Birch pollen-related food allergy: Involved allergens

Birch pollen contains one major allergen, Bet v 1, which is recognized by IgE antibodies from more than 90% of birch pollen-allergic patients (Geroldinger-Simic et al., 2011). Bet v 1 belongs to the pathogenesis-related (PR) 10 protein family. Other members of this protein family have been identified in different foods, such Mal d 1 in apple, Pru p 1 in peach, Pru av 1 in cherry, Pyr c 1 in pear, Cor a 1 in hazelnut, Api g 1 in celery, Dau c 1 in carrot, Gly m 4 in soybean, (all summarized in (Bohle, 2006), Vig r 1 in mungbean (Mittag et al., 2005), Ara h 8 in peanut (Mittag et al., 2004), Act d 8 in kiwi (Oberhuber et al., 2008) and jackfruit (Bolhaar et al., 2004). Although birch pollen contains additional minor allergens, e.g. Bet v 2 (birch profilin), that have homologous proteins in various foods, IgE antibodies specific for Bet v 1 seem to be most relevant for clinical reactions against birch pollen-related foods since a large number of birch pollen-allergic patients with food allergy is exclusively sensitized to the major birch pollen allergen (Geroldinger-Simic et al., 2011).

The identification of the genes encoding various different Bet v 1-homologs in a great variety of food (Table 1) allowed their production as recombinant proteins (Table 1) which were employed to analyse structural and immunological characteristics.

Food	Bet v 1-homolog	GeneBank Acct. No.	Sequence identity (%)
Apple	Mal d 1	AJ417551	56
Hazelnut	Cor a 1	AF136945	67
Nectarine/Peach	Pru p 1	DQ251187	73
Kiwi	Act d 8	AM489568	53
Carrot	Dau c 1	AF456481	37
Apricot	Pru ar 1	U93165	56
Cherry	Pru av 1	U66076	59
Pear	Pyr c 1	AF057030	57
Peanut	Ara h 8	AY328088	46
Celery	Api g 1	Z48967	41
Soybean	Gly m 4	X60043	45
Strawberry	Fra a 1	Q256S2	53
Raspberry	Rub I 1	Q0Z8U9	55

Table 1. Bet v 1-homologs in birch pollen-related foods

Bet v 1-related food proteins display the typical Bet v 1-fold due to their high amino acid sequence similarity with Bet v 1 (Radauer et al., 2008). The highly similar tertiary structure explains why IgE-antibodies specific for conformational epitopes of Bet v 1 can cross-react with its food homologs. In addition to Bet v 1-specific IgE antibodies, Bet v 1-specific T lymphocytes cross-react with related food allergens. This fact has been demonstrated in *in vitro* experiments by employing Bet v 1-specific T cell clones that had been isolated from the blood of birch pollen-allergic patients. The clones were stimulated with recombinant Bet v 1-related food allergens and proliferative and cytokine responses were assessed (Bohle et al., 2003, Bohle et al., 2005, Fritsch et al., 1998). Several Bet v 1-specific clones proliferated in response to different food allergens and produced similar cytokine patterns as compared to stimulation with Bet v 1. In particular, T cells specific for the immunodominant T cell-activating region Bet v $1_{142\text{-}156}$ which is located in a highly conserved amino acid region of the major birch pollen allergen responded to several Bet v 1-related food allergens (Jahn-Schmid et al., 2005). The cellular cross-reactivity is due to the high amino acid sequence similarity between Bet v 1 and its food homologs in this region. In addition to the C-terminal T cell epitope located within Bet v $1_{142\text{-}156}$ (Figure 4), the major birch pollen allergen contains other relevant T cell activating regions spreading its entire amino acid sequence (Jahn-Schmid et al., 2005). Most T cell-activating regions that have been identified in Mal d 1, Cor a 1 and Api g 1 match the amino acid sequences of these epitopes (Bohle et al., 2003, Bohle et al., 2005, Fritsch et al., 1998). Thereby, the receptor of a Bet v 1-specific T cell can cross-react with a peptide derived from antigen-processing of Bet v 1-related food allergens.

```
Bet v 1    GVFNYETETTSVIPAARLFKAFILDGDNLFPKVAPQAISSVENIEGNGGPGTIKKISFPE 60

Mal d 1    GV+ +E E TS IP +RLFKAF+LD DNL PK+APQAI   E +EGNGGPGTIKKI+F E 60
Cor a 1    GVF YE E TSVIP ARLFK+F+LD DNL PKVAPQ  +S EN+EGNGGPGTIKKI+F E 59
Pru p 1    GVF YE+E TS IP  RLFKAF+LD DNL PK+APQAI   E +EG+GGPGTIKKI+F E 61
Act d 8    G   Y+ E  S I A ++FKAF+LDGD + PK  P AI+ V+ +EG+GG GTIK  +F E 61
Dau c 1    G  ++  E TS + A ++F   +LD D + PK A  A  SVE-++G+GG GT++ I+ PE 59
Pru ar 1   GVF YE+E TS IP  RLF AF+L  DNL PK+APQAI   E +EG+GGPGTIKKI+F E 60
Pru av 1   GVF YE+E TS IP  RLFKAF+LD DNL PK+APQAI   E +EG+GGPGTIKKI+F E 60
Pyr c 1    G++ +E E TS IP  RLFKAF+LD DNL PK+APQAI   E +EGNGGPGTIKKI+F E 60
Ara h 8    GVF +E E TS +P A+L+ A + D D++ PK+     + SVE +EGNGGPGTIKK++  E 59
Api g 1    GV  +  E TS + A ++F+ F++D D + PK AP A  SVE-I+G+GGPGT+K I+ P+ 59
Gly m 4    GVF +E E  S +  A L+KA + D DN+ PK-A  +  SVEN+EGNGGPGTIKKI+F E 59
Fra a 1    GV+ YE E TS IPA +LFKAF+LD DNL PK+APQA+   E +EG+GGPGTIKKI+F E 61
Rub i 1              TSVIP  +LFKAF+LD DNL PK+APQA+ SVE IEG+GG GT+KKI   E 61

Bet v 1    GFPFKYVKDRVDEVDHTNFKYNYSVIEGGPIGDTLEKISNEIKIVATPDGGSILKISNKY 120

Mal d 1    G  + YVK R+D +D  ++ Y+Y++IEG  + DT+EKIS E K+VA   G +I  IS+-Y 119
Cor a 1    G  FKY+K +V+E+DH NFKY YS+IEGGP+G TLEKIS EIK+ A P  GGSILKI++K 120
Pru p 1    G  + YVK ++D +D  N  Y+Y++IEG +GD LEKIS E K+VA+P GGSI+K ++ Y 121
Act d 8    G   K VK R+D +D  NF Y+YS+IEGG + D  E IS  IKIVATPDGG I K  + Y 120
Dau c 1    G P   +  R D V+     Y+ +VI+G  +   +E I   + +V T DGGSI K +  + 119
Pru ar 1   G  + YVK ++D +D  N  Y+Y++IEG +G+ LEKIS E K+VA+P GGSI+K ++ Y 120
Pru av 1   G  + YVK ++D +D  N+ Y+Y++IEG +GDTLEKIS E K+VA+P GGSI+K ++ Y 120
Pyr c 1    G  + YVK RVD +D  ++ Y Y++IEG + DT+EKIS E K+VA+  G +I  IS+-Y 119
Ara h 8       K++  +V+ +D  N+ YNYSV+ G  +  T EKI+ E K+V  P+GGSI K++ KY 119
Api g 1    G P   +  R+D V+     ++YSVI+G  +   +E I N + +V T DGGSI K +  + 119
Gly m 4       K+V  +++ +D  N  Y+YSV+ G  + DT EKI+ + K+VA P+GGS  K++ KY 119
Fra a 1    G  + YVK ++  +D  N  Y+YS+IEG  + + +EKI  E K+V+ P GG+I+K ++KY 121
Rub i 1    G    YVK ++D +D  NF Y+YS+ EG  +GD +EKIS EIK+VA+   GSI+K ++ Y 110

Bet v 1    HTKGDHEVKAEQVKASKEMGETLLRAVESYLLAHSDAY  159

Mal d 1    HTKG+ E+K E VK  KE    L + +ESYL  H DAYN 158
Cor a 1    HTKG+  +  E++KA KE    L +AVE+YLLAH DAY  159
Pru p 1    HTKGD E+K E VKA KE    L + +E+YL  H DAYN 160
Act d 8      K D +V  E++KA KE    + + VE+YLLA+ D     157
Dau c 1    HTKGD  V  E +K +      L +A+E+YL+A+       153
Pru ar 1   HTKGD E+K E VKA KE    L + +E+YL  H DAYN 159
Pru av 1   HTKG+ E+K E VKA KE    L + +E+YL  H DAYN 159
Pyr c 1    HTKGD E+K E VKA KE    L + +ESYL  H DAYN 158
Ara h 8    HTKGD +   E++K  K  GE L RA+E Y+LA+   Y  157
Api g 1    HTKGD  V  E +K + E    L +A+E+YL+A+      153
Gly m 4     TKGD E   +++K  K   + L +A+E+YLLAH D-YN 157
Fra a 1    HTKGD E+K E VKA KE    L + +E YL  H   YN 160
Rub i 1    H KG  E+K EQVK  KE    L +              136
```

Fig. 4. Sequence alignment of Bet v 1-related food proteins and Bet v 1. Similar amino acid residues are indicated by +. The immunodominant T cell epitope in the C-terminus of Bet v 1 is underlined.

Resistance to gastrointestinal degradation and to heat treatment is considered to be an important characteristic of food allergens and was investigated by employing recombinant Bet v 1-related food allergens. Simulated gastrointestinal degradation of Mal d 1, Api g 1 and Cor a 1 revealed that these proteins were completely fragmented within a few minutes of exposure to pepsin, the most prominent gastric protease (Kopper et al., 2004, Schimek et al., 2005, Schulten et al., 2011). Proteolytic degradation of Bet v 1-homologous food allergens into small fragments leads to the loss of their IgE-binding capacity because most IgE-epitopes of Bet v 1 are conformational epitopes depending on the tertiary protein structure (Mittag et al., 2006, Neudecker et al., 2003, Scheurer et al., 1999). The rapid and complete degradation of Bet v 1-homologous food allergens explains why systemic IgE-mediated reactions rarely occur after consumption of birch pollen-related foods. At the site of contact with fresh foods, i.e. the oral mucosa, local IgE-mediated immediate allergic reactions are induced by intact food allergens. After swallowing Bet v 1-related food allergens are rapidly degraded in the stomach and cannot be absorbed into the blood stream in a form capable of inducing IgE-mediated effector cell activation. As a consequence, systemic allergic reactions to birch pollen-related foods are rare. However, there are exceptions to this process, for example, the so-called "bio-bar syndrome". This syndrome describes occasional anaphylactic reactions in patients with birch pollen allergy that occur after the consumption of fruit and vegetable smoothies. These drinks are usually prepared from fresh apple and/or raw carrot and drunk very rapidly at so-called bio-bars. We recently found a possible explanation for this phenomenon by performing *in vivo* absorption assays in an animal model (Schulten et al., 2011). We observed that the pH value in the stomach of rats rises to 5 after allergen administration. Similarly, administration of a peanut-based meal initially neutralized the gastric pH value of piglets to approximately 7, which was subsequently acidified by HCl secretion (Kopper et al., 2006). The high pH value renders pepsin inactive. Consequently, Bet v 1-homologous food allergens were not degraded by the protease and could be detected in the rat serum after a time period of 2 hours (Schulten et al., 2011). Deduced from these *in vivo* results from animal models we propose that rapid drinking of freshly prepared smoothies on an relatively empty stomach of birch pollen-allergic individuals will rise the gastric pH value and prevent immediate pepsinolysis of food allergens. Thereby, a dose of IgE-reactive Bet v 1-related food allergens can be absorbed which is sufficient to subsequently cause systemic anaphylaxis. The same cascade of events may also explain the severe anaphylactic reactions observed in birch pollen-allergic patients after ingestion of soy-based foods, in particular soy milk, containing the Bet v 1-homolog Gly m 4 (Kleine-Tebbe et al., 2002).

Recombinant Bet v 1-related food allergens were also employed to investigate the effects of heat treatment on these proteins. Exposure to high temperatures demolishes their 3-dimensional structure, thereby reducing their capacity to bind IgE and consequently, to induce IgE-mediated effector cell activation (Bohle et al., 2006). This biochemical behaviour explained why typically, only fresh fruits and vegetables induce immediate allergic symptoms whereas cooked birch pollen-related foods are usually tolerated by birch pollen-allergic patients.

In summary, Bet v 1-related food allergens lack typical features of primary food allergens, i.e. resistance to gastrointestinal degradation and heat treatment. Therefore, they are considered to be secondary or incomplete food allergens, i.e. incapable of initiating an allergic sensitization in an individual by themselves. However, due to their structural similarity with Bet v 1 and to the high amino acid sequence identity between the major birch pollen allergen and its dietary homologs these proteins can induce allergic symptoms when cross-reactive Bet v 1-specific IgE antibodies and T cells are present in allergic patients. IgE-mediated symptoms appear as OAS immediately after contact with the respective fresh foods in the majority of patients. The activation of Bet v 1-specific T cells by Bet v 1-related food allergens may induce late phase responses in target organs in a minority of birch pollen-allergic patients, for example a worsening of atopic eczema occurring 12-48 hours after consumption of birch pollen-related foods (Bohle et al., 2006, Werfel et al., 1999). In biopsies of such flare ups Bet v 1-specific T cells have been detected (Reekers et al., 1999). This finding indicated that after ingestion and gastrointestinal proteolysis of Bet v 1-related food allergens fragments thereof were absorbed into the blood and induced the activation of Bet v 1-specific T cells. Indeed, several fragments of Bet v 1-homologous food allergens were identified after simulated gastrointestinal degradation that contained T cell activating regions and induced the proliferation and cytokine synthesis of Bet v 1-specific T cell clones *in vitro* (Schimek et al., 2005). *In vivo,* Bet v 1-specific T lymphocytes activated by such cross-reactive peptides may migrate into target organs such as the skin and exert local effector functions, e.g. a worsening of atopic eczema.

Of note, T cell-mediated symptoms induced by Bet v 1-related food allergens can occur independently from IgE-mediated reactions. This means that patients who do not experience an OAS when consuming birch pollen-related foods may still suffer from flare-ups of their atopic eczema several hours after ingestion. For example, when birch pollen-allergic patients were challenged with cooked birch pollen-related foods, these individuals did not experience immediate symptoms but T cell-mediated late phase reactions (Bohle et al., 2006). Together, biochemical and immunological data gained with recombinant Bet v 1-homologous food allergens provide an explanation for this clinical observation. Allergen-recognition differs between IgE antibodies and allergen-specific T cells. In contrast to IgE antibodies which often recognize conformational epitopes depending on the tertiary structure of an allergen T cells recognize small linear peptides generated during antigen processing of proteins (Figure 5). Cooking of Bet v 1-homologs leads to their loss of IgE-binding. Nevertheless, heat-denatured Bet v 1-related food allergens are taken up and processed by antigen-presenting cells and thereafter, presented to T lymphocytes.

N-ALYANLE**PK**AEQPTE**KI**TKVFGDEAEE**V**LKYL-COOH N-ALYANLEPKAEQP**TEKITKVF**GDEAEEVLKYL-COOH

Fig. 5. Antigen-recognition by B and T lymphocytes. Antibodies (indicated as Y) produced by plasma cells often recognize conformational epitopes that depend on the tertiary structure of proteins. The amino acid residues forming the epitope are not neighbouring residues in the primary sequence. In contrast, linear T cell epitopes highlighted as black lines within the amino acid sequence consist of neighbouring amino acid residues.

What may be the consequence of T cell activation by ingested Bet v 1-related food allergens? In allergic individuals, allergen-specific T cells were shown be long-lived and to exist for several years (Bohle et al., 1998, Wedderburn et al., 1993). In order to survive, specific memory T cells seem to require repeated contact with antigen. The ingestion of pollen-related food proteins capable of activating pollen-specific T lymphocytes may represent one way to stimulate these cells, in particular outside of the tree pollen season. In our studies the majority of the food allergen-reactive Bet v 1-specific TCC were Th2-like and synthesized high levels of IL-4 in response to the food allergens (Bohle et al., 2003, Bohle et al., 2005, Fritsch et al., 1998). Therefore, the perennial uptake of pollen-related food could stimulate the survival of T cells and ongoing IL-4 synthesis and thereby contribute to the typical maintenance of high levels of pollen-specific IgE also outside of the tree pollen season. A summary of the consequences of consumption of Bet v 1-related food allergens is provided in Figure 6.

5. Bet v 1 is the primary sensitizer in birch pollen-related food allergy

Clinical, immunological and biochemical data support that birch pollen-related food allergy is a secondary food allergy and results from primary respiratory sensitization to the major birch pollen allergen and subsequent immunological cross-reactivity. From the clinical point of view, the majority of patients develop food-induced allergic symptoms after the onset of respiratory allergy (Geroldinger-Simic et al., 2011). Furthermore, a high number of birch pollen-allergic patients shows IgE-reactivity to Bet v 1-related food allergens without developing clinical reactions to the respective foods whereas only very few food-allergic individuals display IgE-reactivity to Bet v 1-homologous food allergens in the absence of Bet v 1-specific IgE antibodies (Flinterman et al., 2006, Moneo et al., 1999). Finally, patients suffering from allergic reactions to stone-fruits and hazelnuts in birch-free areas are not sensitized to Bet v 1-homologous food allergens but to other plant food allergens, e.g. non-specific lipid transfer proteins (Fernandez-Rivas et al., 2008, Fernandez-Rivas et al., 2006).
Immunologically, Bet v 1 not only cross-reacts with its related dietary proteins but the major birch pollen allergen dominates the IgE and T cell reactivity to its homologs. For example, pre-incubation of patients´ sera with Bet v 1 totally abolishes their IgE-binding to Mal d 1 and Api g 1 whereas pre-incubation of the same sera with Bet v 1-related food allergens reduces IgE-binding to the major birch pollen allergen to only around 50% (Bohle et al., 2003, Kinaciyan et al., 2007). These experimental findings indicate that Bet v 1 contains most IgE-epitopes of its food homologues and binds IgE with higher affinity. Thus, it may be concluded that Bet v 1 initiated the production of specific IgE antibodies *in vivo*. Similar to the IgE level, experimental *in vitro* approaches revealed that Bet v 1 dominates the T cell response to its food-homologs. When T cells reactive with Bet v 1-related food allergens were isolated from the peripheral blood of allergic patients and re-stimulated with either the food allergen or Bet v 1, most cultures responded stronger to the major birch pollen allergen (Bohle et al., 2003, Bohle et al., 2005, Fritsch et al., 1998). This finding indicates that T cells which respond to stimulation with Bet v 1-related food allergens are cross-reactive, Bet v 1-specific clonotypes. Again, these observations support that Bet v 1 was the initial stimulus for an allergic response in birch pollen-related food allergy.
Biochemically, the high susceptibility of Bet v 1-homologous dietary allergens to proteolytic degradation in the stomach and small intestine prevents them from reaching the gut-associated lymphoid tissue (GALT) in an intact form. Therefore, Bet v 1-homologous food allergens are considered to be incapable of sensitizing an individual by themselves after

being taken up through their natural route of exposure. In contrast, the major birch pollen allergen is inhaled and thereby not exposed to the harsh conditions of the gastrointestinal tract. Bet v 1 reaches the respiratory tract in an immunological active form where it can induce IgE-production. Together, clinical and experimental observations support that the major birch pollen allergen is the primary sensitizer in birch pollen-related food allergy.

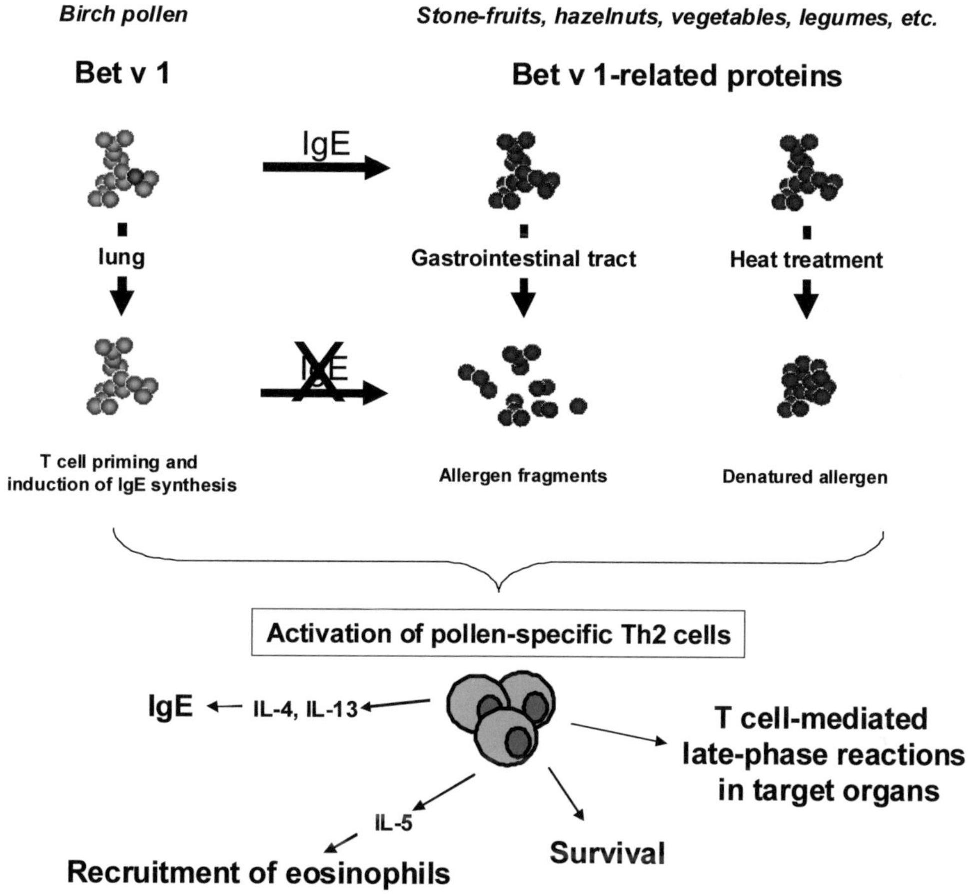

Fig. 6. Proposed pathophysiology of pollen-related food allergy. Bet v 1 initiates respiratory sensitization. Bet v 1-specific IgE antibodies recognize structurally related dietary proteins in various foods which may cause clinical reactions, often directly at the site of allergen contact, e.g. the oral mucosa. After ingestion Bet v 1-related food homologs are degraded when passing through the intestinal tract. Cooking of the respective foods also denatures Bet v 1-related food allergens. The destruction of their 3-dimensional structure leads to the loss of IgE-binding capacity of Bet v 1-homologous food proteins. Nevertheless, allergenic fragments after gastrointestinal degradation as well as heat-denatured Bet v 1-related allergens are still capable of activating Bet v 1-specific T lymphocytes. Upon activation, Bet v 1-specific T cells proliferate and produce cytokines. They also migrate to different target organs where they may exert clinical late-phase reactions, e.g. the worsening of atopic eczema in the skin. Possibly, activation of pollen-specific Th2 cells by ingested food proteins also contributes to their survival and longevity in allergic patients.

Interestingly, a few food-allergic patients have been identified to bear IgE antibodies specific for Bet v 1-related food allergens, e.g. Cor a 1 in hazelnut, without being sensitized to the major birch pollen allergen (Flinterman et al., 2006). This finding suggested that a non-pollen-related route of sensitization to the Bet v 1-homologous hazelnut allergen may be possible. Along these lines, we previously found evidence for a potential sensitizing capacity of Cor a 1 based on the identification of T cell clones that did not cross-react with Bet v 1 (Bohle et al., 2005). However, in simulated gastrointestinal degradation assays pure Cor a 1 lost its IgE-binding ability within a few seconds of incubation with pepsin (Schimek et al., 2005). This discrepancy tempted us to investigate whether the natural matrix embedding Cor a 1 may contribute to its sensitizing capacity. Actually, in simulated gastrointestinal degradation assays, we found that the presence of hazelnut extract protected Bet v 1-related food allergens from gastric proteolysis (Schulten et al., 2011). Since Cor a 1 has been demonstrated to be relatively resistant to simulated degradation by the intestinal protease trypsin (Schimek et al., 2005) we conclude that hazelnuts which provide a food matrix rich in carbohydrates and proteins under certain circumstances may contribute to a sensitizing capacity of the major hazelnut allergen independently from respiratory sensitization to Bet v 1. Most patients showing IgE-reactivity to Cor a 1 but not to Bet v 1 were children (Flinterman et al., 2006). Therefore, the still immature gastrointestinal tract of children may be such an additional precondition for a possible sensitization to Cor a 1.

6. Treatment strategies for birch pollen-related food allergy

6.1 Specific immunotherapy with birch pollen

Together, clinical and immunological observations provide strong evidence that birch pollen-related food allergy is a consequence of cross-reactivity between Bet v 1 and its dietary homologs. Thus, one would assume that successful allergen-specific immunotherapy (SIT) of birch pollen allergy might concomitantly cure birch pollen-related food allergy. SIT consists of a series of continuous administration of increasing doses of allergen extracts to the allergic patient in order to induce clinical tolerance (1993) and is currently the only causative treatment for IgE-mediated allergy that results in long-term clinical tolerance to allergens. Various studies have shown that successful SIT alters the allergen-specific immune response (Larche et al., 2006). In general, SIT induces high levels of allergen-specific IgG antibodies, in particular IgG4, which are considered as "blocking" antibodies because they compete with IgE for allergen-binding and thereby impair IgE-mediated reactions, e.g. allergen-induced activation of basophils and mast cells or IgE-facilitated allergen uptake and presentation to T cells (James et al., 2011, Nouri-Aria et al., 2004, van Neerven et al., 1999, Wachholz et al., 2003). At the T cell level it has been demonstrated that SIT induces a shift from the disease-eliciting T helper (Th) 2- towards a Th1-like response and regulatory $CD4^+$ T (Treg) cells that actively suppress proliferation and cytokine production of allergen-specific effector T cells (Akdis et al., 1998, Bellinghausen et al., 1997, Ebner et al., 1997, Jutel et al., 2003). In addition to the modulation of the adaptive immune response to allergens, SIT also modulates the function of APC and effectors cells (Larche et al., 2006), e.g. reduction of the number of mast cells and their ability to release mediators. The recruitment of eosinophils and neutrophils to sites of allergen exposure is also reduced during SIT.

An overview on the immune mechanisms operative during successful SIT is given in Figure 7. However, it is still not clear which of these immune mechanisms actually translate(s) into clinical tolerance of patients, i.e. improvement of symptoms, and whether one or more of these mechanisms fail those individuals who are not cured by SIT.

SIT with birch pollen has been proven efficient for the treatment of birch pollinosis (Bodtger et al., 2002, Cirla et al., 1996, Winther et al., 2000). However, the clinical benefit of SIT with birch pollen on birch pollen-related food allergy is still debated. Whereas a few studies have described that patients improved their clinical symptoms to birch pollen-related foods after birch pollen-SIT (Asero, 1998, 2003, 2004) others have reported limited curative effects of birch pollen-SIT on birch pollen-related food allergy and some patients even developed allergic reactions to foods during the course of therapy (Bucher et al., 2004, Herrmann et al., 1995, Modrzynski et al., 2002, van Hoffen et al., 2011). It has to be stressed that at present a prospective study investigating food allergic reactions in a sufficient number of birch pollen-allergic patients before and during birch pollen-SIT by means of double-blind placebo controlled food challenges (DBPCFC) is lacking. Nevertheless, the majority of clinicians observe that only approximately one third of birch pollen-allergic patients undergoing birch pollen-SIT concomitantly improve birch pollen-related food allergy. Thus, no effective treatment for this secondary food allergy exists at present. However, because of its high prevalence and the impaired quality of life of the affected individuals, there is a need for an efficient treatment strategy for birch pollen-related food allergy.

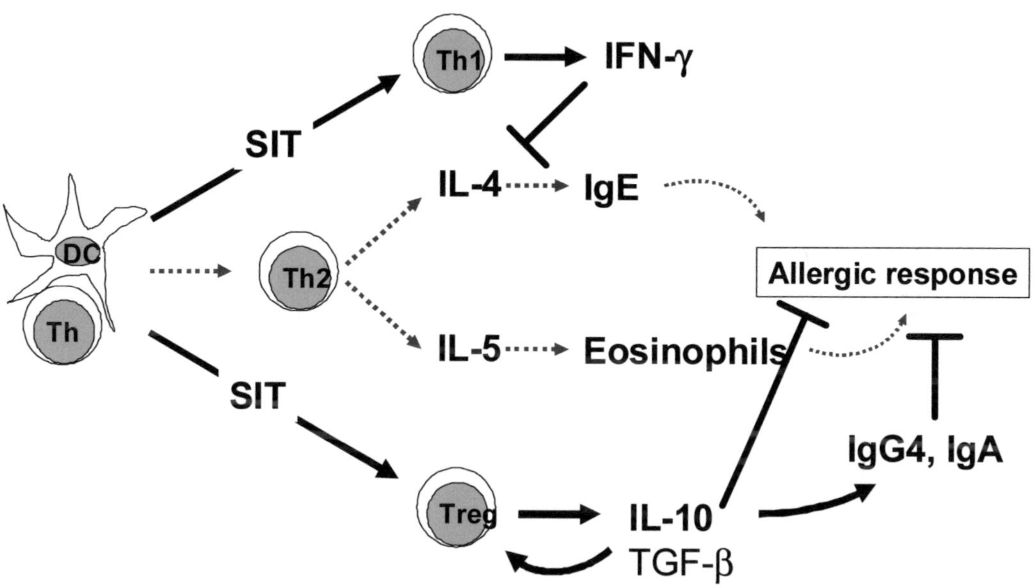

Fig. 7. Immune mechanisms operative during allergen-specific immunotherapy (SIT). An overshooting allergen-specific Th2 response causes allergic diseases. Th2 cells produce IL-4 that triggers B cells to produce allergen-specific IgE antibodies. Th2 cells also synthesize IL-5, which activates eosinophils. IgE and eosinophils mediate the immediate allergic response. SIT induces immune deviation, i.e. the switch from Th2 towards Th1-like cells which produce high levels of IFN-γ, a potent antagonist of IL-4. SIT also promotes the induction of regulatory T (Treg) cells which produce IL-10 and/or TGF-β. These immunosuppressive cytokines induce the production of allergen-specific IgG4 and IgA antibodies which may compete with IgE for allergen-binding ("blocking antibodies". IL-10 promotes further induction of regulatory T cells.

Sublingual immunotherapy (SLIT) has been demonstrated to be an effective and safe alternative for conventional subcutaneous SIT of birch pollen allergy (Horak et al., 1998, Khinchi et al., 2004, Mauro et al., 2007). Similar to subcutaneous immunotherapy SLIT induces allergen-specific IgG1 and IgG4 antibodies and a modulation of the allergen-specific T cell response (O'Hehir et al., 2009, Scadding et al., 2010). Moreover, SLIT induced increased Foxp3+ cells - presumably regulatory T cells - in the sublingual epithelium (Scadding et al., 2010). Speculating that sublingual administration, directly at the site of food-induced allergic symptoms, instead of subcutaneous injections might improve the therapeutic benefit on birch pollen-related food allergy, we have evaluated the effects of SLIT with birch pollen extract on apple allergy in birch pollen-allergic individuals (Kinaciyan et al., 2007). The clinical efficacy of birch pollen SLIT was assessed by means of nasal provocation tests with birch pollen extract and double-blind placebo-controlled food challenges with Golden Delicious apples before and after 1 year of treatment. Nine patients improved in nasal provocation tests to birch pollen and were therefore considered as successfully treated. However, only very few of the nine patients concomitantly improved allergic reactions to apple in double-blind placebo-controlled food challenges. To understand this limited curative effect of birch pollen-SLIT on associated apple allergy, Bet v 1- and Mal d 1-specific antibody and T cell responses were analysed in the successfully treated individuals. All patients developed significantly increased Bet v 1-specific IgG4 antibody levels after 1 year of SLIT. Interestingly, Mal d 1-specific IgG4 antibody levels did not increase significantly in parallel (Kinaciyan et al., 2007). At the T cell level, a significant reduction of Bet v 1-specific T cell proliferation after 4 and 52 weeks of SLIT was found (Bohle et al., 2007). This reduced allergen-specific T cell response could be referred to the induction of IL-10-producing regulatory T cells in the early phase and the switch from Bet v 1-specific Th2 cells towards more Th1 cells in the late phase of SLIT. However, no similar modulation of the Mal d 1-specific T cell response was observed. Together, these findings suggested that birch pollen SLIT induced the characteristic immune mechanisms operative during SIT, such as blocking antibodies, peripheral tolerance, regulatory T cells and immune deviation, specific for Bet v 1 but not for its highly cross-reactive homologue in apple. Along these lines, a more recent study demonstrated that conventional subcutaneous SIT with birch pollen also failed to induce food-reactive IgG4 antibodies (van Hoffen et al., 2011). The sera from 10 birch pollen-allergic patients with associated allergy to hazelnut were investigated for Bet v 1- and Cor a 1-specific IgG4 antibodies before, after 3, 6, 9 and 12 months of birch pollen-SIT. Again, the significant increase of Bet v 1-specific IgG4 antibody titers was not paralleled by a significant increase of Cor a 1-reactive IgG4 antibody levels. Nevertheless, after three months of treatment the sera contained significantly enhanced Cor a 1-reactive IgG levels and the sera obtained after 1 year of treatment showed IgE-blocking capacity in facilitated antigen-binding (FAB) assays (Shamji et al., 2006). Still, SIT with birch pollen extract did not result in clinical improvement of hazelnut allergy in these patients as analyzed by means of double-blind placebo-controlled food challenges at inclusion and after 1 year of treatment (van Hoffen et al., 2011).

Together, these studies imply that the limited clinical effect of SIT with birch pollen may be due to a failure of the induction of cross-reactive IgG and T cell responses. However, it needs to be pointed out that so far in relatively low numbers of birch pollen-allergic individuals were assessed for their antibody and T cell responses to Bet v 1-homologous food allergens during birch pollen-SIT or SLIT. Therefore, we analysed IgG responses specific for Bet v 1, Mal d 1 and Cor a 1 in sera from 49 patients who received birch pollen SIT for 1-3 years and developed Bet v 1-specific IgG4 antibodies. Interestingly, only around 33% of these individuals developed food-reactive IgG4 antibodies. Food-reactive antibodies in general increased later during the course of therapy as compared to Bet v 1-specific IgG4 antibodies and blocked IgE binding to Bet v 1-related food allergens. Similarly, only a limited number of birch pollen-allergic patients developed food-reactive IgG1 antibodies after subcutaneous administration of a recombinant hypoallergenic variant of Bet v 1 (Niederberger et al., 2007). In a recent study including more than 200 birch pollen-allergic individuals we observed that patients tolerating birch pollen-related foods showed higher ratios of serum allergen-specific IgG4/IgE antibody levels than patients with food allergy (Geroldinger-Simic et al., 2011). These naturally occurring allergen-specific IgG4 antibodies were capable of blocking IgE-binding to Bet v 1-related food allergens. These data indicate that the presence of allergen-specific IgG4 antibodies which compete with IgE for allergen-binding may be important for the development of food tolerance. Therefore, SIT or SLIT should induce such antibodies. However, treatment with birch pollen does not effectively induce food-reactive IgG4 antibodies in every patient. Therefore, we propose that vaccines for the treatment of birch pollen-related food allergy should contain the disease-eliciting food allergens. Previously, a randomized, double-blind, placebo-controlled study has demonstrated significant increases in tolerance to hazelnut after sublingual administration of hazelnut extract (Enrique et al., 2005). Tolerance induction was accompanied by increased IgG4 antibody and IL-10 levels after immunotherapy in only the active group. Thus, SLIT with Bet v 1-associated food allergens may be a promising approach for treatment of birch pollen-related food allergy.

Finally, it is an interesting immunological finding that a high number of birch pollen-allergic patients show food-reactive Bet v 1-specific IgE antibodies but fail to develop cross-reactive IgG antibodies during treatment with birch pollen despite developing high levels of Bet v 1-specific IgG antibodies. Therefore, birch pollen-related food allergy is an interesting model to study the question how cross-reactivity of structurally related allergens can cause allergy whereas the immunomodulation of the allergen-specific response in SIT-treated patients who improve their pollinosis does not concomitantly translate into clinical tolerance to associated foods.

6.2 Future concepts for treatment of birch pollen-related food allergy

Although rarely life-threatening birch pollen-related food allergy is highly prevalent and often causes perennial discomfort. Furthermore, this secondary food allergy prevents birch pollen-allergic patients from consuming a great variety of fresh fruits and vegetables which contain vitamins and are considered to be healthy. This situation demands for effective treatment which at present does not exist. Recent developments in the treatment of food allergy suggest oral immunotherapy (OIT) with the disease-eliciting food as an interesting option (Nowak-Wegrzyn and Sampson, 2011). Indeed, results from a double-blind placebo controlled study in peanut-allergic children demonstrated that OIT with peanut induced desensitization and concurrent immune modulation (Varshney et al., 2011). In contrast to the placebo group, the actively treated OIT group showed significant reductions in skin prick reactivity to peanut and significant increases in peanut-specific IgG4 antibodies. Furthermore, the ratio of FoxP3^{hi}: FoxP3^{intermediate} CD4$^+$CD25$^+$ T cells increased in peanut OIT subjects suggesting the induction of regulatory T cells. Similar approaches might be feasible for the treatment of birch pollen-related food allergy. Recently, it was observed that continuous consumption of small amounts of apple induces clinical tolerance in birch pollen-allergic patients with apple allergy (Kopac et al., 2010). In this study, 21 patients daily consumed small amounts of apple, doubling the dose every two weeks. After a regular exposure of in average 22 weeks, 16/21 patients tolerated a complete apple without developing any signs of an OAS. This desensitization was paralleled by a decrease of intradermal reactivity to Mal d 1. This preliminary study indicates that OIT may be a possible approach to treat birch pollen-related apple allergy.

Novel concepts for allergy vaccines for SIT include the use of recombinant allergens instead of crude extracts containing a mixture of allergenic and non-allergenic proteins of an allergen source (Valenta et al., 2011). Although progress has been made to improve the quality and standardization of protein extracts the use of allergen extracts for SIT still bears some disadvantages. The complex protein mixture makes it difficult to determine the exact content of single allergens. Due to the production process the concentration of individual allergens may vary between different batches. Highly labile allergens might even be totally lost during the production process and not be present in the extract. The availability of recombinant allergens with the same immunological characteristics as their natural counterparts can overcome several of these disadvantages. Briefly, recombinant allergens can be produced as molecules with known molecular, immunologic and biological characteristics in consistent quality and unlimited amounts. Thus, the content of individual allergens in a vaccine can precisely be formulated and the potential loss of allergens destroyed during the production process of allergen extracts can be excluded. Regarding the treatment of birch pollinosis, recombinant Bet v 1 has been demonstrated to be as effective as birch pollen extract (Pauli et al., 2008). As discussed above, we propose that vaccines for the treatment of birch pollen-related food allergy should contain the disease-eliciting dietary allergens. Bet v 1-related proteins are known to be easily degraded during the procedures applied for the production of protein extracts. Since the most important and frequently recognized Bet v 1-related food allergens are available as recombinant proteins (Table 1), these proteins should be employed as active component in future vaccines for SIT or SLIT of birch pollen-related food allergy.

In addition to producing well-defined batches of recombinant wild-type allergens with identical features to their natural counterparts, the recombinant DNA technology also offers the possibility to selectively modify certain properties and functions of allergenic proteins (Mutschlechner et al., 2009). Diverse modifications of allergens can be genetically engineered, e.g. variants with reduced IgE-binding capacity, multi-mers of single allergens or hybrids consisting of different allergens. Furthermore, allergens can be genetically fused with proteins that promote immune responses which counter regulate the disease-eliciting Th2-dominated immune response in allergic individuals and may therefore, improve the efficacy of SIT (Bohle et al., 2004, Gerstmayr et al., 2007). All these approaches may also be employed to develop an effective treatment strategy for birch pollen-related food allergy.

We have recently sublingually administered recombinant Mal d 1 to 18 birch pollen-allergic patients with associated apple allergy. The recombinant apple allergen was well tolerated by the individuals and no severe side-effects were observed. This approach may be regarded as a first proof-of-concept for the applicability of recombinant Bet v 1-related food allergens for SLIT. Certainly, several questions regarding the optimum content of a vaccine to treat birch pollen-related food allergy remain open. Most patients react to more than one food and it remains to be determined whether all individual food allergens should be employed for treatment. Moreover, it remains to be investigated whether the vaccine should contain food allergens with or without Bet v 1.

7. Conclusion

Birch pollen-related food allergy is a relevant allergic disease that affects the vast majority of birch pollen-allergic patients and strongly impairs their quality of life. Currently, no effective therapy for this form of food allergy is available. The detailed investigation of the allergic response to Bet v 1-homologous food allergens has provided evidence that birch pollen-related food allergy results from immunological cross-reactivity of the major birch pollen allergen and structurally related dietary proteins. However, it is somehow astonishing that successful SIT or SLIT of birch pollinosis accompanied by the modulation of the Bet v 1-specific immune response does not effectively cure birch pollen-associated food allergy in parallel. Primary sensitization to the major birch pollen allergen and subsequent cross-reactivity can cause food allergy. However, the immunomodulation of Bet v 1-specific antibody and T cell responses during SIT with birch pollen does not concomitantly modulate reactivity to the respective food allergens. Thus, birch pollen-related food allergy is an interesting model to learn more about the consequence of immunological cross-reactivity between related allergens in different sources. The detailed analysis of the immune mechanisms failing in patients who do not improve pollen-associated food allergy during SIT with birch pollen will help to improve the treatment and to develop an efficient therapy for birch pollen-related food allergy.

8. Acknowledgements

The research was funded by the Austrian Science Fund (FWF): SFB B1807-B13.

9. References

(1993). Position paper: Immunotherapy. *Allergy,* 48, 14 Suppl, 9-35, 8342741

Akdis C. A., Blesken T., Akdis M., Wuthrich B.&Blaser K. (1998). Role of interleukin 10 in specific immunotherapy. *J Clin Invest,* 102, 1, (Jul 1), 98-106, 9649562

Asero R. (1998). Effects of birch pollen-specific immunotherapy on apple allergy in birch pollen-hypersensitive patients. *Clin Exp Allergy,* 28, 11, (Nov), 1368-1373, 9824409

Asero R. (2003). How long does the effect of birch pollen injection SIT on apple allergy last? *Allergy,* 58, 5, (May), 435-438, 12752332

Asero R. (2004). Effects of birch pollen SIT on apple allergy: a matter of dosage? *Allergy,* 59, 12, (Dec), 1269-1271, 15507094

Asero R., Massironi F.&Velati C. (1996). Detection of prognostic factors for oral allergy syndrome in patients with birch pollen hypersensitivity. *J Allergy Clin Immunol,* 97, 2, (Feb), 611-616, 8621846

Bellinghausen I., Metz G., Enk A. H., Christmann S., Knop J.&Saloga J. (1997). Insect venom immunotherapy induces interleukin-10 production and a Th2-to-Th1 shift, and changes surface marker expression in venom-allergic subjects. *Eur J Immunol,* 27, 5, (May), 1131-1139, 9174602

Bodtger U., Poulsen L. K., Jacobi H. H.&Malling H. J. (2002). The safety and efficacy of subcutaneous birch pollen immunotherapy - a one-year, randomised, double-blind, placebo-controlled study. *Allergy,* 57, 4, (Apr), 297-305, 11906359

Bohle B. (2006). T-cell epitopes of food allergens. *Clin Rev Allergy Immunol,* 30, 2, (Apr), 97-108, 16645222

Bohle B., Breitwieser A., Zwolfer B., Jahn-Schmid B., Sara M., Sleytr U. B.&Ebner C. (2004). A novel approach to specific allergy treatment: the recombinant fusion protein of a bacterial cell surface (S-layer) protein and the major birch pollen allergen Bet v 1 (rSbsC-Bet v 1) combines reduced allergenicity with immunomodulating capacity. *J Immunol,* 172, 11, (Jun 1), 6642-6648, 15153479

Bohle B., Kinaciyan T., Gerstmayr M., Radakovics A., Jahn-Schmid B.&Ebner C. (2007). Sublingual immunotherapy induces IL-10-producing T regulatory cells, allergen-specific T-cell tolerance, and immune deviation. *J Allergy Clin Immunol,* 120, 3, (Sep), 707-713, 17681368

Bohle B., Radakovics A., Jahn-Schmid B., Hoffmann-Sommergruber K., Fischer G. F.&Ebner C. (2003). Bet v 1, the major birch pollen allergen, initiates sensitization to Api g 1, the major allergen in celery: evidence at the T cell level. *Eur J Immunol,* 33, 12, (Dec), 3303-3310, 14635038

Bohle B., Radakovics A., Luttkopf D., Jahn-Schmid B., Vieths S.&Ebner C. (2005). Characterization of the T cell response to the major hazelnut allergen, Cor a 1.04: evidence for a relevant T cell epitope not cross-reactive with homologous pollen allergens. *Clin Exp Allergy,* 35, 10, (Oct), 1392-1399, 16238801

Bohle B., Schwihla H., Hu H. Z., Friedl-Hajek R., Sowka S., Ferreira F., Breiteneder H., Bruijnzeel-Koomen C. A., de Weger R. A., Mudde G. C., Ebner C.&Van Reijsen F. C. (1998). Long-lived Th2 clones specific for seasonal and perennial allergens can be detected in blood and skin by their TCR-hypervariable regions. *J Immunol,* 160, 4, (Feb 15), 2022-2027, 9469466

Bohle B., Zwolfer B., Heratizadeh A., Jahn-Schmid B., Antonia Y. D., Alter M., Keller W., Zuidmeer L., van Ree R., Werfel T.&Ebner C. (2006). Cooking birch pollen-related food: divergent consequences for IgE- and T cell-mediated reactivity in vitro and in vivo. *J Allergy Clin Immunol,* 118, 1, (Jul), 242-249, 16815162

Bolhaar S. T., Ree R., Bruijnzeel-Koomen C. A., Knulst A. C.&Zuidmeer L. (2004). Allergy to jackfruit: a novel example of Bet v 1-related food allergy. *Allergy,* 59, 11, (Nov), 1187-1192, 15461600

Bruijnzeel-Koomen C., Ortolani C., Aas K., Bindslev-Jensen C., Bjorksten B., Moneret-Vautrin D.&Wuthrich B. (1995). Adverse reactions to food. European Academy of Allergology and Clinical Immunology Subcommittee. *Allergy,* 50, 8, (Aug), 623-635, 7503398

Bucher X., Pichler W. J., Dahinden C. A.&Helbling A. (2004). Effect of tree pollen specific, subcutaneous immunotherapy on the oral allergy syndrome to apple and hazelnut. *Allergy,* 59, 12, (Dec), 1272-1276, 15507095

Cirla A. M., Sforza N., Roffi G. P., Alessandrini A., Stanizzi R., Dorigo N., Sala E.&Della Torre F. (1996). Preseasonal intranasal immunotherapy in birch-alder allergic rhinitis. A double-blind study. *Allergy,* 51, 5, (May), 299-305, 8836333

Duhen T., Geiger R., Jarrossay D., Lanzavecchia A.&Sallusto F. (2009). Production of interleukin 22 but not interleukin 17 by a subset of human skin-homing memory T cells. *Nat Immunol,* 10, 8, (Aug), 857-863, 19578369

Ebner C., Siemann U., Bohle B., Willheim M., Wiedermann U., Schenk S., Klotz F., Ebner H., Kraft D.&Scheiner O. (1997). Immunological changes during specific immunotherapy of grass pollen allergy: reduced lymphoproliferative responses to allergen and shift from TH2 to TH1 in T-cell clones specific for Phl p 1, a major grass pollen allergen. *Clin Exp Allergy,* 27, 9, (Sep), 1007-1015, 9678832

Enrique E., Pineda F., Malek T., Bartra J., Basagana M., Tella R., Castello J. V., Alonso R., de Mateo J. A., Cerda-Trias T., San Miguel-Moncin Mdel M., Monzon S., Garcia M., Palacios R.&Cistero-Bahima A. (2005). Sublingual immunotherapy for hazelnut food allergy: a randomized, double-blind, placebo-controlled study with a standardized hazelnut extract. *J Allergy Clin Immunol,* 116, 5, (Nov), 1073-1079, 16275379

Eriksson N. E. (1978). Food sensitivity reported by patients with asthma and hay fever. A relationship between food sensitivity and birch pollen-allergy and between food sensitivity and acetylsalicylic acid intolerance. *Allergy,* 33, 4, (Aug), 189-196, 717703

Eriksson N. E., Formgren H.&Svenonius E. (1982). Food hypersensitivity in patients with pollen allergy. *Allergy,* 37, 6, (Aug), 437-443, 7137538

Eyerich S., Eyerich K., Pennino D., Carbone T., Nasorri F., Pallotta S., Cianfarani F., Odorisio T., Traidl-Hoffmann C., Behrendt H., Durham S. R., Schmidt-Weber C. B.&Cavani A. (2009). Th22 cells represent a distinct human T cell subset involved in epidermal immunity and remodeling. *J Clin Invest,* 119, 12, (Dec), 3573-3585, 19920355

Fernandez-Rivas M., Benito C., Gonzalez-Mancebo E.&de Durana D. A. (2008). Allergies to fruits and vegetables. *Pediatr Allergy Immunol,* 19, 8, (Dec), 675-681, 19097271

Fernandez-Rivas M., Bolhaar S., Gonzalez-Mancebo E., Asero R., van Leeuwen A., Bohle B., Ma Y., Ebner C., Rigby N., Sancho A. I., Miles S., Zuidmeer L., Knulst A., Breiteneder H., Mills C., Hoffmann-Sommergruber K.&van Ree R. (2006). Apple allergy across Europe: how allergen sensitization profiles determine the clinical expression of allergies to plant foods. *J Allergy Clin Immunol,* 118, 2, (Aug), 481-488, 16890775

Flinterman A. E., Hoekstra M. O., Meijer Y., van Ree R., Akkerdaas J. H., Bruijnzeel-Koomen C. A., Knulst A. C.&Pasmans S. G. (2006). Clinical reactivity to hazelnut in children: association with sensitization to birch pollen or nuts? *J Allergy Clin Immunol,* 118, 5, (Nov), 1186-1189, 17088148

Fritsch R., Bohle B., Vollmann U., Wiedermann U., Jahn-Schmid B., Krebitz M., Breiteneder H., Kraft D.&Ebner C. (1998). Bet v 1, the major birch pollen allergen, and Mal d 1, the major apple allergen, cross-react at the level of allergen-specific T helper cells. *J Allergy Clin Immunol,* 102, 4 Pt 1, (Oct), 679-686, 9802379

Geroldinger-Simic M., Zelniker T., Aberer W., Ebner C., Egger C., Greiderer A., Prem N., Lidholm J., Ballmer-Weber B., Vieths S.&Bohle B. (2011). Birch pollen-related food allergy: Clinical aspects and the role of allergen-specific IgE and IgG4 antibodies. *J Allergy Clin Immunol,* in press,

Gerstmayr M., Ilk N., Schabussova I., Jahn-Schmid B., Egelseer E. M., Sleytr U. B., Ebner C.&Bohle B. (2007). A novel approach to specific allergy treatment: the recombinant allergen-S-layer fusion protein rSbsC-Bet v 1 matures dendritic cells that prime Th0/Th1 and IL-10-producing regulatory T cells. *J Immunol,* 179, 11, (Dec 1), 7270-7275, 18025169

Ghunaim N., Gronlund H., Kronqvist M., Gronneberg R., Soderstrom L., Ahlstedt S.&van Hage-Hamsten M. (2005). Antibody profiles and self-reported symptoms to pollen-related food allergens in grass pollen-allergic patients from northern Europe. *Allergy,* 60, 2, (Feb), 185-191, 15647039

Hannuksela M.&Lahti A. (1977). Immediate reactions to fruits and vegetables. *Contact Dermatitis,* 3, 2, (Apr), 79-84, 872578

Herrmann D., Henzgen M., Frank E., Rudeschko O.&Jager L. (1995). Effect of hyposensitization for tree pollinosis on associated apple allergy. *J Investig Allergol Clin Immunol,* 5, 5, (Sep-Oct), 259-267, 8574432

Horak F., Stubner P., Berger U. E., Marks B., Toth J.&Jager S. (1998). Immunotherapy with sublingual birch pollen extract. A short-term double-blind placebo study. *J Investig Allergol Clin Immunol,* 8, 3, (May-Jun), 165-171, 9684190

Jahn-Schmid B., Radakovics A., Luttkopf D., Scheurer S., Vieths S., Ebner C.&Bohle B. (2005). Bet v 1142-156 is the dominant T-cell epitope of the major birch pollen allergen and important for cross-reactivity with Bet v 1-related food allergens. *J Allergy Clin Immunol,* 116, 1, (Jul), 213-219, 15990797

James L. K., Shamji M. H., Walker S. M., Wilson D. R., Wachholz P. A., Francis J. N., Jacobson M. R., Kimber I., Till S. J.&Durham S. R. (2011). Long-term tolerance after allergen immunotherapy is accompanied by selective persistence of blocking antibodies. *J Allergy Clin Immunol,* 127, 2, (Feb), 509-516 e501-505, 21281875

Juhlin-Dannfelt C. (1948). About the occurrence of various forms of pollen allergy in Sweden. *Acta Med Scand,* 131, Suppl 206, 563-577, 18881184

Jutel M., Akdis M., Budak F., Aebischer-Casaulta C., Wrzyszcz M., Blaser K.&Akdis C. A. (2003). IL-10 and TGF-beta cooperate in the regulatory T cell response to mucosal allergens in normal immunity and specific immunotherapy. *Eur J Immunol,* 33, 5, (May), 1205-1214, 12731045

Khinchi M. S., Poulsen L. K., Carat F., Andre C., Hansen A. B.&Malling H. J. (2004). Clinical efficacy of sublingual and subcutaneous birch pollen allergen-specific immunotherapy: a randomized, placebo-controlled, double-blind, double-dummy study. *Allergy,* 59, 1, (Jan), 45-53, 14674933

Kinaciyan T., Jahn-Schmid B., Radakovics A., Zwolfer B., Schreiber C., Francis J. N., Ebner C.&Bohle B. (2007). Successful sublingual immunotherapy with birch pollen has limited effects on concomitant food allergy to apple and the immune response to the Bet v 1 homolog Mal d 1. *J Allergy Clin Immunol,* 119, 4, (Apr), 937-943, 17204315

Kleine-Tebbe J., Vogel L., Crowell D. N., Haustein U. F.&Vieths S. (2002). Severe oral allergy syndrome and anaphylactic reactions caused by a Bet v 1- related PR-10 protein in soybean, SAM22. *J Allergy Clin Immunol,* 110, 5, (Nov), 797-804, 12417891

Kopac P., Gentinetta T., Gerber R., Rudin M., Pichler C., Hausmann O.&Pichler W. J. (2010). Clinical effective apple desensitization in birch allergic patients with oral allergy syndrome. *Annual congress of the Austrian Society for Allergology and Immunology,*

Kopper R. A., Odum N. J., Sen M., Helm R. M., Steve Stanley J.&Wesley Burks A. (2004). Peanut protein allergens: gastric digestion is carried out exclusively by pepsin. *J Allergy Clin Immunol,* 114, 3, (Sep), 614-618, 15356566

Kopper R. A., West C. M.&Helm R. M. (2006). Comparison of physiological and in vitro porcine gastric fluid digestion. *Int Arch Allergy Immunol,* 141, 3, 217-222, 16926541

Larche M., Akdis C. A.&Valenta R. (2006). Immunological mechanisms of allergen-specific immunotherapy. *Nat Rev Immunol,* 6, 10, (Oct), 761-771, 16998509

Lin R. Y., Clauss A. E.&Bennett E. S. (2002). Hypersensitivity to common tree pollens in New York City patients. *Allergy Asthma Proc,* 23, 4, (Jul-Aug), 253-258, 12221895

Mauro M., Russello M., Incorvaia C., Gazzola G. B., Di Cara G.&Frati F. (2007). Comparison of efficacy, safety and immunologic effects of subcutaneous and sublingual immunotherapy in birch pollinosis: a randomized study. *Eur Ann Allergy Clin Immunol,* 39, 4, (Apr), 119-122, 17523385

Mittag D., Akkerdaas J., Ballmer-Weber B. K., Vogel L., Wensing M., Becker W. M., Koppelman S. J., Knulst A. C., Helbling A., Hefle S. L., Van Ree R.&Vieths S. (2004). Ara h 8, a Bet v 1-homologous allergen from peanut, is a major allergen in patients with combined birch pollen and peanut allergy. *J Allergy Clin Immunol,* 114, 6, (Dec), 1410-1417, 15577846

Mittag D., Batori V., Neudecker P., Wiche R., Friis E. P., Ballmer-Weber B. K., Vieths S.&Roggen E. L. (2006). A novel approach for investigation of specific and cross-reactive IgE epitopes on Bet v 1 and homologous food allergens in individual patients. *Mol Immunol,* 43, 3, (Feb), 268-278, 16199263

Mittag D., Vieths S., Vogel L., Wagner-Loew D., Starke A., Hunziker P., Becker W. M.&Ballmer-Weber B. K. (2005). Birch pollen-related food allergy to legumes: identification and characterization of the Bet v 1 homologue in mungbean (Vigna radiata), Vig r 1. *Clin Exp Allergy,* 35, 8, (Aug), 1049-1055, 16120087

Modrzynski M., Zawisza E., Rapiejko P.&Przybylski G. (2002). [Specific-pollen immunotherapy in the treatment of oral allergy syndrome in patients with tree pollen hypersensitivity]. *Przegl Lek,* 59, 12, 1007-1010, 12731377

Moneo I., Gomez M., Sanchez-Monge R., Alday E., de las Heras M., Esteban I., Bootello A.&Salcedo G. (1999). Lack of crossreaction with Bet v 1 in patients sensitized to Dau c 1, a carrot allergen. *Ann Allergy Asthma Immunol,* 83, 1, (Jul), 71-75, 10437820

Mutschlechner S., Deifl S.&Bohle B. (2009). Genetic allergen modification in the development of novel approaches to specific immunotherapy. *Clin Exp Allergy,* 39, 11, (Nov), 1635-1642, 19624521

Neudecker P., Lehmann K., Nerkamp J., Haase T., Wangorsch A., Fotisch K., Hoffmann S., Rosch P., Vieths S.&Scheurer S. (2003). Mutational epitope analysis of Pru av 1 and Api g 1, the major allergens of cherry (Prunus avium) and celery (Apium graveolens): correlating IgE reactivity with three-dimensional structure. *Biochem J,* 376, Pt 1, (Nov 15), 97-107, 12943529

Niederberger V., Reisinger J., Valent P., Krauth M. T., Pauli G., van Hage M., Cromwell O., Horak F.&Valenta R. (2007). Vaccination with genetically modified birch pollen allergens: immune and clinical effects on oral allergy syndrome. *J Allergy Clin Immunol,* 119, 4, (Apr), 1013-1016, 17292956

Nouri-Aria K. T., Wachholz P. A., Francis J. N., Jacobson M. R., Walker S. M., Wilcock L. K., Staple S. Q., Aalberse R. C., Till S. J.&Durham S. R. (2004). Grass pollen immunotherapy induces mucosal and peripheral IL-10 responses and blocking IgG activity. *J Immunol,* 172, 5, (Mar 1), 3252-3259, 14978133

Nowak-Wegrzyn A.&Sampson H. A. (2011). Future therapies for food allergies. *J Allergy Clin Immunol,* 127, 3, (Mar), 558-573; quiz 574-555, 21277625

Oberhuber C., Bulley S. M., Ballmer-Weber B. K., Bublin M., Gaier S., DeWitt A. M., Briza P., Hofstetter G., Lidholm J., Vieths S.&Hoffmann-Sommergruber K. (2008). Characterization of Bet v 1-related allergens from kiwifruit relevant for patients with combined kiwifruit and birch pollen allergy. *Mol Nutr Food Res,* 52 Suppl 2, (Nov), S230-240, 18925615

O'Hehir R. E., Gardner L. M., de Leon M. P., Hales B. J., Biondo M., Douglass J. A., Rolland J. M.&Sandrini A. (2009). House dust mite sublingual immunotherapy: the role for transforming growth factor-beta and functional regulatory T cells. *Am J Respir Crit Care Med,* 180, 10, (Nov 15), 936-947, 19696440

Ortolani C., Ispano M., Pastorello E., Bigi A.&Ansaloni R. (1988). The oral allergy syndrome. *Ann Allergy,* 61, 6 Pt 2, (Dec), 47-52, 3264668

Osterballe M., Hansen T. K., Mortz C. G., Host A.&Bindslev-Jensen C. (2005). The prevalence of food hypersensitivity in an unselected population of children and adults. *Pediatr Allergy Immunol,* 16, 7, (Nov), 567-573, 16238581

Pauli G., Larsen T. H., Rak S., Horak F., Pastorello E., Valenta R., Purohit A., Arvidsson M., Kavina A., Schroeder J. W., Mothes N., Spitzauer S., Montagut A., Galvain S., Melac M., Andre C., Poulsen L. K.&Malling H. J. (2008). Efficacy of recombinant birch pollen vaccine for the treatment of birch-allergic rhinoconjunctivitis. *J Allergy Clin Immunol,* 122, 5, (Nov), 951-960, 19000581

Radauer C., Lackner P.&Breiteneder H. (2008). The Bet v 1 fold: an ancient, versatile scaffold for binding of large, hydrophobic ligands. *BMC Evol Biol,* 8, 286, 18922149

Reekers R., Busche M., Wittmann M., Kapp A.&Werfel T. (1999). Birch pollen-related foods trigger atopic dermatitis in patients with specific cutaneous T-cell responses to birch pollen antigens. *J Allergy Clin Immunol,* 104, 2 Pt 1, (Aug), 466-472, 10452773

Scadding G. W., Shamji M. H., Jacobson M. R., Lee D. I., Wilson D., Lima M. T., Pitkin L., Pilette C., Nouri-Aria K.&Durham S. R. (2010). Sublingual grass pollen immunotherapy is associated with increases in sublingual Foxp3-expressing cells and elevated allergen-specific immunoglobulin G4, immunoglobulin A and serum inhibitory activity for immunoglobulin E-facilitated allergen binding to B cells. *Clin Exp Allergy,* 40, 4, (Apr), 598-606, 20184605

Scheurer S., Son D. Y., Boehm M., Karamloo F., Franke S., Hoffmann A., Haustein D.&Vieths S. (1999). Cross-reactivity and epitope analysis of Pru a 1, the major cherry allergen. *Mol Immunol,* 36, 3, (Feb), 155-167, 10403481

Schimek E. M., Zwolfer B., Briza P., Jahn-Schmid B., Vogel L., Vieths S., Ebner C.&Bohle B. (2005). Gastrointestinal digestion of Bet v 1-homologous food allergens destroys their mediator-releasing, but not T cell-activating, capacity. *J Allergy Clin Immunol,* 116, 6, (Dec), 1327-1333, 16337467

Schulten V., Lauer I., Scheurer S., Thalhammer T.&Bohle B. (2011). A food matrix reduces digestion and absorption of food allergens in vivo. *Mol Nutr Food Res, 55,* (Oct 10), 1484-1491, 21984443

Shamji M. H., Wilcock L. K., Wachholz P. A., Dearman R. J., Kimber I., Wurtzen P. A., Larche M., Durham S. R.&Francis J. N. (2006). The IgE-facilitated allergen binding (FAB) assay: validation of a novel flow-cytometric based method for the detection of inhibitory antibody responses. *J Immunol Methods,* 317, 1-2, (Dec 20), 71-79, 17070537

Stevens W. J., Ebo D. G., Hagendorens M. M., Bridts C. H.&De Clerck L. S. (2003). Is the prevalence of specific IgE to classical inhalant aeroallergens among patients with respiratory allergy changing? Evidence from two surveys 15 years apart. *Acta Clin Belg,* 58, 3, (May-Jun), 178-182, 12945477

Valenta R., Niespodziana K., Focke-Tejkl M., Marth K., Huber H., Neubauer A.&Niederberger V. (2011). Recombinant allergens: what does the future hold? *J Allergy Clin Immunol,* 127, 4, (Apr), 860-864, 21458656

van Hoffen E., Peeters K. A., van Neerven R. J., van der Tas C. W., Zuidmeer L., van Ieperen-van Dijk A. G., Bruijnzeel-Koomen C. A., Knol E. F., van Ree R.&Knulst A. C. (2011). Effect of birch pollen-specific immunotherapy on birch pollen-related hazelnut allergy. *J Allergy Clin Immunol,* 127, 1, (Jan), 100-101, 101 e101-103, 20933256

van Neerven R. J., Wikborg T., Lund G., Jacobsen B., Brinch-Nielsen A., Arnved J.&Ipsen H. (1999). Blocking antibodies induced by specific allergy vaccination prevent the activation of CD4+ T cells by inhibiting serum-IgE-facilitated allergen presentation. *J Immunol,* 163, 5, (Sep 1), 2944-2952, 10453043

van Zuuren E. J., Terreehorst I., Tupker R. A., Hiemstra P. S.&Akkerdaas J. H. (2010). Anaphylaxis after consuming soy products in patients with birch pollinosis. *Allergy,* 65, 10, (Oct), 1348-1349, 20219061

Varshney P., Jones S. M., Scurlock A. M., Perry T. T., Kemper A., Steele P., Hiegel A., Kamilaris J., Carlisle S., Yue X., Kulis M., Pons L., Vickery B.&Burks A. W. (2011). A randomized controlled study of peanut oral immunotherapy: clinical desensitization and modulation of the allergic response. *J Allergy Clin Immunol,* 127, 3, (Mar), 654-660, 21377034

Veldhoen M., Uyttenhove C., van Snick J., Helmby H., Westendorf A., Buer J., Martin B., Wilhelm C.&Stockinger B. (2008). Transforming growth factor-beta 'reprograms' the differentiation of T helper 2 cells and promotes an interleukin 9-producing subset. *Nat Immunol,* 9, 12, (Dec), 1341-1346, 18931678

Wachholz P. A., Soni N. K., Till S. J.&Durham S. R. (2003). Inhibition of allergen-IgE binding to B cells by IgG antibodies after grass pollen immunotherapy. *J Allergy Clin Immunol,* 112, 5, (Nov), 915-922, 14610480

Wedderburn L. R., O'Hehir R. E., Hewitt C. R., Lamb J. R.&Owen M. J. (1993). In vivo clonal dominance and limited T-cell receptor usage in human CD4+ T-cell recognition of house dust mite allergens. *Proc Natl Acad Sci U S A,* 90, 17, (Sep 1), 8214-8218, 8367485

Werfel T., Reekers R., Busche M., Schmidt P., Constien A., Wittmann M.&Kapp A. (1999). Association of birch pollen-related food-responsive atopic dermatitis with birch pollen allergen-specific T-cell reactions. *Curr Probl Dermatol,* 28, 18-28, 10374046

Winther L., Malling H. J., Moseholm L.&Mosbech H. (2000). Allergen-specific immunotherapy in birch- and grass-pollen-allergic rhinitis. I. Efficacy estimated by a model reducing the bias of annual differences in pollen counts. *Allergy,* 55, 9, (Sep), 818-826, 11003445

Wong M. T., Ye J. J., Alonso M. N., Landrigan A., Cheung R. K., Engleman E.&Utz P. J. (2010). Regulation of human Th9 differentiation by type I interferons and IL-21. *Immunol Cell Biol,* 88, 6, (Aug), 624-631, 20421880

Part 2

Clinical Allergy

7

Anaphylaxis: Etiology, Clinical Manifestations, Diagnosis and Management

Aslı Gelincik and Suna Büyüköztürk
Istanbul University, Istanbul Faculty of Medicine, Turkey

1. Introduction

Anaphylaxis is an acute systemic allergic reaction that can potentially be life-threatening. Therefore it has to be diagnosed and treated promptly. It can occur after exposure to various triggers or spontaneously and can potentially affect multiple organ systems and prompt and definite treatment may be life saving. In this chapter, possible triggers of anaphylaxis, clinical manifestations, diagnosis and management will be discussed.

2. Epidemiology

Anaphylaxis is defined as a "severe, potentially fatal, systemic allergic reaction that occurs suddenly after contact with an allergy-causing substance" (Sampson et al., 2006). As there is no unified method of obtaining data about anaphylaxis, its incidence is very difficult to evaluate clearly. A substantial portion of the existing data on the epidemiology of anaphylaxis has come from investigations that have limited scope population sources, such as surveys and volunteer registries (Harduar-Morano et al., 2011). Lifetime prevalence is estimated as 0.05% to 2% (Simons, 2008). Recent studies confirm that the incidence of anaphylaxis, particularly food-induced anaphylaxis, is increasing world-wide (Chiu & Kelly, 2005). A very recent study investigated a large diverse population with anaphylaxis diagnosed in emergency departments using rigorous descriptive and analytic evaluation of risk factors, such as sex, race, ethnicity, and age (Harduar-Morano et al., 2011). In this study the highest observed rates were among the youngest male subjects (8.2/100,000 aged 0-4 years) and among adult female subjects (15-54 years) grouped in 10-year age categories (9,9-10.9/100,000). Previous epidemiologic studies also suggested that until age 15 years, there is a predilection for males, but after age 15 years, there is a predilection for females. Different trigger factors predominate in different age groups; for example, fatalities from food-induced anaphylaxis peak in adolescents and young adults, and fatalities from anaphylaxis triggered by insect stings, diagnostic agents, and medications predominate in middle-aged and older adults (Simons, 2008). Atopy is an associated risk factor for anaphylaxis triggered by food, exercise, and latex but not for anaphylaxis triggered by insect stings, β-lactam antibiotics (Chiu and Kelly, 2005). In addition, asthma was reported in 23% of 142 patients with anaphylaxis who presented to an emergency department from 1998 to 1999 (Brown et al., 2001).

3. Pathogenesis

The underlying pathogenesis of human anaphylaxis commonly involves an immunologic mechanism in which IgE is synthesized in response to allergen exposure and becomes fixed to high affinity receptors for IgE (FcεRI receptors) on the surface membranes of mast cells and basophils (Simons, 2010). Other potential immunologic mechanisms in anaphylaxis include involvement of immune aggregates, IgG, IgM, platelets, and T cells; shift in eicosanoid metabolism toward leukotriene formation; and activation of the complement or coagulation systems (Simons, 2008).

The mast cells and basophils are central players in allergic reaction (Rivera & Gilfillan, 2006). Activation of these cells induces the release of preformed inflammatory mediators localized in specialized granules and the de novo synthesis and secretion of cytokines, chemokines, and eicosanoids. Appropriate activation of mast cells is mediated by a number of factors, including the cells' ability to distinguish activating or inhibiting stimuli and the strength and duration of stimulus. FcεRI on mast cells is comprised of an IgE- binding α chain, a 4-transmembrane spanning β chain and a monodimer of γ chains. The β chain functions as an amplifying modul for this receptor. The γ chain monodimer imports signaling competence to this receptor. It has been demonstrated that both the β and γ chains function to generate positive signals that are key in initiating and amplifying the mast cells' effector responses. However, recent evidence suggests that these two chains can also function to negatively regulate cell activation and effector responses (Rivera & Gilfillan, 2006).

Current knowledge suggests that mast cell's response to a stimulus is very complex. A number of molecules play role in the coordination and control of degranulation. FcεRI-mediated activation of mast cells requires both Lyn and the related Src PTK Fyn as receptor-proximal kinases. Fyn-deficient and Lyn/Fyn double deficient mice showed defective passive systemic anaphylaxis responses indicating a positive role for Fyn in promoting mast cell degranulation in vivo (Rivera & Gilfillan, 2006).

Recent investigations showed that stem cell factor and its receptor Kit are fundamentally important in IgE/antigen-induced mast cell activation, and concurrent inhibition of Kit- and FcεRI-mediated signaling achieves coordinated suppression of human mast cell activation (Jensen et al., 2007). Inhibitory sialic acid-binding immunoglobulin-like lectins are expressed on human mast cells, on which Siglec-8 engagement results in inhibition of FcεRI-dependent mediator release without apoptosis (Yokoi et al., 2006). Sphingosine kinases are reported to be determinants of mast cell responsiveness (Olivera et al., 2007).

In some individuals described as having idiopathic anaphylaxis, FcεRI receptors may be aggregated through autoimmune mechanisms (Simons, 2010). Nonimmunological factors, which activate mast cells by mechanisms not yet fully understood, include exercise, cold air or water exposure, radiation, ethanol, insect venom, constituents, radiocontrast media and medications such as opioids and vancomycin (Simons, 2010). Regardless of the immunologic or nonimmunologic triggering mechanism, and regardless of whether FcεRI or other receptors such as G protein-coupled receptors or Toll-like receptors are activated, mast cells and basophils play an important role in initiating and amplifying the acute allergic response. They release mediators of inflammation including histamine, proteases such as tryptase, mast cell carboxypeptidase A3 and chymase, lipids such as platelet activating factor (PAF), prostaglandines (PGD2) and leukotrienes (LTC4) as well as chemokines and cytokines (Simons, 2008).

3.1 Animal models

Studies with murine models demonstrate 2 pathways of systemic anaphylaxis: one mediated by IgE, FcεRI, mast cells, histamine, and platelet-activating factor (PAF), and the other mediated by IgG, FcγRIII, macrophages, and PAF. The former pathway requires much less antibody and antigen than the latter. As a result, IgG antibody can block IgE-mediated anaphylaxis induced by small quantities of antigen without mediating FcγRIII-dependent anaphylaxis (Finkelman et al., 2005).

The IgE pathway is most likely responsible for most human anaphylaxis, which generally involves small amounts of antibody and antigen; similarities in the murine and human immune systems suggest that the IgG pathway might mediate disease in persons repeatedly exposed to large quantities of antigen. Antigen cross-linking of antigen specific IgE bound to mast cell FcεRI stimulates mast cell degranulation, with the rapid release of histamine and serotonin and the synthesis and secretion of platelet activation factor (PAF) and leukotrienes. These mediators act on target cells to increase vascular permeability which cause depletion of intravascular volume. The resulting decrease in vital organ perfusion is the primary cause of the symptoms that characterize murine anaphylaxis (Finkelman et al., 2005).

The other pathway in mouse is Ig-E independent pathway. As contrary of clasical pathway, at first immunized and antigen challenged mice had anaphylaxis despite the absence of mast cells, FcεRI and IgE. This pathway is also complement independent but requires IgG antibody, macrophages, FcγRIII and PAF. Regardless which pathway takes place, mouse anaphylaxis occurs in very short time and displays similar symptoms. Potentially important differences between mouse and human anaphylaxis are proposed as follows: 1. Mouse IgG has some ability to activate mast cells, an effect that is not shared by any human IgG isotype, 2. IgE binds weakly to murine, but not human low-affinity FcγRs, 3. Human but not mouse macrophages, Langerhans cells and dendritic cells can express FcεRI, and 4. Human platelets, B cells and natural killer cells, and neutrophils express low affinity IgG receptor (FcγRIIA, FcγRIIC, and FcγRIIIB, respectively) that are not expressed in mouse (Finkelman et al., 2005).

Less antibody and antigen are required to trigger IgE dependent anaphylaxis then IgG mediated anaphylaxis. IgG and IgA blocking antibodies inhibit the ability of small quantities of antigen to induce IgE dependent anaphylaxis by neutralizing antigen before it can cross link mast cell associated IgE. IgG antibodies also inhibit IgE-dependent anaphylaxis by mediating an interaction between FcεRI and FcγRIIb on mast cells. In mice the predominant determinants that influence whether IgE dependent anaphylaxis is induced appear to be the quantity of antigen specific IgG antibody produced and the quantity of antigen used to challenge immunized mice. This suggests that IgG antibodies, in addition to mediating IgE- independent anaphylaxis, can block IgE-dependent anaphylaxis and provide the rationale for investigating the function of blocking antibody. Gastrointestinal anaphylaxis is induced by IgE/ FcεRI/mast cell/PAF plus serotonin pathway and can cause systemic symptoms if levels of blocking antibodies are low (Finkelman et al., 2005).

3.2 Cytokines

The development and severity of anaphylaxis depend not only on the presence of the required IgE or IgG antibodies, inflammatory cells that express receptor for these antibodies and mediators that are released by these cells but also on the responsiveness of cells that are targeted by these mediators. This last factor is influenced by IL-4 and IL-13, cytokines that are also important in the initial generation of the antibody and inflammatory cell responses that mediate anaphylaxis to a considerable extent. These effects depend on IL-4Rα-dependent IL4/IL13 activation of transcription factor signal transducer and activator of transcription 6 and thus likely depend on new gene expression and protein synthesis even though they develop within 1-2 hours after mice are treated with either cytokine. The most dramatic and rapid effect of IL-4 on anaphylaxis is a 3-to-6 fold enhancement of responsiveness of targeted cells to vasoactive mediators, including histamine, serotonin, PAF and cysteinyl lekotrienes (Finkelman et al., 2005).

4. Clinical aspects

Currently, there is no universally accepted clinical definition of anaphylaxis. Because of large variability in presenting clinical signs and symptoms, a clear definition of anaphylaxis is difficult. It is likely that anaphylaxis is under diagnosed, especially if it is a patient's first episode, if there is a hidden or previously unrecognized trigger, or if symptoms are mild, transient, or skin signs are absent. Patients might not be able to describe their symptoms if awareness, recognition, and judgment are impaired or if they are dyspneic or becoming unconscious. Symptoms may be suppressed by other medications such as first-generation H1- antihistamines. Health care providers may fail to recognize symptoms of anaphylaxis without obtaining a detailed history and full physical examination. Even after a detailed history and examination, the diagnosis may be overlooked when hives or other skin manifestations are absent. The guidelines published in 2006 by the National Institute of Allergy and Infectious Disease (NIAID) and the Food Allergy and Anaphylaxis Network (FAAN) have partially responded to this difficulty (Sampson et al., 2006) (Table 1). However, new large studies are necessary to evaluate current situation.
For the diagnosis of anaphylaxis, a detailed and comprehensive clinical history is essential. Such a history may disclose exposure to potential triggering agents or events, time elapsed between exposure and symptom onset, and evolution of the episode over minutes or hours.

5. Anaphylaxis triggers

The triggering factors of anaphylaxis are listed on Table 2. Foods, medications, and venom continue to be leading causes of anaphylaxis (Boden & Burks, 2011).

5.1 Foods

Food allergy is the most common trigger of children presenting with anaphylaxis (Boden & Burks, 2011). Although most episodes of food-induced anaphylaxis occur within minutes of ingestion, anaphylaxis triggered by mammalian meat may be delayed by several hours. Although, the most common food triggers are reported to be peanut, tree nuts, shellfish, fish, milk, egg, and sesame; there are important variations between the populations from different geographic regions (Sicherer & Sampson, 2006). Any food can potentially trigger anaphylaxis, including previously unrecognized triggers, or some fresh red meats containing carbohydrates. Food triggers can be hidden (eg, substituted foods, cross-reacting foods, and cross-contacting foods). Food triggers also include additives, such as spices, vegetable gums, and colorants (eg, carmine [cochineal]); contaminants, such as dust mites; and parasites, such as the live sea fish nematode Anisakis simplex. Although some food allergies resolve with age others persist. An estimated 80% of children with anaphylaxis to milk or egg are able to tolerate ingestion by age 16 years (Sampson & Burks, 2009).

Anaphylaxis is highly likely when any 1 of the following 3 criteria is fulfilled:	
1.	Acute onset of an illness (minutes to several hours) with involvement of the skin, mucosal tissue, or both (eg, generalized hives, pruritus or flushing, and swollen lips-tongue-uvula) AND at least 1 of the following:
	A. Respiratory compromise (eg, dyspnea, wheeze-bronchospasm, stridor, reduced PEF, hypoxemia)
	B. Reduced blood pressure or associated symptoms of end-organ dysfunction (eg, hypotonia [collapse], syncope, incontinence)
2.	Two or more of the following that occur rapidly after exposure to a likely allergen for that patient (minutes to several hours):
	A. Involvement of the skin–mucosal tissue (eg, generalized hives, itch-flush, swollen lips-tongue-uvula)
	B. Respiratory compromise (eg, dyspnea, wheeze-bronchospasm, stridor, reduced PEF, hypoxemia)
	C. Reduced blood pressure or associated symptoms (eg, hypotonia [collapse], syncope, incontinence)
	D. Persistent gastrointestinal symptoms (eg, cramping abdominal pain, vomiting)
3.	Reduced blood pressure after exposure to a known allergen for that patient (minutes to several hours):
	A. Infants and children: low systolic blood pressure (age-specific) or greater than 30% decrease in systolic blood pressure
	B. Adults: systolic blood pressure of less than 90 mm Hg or greater than 30% decrease from that person's baseline

Table 1. Clinical criteria for diagnosing anaphylaxis (Sampson et al., 2006 with permission)

Immunologic mechanisms (IgE dependent)
Foods and food additives Medications Venoms, such as stinging insects (Hymenoptera) Natural rubber latex Occupational allergens Seminal fluid (prostate-specific antigen) Inhalants, such as horse, hamster, and other animal danders and grass pollen (rare) Radiocontrast media Immunologic mechanisms (IgE independent, formerly classified as anaphylactoid reactions) Dextran, such as high-molecular-weight iron dextran Infliximab
Nonimmunologic mechanisms
Physical factors, such as exercise, cold, heat, and sunlight/UV radiation Ethanol Medications, such as opioids Idiopathic anaphylaxis Consider the possibility of hidden or previously unrecognized allergens Consider the possibility of mastocytosis/clonal mast cell disorder

Table 2. Mechanisms and triggers of anaphylaxis in the community (Simons, 2010 with permission)

5.2 Drugs

Many drugs may induce anaphylaxis as a consequence of drug allergy/hypersensitivity. The parenteral use of drugs increases the risk and severity of anaphylactic reactions, and most fatal reactions have occurred with intramuscular or intravenous administration (Chiu & Kelly, 2005). Although drug related anaphylaxis may occur at any age , it is particularly common in middle-aged and older adults. Atopy appears to be associated with a substantially increased risk of serious allergic reactions (including anaphylaxis) once an IgE antibody response to any drug has developed (Lieberman et al., 2010). Antibiotics, especially β-lactam antibiotics including penicillin, semi-synthetic penicillins (eg, amoxicillin), cephalosporins, carbapenems (eg, imipenem), monobactams (eg, aztreonam), and carbecephems, and nonsteroidal anti-inflammatory drugs (NSAIDs), including aspirin, ibuprofen, and other agents, are the most often implicated drugs. In the retrospective review of pediatric cases of anaphylaxis, the incidence of drug-induced anaphylaxis was 11%, with nonsteroidal anti-inflammatory drugs causing 50%, antibiotics 40%, and muscle relaxants 10% of reactions (Novembre et al., 1998). In another study, the incidence of medications inducing anaphylaxis was 16%, with antibiotics causing 9%, and other drugs causing 7% of reactions (Dibs & Baker, 1997). In a review of fatal reactions, over four fifths of victims of fatal drug anaphylaxis had no previous awareness or indication of their drug allergy (Chiu and Kelly, 2005). Other common drugs that cause such reactions are insulin, enzymes (streptokinase and chymopapain), heterologous antisera (equine antitoxins and, antilymphocyte globulin), monoclonal antibodies (such as cetuximab, infliximab, and omalizumab), protamine, and heparin. However a great number of medications are known to cause anaphylactic reactions including chemotherapeutic agents, anesthetic agents, radioconrast media etc. Vaccines to prevent infectious diseases seldom trigger anaphylaxis (Simons, 2010). Allergic Type 1 reactions also have been reported after exposure to excipients such as eugenol, carmine, vegetable gums, paraben, thiomerosal, sodium metabisulfite, formaldehyde, and sulfonechloramide.

5.3 Venom

Hymenoptera stings can cause systemic and occasionally fatal anaphylaxis (Bilo & Bonifazi, 2009). Epidemiological population-based studies over the last decade show a prevalence of systemic reaction from hymenoptera stings ranging from 0.3% to 8.9%, with the lowest occurrence in children (Chiu & Kelly, 2005). Order Hymenoptera, family Apidae [honeybees]; family Vespidae [eg, yellow jackets, yellow hornets, white-faced hornets, and paper wasps]; and family Formicidae [eg, ants]) are well known causes. Factors determining the severity of reaction to hymenoptera sting include history of previous severe systemic reaction, insect type, older age, pre-existing cardiovascular and respiratory disease, and use of some medications. Mastocytosis and monoclonal mast cell activation syndrome are a risk factor for severe systemic reactions in allergic patients (Brockow & Ring, 2011).

5.4 Latex

Latex-induced anaphylaxis is due to IgE-mediated mechanisms and may occur in latex sensitive individuals due to direct contact with latex, usually gloves, or instruments, or with aerosolization of latex antigen adherent to the cornstarch powder of latex gloves (Lieberman et al., 2010). Anaphylaxis to natural rubber latex (NRL) became one of the most pervasive problems in medical and surgical care in the early 1990s in children with spina bifida (Chiu

& Kelly, 2005). Latex reactions may occur immediately with latex contact or may be delayed from 30 to 60 minutes. Latex has been reported to account for up to 17% of intraoperative anaphylaxis (Lieberman et al., 2010). Intraoperative latex anaphylaxis may be related to the administration of drug through a latex port prior to surgery, or during the surgical procedure itself. Latex reactions have also been reported to occur during dental procedures from latex gloves or dams, during obstetrical or gynecologic examinations and during latex condom use. Spina bifida patients are potentially at risk during each surgical procedure because of the number of procedures they undergo. Latex sensitization is due to IgE-mediated reactivity to any number of antigens from *Hevea brasiliensis*, the source of latex. Sensitization occurs in up to 12 percent of health care workers, up to 75 percent of patients with spina bifida and in patients undergoing multiple surgical procedures (Lieberman et al., 2010).

5.5 Perioperative anaphylaxis

The incidence of anaphylaxis during anesthesia has been reported to range from 1 in 4000 to 1 in 25,000 (Lieberman et al., 2005). The causes of anaphylaxis in this setting are varied, as are the mechanisms responsible for the reaction. The most common cause of anaphylaxis during general anesthesia or postoperatively is neuromuscular blocking agents (muscle relaxants), which are responsible for sixty to seventy percent of episodes of anaphylaxis occurring during this period. Most of the muscle relaxants cause direct release of mast cell histamine without the requirement for specific antibody. However, life-threatening reactions usually are IgE- mediated. The tertiary or quaternary ammonium group, common to all muscle relaxants, is likely the immunodominant determinant recognized by IgE. The antigenicity of the shared ammonium structures may be responsible for cross-reactivity among the muscle relaxants. Cross-reactivity occurs most consistently between pancuronium and vecuronium. Cross-reactions also may occur between muscle relaxants and other classes of pharmaceuticals, based upon in vitro inhibition of specific-IgE binding to the muscle relaxants. Agents that potentially cross-react with muscle relaxants include: acetylcholine, choline, morphine, neostigmine, and pentolinium. Cross-inhibition suggests that previous exposure to these non-anesthetic drugs may sensitize individuals to muscle-relaxing agents, resulting in reactions among patients without prior anesthesia (Lieberman et al., 2005).

5.6 Exercise anaphylaxis

In some individuals anaphylaxis can be triggered by exercise (exercise-induced anaphylaxis EIA); this phenomenon usually preceded by a causative food ingestion (food-dependent, exercise-induced anaphylaxis (FDEIA) (Barg et al., 2011) . Both are rare but potentially life-threatening clinical syndromes. The symptoms of FDEIA may vary in severity but, reassuringly, fatalities are rare. EIA occurs in all ages, in both sexes, and is more common in atopic individuals. Typical early signs and symptoms begin a few minutes into exercise, and include diffuse warmth, flushing, pruritus, urticaria, and fatigue. If exercise continues, there may be progression to angioedema of the face and extremities, gastrointestinal symptoms, laryngeal edema, hypotension, or collapse. Wheezing can occur, although it is less common than other symptoms. Some patients experience disabling headache that persists for several days after an episode. Attacks occur sporadically and unpredictably, even though most patients with this disorder exercise regularly. Vigorous exercises, such as jogging, racquet sports, dancing, and aerobics, are most often implicated, although lower levels of exertion, such as brisk walking or yard work, are capable of triggering attacks in some patients. Cessation of exercise usually results in improvement or resolution of symptoms, although, patients often do not instinctively stop exercising when they first experience symptoms. Instead, many try to run for help or sprint home, and this precipitates a dramatic worsening of symptoms. Although wheat is the most commonly reported food allergen associated with FDEIA many other food allergens such as grains, nuts, and seafood, have also been reported (Barg et al., 2011).

5.7 Idiopathic anaphylaxis

Idiopathic anaphylaxis is diagnosed when no triggers can be identified based on history, skin tests are negative, and serum specific IgE levels are absent or undetectable (Greenberger, 2007). Before this diagnosis is made, however, the possibility of a hidden or previously unrecognized trigger should be ruled out and the patients should be evaluated for mastocytosis and clonal mast cell disorders. Idiopathic anaphylaxis has been classified into two categories. When there is a sudden episode that includes urticaria and angioedema associated with acute bronchoconstriction, voice change or stridor, syncope or proven hypotension with or without abdominal pain and diarrrhea, it is then considered as idiopathic anaphylaxis generalized (IA-G). Anaphylaxis that is characterized by marked upper airway obstruction attributable to massive tongue enlargement or a severely edematous larynx or pharynx is categorized as anaphylaxis angioedema (IA-A) (Greenberger, 2007).

5.8 Mastocytocic and anaphylaxis

In adults with mastocytosis, the cumulative prevalence of anaphylaxis has been reported to be 22% to 49%, and in children 6% to 9%. Those with systemic disease have an increased risk of anaphylaxis as compared with patients with cutaneous disease only. As in patients without mastocytosis, the most frequently reported elicitors of anaphylaxis are insect venoms, drugs, and food. Severe and fatal reactions to hymenoptera venom have been described in patients with mastocytosis (Brockow & Ring, 2011).

A variety of drugs have been reported to elicit anaphylaxis in patients with mastocytosis. Every year, reports have been published regarding patients with mastocytosis in whom the diagnosis of systemic mastocytosis was made following anaphylaxis to muscle relaxants or other drugs used during general anesthesia. Other medications leading to reactions in patients with mastocytosis are opiates (including morphine and codeine), acetylsalicylic acid, other NSAIDs, antibiotics, and radiocontrast media. In some patients with mastocytosis, anaphylaxis remains idiopathic despite an extensive search for elicitors (Brockow & Ring, 2011).

The intensity of anaphylaxis in patients with mastocytosis has been described to be particularly severe. Among 55 patients with insect sting allergy and confirmed mastocytosis, 81% experienced severe anaphylaxis with shock or cardiopulmonary arrest (Brockow & Metcalfe, 2010). In another study in which the severity of anaphylaxis was rated, 60% of patients reported severe symptoms and 43% experienced loss of consciousness. Fatal reactions may occur. This is in agreement with the observation that baseline serum tryptase levels are the best known predictor of the severity of anaphylaxis in insect sting–allergic patients (Brockow & Ring, 2011) .

5.9 Rare causes of anaphylaxis

Although rare, anaphylaxis due to coital exposure to human seminal fluid is a known occurrence. Since the initial report in 1958, approximately 30 cases of seminal fluid induced anaphylaxis have been described. All reactions have occurred in female patients during or after sexual intercourse. The vast majority of such reactions are caused by IgE-mediated sensitization to human seminal plasma proteins with molecular weights ranging from 12-75 kD (Lieberman et al., 2010).

Subcutaneous allergen immunotherapy (AIT) injections may rarely cause systemic reactions. Its rate has been estimated at 0.25-1.3%. Fatal anaphylaxis to AIT injections occurs at an estimated rate of 1 in 2.5 million injections and near-fatal anaphylactic reactions at a rate of 1 in every 1 million injections. Patients with asthma, particularly poorly controlled asthma are at higher risk for serious systemic reactions to AIT injections (Lieberman et al., 2005).

In the patients having anaphylaxis attacks without any apparent trigger hydatid cyst ruptures must be kept in mind. Hydatid cysts can rupture as a result of trauma or sometimes spontaneously, and anaphylaxis can be a complication. However, several case reports indicate that anaphylaxis can also occur without macroscopic hydatid cyst rupture (Gelincik et al., 2007).

6. Clinical presentation

Although most definitions specify the need for more than one organ system involvement in the syndrome, it is more important to understand the systemic nature of the clinical symptoms. The first symptoms and signs of anaphylaxis often appear within seconds to minutes after exposure to an offending trigger, however sometimes they may develop later. Late phase or biphasic reactions could also arise 8-12 hours after the initial attack (Lieberman et al., 2010). Each exposure to antigen is unique, and past episodes of anaphylaxis do not predict future events (Boden & Burks, 2011). Among individuals recognized as having anaphylaxis, typical initial symptoms are palmar and/or plantar itch with or without urticaria and/or angioedema. Target organs include skin (90% of episodes), respiratory tract (70%), gastrointestinal tract (30% to 45%), cardiovascular system (10% to 45%), and central nervous system (CNS; 10% to 15%) (Simons, 2008). Accordingly, there may be nausea, abdominal pain, vomiting, or diarrhea. There may also be rhinoconjunctivitis, obstructive respiratory symptoms, tachycardia, arrhythmia, altered mental state, and fainting. Severe respiratory and cardiovascular signs and symptoms such as arterial hypotension and cardiovascular collapse may be the primary manifestations, particularly in perioperative reactions (Schnyder, 2009).

Urticaria and angioedema are the most common and usually the first manifestations of anaphylaxis (Greenberger, 2006). Angioedema was found in 40% and urticaria in 49.3% of 142 patients presenting to an ER with anaphylaxis (Brown et al., 2001). Laryngeal edema was present in 25% of such patients. In 67 patients referred to an outpatient service for evaluation of anaphylaxis, 44.8% of patients had experienced angioedema compared with 58.2% for urticaria. Dyspnea, which may have included oropharyngeal or laryngeal swelling, was noted in 59.7% of patients (Thong et al., 2005). In patients with idiopathic anaphylaxis, 335 patients, ages 5 to 83, were categorized based on whether the acute episode was generalized (urticaria or angioedema with bronchospasm, hypotension, syncope, or gastrointestinal symptoms with or without upper airway obstruction) or angioedema (urticaria or angioedema with upper airway compromise without other systemic symptoms such as shock) (Ditto et al., 1996). From the 335 patients, 201 (60%) were classified as IA-G and 119 (35.5%) were designated as IA-A. In this series, urticaria or angioedema occurred in all 335 patients, but anaphylaxis, implying a life-threatening emergency, involved angioedema of the upper airway in over a third of patients. Indeed, these patients had experienced laryngeal or pharyngeal edema or "massive tongue edema". Perhaps, most persuasively, in this series of 335 patients, upper airway obstruction occurred in 210 (63%) patients (Ditto et al., 1996).

However, skin and mucosal symptoms and signs are absent or unrecognized in 10% to 20% of all anaphylactic episodes (Simons, 2010). These are rather more severe forms of anaphylaxis arising suddenly with either respiratory compromises or cardiovascular collapse. The lack of cutaneous signs reflects that anaphylaxis episode is likely to become fatal.

There are some differences in the presentation of anaphylaxis in the pediatric population compared with the adult population, including smaller numbers having cardiovascular signs and symptoms (21% compared with 41%). Other features noted in pediatric anaphylaxis include skin and respiratory signs appearing with an earlier onset compared with gastrointestinal and cardiovascular signs. Most children had a personal history of atopy (Dibbs & Baker, 1997).

The symptoms and signs of anaphylaxis are shown in Table 3.

Cutaneous/subcutaneous/mucosal tissue
Flushing, pruritus, hives (urticaria), swelling, morbilliform rash, pilor erection Periorbital pruritus, erythema and swelling, conjunctival erythema, tearing Pruritus and swelling of lips, tongue, uvula/palate Pruritus in the external auditory canals Pruritus of genitalia, palms, soles
Respiratory
Nose: pruritus, congestion, rhinorrhea, sneezing Larynx: pruritus and tightness in the throat, dysphonia and hoarseness, dry staccato cough, stridor, dysphagia Lung: shortness of breath, chest tightness, deep cough, wheezing/bronchospasm (decreased peak expiratory flow) Cyanosis
Gastrointestinal
Nausea, cramping abdominal pain, vomiting (stringy mucus), diarrhea
Cardiovascular
Chest pain, palpitations, tachycardia, bradycardia, or other dysrhythmia Feeling faint, altered mental status, hypotension, loss of sphincter control, shock, cardiac arrest
CNS
Aura of impending doom, uneasiness, throbbing headache, dizziness, confusion, tunnel vision; in infants and children, sudden behavioral changes, such as irritability, cessation of play, and clinging to parent
Other
Metallic taste in the mouth
Dysphagia
Uterine contractions in postpubertal female patients

Table 3. Symptoms and signs of anaphylaxis (Simons, 2010 with permission)

7. Laboratory tests

No optimal and readily available laboratory test can confirm the clinical diagnosis of an anaphylactic episode. Nevertheless, in some patients the clinical diagnosis of anaphylaxis can be confirmed by means of a blood test; for example, an increased plasma histamine level or serum total tryptase level (Simons, 2010). These tests are not specific for anaphylaxis. Plasma histamine levels should optimally be measured 15 to 60 minutes after onset of symptoms of anaphylaxis. Special handling of the blood sample is required. Histamine and its metabolite, N-methylhistamine, can also be measured in a 24-hour urine sample. Because tryptase is selectively and abundantly produced by mast cells, tryptase levels in biologic fluids should provide a more precise measure of local or systemic involvement of these cells than is possible to ascertain by clinical presentation or documentation of antigen-specific IgE. Basophils, the only other cell type that normally expresses tryptase, contain approximately 1/500th the amount mature β tryptase levels generally reflect the magnitude of mast cell activation and are elevated during most cases of systemic anaphylaxis, particularly with parenteral exposure to the inciting agent (Schwartz, 2006). Not all hypotensive reactions that clinically seem to be anaphylactic are associated with elevated levels of mature tryptase, however. For example, victims of fatal and near-fatal food-induced anaphylaxis often show no mature tryptase elevation, raising the possibility that some of these events may not be dependent on mast cell activation. Basophils have been suggested as an alternative effector cell, but direct evidence for this has not yet emerged. Other considerations might include overproduction through non-mast cell pathways of vasoactive mediators, such as complement anaphylatoxins, kinins, or lipids (Schwartz, 2006).

Serum total tryptase levels should optimally be measured from 15 minutes to 3 hours after onset of symptoms. No special handling of the blood sample is required. The total tryptase level is typically increased in patients with anaphylaxis triggered by an injected medication or an insect sting and in those with hypotension and shock but is less likely to be increased in those with anaphylaxis triggered by food or in those who are normotensive. Serial measurements of serum total tryptase and comparison with baseline levels obtained after the acute episode or available in stored serum might be more helpful than measurement at a single point in time. Other biomarkers reported to be useful in confirming an acute episode of anaphylaxis include serum mature β-tryptase; mast cell carboxypeptidase A3; chymase; platelet-activating factor; bradykinin; C-reactive protein; cytokines, such as IL-2, IL-6, IL-10, IL-33, and TNF-receptor I; and urinary cysteinyl leukotriene E4 and 9-a-11-b prostaglandin F2 (Simons, 2010).

It was shown that serum PAF levels were directly correlated and serum PAF acetylhydrolase activity was inversely correlated with the severity of anaphylaxis. PAF acetylhydrolase activity was significantly lower in patients with fatal anaphylactic reactions to peanuts than in patients in any of the control groups. Failure of PAF acetylhydrolase to inactivate PAF may contribute to the severity of anaphylaxis (Vadas et al., 2008).

8. Diagnosis

All individuals who have had a known or suspected anaphylactic episode require a careful and complete review of their clinical history. This history may elicit manifestations such as urticaria, angioedema, flushing, pruritus, upper airway obstruction, gastrointestinal symptoms, syncope, hypotension, lower airway obstruction, and/or other less common manifestations (Lieberman et al., 2010).

Other conditions that should be considered in the differential diagnosis include: (1) vasodepressor (vasovagal/neuro-cardiogenic) syncope; (2) syndromes that can be associated with flushing (e.g., metastatic carcinoid); (3) postprandial syndromes (e.g., scombroid poisoning); (4) systemic mastocytosis; (5) psychiatric disorders that can mimic anaphylaxis such as panic attacks or vocal cord dysfunction syndrome; (6) angioedema (e.g., hereditary angioedema); (7) other causes of shock (e.g., cardiogenic); and (8) other cardiovascular or respiratory events (Lieberman et al., 2005).

The history is the most important tool to establish the cause of anaphylaxis and takes precedence over diagnostic tests. A detailed history of all food consumed and drugs taken over the four to six hours prior to the episode should be obtained. In addition, the labels for all packaged foods ingested by the patient in this period of time should be reviewed since a substance added to the food could be responsible. A history of any preceding bite or sting should be obtained. The patient's activities (e.g., exercise, sexual activity) preceding the event should be reviewed. Patient diaries may be a useful adjunct in confirming or identifying the cause of anaphylaxis (Lieberman et al., 2010).

A detailed history of all potential causes should be obtained. This includes a list of ingestants consumed and/or medications taken within six hours of the event, any sting or bite occurring prior to the event, if the event occurred during exercise, location of the event (e.g., work versus home), and whether or not the event was related to exposure to heat, cold, or occurred during sexual activity. The patient's atopic status should be noted since food-induced, seminal fluid and idiopathic anaphylaxis are more common in atopic than non-atopic individuals. In women, the history should include any relationship between the attack and their menstrual cycle. A return of symptoms following a remission should be noted since this may indicate a late phase reaction, which might require a prolonged period of observation if subsequent events occur (Lieberman et al., 2010).

8.1 Confirmation of the triggers of anaphylaxis

The next step in the evaluation of a patient experienced anaphylaxis is confirmation of the trigger or triggers identified or suspected through the history (Simons, 2010). So that the relevant specific trigger or triggers can be avoided and recurrences of anaphylaxis can be prevented. Skin tests should be performed with validated instruments, techniques, and recording systems, preferably at least 3 to 4 weeks after the anaphylactic episode, to allow time for rearming of skin mast cells and recovery of mast cell releasability. When possible, standardized extracts for skin testing should be used, although occasionally fresh food extracts will be superior to available standardized extracts. If the skin testing extract has not been standardized (e.g., latex, protamine, or antibiotics other than penicillin), the clinical relevance of the results may be uncertain. Skin tests or in vitro tests can determine the presence of specific IgE antibodies to foods, medications (e.g., penicillin and insulin), and stinging insects as a cause of anaphylaxis (Lieberman et al., 2010). Measurement of allergen-specific IgE levels by using a quantitative method can be performed at any time during or after the acute anaphylactic episode; however, if the blood sample is obtained during or shortly after the episode from patients who have received intravenous fluid resuscitation, levels can be falsely undetectable or low because of the dilutional effect on circulating IgE. Negative tests for sensitization to a trigger in a patient with a convincing history of anaphylaxis from that trigger should be repeated weeks or months later. It is important to note that both positive skin tests and increased specific IgE levels indicate sensitization to the allergens tested but are not diagnostic of anaphylaxis or any other disease (Lieberman et al., 2010). The clinical significance of skin testing or in vitro test depends on the ability to correlate the results of such testing with the patient's history. If tests for specific IgE antibodies (i.e., skin tests, in vitro tests, or both) do not provide conclusive evidence of the cause of anaphylaxis, challenge with the suspected agent can be considered. If indicated, incremental challenge/provocation tests should be conducted in appropriately equipped health care facilities by professionals trained and experienced in patient selection, timing of the challenge, use of challenge protocols, and diagnosing and treating anaphylaxis. Before a challenge is performed, the potential risks and benefits should be discussed with the patient (or, for children, the caregivers) and documented in the medical record. Challenge procedures may also be appropriate in patients who develop non-IgE-mediated reactions (e.g., reactions to aspirin (ASA) or other nonsteroidal anti-inflammatory drugs. Challenge with suspected agents must be done carefully by individuals knowledgeable in the challenge procedure and with expertise in managing reactions to the challenge agent if they should occur (Lieberman et al., 2010).

8.2 Assessment of patients with food-triggered anaphylaxis

Skin prick tests with foods that elicit a wheal of 3 mm larger than that caused by the negative control (eg. saline) are considered positive (Simons, 2010). Commercially available food allergen extracts do not contain standardized allergens. Some food allergens, such as fruits and vegetables, are labile and degrade in glycerinated extracts during manufacture and storage; therefore skin prick tests with these allergens are often performed with fresh foods.

Intradermal tests to foods are contraindicated because of lack of specificity (false-positive tests) and their potential for triggering anaphylaxis (Lieberman et al., 2010). An exception to this might be use of intradermal tests to assess sensitization to fresh meat containing the carbohydrate galactose-alpha-1,3-galactose. In food-sensitized patients specific IgE levels have predictive values for positive (failed) or negative (passed) food challenge tests. Allergen-specific IgE levels with greater than 95% predictive risk values of a positive (failed) food challenge result have been identified by using the ImmunoCAP (Phadia, Uppsala, Sweden). These levels are defined for cow's milk (15 kU/L), egg (7 kU/L), peanut (14 kU/L), tree nuts (15 kU/L), and fish (20 kU/L); in infants lower values have been established for milk (5 kU/L) and egg (2 kU/L) (Boden & Burks, 2011). Predictive values for allergen-specific IgE levels potentially differ from one immunoassay to another, and this can affect management decisions.

A positive skin test, an increased serum IgE level, or both to a specific food document sensitization to that food. Such tests are not diagnostic of anaphylaxis because sensitization to 1 or more food allergens is common in the general population of healthy people who have no history of anaphylaxis. For example, 60% of young people have a positive skin prick test to 1 or more foods, yet most of those with positive tests have never experienced anaphylaxis from a food. In addition, although positive skin tests and increased allergen-specific IgE levels correlate with an increased probability of clinical reactivity to specific foods, the results of these tests do not necessarily correlate with the risk of future anaphylactic episodes or with the severity of such episodes (Simons, 2010).

Oral food challenge testing is accepted as a gold standard for detection of a food allergy/hypersensitivity (Sampson & Burks, 2009). Patients with a convincing history of anaphylaxis to a specific food and evidence of sensitization to that food should not undergo oral food challenge tests because of their high risk of anaphylaxis from such tests. Others, such as those with an equivocal history, low or moderate evidence of sensitization, or both, might benefit from a physician-monitored incremental oral food challenge. A positive (failed) challenge provides a basis for continued avoidance of the food. A negative (passed) challenge allows introduction or reintroduction of the specific food into the patient's diet.

8.3 Assessment of medication- or biological agent –triggered anaphylaxis

Any medication or biological agent can potentially trigger anaphylaxis. In cases with severe anaphylactic reactions, it is advisable to first perform skin tests with the presumably causative drugs only by prick (Schnyder & Pichler, 2009). If responses are negative and the involved drug is available as a parenteral formulation, negative skin tests do not have sufficient sensitivity to exclude an immune-mediated hypersensitivity in the case of a suggestive history. For most agents, the antigenic determinants have not been characterized or validated; indeed, the relevant immunogenic prodrugs, haptens, metabolites, and unidentified degradation products or contaminants are often unknown. For most medications, with the exception of some β-lactam antibiotics, appropriate reagents are not commercially available for use in skin tests, measurement of medication-specific IgE levels, or other in vitro tests. In penicillin allergies, standardized preparations with penicilloylpolylysine and minor determinant mixture may be used (Lieberman et al., 2010). Penicillin allergy may also be evaluated by in vitro tests for specific IgEs; however, these tests have a low sensitivity. Additionally, assays for a few drugs such as suxamethonium, rocuronium, morphine, sulfamethoxazole, and chlorhexidine, are offered, some with potentially higher sensitivity (Schnyder, 2009). A further in vitro test to identify the relevant drug may be the basophil activation test. This test is based on flow cytometric quantification of drug-induced CD63 expression or CD203c up-regulation or measurement of sulfo-leukotriene release by ELISA. The sensitivity in IgE-mediated reactions appears to be superior to CAP-based IgE determinations and comparable with skin tests. Customized tests and physician-monitored challenge/provocation tests performed in specialized centers therefore play a central role in assessment of patients with a history of anaphylaxis triggered by a medication. A drug provocation test (DPT) is defined as controlled administration of a drug to diagnose immune-mediated and non–immune-mediated drug hypersensitivity. Its advantage is that it permits testing of a patient with his or her individual metabolism and immunogenetic background. A DPT reproduces not only symptoms of allergy but other adverse clinical manifestations, irrespective of their mechanism. A DPT is currently the "gold standard," but its use is limited by the possibility of severe and uncontrollable relapse of the reaction (Aberer et al., 2010). Therefore, a DPT should be reserved for specific situations when a significant drug is suspected to have provoked an intolerance reaction and alternative test methods have failed to yield conclusive results. The patient being tested has to be in stable condition, and an anticipated positive reaction must be controllable by adequate measures. Because of these restrictions, only physicians experienced in drug allergy should perform this test. The two main indications for a DPT with the suspected drug are the following: to exclude hypersensitivity in the presence of unconvincing histories of drug hypersensitivity or in patients with nonspecific conditions, such as subjective symptoms under local anesthesia, or to establish a distinct diagnosis in suggestive histories of drug hypersensitivity with inconclusive, negative, or nonavailable allergy test results. A positive DPT result optimizes the avoidance of certain drugs, whereas a negative one permits the clinician to rule out a false diagnosis of drug hypersensitivity.

For assessment of anaphylaxis triggered by vaccines to prevent allergic diseases, skin prick tests should be performed not only with the immunizing agent but also with the relevant excipients in the culprit vaccine, such as gelatin in measles vaccines or egg in some influenza vaccines and in yellow fever vaccine (Simons, 2010).

8.4 Assessment of stinging insect-triggered anaphylaxis

Standardized Hymenoptera venoms, such as honeybee, yellow jacket, yellow hornet, white-faced hornet, and Paper wasp, are available for skin testing. Skin prick tests, if negative, should be followed by intradermal tests (Bilo & Bonifazi, 2009). Use of dialyzed venoms in skin tests is reported to improve the identification of venom-sensitized patients (Golden et al., 2009). For fire ant-triggered anaphylaxis, whole-body extracts are used as skin test reagents. Measurements of venom-specific IgE levels are commercially available (Freeman, 2004). Some patients with a history of Hymenoptera sting–triggered anaphylaxis have negative skin test responses to insect venoms but increased specific IgE levels to venoms and vice versa (Simons, 2010). Positive intradermal tests to stinging insect venoms, increased venom-specific IgE levels, or both occur in up to 28.5% of the general adult population, most of whom do not have systemic symptoms after an insect sting (Simons, 2010). It is therefore critically important that the test results be interpreted in the context of the clinical history. In some centers additional tests used to assist in interpretation of positive test results include consideration of total IgE levels as well as venom-specific IgE levels, and measurement of basophil activation markers, such as CD63 or CD203c after incubation with different concentrations of venom (Simons, 2010). Conversely, venom skin tests might be negative and venom specific IgE levels might be absent or undetectable in patients with a convincing history of insect sting–triggered anaphylaxis (Simons, 2010).

8.5 Perioperative anaphylaxis

Skin testing may be useful to determine the safest alternative for subsequent anesthesia following a suspected reaction. Skin testing with neuromuscular blocking agents, hypnotics and opioids is used. Antibiotics frequently are administered before, during, or immediately after anesthesia and surgery. Allergic reactions to antibiotics, particularly anaphylaxis, may occur during the perioperative period. For this reason, following a suspected reaction during anesthesia, skin tests with antibiotics should also be done. It should be noted that nonimmunologic reactions are not identified by this diagnostic method. Skin testing is not recommended for preanesthetic screening of subjects without a history of suspected reactions (Lobera et al., 2008).

8.6 Assessment of anaphylaxis triggered by natural rubber latex

Skin prick tests should be performed with commercial latex allergens, where available, or with extracts of rubber products, such as natural rubber latex gloves, where commercial allergens are not available. In vitro tests have highly variable sensitivity and specificity characteristics (Lieberman et al., 2010). Consideration should be given to testing with foods that cross-react with latex, such as banana, kiwi, papaya, avocado, potato, and tomato. Latex-specific IgE antibodies can also be measured.

8.7 Assessment of exercise-triggered anaphylaxis

These should be done: meticulous clinical history, skin or in vitro testing for potential food allergen co triggers, and occasionally, documenting mast cell activation if this can be determined in the minutes or hours following an attack (Lieberman et al., 2010). The diagnosis of EIA can be confirmed by eliciting symptoms with treadmill testing. However, symptoms are difficult to reproduce. The differential diagnosis includes arrhythmias and other cardiovascular events, but such events do not include pruritus, urticaria, angioedema, or upper airway obstruction. Exercise induced bronchoconstriction presents with symptoms that are limited to the airways. Exercise-associated gastroesophageal reflux could mimic mild symptoms of EIA, although, urticaria and/or pruritus are not observed (Feldweg & Sheffer, 2011).

8.8 Assessment of idiopathic anaphylaxis

When a meticulous history of antecedent exposures and events does not yield any clues about potential triggers and when allergen skin tests are negative and specific IgE measurements are absent or undetectable to selected common allergens, patients are said to have idiopathic anaphylaxis (Greenberger, 2007). The diagnosis of idiopathic anaphylaxis is based on exclusion. Before making this diagnosis, physicians should consider the possibility of a hidden or previously unrecognized trigger. Sensitization to a novel trigger for which there is no commercially available test material, can be identified through a history of the event and confirmed by objective tests.

Patients with idiopathic anaphylaxis should receive careful evaluation for possible causes, with emphasis on the history of events in the 3 hours prior to an episode. Selective skin testing with foods (and if indicated to fresh food extracts) may be of value. Indolent systemic mastocytosis must be excluded. Consistently elevated serum tryptase levels suggest the presence of indolent systemic mastocytosis since the serum tryptase will be elevated in the absence of episodes of anaphylaxis. In contrast, serum tryptase levels will be normal in quiescent idiopathic anaphylaxis. A bone marrow examination may be indicated in patients with a diagnosis of idiopathic anaphylaxis even in the absence or elevated tryptase levels if salmon colored, hyperpigmented macules and papules consistent with urticaria pigmentosa are found (Akın et al., 2007). The differential diagnosis of idiopathic anaphylaxis includes hereditary angioedema or acquired C1 inhibitor deficiency. Some patients with idiopathic anaphylaxis present with massive enlargement of the tongue and/or life-threatening upper airway obstruction due to pharyngeal or laryngeal angioedema, but their C4 concentration is not reduced.

9. Management

Anaphylaxis, as a potentially life-threatening condition must be diagnosed and managed promptly. Although the etiology may be various or indefinite and there is lack of rapid diagnostic tests, the diagnosis relies mostly on clinical symptoms, therefore requires a high index of suspicion. Irrespective of the trigger or mechanism of anaphylaxis, the initial management is the same and is based on basic therapeutic agents that all healthcare professionals should be able to provide, even in a low resource environment (Lee & Vadas, 2011; Simons et al., 2011). Prompt and definitive management can be life saving whereas the delay in the management may result in a fatal outcome (Lieberman et al., 2010).

Anaphylaxis can potentially affect cardiovascular and respiratory systems and be presented as a multisystem emergency. The trigger has to be removed, if possible and the patient's circulation, airway, breathing, level of consciousness, and skin should be rapidly assessed (Simons et al., 2011). According to the consensus of experts, in general the treatment in order of importance includes epinephrine (adrenaline), patient position, oxygen, intravenous fluids, nebulized therapy, vasopressors, antihistamines, corticosteroids, and other agents (Lieberman et al., 2010).

In a series of over 200 anaphylaxis deaths the median time from onset of symptoms to fatal cardiopulmonary arrest was reported as <30 minutes (Pumphrey, 2000). In the same paper the median times to cardiopulmonary arrest were 5 minutes after administration of a diagnostic or therapeutic intervention, 15 minutes after an insect sting, and 30 minutes after food ingestion. As soon as the need is recognized, supplemental oxygen at a flow rate of 6-8 L/min, intravenous fluid resuscitation must be administered and the cardiopulmonary resuscitation with continuous chest compressions before giving rescue breathing must be initiated (Simons et al., 2011). Patients should be kept supine with legs raised to prevent death due to 'empty vena cava/ empty ventricle syndrome' with pulseless electrical activity (Pumphrey, 2003). In this syndrome patients in shock suddenly sit, stand, or are placed upright, the vena cava empties within seconds, and epinephrine is prevented from circulating the body (Pumphrey & Gowland, 2007). The patient must be kept in a comfortable position if vomiting or respiratory distress is present (Simons et al., 2011).

Supplemental oxygen should be given by face mask or oropharyngeal airway to all patients with concomitant asthma, other chronic respiratory disease, or cardiovascular disease and those having prolonged reactions or those who are receiving inhaled β-agonists as part of the treatment for anaphylaxis or repeated doses of epinephrine (Lieberman et al., 2010; Simons et al., 2011). Oxygen supplementation should be guided with continuous pulse oximetry and/or arterial blood gas determination (Lieberman et al., 2010).

The fluid management is critical as massive fluid shifts can occur due to increased vascular permeability within minutes (Brown et al., 2004). Saline stays in the intravascular space longer than dextrose and contains no lactate which may exacerbate metabolic acidosis. Therefore one to 2 L of 0.9% isotonic saline as a preferred solution should be commenced as 5-10 mL/kg in the first 5-10 minutes to an adult or 10 mL/kg to a child as soon as the need for it is recognized (Lieberman et al., 2010; Simons et al., 2011). The rate of administration should be titrated according to the blood pressure, cardiac rate and function and urine output. Caution should be undertaken for volume overload (Simons et al., 2011). In some cases fluid replacement may not be so effective when considered with other indications. It is possible that the replaced fluid during management can also shift from the vasculature to tissues. Therefore the cornerstone of management is a non-selective adrenergic agonist agent, epinephrine which acts on α-1, β-1 and β-2 adrenergic receptors and is highly effective to reverse the clinical symptoms mainly with vasoconstriction, cardiac stimulation and bronchodilatation (Lee & Vadas, 2011; Simons et al., 2009a). The World Health Organization (WHO) classifies epinephrine as an essential medication for the treatment of anaphylaxis (Simons et al., 2011). The evidence base for prompt epinephrine injection in the initial treatment of anaphylaxis is stronger than the evidence base for the use of antihistamines and glucocorticoids in anaphylaxis (Simons et al., 2011). Therefore overt signs of distributive shock or cardiovascular compromise should not be waited to administer epinephrine. It is recommended that epinephrine be given as soon as possible (Lee & Vadas, 2011). Although there is any doubt in recognition of the clinical situation as anaphylaxis, it is generally better to administer epinephrine (Lieberman et al., 2010).

Pharmacokinetic studies have shown that the intramuscular route of administration into the mid-anterolateral thigh (the vastus lateralis muscle) is preferable with a faster onset of action and more sustained levels as compared with the subcutaneous route (Lee & Vadas,

2011; Simons, 2009b). The rationale for intramuscular injection is that the striated muscle is well vascularized, facilitating rapid systemic absorption and prompt achievement of peak epinephrine pharmacologic effects. In contrast subcutaneous tissue consisting mostly of poorly vascularized adipose tissue provides the slow absorption of epinephrine with variable time intervals for peak pharmacologic effects (Simons, 2009b). Significantly faster peak plasma concentrations are achieved via the intramuscular route (8 ± 2 min) than the subcutaneous route of administration (34 ± 14 min) in children, and in adults (Frew, 2010). Intramuscular epinephrine injections into the thigh have been reported to provide more rapid absorption and higher plasma epinephrine levels in both children and adults than intramuscular or subcutaneous injections administered in the arm (Lieberman et al., 2010). Alternative routes of administration have been anecdotally tried. For example sublingual delivery of 40 mg epinephrine has been shown to lead to plasma concentrations that are not significantly different to those following intramuscular administration of 0.3 mg epinephrine (Frew, 2010).

The recommended dose of epinephrine for children is 0.01 mg/kg body weight of a 1:1,000 (1 mg/mL) solution, to a maximum initial dose of 0.3 mg in a 30 kg child (Simons, 2009b). In the recent guideline of World Allergy Organization (WAO) the same dose of epinephrine in adults with a maximum initial dose of 0.5 mg is recommended (Simons et al., 2011). In the recent Practice Parameter on the Diagnosis and Management of Anaphylaxis, the dose is defined as 0.2-0.5 ml of aqueous epinephrine of a 1:1,000 dilution in adults and as 0.01mg/kg of the same dilution in children (Lieberman et al., 2010). The dose can be repeated every 5-15 minutes, as needed depending on the severity of the episode and the response to the initial injection (Lieberman et al., 2010; Simons et al., 2011). Approximately 20% of cases in the community require a second dose because of lack of response to the first dose, or development of a biphasic reaction (Simons, 2009b).

The patient has to be monitored with blood pressure, cardiac rate and function, respiratory status at regular intervals and oxygenation continuously, if possible (Simons et al., 2011). The duration of monitoring should be individualized. Patients with moderate respiratory or cardiovascular compromise should be monitored in a medically supervised setting for at least 4 hours and if indicated 8-10 hours or longer, and patients with severe or protracted anaphylaxis might require monitoring and interventions for days (Simons et al., 2011).

In patients who remain hypotensive and unresponsive to intramuscular epinephrine and fluid resuscitation, the ones who have progressed to shock or cardiac arrest intravenous epinephrine is recommended (Lee & Vadas, 2011; Simons et al., 2011). Ideally, this route should be administered only by trained, experienced physicians who are equipped to give vasopressors through an infusion pump and titrate the dose frequently according to noninvasive continuous monitoring of cardiac rate and function. A controlled infusion is safer than bolus administration (Soar et al., 2008). If cardiac arrest is imminent or has already occurred, an intravenous bolus dose of epinephrine is indicated according to Resuscitation Guidelines (Simons et al., 2011). An intravenous epinephrine infusion is prepared by adding 1 mg (1 mL) of 1:1,000 dilution of epinephrine to 250 mL of 5% dextrose to yield a concentration of 4.0 μg/mL. This 1:250,000 solution is infused at a rate of 1μg/mL, titrated to a maximum of 10.0μg/min for adults. In children, a dosage of 0.01 mg/kg (0.1 mL/kg of a 10,000 solution up to 10μg/min; maximum dose, 0.3 mg is administered (Lieberman et al., 2010). Other protocols for intravenous administration are also suggested (Lieberman et al., 2010).

Dopamine as a vasopressor agent is recommended when epinephrine and fluid resuscitation fail to alleviate hypotension in a dose of 2-20μg/kg/min, titrated to maintain systolic blood pressure greater than 90 mmHg. During cardiopulmonary resuscitation intravenous high-dose epinephrine is recommended. A common sequence is 1 to 3 mg (1:10,000 dilution) intravenous slowly administered over 3 min, 3 to 5 mg intravenous over 3 min, and then 4-10 μg/min infusion. For children, the recommended initial resuscitation dosage is 0.01 mg/kg (0.1 ml/kg of a 1:10,000 solution up to 10 μg/min rate of infusion), repeated every 3 to 5 min for ongoing arrest. Higher subsequent dosages (0.1-0.2 mg/kg: 0.1 ml/kg of a 1:1,000 solution) may be considered for unresponsive asystole or pulseless electrical activity (Lieberman et al., 2010).

The common adverse effects of epinephrine include anxiety, dizziness, restlessness, headache, palpitations, tremor, and pallor and indicate that a therapeutic dose has been given (Lee & Vadas, 2011; Simons, 2009b). Rare side effects of epinephrine more commonly related with high or rapid doses of intravenous administration include ventricular arrhythmias, angina, myocardial infarction, pulmonary edema, hypertensive emergency, and intracranial haemorrhage (Lee & Vadas, 2011; Simons et al., 2011). It was demonstrated that the heart is the target organ of anaphylaxis and acute coronary syndrome can occur in anaphylaxis in the absence of epinephrine administration in patients with known coronary artery disease, and those in whom subclinical coronary artery disease is unmasked by the anaphylactic episode (Simons et al., 2011). Concerns about adverse effects, especially potential myocardial infarction and cardiac arrhythmias, need to be weighed against the cardiac risks of untreated anaphylaxis (Simons, 2009b; Simons et al., 2011). As there is no controlled trials mainly because of ethical concerns, there is no way to estimate the risk in relation to benefit of epinephrine, but on the basis of current evidence, the benefit of using appropriate doses of intramuscular epinephrine is likely to far exceed the risk (Sheikh et al., 2009). According to the recent WAO guidelines epinephrine is not contraindicated in the treatment of anaphylaxis in patients with known or suspected cardiovascular disease, or in elderly patients without known coronary artery disease who are at risk of acute coronary syndrome only because of their age (Simons et al., 2011). However, careful monitoring and avoidance of an adrenaline overdose are necessary in these patients (Sheikh et al., 2009).

In a recent systematic Cochrane review, it was emphasized that there are no absolute contraindications to epinephrine use in anaphylaxis and in the absence of appropriate trials, and suboptimal evidence, epinephrine administration is recommended to be regarded as the first-line treatment for the management of anaphylaxis (Sheikh et al., 2009). Some relative contraindications include patients using mono-amine oxidase inhibitors, tricyclic anti-depressants, or stimulant medications or illicit substances, all of which are possibly increasing the risk of adverse effects of epinephrine (Lee & Vadas, 2011). Caution is needed in patients with recent intracranial surgery, aortic or cerebral aneurism(s), uncontrolled hyperthyroidism, or hypertensive emergencies (Lee & Vadas, 2011).

H1-antihistamines are frequently used in anaphylaxis, but they cannot be substituted for epinephrine as first line treatment (Sheikh et al., 2007). A Cochrane systematic review of the literature has found no high quality evidence either for or against the use of H1-antihistamines in anaphylaxis; therefore randomized controlled trials are needed (Sheikh et al., 2007). These agents do not prevent or reverse life-threatening upper and lower respiratory tract obstruction, hypotension or shock (Simons et al., 2009a), but they relieve itching, flushing, urticaria, angioedema and nasal and eye symptoms (Simons, 2009b;

Simons et al., 2011). As a second line medication, for example diphenhydramine 1 mg/kg, approximately 25-50 mg in adults, maximum 50 mg in children is recommended by slow intravenous infusion over 10-15 minutes. The route of administration depends on the severity of the attack. Only the first generation H1-antihistamines are available for intravenous use and they potentially increase vasodilation and hypotension if given rapidly (Simons et al., 2011). H2-antihistamines in combination with H1-antihistamines are sometimes used for anaphylaxis treatment in the US and Canada (Lieberman et al., 2010; Simons et al., 2011). When an oral H1-antihistamine is indicated, a low sedating medication such as cetirizine is preferable to a sedating H1-antihistamine (Simons et al., 2011).

Glucagon is preferred in patients who are already using β- blockers therefore experiencing a relative bradycardia and refractory hypotension and are not fully responding to epinephrine (Gallagher et al., 2011; Thomas & Crawford, 2005). It shows its effects independent of β-receptors by directly activating adenyl cyclase. The recommended dose is 1 to 5 mg in adults and 20-30 μg/kg (maximum of 1 mg) administered intravenously over 5 min as a bolus. The bolus dose can be repeated or followed by an infusion of 5-15μg/min, titrated to clinical response (Lieberman et al., 2010). The common side effect is emesis, particularly related with rapid infusion and therefore protection of the airways to prevent aspiration in severely drowsy patients is important (Lee & Vadas, 2011; Lieberman et al., 2010).

A recent Cochrane systematic review concluded that there is insufficient high-quality evidence to either support or not to support the use of glucocorticosteroids in the management of anaphylaxis (Choo et al., 2010). The existing evidence consists mainly of retrospective studies, case reports, and other descriptive literature. The recent WAO anaphylaxis guideline recommends glucocorticosteroid use in anaphylaxis management as a second line medication. It is used to prevent biphasic or protracted symptoms, although there is weak evidence for it (Simons et al., 2011). It doesn't provide rapid relief of upper or lower airway obstruction, shock, or other symptoms of anaphylaxis (Simons, 2009b). The route of administration depends on the severity of the attack (Simons et al., 2011). The recommended dose of methylprednisolone by WAO anaphylaxis guideline is 1-2mg/kg/day, approximately 50-100 mg or equivalent for 3-4 days in adults, at a maximum dose of 50 mg in children (Lee & Vadas, 2011; Simons et al., 2011). Other guidelines recommend hydrocortisone, triamcinolone, prednisone by intravenous, intramuscular, or oral routes using different doses and dose regimens (Soar, 2005, Brown et al., 2006, Alrasbi & Sheikh, 2007, Muraro et al., 2007, as cited in Choo et al., 2010). Short term glucocorticoid treatment is seldom associated with adverse effects (Choo et al., 2010).

Additionally short and rapid acting β2-adrenergic agonist, salbutamol is recommended in nebulised form in doses of 2.5 mg/3 mL in children or 5 mg/3 mL in adults to treat bronchoconstriction with combination of oxygen supplementation (Simons et al., 2011). Tremor, tachycardia dizziness are potential side effects in usual doses, where as headache, hypokalemia, vasodilation can be seen in overdoses (Simons et al., 2011). Vasopressors such as dopamine can be used to correct hypotension despite other interventions.

It should be pointed out that the time taken by draw up and administration of a second-line medication such as H1- antihistamines, corticosteroids, β2-adrenergic agonists should not cause a delay in the administration of the first line treatment of epinephrine, supplementation of oxygen or intravenous fluid resuscitation (Simons et al., 2011).

In refractory anaphylaxis methylene blue is used in a number of case reports. In anaphylactic shock endothelial nitric oxide synthase-derived NO appears to be the principal vasodilator. Therefore methylene blue by inhibiting nitric oxide synthesis inhibition blocks nitric oxide (NO)-mediated vascular smooth muscle relaxation and seems to be effective in these cases (Lieberman et al., 2010). Tranexamic acid was used to treat anaphylactic episodes associated with disseminated intravascular coagulation (Lieberman et al., 2010).

The management of anaphylaxis in pregnancy is similar to the management of non-pregnant patients. The correct posture of the patient is also important. She has to be placed semi recumbent on her left side with the lower extremities elevated, to prevent positional hypotension resulting from compression of the inferior vena cava by gravid uterus (Simons et al., 2011).

10. Prevention

Long-term preventive measures to reduce the risk of fatality of anaphylaxis include avoidance of triggers, optimal management of relevant comorbidities such as asthma, cardiovascular diseases, mastocytosis and immunomodulation (Simons, 2009b).

When anaphylaxis has occurred because of exposure to a specific trigger, patients should be educated about agents or exposures that would place them at risk for future reactions and be counseled on avoidance measures that may be used to reduce risk for such exposures (Lieberman et al., 2010). Triggers should be identified with a detailed history, and the sensitization to the triggers should be confirmed by using allergen skin tests and/or measurement of allergen-specific IgE levels in serum or challenge tests especially for therapeutic agents or foods. Optimally the patients can be tested for IgE sensitizations approximately 3-4 weeks after an acute anaphylactic episode. The time interval has not been definitely identified for most of the allergens, preferably patients with a convincing history of anaphylaxis and a negative test result should be retested afterwards. Challenge tests should be conducted in an appropriately equipped healthcare setting staffed by trained and experienced healthcare professionals as a supervised, graded test in order to diagnose and to assess risk of future anaphylactic episodes further. Before a challenge is performed the potential risk versus the potential benefit should be discussed with the patient and documented in the medical record (Simons et al., 2011).

Absolute avoidance of triggers such as allergens like latex, foods, or a medication is life saving, but as an example lifelong avoidance of a food may disrupt daily life and may lead to anxiety or decrease the quality of life of the patients and their families or may lead to nutritional deficiencies, especially in children (Simons, 2009b). Additionally avoidance is difficult to perform in some situations. For example hidden, substituted, and cross-reacting foods, or foods that are contaminated and mislabeling or confusing labels on packaged foods are some of the reasons of difficulties in avoidance of triggers. So patients with food anaphylaxis should be informed about all of these possibilities, regularly provided personalized written instructions for avoidance of the confirmed specific triggers (Simons et al., 2011). Biphasic reactions appear to be more common in food-induced anaphylaxis when compared to other reasons of anaphylaxis and it is reported in up to 25% of fatal or near fatal reactions (Lieberman, 2005, as cited in Lieberman et al., 2010). Although it is rare for patients with oral allergy syndrome to develop anaphylaxis, they may be at increased risk. Therefore these patients may be prescribed epinephrine auto-injectors (Kleine-Tebbe et al., 2002, as cited in Lieberman et al., 2010). Another important trigger to which avoidance is difficult is the stinging insects. Beekeepers, gardeners, others with occupational exposure may find it difficult to follow this advice (Lieberman et al., 2010; Simons et al., 2011). In patients with a history of anaphylaxis triggered by a medication should not be given the offending drug, and if available a safe, non-reacting alternative medication should be substituted. Patients should be informed about the offending drug, related and cross-reactive drug with written documents (Simons et al., 2011). During anesthesia patients are under drapes and are unconscious, so early cutaneous signs are often unrecognized (Brock-Utne, 2003). Therefore the staff has to be prepared and ready for unexpected anaphylaxis. Patients who experience anaphylaxis during the peri-operative period should be carefully evaluated to elucidate the responsible agent and be examined by an allergist prior future procedure. In the case of anaphylaxis due to radiocontrast agents, non-ionic radiocontrast agents should be considered as alternatives (Lieberman et al., 2010; Simons et al., 2011).

In exercise-induced anaphylaxis avoidance of relevant co-triggers such as foods, medications, cold or hot air exposure, or other concomitant factors should be considered (Simons, 2009b). Exercise under ambient conditions of high humidity, extreme heat or cold or high pollen counts should be avoided (Simons et al., 2011). These patients should never exercise alone, should stop exercise immediately with the first symptom of anaphylaxis, and should carry a mobile phone and an epinephrine auto-injector during every exercise (Lieberman et al., 2010; Simons et al., 2011).

In latex induced anaphylaxis avoidance of latex and if relevant, also the avoidance of cross-reactive fruits, vegetables is extremely important (Lieberman et al., 2010; Simons et al., 2011). Latex can enter the body through different routes including, mucous membranes, contact with the skin, parenteral exposure, and contact with internal organs as in surgery and with inhalation of latex powder. Therefore avoidance measures for latex allergy should be intensively applied to establish a latex-safe environment for the patients. Both latex-sensitive healthcare workers and their co-workers should wear non-latex or non-powdered gloves and all non-glove latex devices should be replaced by non-latex devices. The most important procedures during which latex avoidance should be instituted in latex-sensitive patients include surgical procedures, obstetrical or gynecologic examinations or dental care (Lieberman et al., 2010). The problem can also manifest itself when latex sensitive patients experience anaphylaxis with related foods. These patients should be informed about the possible foods known to be cross-reactive latex. For anaphylaxis induced by some nonimmune triggers such as cold, heat, sunlight or ethanol, avoidance of the trigger is the key to prevention of recurrence (Simons et al., 2011).

Anaphylaxis due to allergen specific immunotherapy is another important cause of anaphylaxis which can be strongly avoided when this treatment is administered by healthcare professionals trained in the recognition and treatment of anaphylaxis. In patients using β-blockers the beneficial therapeutic effects of epinephrine may be diminished. Therefore a cautious attitude should be adopted in patients receiving concomitant β-blockers and allergen specific immunotherapy (Lieberman et al., 2010).

Seminal fluid anaphylaxis is a rare condition, which can not be generally prevented with antihistamines or intravaginal cromolyn sodium taken as precoital medications, where as barrier condoms are successful options for prevention. When these therapies are not effective or unacceptable, immunotherapy with seminal plasma fractions can be instituted in specialized centers (Lieberman et al., 2010).

The accompanying medications which can interfere with anaphylaxis and management such as β-blockers, angiotensin-converting enzyme inhibitors, NSAIDs, aspirin should be given weighing the risks and benefits of each medication (Lee & Vadas, 2011).

Oral desensitization to a specific food, subcutaneous anti-IgE injections, Food Allergy Herbal Formula-2, a well-characterized Chinese herbal formulation are investigational immunomodulator interventions being studied in humans for the prevention of anaphylaxis (Simons, 2009b). Desensitization strategies with the offending drug, where an alternative drug is not available are safe and effective immunomodulatory approaches particularly in patients with anaphylaxis due to β-lactam or other antibiotics, aspirin, or other nonsteroidal anti-inflammatory drugs, and chemotherapy agents. This procedure should be conducted by trained and experienced healthcare professionals in healthcare settings where all facilities for the management of anaphylaxis are available. This method provides protection only during the procedure as a temporary state of tolerance (Simons et al., 2011). Where as long-lasting protection against anaphylaxis can only be achieved with successful allergen specific immunotherapy which is mostly seen in subcutaneous venom immunotherapy (Simons, 2009b). It protects up to 80-90% of adults and 98% of children, in whom it lasts for decades (Simons et al., 2011). Latex sublingual immunotherapy has been shown to be an effective treatment in double blind placebo controlled studies both in children and adults, but according to our experience in the dose incremental phase precautions should be taken (Bernardini et al., 2008; Buyukozturk et al. , 2010).

In patients with frequent recurrent episodes of idiopathic anaphylaxis, empiric use of prednisone in a daily dose of 60-100 mg in combination with H1-antihistamines for 1-2 weeks followed by decreasing alternate day prednisone over 3 months as prophylaxis is recommended by the experts and has been demonstrated to reduce the frequency or severity of episodes (Lieberman et al., 2010). This treatment is considered in patients experiencing 6 or more episodes per year or 2 episodes in 2 months (Lieberman et al., 2010). Anti-IgE treatment is also promising (Simons, 2009b; Simons et al., 2011). These patients should carry their epinephrine auto-injectors at all times. Pretreatment strategies with antihistamines and corticosteroids have been used successfully to prevent anaphylaxis due to radiocontrast agents, cold-induced anaphylaxis and fluorescein (Lee & Vadas, 2011; Simons, et al., 2011).

Despite these preventive measures anaphylaxis sometimes recurs. Therefore, those at risk, should be prepared to recognize and treat unexpected episodes and be educated. Anaphylaxis education should begin before patients are discharged from the emergency department or other healthcare facility where the anaphylaxis was treated (Simons et al., 2011). Patients should be informed about the importance of the reactions that they have experienced. For this purpose, patients should carry medical identification prepared as a bracelet or a wallet card listing their diagnosis of anaphylaxis, confirmed trigger factors, relevant comorbidities, and concurrent medications (Simons, 2009b; Simons et al., 2011). They should be also advised that they are at increased risk for future episodes of anaphylaxis and therefore need follow-up, preferably by an allergy/immunology specialist (Simons et al., 2011) and prescribed for epinephrine auto-injectors and have their personalized written anaphylaxis emergency action plans (Simons 2009b; Liebermann et al., 2010). If epinephrine auto-injectors are not available or affordable, a substitute epinephrine formulation should be recommended, such as an ampoule of epinephrine, a 1 ml syringe, and written instructions about drawing up the correct dose. In emergency action plans, patients should be briefly informed about how to recognize anaphylaxis symptoms, instructed to inject epinephrine promptly and then admit to emergency to seek medical assistance (Simons et al., 2011).

Delayed injection or non-injection of epinephrine has been shown to be a risk factor for severe and biphasic reactions and fatal outcome (Gallagher et al., 2011; Lee & Vadas, 2011; Simons et al., 2010). Therefore patients are commonly prescribed at least two auto-injector devices for the administration of epinephrine in the community settings for this sudden, rapid, and usually unexpected clinical situation (Gallagher et al., 2011; Kemp et al., 2007). There is clear consensus in the research literature that these auto-injectors are under-used by patients of all-ages (Gallagher et al., 2011; Simons, 2009b, Simons et al., 2011). A recent paper suggested that auto-injector under-use is commonly due to patients preferring to take other medications most commonly antihistamines, not having auto-injector prescriptions, lack of severity of previous episodes or spontaneous recovery from previous episodes (Simons et al., 2009a). A recent study demonstrated that in addition to demonstrating injection technique, several other points must also be elucidated to the patients (Gallagher et al., 2011). They should be informed that auto-injectors should be used swiftly rather than waiting. They should be trained in recognizing anaphylaxis, taking into account the wide variability of symptoms and the side effects of epinephrine, offering reassurance about its safety if used unnecessarily (Gallagher et al., 2011). It should also be pointed out that an anaphylactic episode doesn't possess a predictive value for the severity of future episodes because of variable target organ involvement and the influence of comorbid illness and concurrently medications (Simons et al., 2009a).
The currently available epinephrine auto-injectors have some structural limitations (Frew, 2010). There are two types of delivery systems either as cartridge-based or a syringe delivery system used in the currently available auto-injectors (Frew, 2010). Evidence suggests there are several clear advantages of auto-injectors that utilize a cartridge system compared with a syringe system, but they are found in only 2 fixed doses as 0.15 mg which may be too high for infants and young children weighing less than 15 kg and 0.3 mg which can be a low dose for some children and adults, especially those who are overweight or obese (Frew, 2010; Simons, 2009b). Additionally the needle is 1.43 cm, not allowing optimal intramuscular injection in especially obese patients. New compact, lightweight, auto-injectors providing a 0.5 mg dose per injection, with a needle length of 2.54 cm are being designed and noninjectable epinephrine preparations for sublingual or transdermal administrations are also in development (Frew, 2010; Simons, 2009b).
The reasons for lack of response to epinephrine can be summarized as the error in the diagnosis, the wrong position of the patient after the injection, the rapid progression of anaphylaxis, the presence of a beta-adrenergic blocker or interfering drugs in the patient's medications, the low dose or the delayed injection of epinephrine, and the suboptimal route or injection site (Simons et al., 2011). Therefore the aim of every physician should be to teach their patients when and how to inject epinephrine and to educate them about anaphylaxis and save their lives.

11. Conclusion

Anaphylaxis is a serious acute allergic reaction and has to be recognized with signs and symptoms involving various organ systems and treated promptly. To diminish the risk for further attacks detailed history has to be taken carefully from the patients including the potential triggers or events, the clinical signs and symptoms. Laboratory tests most importantly an elevated serum tryptase level sometimes but not always support the diagnosis. The trigger has to be removed, if possible and the patient's circulation, airway, breathing, level of consciousness, and skin should be rapidly assessed. Epinephrine is the cornerstone of the treatment. Patients should be kept in the correct position, oxygen and fluid supplementation should be given. Antihistamines, corticosteroids, and other agents are the second-line treatment agents. Patients should be informed about the potential risk for the future attacks and be educated and prepared. For this purpose, patients should carry medical identification and be prescribed for epinephrine auto-injectors and have their personalized written anaphylaxis emergency action plans.

12. References

Aberer, W., Bircher, A., Romano, A., Blanca, A., Campi, P., Fernandez, J., Brockow, K., Pichler, WJ., Demoly, P. (2003). Position paper. Drug provocation testing in the diagnosis of drug hypersensitivity reactions: general considerations. *Allergy* Vol.58, pp.854-863, ISSN 0105-4538.

Akin, C., Scott, LM., Kocabas CN., Kushnir-Sukhov, N., Brittain, E., Noel, P. & Metcalfe, DD. (2007). Demonstration of an aberrant mast-cell population with clonal markers in a subset of patients with "idiopathic" anaphylaxis. *Blood* Vol. 110, pp.2331-3, ISSN 0006-4971.

Barg, W., Medrela, W. & Wolanczyk-Medrala, A. (2011). Exercise-Induced Anaphylaxis: An Update on Diagnosis and Treatment. *Current Allergy & Asthma Reports* Vol.11, pp. 45–51, ISSN 1529-7322.

Bernardini, R., Pecora, S., Milani, M. & Burastero, SE. (2008). Natural rubber latex allergy in children: clinical and immunological effects of 3-years sublingual immunotherapy. *European Annals of Allergy and Clinical Immunology* Vol. 40, pp. 1-6, ISSN 1764-1489.

Bilo, MB. & Bonifazi, F. (2009). The natural history and epidemiology of insect venom allergy: clinical implications. Clin Exp Allergy 2009,39:1467–1476 *Clinical & Experimental Allergy*, Vol.39, pp. 1467-1476, ISSN 0954-7894.

Boden, SR. & Burks, AW. (2011). Anaphylaxis: a history with emphasis on food allergy. *Immunological Reviews* Vol. 242, pp. 247–257, ISSN 0105-2896.

Brockow, K. & Ring J. (2011). Update on diagnosis and treatment of mastocytosis. *Current Allergy and Asthma Reports* Vol 11, No 4, pp.292-9, ISSN 1529-7322.

Brock-Utne, JG. (2003). Clinical manifestations of latex anaphylaxis during anesthesia differ from those not anesthesia/surgery-related. *Anesthesia & Analgesia* Vol. 97, pp. 1195-1207, ISSN 0003-2999.

Brown, AFT., McKinnon, D. & Chu, K. (2001). Emergency department anaphylaxis: a review of 142 patients in a single year. *Journal of Allergy & Clinical Immunology* Vol. 108, pp. 861-6, ISSN 0091-6749.

Brown, SG., Blackman, KE., Stenlake, V. & Heddle, RJ. (2004). Insect sting anaphylaxis: prospective evaluation of treatment with intravenous adrenaline and volume resuscitation. *Emergency Medicine Journal* Vol. 21, pp.149-54, ISSN 1472-0205.

Buyukozturk, S., Gelincik, A., Ozseker, F., Colakoglu, B. & Dal, M. (2010). Latex sublingual immunotherapy: can its safety be predicted? *Annals Allergy Asthma & Immunology* Vol. 104, pp. 339-42, ISSN 1081-1206.

Chiu, AM. & Kelly, KJ. (2005). Anaphylaxis: Drug Allergy, Insect Stings, and Latex. *Immunology and Allergy Clinics of North America* Vol.25, pp. 389– 405, ISSN 0889-8561

Choo, KJL., Simons, E. & Sheikh, A. (2010). Glucocorticoids for the treatment of anaphylaxis: Cochrane systemic review. *Allergy*, Vol. 65, pp. 1205-11, ISSN 0105-4538.

Dibs, SD. & Baker, MD. (1997). Anaphylaxis in children: a 5- year experience. *Pediatrics*, Vol 99, No.1, pp. E7, ISSN 1884-426X.

Ditto, AM., Harris, KE., Krasnick, J., Miller, MA. & Patterson R (1996). Idiopathic anaphylaxis: a series of 335 cases. *Annals Allergy Asthma & Immunology* Vol. 77, No.4, pp. 285-91, ISSN 1081-1206.

Feldweg, AM., Sheffer, AL. (2011). Exercise-induced anaphylaxis and food-dependant exercise-induced anaphylaxis in Castells MC. *Anaphylaxis and Hypersensitivity Reactions*, Springer, New York, pp.235-243, ISBN 978-1-60327-950-5

Finkelman, FD., Rothenberg, ME., Brandt, EB., Morris, SC. & Strait, RT. (2005). Molecular mechanisms of anaphylaxis: lessons from studies with murine models. *Journal of Allergy & Clinical Immunology* Vol. 115, pp. 449-57, ISSN 0091-6749.

Freeman, TM.(2004). Clinical practice. Hypersensitivity to hymenoptera stings. *New England Journal of Medicine* Vol. 351, pp. 1978-84, ISSN 0028-4793.

Frew, AJ. (2011). What are the 'ideal' features of an adrenaline (epinephrine) auto-injector in the treatment of anaphylaxis? *Allergy* Vol.66, pp. 15-24, ISSN 0105-4538.

Gallagher, M., Worth, A., Cunningham -Burley, S. & Sheikh, A. (2011). Epinephrine auto-injector use in adolescents at risk of anaphylaxis: a qualitative study in Scotland, UK. *Clinical & Experimental Allergy*, Vol.41, pp. 869–77, ISSN 0954-7894.

Gelincik, A., Ozşeker, F., Büyüköztürk, S., Colakoğlu, B., Dal, M. & Alper, A. (2007). Recurrent anaphylaxis due ton on-ruptured hepatic hydatid cystc. *International Archives of Allergy and Clinical Immunology* Vol 143, No. 4, pp. 296-8, ISSN 1018-2438.

Golden, DBK., Kelly, D., Hamilton, RG., Wang, NY. & Kagey-Sobotka, A. (2009). Dialyzed venom skin tests for identifying yellow jacket-allergic patients not detected using standard venom. *Annals Allergy Asthma & Immunology* Vol. 102, pp. 47-50, ISSN 1081-1206.

Greenberger, PA. (2006). Anaphylactic and Anaphylactoid Causes of Angioedema. *Immunology and Allergy Clinics of North America* Vol.26, pp.753-67, ISSN 0889-8561.

Greenberger, PA. (2007). Idiopathic anaphylaxis. *Immunology and Allergy Clinics of North America* Vol. 27, pp.273-93, ISSN 0889-8561.

Harduar-Morano, L., Simon, MR., Watkins, S. & Blackmore, C. (2011). A population-based epidemiologic study of emergency department visits for anaphylaxis in Florida. *Journal of Allergy & Clinical Immunology* (in pres), ISSN 0091-6749.

Jensen, BM., Metcalfe, DD. & Gilfillan AM. (2007). Targeting kit activation: a potential therapeutic approach in the treatment of allergic inflammation. *Inflammation & Allergy Drug Targets* Vol.6, pp. 57-62, ISSN 1871-5281.

Kemp, SF., Lockey, RF. & Simons FE. (2008) World Allergy Organization ad hoc Committee on Epinephrine: the drug of choice for anaphylaxis. A statement of World Allergy Organization. *Allergy* Vol.63, pp. 1061-70, ISSN 0105-4538.

Lee, JK., Vadas, P. (2011). Anaphylaxis: mechanisms and management. *Clinical & Experimental Allergy* Vol. 41, pp. 923-38, ISSN 095 4-7894.

Lieberman, P., Kemp, SF., Oppenheimer, J., Lang, DM., Bernstein, L., Nicklas, RA. & Workgroup Contributors (2005). The diagnosis and management of anaphylaxis: An updated practice parameter. *Journal of Allergy & Clinical Immunology*, Vol. 115, pp. S483523, ISSN 0091-6749.

Lieberman, P., Nicklas, RA., Oppenheimer, J., Kemp, SF., Lang DM. & Workgroup Contributors (2010). The diagnosis and management of anaphylaxis practice parameter: 2010 update. *Journal of Allergy & Clinical Immunology*, Vol. 126, pp. 477-80, ISSN 0091-6749.

Lobera, T., Audicana, MT., Pozo, MD., Blasco, A., Fernández, E., Cañada, P., Gastaminza, G., Martinez-Albelda, I., González-Mahave, I. & Muñoz, D. (2008). Study of hypersensitivity reactions and anaphylaxis during anesthesia in Spain. *Journal of Investigational Allergology & Clinical Immunology* Vol. 18, No. 5, 350-356, ISSN 1018-9068.

Novembre, E., Cianferoni, A., Bernardini, R., Mugnaini, L., Caffarelli, C., Cavagni, G., Giovane, A. & Vierucci, A. (1998). Anaphylaxis in children: clinical and allergologic features. *Pediatrics* Vol101, No 4, pp. E8, ISSN 1884-426X.

Olivera, A., Mizugishi, K., Tikhonova, A., Ciaccia, L., Odom, S., Proia, RL. & Rivera, J (2007). The sphingosine kinase-sphingosine-1-phophate axis is a determinant of mast cell function and anaphylaxis. *Immunity* Vo. 26, pp. 287-297. ISSN 1074-7613.

Pumphrey, RS. (2000). Lessons for the management of anaphylaxis from a study of fatal reactions. *Clinical & Experimental Allergy* Vol. 30, pp. 1144-50, ISSN 0954-7894.

Pumphrey, RS. (2003). Fatal posture in anaphylactic shock. *Journal of Allergy & Clinical Immunology* Vol. 112, pp. 451-2, ISSN 0091-6749.

Pumphrey, RSH. & Gowland, MH. (2007). Further fatal allergic reactions to food in the United Kingdom, 1999-2006. *Journal of Allergy & Clinical Immunology* Vol.119, pp. 1018-9, ISSN 0091-6749.

Brockow, K., Metcalfe, DD. (2010). History and classification of anaphylaxis in Ring, J., Blaser, K., Capron, M., Denburg, JA., Holgate, ST., Marona, G., Saito, H. (eds.) *Anaphylaxis. Chem. Immunol. Allergy* , Karger Publishers, Basel, Vol. 95, pp. 10-124, ISSN 1660-2242

Rivera, .J, Gilfillan, AM. (2006). Molecular regulation of mast cell activation. *Journal of Allergy & Clinical Immunology* Vol. 117, pp. 1214-25, ISSN 0091-6749.

Sampson, HA., Munoz-Furlong, A., Campbell, RL., Adkinson, NF. Jr., Bock, SA., Branum. A., Brown, SG., Camargo,CA.Jr., Cydulka, R., Galli, SJ., Gidudu, J., Gruchalla, RS., Harlor, AD. Jr., Hepner, DL., Lewis, LM., Lieberman, PL., Metcalfe, DD., O'Connor, R., Muraro, A., Rudman, A., Schmitt, C., Scherrer, D., Simons, FE., Thomas, S., Wood, JP., & Decker, WW. (2006). Second symposium on the definition and management of anaphylaxis: summary report—Second National Institute of Allergy and Infectious Disease/ Food Allergy and Anaphylaxis Network symposium. *Journal of Allergy & Allergy Clinical Immunology* Vol. 117, pp. 391-7, ISSN 0091-6749.

Sampson, HA. & Burks, AW. (2009). Adverse reactions to foods. In: *Middleton's allergy: principles and practice* Adkinson NF Jr, BochnerBS, Busse WW, Holgate ST, Lemanske RF Jr, Simons FER, editors . 7th ed. p. 1139-67. Mosby Elsevier Inc , ISBN: 978-0-323-05659-5, St Louis.

Schwartz, LB. (2006). Diagnostic Value of Tryptase in Anaphylaxis and Mastocytosis. *Immunology and Allergy Clinics of North America* Vol.26, pp. 451-63, ISSN 0889-8561

Schnyder, B. (2009). Approach to the Patient with Drug Allergy. *Immunology and Allergy Clinics of North America* Vol.29, pp. 405-18, ISSN 0889-8561.

Schnyder, B. & Pichler, WJ. (2009). Clinical manifestations of allergic diseases: Drug hypersensitivity in Rawankar, R, Holgate, ST & Rosenwasser LJ (eds.) *Allergy*

Frontiers: Diagnosis & Health Economics, Springer, Germany, Vol.4, pp. 403-422, ISBN978-4-431-98293-7.

Sheikh, A., Ten Broek, V., Brown, SGA. & Simons, FER. (2007). H1-antihistamines for the treatment of anaphylaxis: Cochrane systemic review. *Allergy,* Vol.62, pp. 830-7, ISSN 0105-4538.

Sheikh, A., Shehata, YA., Brown, SGA., Simons, FER. (2009). Adrenaline for the treatment of anaphylaxis: Cochrane systematic review. *Allergy* Vol. 64, pp. 204-212, ISSN 0105-4538.

Sicherer, SH., Sampso,n HA.(2006). Food allergy. *Journal of Allergy & Clinical Immunology* Vol. 117, pp. S470-5, ISSN0091-6749.

Simons, FER. (2008). Anaphylaxis. *Journal of Allergy & Clinical Immunology,* Vol.121, pp. S402-7 ISSN 0091-6749.

a Simons, FER., Clark, S., Camargo, CA. (2009). Anaphylaxis in the community: learning from the survivors. *Journal of Allergy & Clinical Immunology* Vol.124, pp. 301–6, ISSN 0091-6749.

b Simons, FER. (2009). Anaphylaxis: recent advances in assessment and treatment. *Journal of Allergy & Clinical Immunology* Vol.124, pp. 625-36, ISSN 0091-6749.

Simons, FER. (2010). Anaphylaxis. *Journal of Allergy & Clinical Immunology* Vol. 125, pp. 4S161-81, ISSN 0091-6749.

Simons, FER., Ardusso, LRF., Bilo, B., El-Gamal, YM., Ledford, DK., Ring, J., Sanchez-Borges, M., Senna., GE., Sheikh, A. & Thong, BY. (2011). World Allergy Organization anaphylaxis guidelines: Summary. *Journal of Allergy & Clinical Immunology* Vol. 127, pp. 587-93, ISSN 0091-6749.

Soar, J., Pumphrey, R., Cant, A., Clarke, S., Corbett, A., Dawson, P. et al., for the Working Group of the Resuscitation Council (UK). (2008). Emergency treatment for anaphylactic reactions: guidelines for healthcare providers. *Resuscitation* Vol.77, pp. 157-69, ISSN 0300-9572.

Thomas, M. & Crawford, I. (2005). Best evidence topic report. Glucagon infusion in refractory anaphylactic shock in patients on beta-blockers. *Emergency Medicine Journal* Vol.22, pp. 272-3, ISSN 1472-0205.

Thong, BY., Cheng, YK., Leong, KP., Tang, CY. & Chng, HH. (2005). Anaphylaxis in adults referred to a clinical immunology/allergy center in Singapore. *Singapore Medical Journal* Vol.46, No. 10, pp. 529–34, ISSN 0037-5675.

Vadas, P., Gold, M., Perelman, B., Liss, G., Lack, G., Blyth, T., Simons, FE., Simons, KJ, Cass, D. & Yeung, J. (2008). Platelet-activating factor, PAF-acetylhydrolase and severe anaphylaxis. *New England Journal of Medicine* Vol.358, pp. 28-35, ISSN 0028-4793.

Yokoi, H., Myers, A., Matsumoto, K., Crocker, PR., Saito, H. & Bochner BS. (2006). Alteration and acquisition of Siglecs during in vitro maturation of CD341 progenitors into human mast cells. *Allergy* Vol. 61, pp. 769-76, ISSN 0105-4538.

8

Allergic Airway Inflammation

Gabriel Morán[1], Claudio Henriquez[2] and Hugo Folch[2]
[1]*Department of Pharmacology, Universidad Austral de Chile,*
[2]*Department of Immunology, Universidad Austral de Chile,*
Chile

1. Introduction

Allergic airway inflammation is one characteristic feature of asthma disease, with additional pathology including a reversible airway obstruction, airway hyperresponsiveness (AHR), infiltration of eosinophils and T-helper type 2 (Th2) cells into the airway submucosa, mucus hypersecretion, and airway remodeling (Agrawal & Shao 2010). Allergic airway diseases are inflammatory disorders in which aberrant immune regulation occurs and susceptible individuals mount allergen specific responses. Inflammatory cells are recruited to the asthmatic airways or are activated in situ. The inflammatory cells include mast cells, macrophages, eosinophils, T lymphocytes, dendritic cells, basophils, neutrophils, and platelets (Barnes et al. 1998). Structural cells may also be important sources of inflammatory mediators in asthma. Airway epithelial cells, smooth muscle cells, endothelial cells, and fibroblasts are all capable of synthesizing and releasing inflammatory mediators (Levine, 1995; Saunders et al. 1997; John et al. 1997). Moreover, these cells may become the major source of inflammatory mediators in the airway, which may explain how asthmatic inflammation persists even in the absence of activating stimuli. A majority of patients with asthma have an atopic, allergic background (Robinson 2000). The prevailing consensus in regards to these patients is that the immunological basis of atopic sensitization and allergic disease results from inappropriate Th2 cell responses to common environmental proteins termed allergens (Robinson 2009).
Here, we summarize recent findings regarding how immune response and inflammatory cells contribute to allergic airway inflammation and discuss recent progress in the regulation of these cells.

2. Immune mechanism

In general, airway inflammation involves the activation of pathogenic-specific inflammatory cells, modulation of transcription factors and release of inflammatory mediators (Barnes et al. 1998). Allergic asthma, classified as a type 1 hypersensitivity reaction, involves allergen-specific immunoglobulins of the IgE class bound to high-affinity Fcε receptors (FceR) on the surface of basophils and mast cells present in the subepithelial layer of the airways. Cross-linking of the receptor initiates a coordinated sequence of biochemical and morphological events that results in exocytosis (figure 1) of secretory granules containing histamine or other pre-formed inflammatory mediators; synthesis and secretion of newly formed lipid mediators, such as prostaglandins and leukotrienes; and synthesis and secretion of cytokines (Will-Karp et al. 1999). Many mediators are released in asthma, and it is clear that these mediators interact with each other in some way. Mediators may act synergistically to enhance each other's effects, or one mediator may modify the release or action of another mediator. Although the involved signaling pathways have been extensively studied, the precise sequence of events is still not well understood (Turner et al. 1999; Kim et al. 1997; Ali., et al. 2001; Ching et al., 2001; Siraganian 2003; Galli et al. 2008; Kim et al. 2008; Saini et al. 2009; Moran et al. 2010a,b; Colgan & Hankel 2010). The inflammatory mediators are capable of contracting airway smooth muscle cells, inducing edema and mucus secretion, which leads to narrowed, constricted airways. Furthermore, locally produced chemokines stimulate the recruitment of eosinophils, macrophages, neutrophils, and T lymphocytes (Broide 2001).

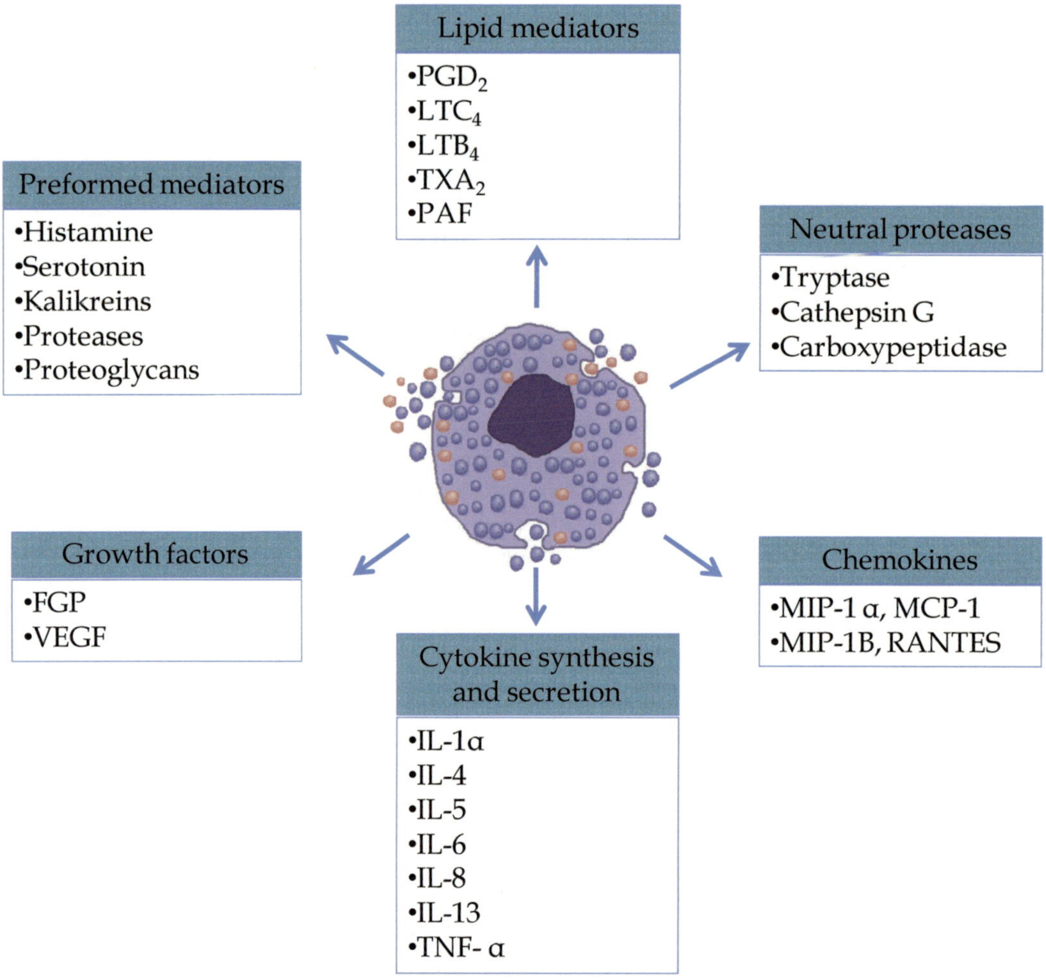

Fig. 1. Products of Mast Cells. PGD2, prostaglandin D2; LTC4, leukotriene C4; PAF, platelet-activating factor; FGP, fibroblast growth factor; VEGF, vascular endothelial growth factor, MIP; macrophage inflammatory protein; RANTES, regulated on activation, normal T-cell expressed and secreted MCP-1, monocyte chemotactic protein-1.

2.1 Role of T cells in airways allergy disease

T cells play an important role in the modulation of the immune response and are critical during allergy airway pathogenesis. Since 1986, the Th1/Th2 paradigm has dominated the understanding of the pathophysiology of asthma and allergic disease (Akbari et al. 2003). It is generally accepted that allergic respiratory disease in adults is associated with active T-cell immune responses to inhaled allergens that are skewed toward the Th2 phenotype, which is in contrast to a Th1-skewed immunity in healthy individuals (Agrawal and Shao 2010). Experimental animals model have been useful in the immunological delineation of the role of T cells and T cell-derived cytokines in the pathogenesis of airway allergy disease. In these animal models, sensitization with various allergens, such as ovalbumin, house dust mite, and aspergillus, induce a phenotype closely resembling that observed in human asthma (Hausding et al. 2008; Humar et al. 2008; Allen 2009; Bates et al. 2009; Qarcoo et al. 2009; Moran & Folch 2011).

Th2-associated cytokines such as IL-4 are important in driving IgE production to allergens and are essential in the initiation of an allergic airway response (Coyle et al. 1995). IL-5 contributes to the development, recruitment and activation of eosinophils at the site of the Th2 inflammatory response, which characterizes allergic disease. IL-9 is an important regulator of mast-cell activation. Studies suggest that IL-13 has an important role in the effector phase of the allergy response, specifically airway inflammation, bronchial hyperresponsiveness and mucus cell hypersecretion (Wills-Karps et al. 1998; Wills-Karps et al. 1999). The involvement of each the specific Th2 cytokines in atopic airway response has been demonstrated in studies in which IL-4, IL-5, IL-9 and IL-13 have been manipulated through either antibody blockade (Kung et al. 1995; Gavet et al. 1997) or gene targeting (Brusselle et al. 1995; Foster et al. 1996; Spergel et al. 1999). Additionally, IL-21 has been shown to be important in the development of Th2 immune response (Frohlich et al. 2007). Frohlich and colleagues (2007) suggest that although the mechanisms by which IL-21 regulates allergy inflammation are unknown, IL-21 may be important for Th2-cell survival or migration to peripheral tissues. On the other hand, Th1 cells are also pro-inflammatory, and the development of a Th1-associated inflammatory response can exacerbate asthma and allergic disease. IFN-γ is often present at sites of allergic inflammation and is thought to contribute to the disease. Th1 cells cross-regulate Th2 cells in some systems, and it was thought that Th1 cells downmodulated the effects of Th2 cells. However, recent advances in immunology have raised the possibility that other mechanisms may drive or co-exist with pathology in some patients with Th2-type allergy airway inflammation. New effector T-cell lineages have recently been identified. Th17 cells, which differentiate from naïve CD4+ T cells under the influence of IL-6/IL-21/IL-23 and transforming growth factor (TGF)-β via the signal transducer and activator of transcription 3 (STAT3)-RORγt pathway, are mainly responsible for neutrophilia in allergic severe asthma (Louten et al. 2009). Moreover, a variety of cytokines derived from epithelium, fibroblasts and other airway structural cells have recently been shown to have an important potential for interaction with Th1, Th2, Th17, eosinophil and mast cells. These cytokines include the following: proinflammatory cytokines [IL-1β, IL-6, IL-11, tumor necrosis factor (TNF)-α, and granulocyte/macrophage colony-stimulating factor (GMCSF)], which are involved in innate host defense; anti-inflammatory cytokines [IL-10, IFN-γ, IL-12, and IL-18]; growth factors [platelet derived growth factor (PDGF), TGF-β, fibroblast growth factor (FGF), and epidermal growth factor (EGF)]; and chemotactic cytokines or chemokines [RANTES, monocyte chemoattractant protein (MCP)-1–MCP-5, eotaxin, and IL-8] (Hamid and Tulic 2009).

Conversely, investigations into the contribution of cytotoxic CD8+ T cells towards the development of allergic airway inflammation are not well understood. The depletion of CD8+ T cells does not affect airway response to allergen challenge in mice (Gonzalo et al. 1996). However, a subset of CD8+ T cells, named *Tc2* cells, can produce Th2 cytokines such as IL-4, IL-5, and IL-13, which are increased in the bronchoalveolar lavage fluids (BALF) of allergic asthmatic patients in studies. This rise of cytokine production suggests that the immune responses to virus infections are characterized by an increase in the frequency of type 2 cytokine-producing T cells when they take place in an allergic environment in animal models (Coyle et al. 1995; Makela et al. 2003). Human studies show that CD8+ T cells from both normal and asthmatic subjects have the capacity to produce type 2 cytokines (Stanciu et al. 1996; Stanciu et al. 1997). In addition, the stimulation of CD8+ T cells from normal, healthy subjects in an IL-4 rich milieu significantly increased the number of IL-5-positive CD8+ T cells (Stanciu et al. 2001). Additionally, studies suggest that during a respiratory virus infection activated CD8+ T cells from asthmatic subjects may produce excess type 2 cytokines and may contribute to asthma exacerbation by augmenting allergic inflammation (Stanciu et al. 2005). These studies thus demonstrate that the frequency of airway CD8+ T cells producing type 2 cytokines are as great as those of airway CD4+ T cells are and that both are increased in asthma and are related to disease severity (Cho et al. 2005).

2.1.1 Transcription factors responsible for the Th1/Th2/Th17 cells and inflammatory mediators

Transcription factors are DNA-binding proteins that regulate the expression of inflammatory genes, including enzymes involved in the synthesis of inflammatory mediators as well as protein and peptide mediators (Barnes et al. 1998). Inflammation associated with hypersensitivity results from an exaggerated expression of inflammatory genes, and a number of researchers have explored the mechanisms implicated in inflammatory gene induction (Barnes and Karin, 1997; Barnes and Adcock, 1998). Many transcription factors are cell-specific and are crucial in cell differentiation and the regulation of specific cellular processes such as proliferation, enzymes, and cytokine expression. In animal models of airway diseases, such as atopic asthma, nuclear factor NF-(kB), activator protein-1 (AP-1), GATA-3, JunB and c-Maf play a central role in the control of airway inflammation (Finotto et al. 2001; Nguyen et al. 2003; Yamashita et al. 2007). In humans, there is evidence that NF-kB, AP-1 and GATA-3 expression is increased in asthmatic airways (Hart et al., 1998; Taha et al. 2003). Furthermore, these transcription factors are key downstream regulators of Th1/Th2/Th17 cytokine function and are phosphorylated/dephosphorylated in the asthmatic airway (Pernis and Rothman, 2002). The Th1 master regulator, T-box transcription factor (T-bet), is extensively expressed in polarized Th1 cells, and its expression and activity are induced by IL-12 via STAT4 or by IFN-γ via STAT1. IL-4 drives differentiation of IL-4-producing Th2 cells through STAT6, which is necessary and sufficient for the induction of the Th2 master regulator, GATA-3. Moreover, transcription factor c-Maf is selectively expressed in Th2 cells as a downstream effector of the IL-4/IL-4R/STAT6 signal transduction pathway, primarily regulating IL-4 expression in Th2 cells (Agrawal & Shao 2010).

2.1.2 Role of regulatory T cells in allergy airway diseases

As mentioned previously, allergic airway diseases show complex genetic associations and have a hereditary component (Cookson & Moffat 2004). However, the rapid and geographically localized nature of the increase in the incidence of allergic diseases indicates compounding effects of recent changes in environment and lifestyle in the Western world. How these factors impact disease by promoting immune responses to allergens is a subject of considerable debate, which has led to the "hygiene hypothesis" (Wills-Karp et al. 2001; Liu & Murphy 2003). According to the theory, in its simplest iteration, the increase in hygienic living conditions and in the use of antibiotic and sterile food preparations resulted in the separation of the immune system from positive microbial exposure early in life (Martinez and Holt, 1999). The immunoregulatory mechanisms remain underdeveloped, and an imbalance in immune homeostasis predisposes to the development of T helper type 2-biased immune responses and, consequently, allergic disease (Feleszko et al. 2005).

Recent studies indicate that Th2 responses that are characteristic of allergic manifestations can be regulated by naturally occurring CD4+CD25+ regulatory T (nTreg) cells. These cells are a functionally mature T-cell subpopulation, which play key roles in the maintenance of immunologic self-tolerance and negative control of a variety of physiological and pathological immune responses (Sakagushi et al. 2006). They also constitutively express transcription factor forkhead box P3 (FoxP3), which prevents the deviation of Tregs into effector T cells (Burchill et al. 2007). These cells originate in the thymus, but inducible Treg (iTreg) cells, which have similar properties and characteristics, can also be induced in the periphery. Regulatory T cells appear to control the development of autoimmune disease and transplant rejection and may play a critical role in controlling asthma and allergy (Akdis et al. 2005). Several studies indicate that the function of naturally occurring Treg cells is impaired or altered in patients with allergies compared with normal healthy individuals. The adoptive transfer of antigen-specific CD4+CD25+ T-regs attenuates acute allergic airway inflammation, AHR, and airway remodeling. The capacity of Treg cells to inhibit the proliferation of naive T cells *in vitro* requires cell–cell contact (induction of an inhibitory signals on CD4+ and CD8+ T cells); however, *in vivo*, these cells can also function through induction of inhibitory cytokines (such as TGF-β and IL-10) and inhibition of antigen-presenting capacity (Zheng et al. 2006; Kearly et al. 2008). These data suggest that one potential treatment option would be to enhance CD4+CD25+ Tregs in addition to targeting decreased Th2 populations. An example of this therapeutic strategy would be allergen desensitization immunotherapy, which has been in use for almost a century and is one of the few specific immunomodulatory treatments that are commonly used for allergic asthma (Akbari et al. 2003; Kearly et al. 2008). Understanding the immune mechanisms that underlie successful allergen immunotherapy offers the potential to improve current allergen-immunotherapy regimens. Some authors suggest that this therapy might function, at least in part, to promote the generation of IL-10 and TGF-β-secreting regulatory T cells (Hawrylowicz & Garra 2005; Shevach et al. 2008).

3. Apoptosis regulation in allergy airway disease

Apoptosis is defined as a genetic program that eliminates unneeded, senescent, or damaged cells (Thompson 1995). Moreover, apoptosis is an important regulatory mechanism in the selection and containment of an immunocompetent T cell population, in T cell development and during immune responses. Dysregulation of apoptosis has been implicated in a range of diseases including tumors, neurodegenerative disorders, autoimmunity (Cohen 1999) and, perhaps, allergic asthma (Vignola et al. 1999; Woolley et al. 1996). Studies in human patients have demonstrated that reduced T cell apoptosis plays an important role in the pathogenesis of allergic bronchial asthma (Cormican et al. 2001; Vignola et al. 1999; De Rose et al. 2004). These findings are also consistent in murine models of asthma (Jayaraman et al. 1999; Tong et al. 2006; Finotto et al. 2007). In addition, increasing lines of evidence suggest that changes in programmed cell death mechanisms in both mobile and resident cells of the airway may directly contribute to the development and clinical severity of allergy airway inflammation (Vignola et al. 2000).

Apoptosis has emerged as a major mechanism in the clearance of activated T cells during the resolution of an inflammatory response (Akbar and Salmon 1997). Inadequate T cell apoptosis in asthma patients appears to interfere with normal T cell elimination, resulting in T cell accumulation, which contributes to chronic inflammation and may be the major underlying cause for tissue damage, remodeling and repair (Müller et al. 2006; Vignola et al. 2000). Spinozzi et al. (1998) reported that pulmonary T cells isolated from the BALF of atopic asthma patients showed hypoexpression of Fas and FasL; this result may explain the low frequency of apoptosis in this group of patients. In contrast, horses with acute airway allergy have increased apoptosis of airway lymphocytes, which may partially explain the rapid resolution of the pathology once the allergen is removed in this allergy model (Moran et al. 2011). However, these authors suggest additional studies to examine apoptosis and cytokine profiles in other stages of the disease. In addition, basal levels of apoptotic activity were significantly lower in BALF lymphocytes from asthmatic subjects compared with peripheral blood lymphocytes from the same subjects. These data indicate that airway inflammation in asthma is associated with a reduced susceptibility to apoptosis, which may lead to enhanced survival of lymphocytes in the bronchial mucosa and prolonged inflammation (Müller et al. 2006). Other molecules are involved in the programmed cell death process, including members of the Bcl-2 gene family, which are known to inhibit apoptosis. Studies have shown that Bcl-2 expression is increased in lymphoid cells obtained from the airways of asthmatic patients and that neutralization of IL-10, an important inducer of Bcl-2, decreases Bcl-2 expression and apoptosis of cells from the respiratory tract of asthmatic patients (Hamzaoui et al. 1999a; Hamzaoui et al. 1999b).

4. Airway remodeling

Recently, airway remodeling has become a field of special interest in chronic asthma, chronic bronchitis, chronic obstructive pulmonary disease (COPD) and cystic fibrosis research as the process that causes patients to become largely resistant to medication and is an important factor in the development of irreversible airflow limitation (James et al., 1989; Lange et al., 1998; Jeffery et al., 2000; Kranenburg et al., 2002 Wegmann, 2008). In tissues from human with these diseases, remodeling changes include goblet cell and mucous gland hyperplasia, subepithelial fibrosis, neovascularization, airway smooth muscle (ASM) growth as well as increased deposition of extracellular matrix (ECM) proteins such as collagens, elastin, laminin, and proteoglycans around the smooth muscle and an overall thickening of the airway wall (Roche et al 1989; Laitinen et al., 1997; Davies et al., 2003). The molecular mechanisms that drive remodeling remain undefined, but many growth factors and cytokines, including fibroblast growth factor (FGF)-1, FGF-2, and transforming growth factor (TGF)-β1, that are released from the airway wall have the potential to contribute to airway remodeling, revealed by enhanced ASM proliferation and increased ECM protein deposition (Parameswaran et al., 2006; Kariyawasam and Robinson 2007). TGF-β1 is an important fibroblast chemotactic factor. Fibroblast numbers have been shown to correlate with TGF-β1 expression. TGF-β1 also induces the differentiation of fibroblasts to myofibroblasts (Postlethwaite and Seyer, 1995; Vignola et al., 1997; Thannickal et al., 2003). Morover, TGF-β1 and FGF-1 stimulate mRNA expression of collagen I and III in ASM cells, suggesting their role in the deposition of extracellular matrix proteins by ASM cells in the airways of patients with chronic lung diseases. Furthermore, ECM proteins promote the survival, proliferation, cytokine synthesis, migration, and contraction of human ASM cells contributing to airway wall remodeling (Parameswaran et al., 2006)

5. Conclusion

Asthma allergy disease is multifactorial, characterized by allergy airway inflammation and increased bronchoconstrictory response to nonspecific stimuli. The current body of knowledge suggests that the inflammatory component of asthma results from a combination of elements from both the innate and adaptive immune responses. Expression of cytokine patterns consistent with Th1, Th2 and Th17 cell activation has been identified and determined to vary based on the chronic condition of the disease. Activation of transcription factors plays a pivotal role in regulating cellular signaling pathways through dynamic modulation of cytokines, chemokines, and similar molecules. The regulation of the apoptosis of inflammatory cells, fibroblasts, and myocytes through Bcl-2 expression contributes to the establishment of chronic disease and remodeling. Tregs seem to play a pivotal role in balancing tolerance versus immunologic response to allergens. Therapy with immunomodulators that enhance tolerance to allergens and increase Tregs would be most effective in the treatment of allergy airway disease.

6. Acknowledgment

The author acknowledges the support of Fondecyt grants (Chilean governments), 11100196.

7. References

Agrawal, D.K & Shao Z. (2010).Pathogenesis of allergic airway inflammation. *Current Allergy and Asthma Reports* 10, 39-4; ISSN 1529-7322

Ali, H; Maeyama, K; Sagi-Eisenberg, R & Beaven, M.A. (2001). Antigen and thapsigargin promote influx of Ca^{2+} in rat basophilic RBL-2H3 cells by ostensibly similar mechanisms that allow filling of inositol 1,4,5-triphosphate-sensitive and mitochondrial Ca^{2+} stores. *The Biochemical journal* 304, 431-440; ISSN 0264-6021

Allen, I.C. (2009). Searching for an improved mouse model of allergic airway disease using dual allergen exposures. *Disease Models & Mechanism*. 12, 519-520; ISSN 1754-8403

Akbar, A.N & Salmon, M. (1997). Cellular environments and apoptosis: tissuemicroenvironments control activated T cell death. *Immunology Today* 18, 726-6; ISSN 0167-5699

Akbari, O; Stock, P; DeKruyff, R.H & Umetsu DT.(2003). Role of regulatory T cells in allergy and asthma. *Current Opinion in Immunology* 15, 627-633; ISSN 0952-7915

Akdis, M; Blaser, K & Akdis C.A (2005). T regulatory cells in allergy: novel concepts in the pathogenesis, prevention, and treatment of allergic diseases. *The Journal of Allergy Clinical Immunology* 116, 961-968; ISSN 0091-6749

Barnes, PJ; Fan, K & Chung, C. (1998). Inflammatory mediators of asthma: An Update. *Pharmacological Reviews* 50, 515-596; 0031-6997

Barnes, P.J & Adcock, I.M (1998). Transcription factors and asthma. *The European Respiratory Journal* 2, 221–234; ISSN 0903-1936

Barnes, P.J & Karin, M. (1997). Nuclear factor-kB: A pivotal transcription factor in chronic inflammatory diseases. *The New England Journal Medicine* 336,1066–1071; ISSN 0028-4793

Bates, J.H; Rincon, M & Irvin C.G. (2009). Animal models of asthma. *American Journal of Physiology. Lung and Cellular and Molecular Physiology* 297, L401-1; ISSN 1040-0605

Broide D.H. (2001). Molecular and cellular mechanisms of allergic disease. *The Journal of Allergy Clinical Immunology* 108, S65–S71; ISSN 0091-6749

Brusselle, G; Kips, J; Joos, G; Bluethmann, H & Pauwels R (1995). Allergen-induced airway inflammation and bronchial responsiveness in wild-type and interleukin- 4-deficient mice. *American Journal of Respiratory Cell and Molecular Biology* 12, 254–259; ISSN 1044-1549

Burchill, M.A; Yang, J; Vogtenhuber, C; Blazar B.R & Farrar, M.A. (2007). IL-2 receptor betadependentSTAT5 activation is required for the development of Foxp3+ regulatory T cells. *The Journal of Immunology* 178, 280–290; ISSN 0022-1767

Cohen J.J. (1999). Apoptosis: mechanisms of life and death in the immune system. *The Journal of Allergy and Clinical Immunology* 103, 548–54; ISSN 0091-6749

Ching T.T; Hsu, AL; Johnson A.J & Chen C.S. (2001). Phosphoinositide 3-kinase facilitates antigen-stimulated Ca(2+) influx in RBL-2H3 mast cells via a phosphatidylinositol 3,4,5-trisphosphate-sensitive Ca(2+) entry mechanism. *The Journal of Biological Chemistry* 276, 14814-14820; ISSN 0021-1767

Cho, S.H; Stanciu, L.A; Holgate, S.T & Johnston SL (2005). Increased interleukin-4, interleukin-5, and interferon-gamma in airway CD4+ and CD8+ T cells in atopic asthma. *American Journal of Respiratory Critical and Care Medicine* 171:224–230; ISSN 1073-449X

Colgan JD, Hankel IL. (2010). Signaling pathways critical for allergic airway inflammation. *Current in Opinion and Allergy Clinical Immunology* 10, 42-47; ISSN 1528-4050

Cormican, L; O'Sullivan S; Burke, C.M & Poulter, L.W. (2001). IFNgamma but not IL-4 T cells of the asthmatic bronchial wall show increased incidence of apoptosis. *Clinical and Experimental Allergy* 31, 731–739; ISSN 0954-7894

Cookson, W & Moffatt M. (2004). Making sense of asthma genes. *The New England Journal of Medicine* 51, 1794-6; ISSN 0028-4793

Coyle, A.J; Erard, F; Bertrand, C; Walti, S; Pircher, H & Le Gros G. (1995). Virusspecific CD8+ cells can switch to interleukin 5 production and induce airway eosinophilia. The *Journal of Experimental Medicine*, 181,1229-1233; ISSN 022-1007

Davies, D.E; Wicks, J; Powell, R.M; Puddicombe, S.M & Holgate ST. (2003). Airway remodeling in asthma: new insights. *The Journal of Allergy and Clinical Immunology* 111, 215-25; ISSN 0091-6749

De Rose, V; Cappello, P; Sorbello, V; Ceccarini, B; Gani, F; Bosticardo, M; Fassio, S & Novelli, F. (2004). IFN-gamma inhibits the proliferation of allergen-activated T lymphocytes from atopic, asthmatic patients by inducing Fas/FasL-mediated apoptosis. *Journal of Leukocyte Biology* 76, 423-32; ISSN 0741-5400

Feleszko, W; Jaworska, J & Hamelmann, E. (2006). Toll-like receptors—novel targets in allergic airway disease (probiotics, friends and relatives). *European Journal of Pharmacology* 533, 308-318; ISSN 0014-2999

Finotto, S; De Sanctis, G; Lehr, H; Herz, U; Buerke, M; Schipp, M; Bartsch, B; Atreya, R; Schmitt, E; Galle, P; Renz, H & Neurath M. (2001). Treatment of allergic airway inflammation and hyperresponsiveness by antisense-induced local blockade of GATA-3 expression. *Journal of Experimental Medicine* 193, 1247–1260; ISSN 022-1007

Finotto, S; Eigenbrod, T; Karwot, R; Boross, I; Doganci, A; Ito, H; Nishimoto, N; Yoshizaki, K; Kishimoto, T; Rose-John, S; Galle, P.R & Neurath, M.F. (2007). Local blockade of IL-6R signaling induces lung CD4+ T cell apoptosis in a murine model of asthma via regulatory T cells. *International Immunology* 19, 685-93; ISSN 0953-8178

Foster, P.S; Hogan, S.P; Ramsay, A.J; Matthaei, K.I & Young IG (1996). Interleukin 5 deficiency abolishes eosinophilia, airways hyperreactivity, and lung damage in a mouse asthma models. *The Journal of Experimental Medicine* 183, 195-201; ISSN 022-1007

Fröhlich, A; Marsland, B.J; Sonderegger, I; Kurrer, M; Hodge, MR; Harris, N.L & Kopf M. (2007). IL-21 receptor signaling is integral to the development of Th2 effector responses in vivo.*Blood* 109, 2023-2031; ISSN 0006-4971

Galli, S.J; Grimbaldeston, M & Tsai M. (2008). Immunomodulatory mast cells: negative, as well as positive, regulators of immunity. *Nature Review Immunology* 8, 478–486; ISSN 1474-1733

Gonzalo JA, Lloyd CM, Kremer L, Finger E, Martinez-A C, Siegelman MH, Cybulsky M,

Gutierrez-Ramos JC (1996). Eosinophil recruitment to the lung in a murine model of allergic inflammation. The role of T cells, chemokines, and adhesion receptors. *The Journal of Clinical Investigation* 98, 2332-2345; ISSN 0021-9738

Gavett, SH; O'Hearn, D.J; Karp, C.L Patel EA, Schofield, B.H; Finkelman F.D & Wills-Karps M (1997). Interleukin-4 receptor blockade prevents airway responses induced by antigen challenge in mice. *American Journal of Physiology* 272, L253–L261; ISSN 0002-9513

Hamid, Q & Tulic M. (2009). Immunobiology of asthma. *Annual Review Physiology* 71, 489-507; ISSN 0066-4278

Hamzaoui, A; Hamzaoui, K; Salah, H & Chabbou, A. (1999a). Lymphocytes apoptosis in patients with acute exacerbation of asthma. *Mediators of Inflammation* 8, 237–243; ISSN 0962-9351

Hamzaoui, K; Hamzaoui, A.; Zakraoui, L & Chabbou, A. (1999b). Expression of Bcl-2 in inflammatory sites from patients with active Behçet's disease. *Mediators of Inflammation* 8, 101–106; ISNN 0962-9351

Hart, L; Krishman, V; Adcock, I; Barnes, P & Chung K. (1998). Activation and localization of transcription factor, nuclear factor-kappaB, in asthma. *American Journal of Respiratory and Critical Care Medicine* 158, 1585–1592; ISSN 1073-449X

Hausding, M; Sauer, K; Maxeiner, J.H & Finotto S. (2008) Transgenic models in allergic responses. *Current Drug Targets* 9, 503-10; ISSN 1389-4501

Hawrylowicz, C.M & O'Garra A (2005). Potential role of interleukin-10-secreting regulatory T cells in allergy and asthma. *Nature Reviews Immunology* 5, 271-283; 1474-1733

James, AL; Pare, PD & Hogg JC. (1989). The mechanics of airway narrowing in asthma. *The American Review of Respiratory Disease* 139, 242 246; ISSN 0003-0805

Jayaraman, S; Castro, M; O'Sullivan, M; Bragdon, M.J & Holtzman, M.J. (1999) Resistance to Fas-mediated T cell apoptosis in asthma. *The Journal of Immunology* 162, 1717–22; ISSN 0022-1767

Jeffery, PK; Laitinen, A & Venge P. (2000). Biopsy markers of airway inflammation and remodelling. *Respiratory Medicine* 94, S9–S15; ISSN 0954-6111

John, M; Hirst, S.J; Jose, P; Robichaud, A; Witt, C; Twort, C; Berkman, N; Barnes, P.J & Chung KF. (1997). Human airway smooth muscle cells express and release RANTES in response to Th1 cytokines: Regulation by Th2 cytokines. The *Journal of Immunology* 158:1841–1847; ISSN 0022-1767

Kariyawasam; H.H & Robinson D.S. (2007). The role of eosinophils in airway tissue remodelling in asthma. *Current Opinion in Immunology* 19, 681–686; ISSN 0952-7915

Kearley, J; Robinson, D.S & Lloyd C.M. (2008). CD4+CD25+ regulatory T cells reverse established allergic airway inflammation and prevent airway remodeling. *Journal of Allergy Clinical Immunology* 122, 617–624; ISSN 0091-6749

Kim, T.D; Eddlestone, G.T; Mahmoud, S.F; Kuchtey, J & Fewtrell C. (1997). Correlating Ca2+ responses and secretion in individual RBL-2H3 mucosal mast cells. *The Journal of Biological Chemestry 272, 31225-31229; ISSN 0021-9258*

Kim, M.S; Radinger, M & Gilfillan AM. (2008). The multiple roles of phosphoinositide 3-kinase in mast cell biology. *Trends in Immunology* 29, 493–501; ISSN 1471-4906

Kranenburg, A. R., Willems-Widyastuti, A., Saxena, P. R., Sterk, P. J., de Boer, W. I. & Sharma, H. S. (2002). Enhanced pulmonary expression of extracellular matrix proteins in central airways of COPD patients. *American Journal of Respiratory Critical and Care Medicine* 165, A600; ISNN 1073-449X

Kung, T.T; Stelts, D.M; Zurcher, J.A; Adams, G.K 3rd; Egan, R.W; Kreutner, W; Watnick, A.S; Jones, H & Chapman R.W (1995). Involvement of IL-5 in a murine model of allergic pulmonary inflammation: prophylactic and therapeutic effect of an anti-IL-5 antibody.. *American Journal of Respiratory and Cell Molecular Biology*. 13, 360-365; ISSN 1044-1549

Kumar, R.K; Herbert, C & Foster PS. (2008). The "classical" ovalbumin challenge model of asthma in mice. *Current Drug Targets* 9, 485-94; ISSN 1389-4501

Lang, P; Parner, J; Vestbo, J; Schnohr, P & Jensen G. (1998). A 15-year followup study of ventilatory function in adults with asthma. *The New England Journal of Medicine* 339, 1194-1200; ISSN 0028-4793

Laitinen, A., Altraja, A., Kampe, M., Linden, M., Virtanen, I. & Laitinen, L. A. (1997) Tenascin is increased in airwaybasement membrane of asthmatics and decreased by an inhaled steroid. *American Journal of Respiratory Critical and Care Medicine* 156, 951–958; ISSN 1073-449X

Levine, S.J (1995). Bronchial epithelial cell-cytokine interactions in airway epithelium. *Journal of Investigative Medicine* 43, 241–249; 1081-5589

Liu, A.H & Murphy J.R (2003). Hygiene hypothesis: fact or fiction?*Journal of Allergy Clinical Immunology* 111, 471-8; ISSN 0091-6749

Louten, J; Boniface, K & de Waal Malefyt R. (2009). Development and function of Th17 cells in health and disease. *Journal of Allergy Clinical Immunology* 123, 1004–1011; ISSN 0091-6749

Martinez, F.D & Holt PG. (1999). Role of microbial burden in aetiology of allergy and asthma..*Lancet* 354, SII12-5; ISSN 0140-6736

Makela, M.J; Tripp, R; Dakhama, A; Park, J.W; Ikemura, T; Joetham, A; Waris, M; Anderson, L.J & Gelfand EW. (2003). Prior airway exposure to allergen increases virus-induced airway hyperresponsiveness. *Journal of Allergy Clinical Immunology* 112, 861-869 ; ISSN 0091-6749

Morán, G; Burgos, R; Araya, O & Folch H. (2010a). *In vitro* bioassay to detect reaginic antibodies from the serum of horses affected with Recurrent Airway Obstruction. *Veterinary Research Communications* 34, 91-99; ISSN 0165-7380

Morán, G; Folch, H; Burgos, R; Araya, O & Barria M. (2010b): Detection of reaginic antibodies against *Faenia rectivirgula* from the serum of horses affected with Recurrent Airway Obstruction by an in *vitro* bioassay. *Veterinary Research Communications* 34, 719-726; ISSN 0165-7380

Morán, G & Folch H. 2011. Recurrent airway obstruction in horses - an allergic inflammation: a review. *Veterinarni Medicina* 56, 1-13; ISSN 0375-8427

Moran, G; Buechner-Maxwell, V.A; Folch, H; Henriquez, C; Galecio, J.S; Perez, B; Carrasco, C & Barria (2011). Increased apoptosis of CD4 and CD8 T lymphocytes in the airways of horses with recurrent airway obstruction..*Veterinary Research Communications 35, 447-456;* ISSN 0165-7380

Müller, M; Grunewald, J; Olgart Höglund, C; Dahlén, B; Eklund, A & Stridh, H. 2006 Altered apoptosis in bronchoalveolar lavage lymphocytes after allergen exposure of atopic asthmatic subjects. *The European Respiratory Journal* 28, 513-22; ISSN 0903-1936

Nguyen, C; Teo, J.L; Matsuda, A; Eguchi, M; Chi, E; Henderson, Jr W & Kahn M. (2003). Chemogenomic identification of Ref-1/AP-1 as a therapeutic target for asthma. *Proceedings of the National Academy of Sciences of the United States of America* 100, 1169–1173; ISSN 0027-8424

Parameswaran, K; Willems-Widyastuti, A; Alagappan, VK; Radford, K; Kranenburg, A.R. & Sharma HS. (2006). Role of extracellular matrix and its regulators in human airway smooth muscle biology. *Cell Biochemistry* and *Biophysics* 44, 139-146; ISSN 1085-9195

Pernis, A.B & Rothman PB. (2002). JAK-STAT signaling in asthma. The *Journal of Clinical Investigation* 109, 1279–1283; ISSN 0021-9738

Postlethwaite, AE & Seyer JM. (1995). Identification of a chemotactic epitope in human transforming growth factor-beta 1 spanning amino acid residues 368–374. *Journal of Cellular Physiology* 164, 587-592; ISSN 0021-954

Quarcoo, D; Pavlovic, S & Joachim RA. (2009). Stress and airway reactivity in a murine model of allergic airway inflammation. *Neuroimmunomodulation*. 16, 318-24; ISSN 1021-7401

Robinson, D. S. (2000). TH2 cytokines in allergic disease. *British Medical Bulletin* 56, 956–968; ISNN 0007-1420

Robinson D.S. (2010). Regulatory T cells and asthma. *Clinical and Experimental of Allergy* 39, 1314–1323; ISSN 0954-7894

Roche, W. R., Beasley, R., Williams, J. H. & Holgate, S. T.(1989) Subepithelial fibrosis in the bronchi of asthmatics. *Lancet* 1, 520–524; ISSN 0140-6736

Sakaguchi, S; Ono, M; Setoguchi, R; Yagi, H; Hori, S; Fehervari, Z; Shimizu, J; Takahashi, T & Nomura T. (2006). Foxp3+ CD25+ CD4+ natural regulatory T cells in dominant self-tolerance and autoimmune disease. *Immunological Reviews* 212, 8-27; ISSN 0105-2896

Saini, S.S; Paterniti, M; Vasagar, K; Gibbons, S.P; Jr Sterba, P.M & Vonakis BM. (2009). Cultured peripheral blood mast cells from chronic idiopathic urticaria patients spontaneously degranulate upon IgE sensitization: Relationship to expression of Syk and SHIP-2. *Clinical Immunology* 132, 342–348; ISSN 1521-6616

Saunders, M.A; Mitchell, J.A; Seldon, P.M; Barnes, P.J; Giembycz, M.A & Belvisi MG. (1997). Release of granulocyte-macrophage colony-stimulating factor by human cultured airway smooth muscle cells: Suppression by dexamethasone. *British Journal of Pharmacology* 120, 545–546; ISSN 0007-1188

Shevach, E.M; Tran, D.Q; Davidson, T.S & Andersson J. (2008). The critical contribution of TGF-beta to the induction of Foxp3 expression and regulatory T cell function. *European Journal of Immunology* 38, 915–917; ISSN 0022-1767

Siraganian RP. (2003). Mast cell signal transduction from the high-affinity IgE receptor.*Current Opinion in Immunology* 15, 639-46; ISSN 0952-7915

Spergel, J.M; Mizoguchi, E; Oettgen, H; Bhan, AK & Geha RS. (1999).Roles of TH1 and TH2 cytokines in a murine model of allergic dermatitis. *The Journal of Clinical Investigation* 103, 1103-11; ISSN 0021-9738

Spinozzi, F; Fizzotti, M; Agea, E; Piattoni, S; Droetto, S; Russano, A; Forenza, N; Bassotti, G; Grignani, F & Bertotto A. (1998). Defective expression of Fas messenger RNA and FAS receptor on pulmonary T cells from patients with asthma. *Annals of Internal Medicine* 128, 363–9; ISSN 0003-4819

Stanciu, L.A; Shute, J; Holgate, S.T & Djukanovic R. (1996). Production of IL-8 and IL-4 by positively and negatively selected CD4+ and CD8+ human T cells following a four-step cell separation method including magnetic cell sorting (MACS). *Journal of Immunological Methods* 189, 107-115; ISSN 0022-1759

Stanciu, L.A; Shute, J; Promwong, C; Holgate, S.T & Djukanovic R. (1997). Increased levels of IL-4 in CD8+ T cells in atopic asthma. *Journal of Allergy Clinical Immunology* 100,373-378; ISSN 0091-6749

Stanciu, L.A; Roberts, K; Lau, L.C.K; Coyle, A.J & Johnston SL. (2001). Induction of type 2 activity in adult human CD8 Tcells by repeated stimulation an IL-4. *International Immunology* 13, 341-348; ISSN 0953-8178

Stanciu, L.A; Roberts, K; Papadopoulos, N.G; Cho, S.H; Holgate, S.T; Coyle, A.J & Johnston SL. (2005). IL-4 increases type 2, but not type 1, cytokine production in CD8+ T cells from mild atopic asthmatics. *Respiratory Research* 7; 6: 67; ISSN 1465-9921

Taha, R; Hamid, Q; Cameron, L & Olivenstein R. (2003). T helper type 2 cytokine receptors and associated transcription factors GATA-3, c-MAF, and signal transducer and activator of transcription factor-6 in induced sputum of atopic asthmatic patients. *Chest* 123, 2074–2082; ISSN 0012-3692

Thannickal, V.J; Lee, D.Y; White, E.S; Cui, Z; Larios, J.M; Chacon, R; Horowitz, J.C; Day, R.M & Thomas PE. (2003). Myofibroblast differentiation by transforming growth factor-beta1 is dependent on cell adhesion and integrin signaling via focal adhesion kinase. *The Journal of Biological Chemestry* 278, 12384-12389; ISSN 0021-9258

Thompson, C.B. (1995). Apoptosis in the pathogenesis and treatment of disease. *Science* 267, 1456–1462; ISSN 0036-8075

Tong, J; Bandulwala, H.S; Clay, B.S; Anders, R.A; Shilling, R.A; Balachandran, D.D; Chen, B; Weinstock, J.V; Solway, J; Hamann, K.J & Sperling, A.I. (2006) Fas-positive T cells regulate the resolution of airway inflammation in a murine model of asthma. *The Journal of Experimental Medicine* 203, 1173-84; ISSN 022-1007

Turner, H & Kinet J.P. (1999) Signalling through the high-affinity IgE receptor Fc epsilonRI.. *Nature* 402, B24-30; ISSN 0028-0836

Vignola, A.M; Chanez, P; Chiappara, G; Merendino, A; Pace, E; Rizzo, A; la Rocca, A.M; Bellia, V; Bonsignore, G & Bousquet J. (1997). Transforming growth factor-beta expression in mucosal biopsies in asthma and chronic bronchitis. *American Journal of Respiratory and Critical Care Medicine* 156, 591-599; ISSN 1044-1549

Vignola, A.M; Chanez, P; Chiappara, G; Siena, L; Merendino, A; Reina, C; Gagliardo, R; Profita, M; Bousquet, J & Bonsignore, G. 1999 Evaluation of apoptosis of eosinophils, macrophages, and T lymphocytes in mucosal biopsy specimens of patients with asthma and chronic bronchitis. *The Journal of Allergy Clinical Immunololy*. 103, 563–573; ISSN 0091-6749

Vignola, A.M; Chiappara, G; Gagliardo, R; Gjomarkaj, M; Merendino, A; Siena, L; Bousquet J & Bonsignore G. (2000). Apoptosis and airway inflammation in asthma. *Apoptosis* 5, 473-85; ISSN 1360-8185

Wegmann M. (2008). Animal models of chronic experimental asthma —strategies for the identification of new therapeutic targets. *Journal of Occupational Medicine and Toxicology* 3, S4; ISSN 1745-6673

Wills-Karp, M; Luyimbazi, J; Xu, X; Schofield, B; Neben, T.Y; Karp, C.L & Donaldson D.D. (1998). Interleukin-13: central mediator of allergic asthma. *Science* 282:2258–61; ISSN 0036-8075

Wills-Karp, M. (1999). Immunologic basis of antigen-induced airway hyperresponsiveness. *Annual Review in Immunology* 17, 255-281; ISSN 1545-3278

Wills-Karp, M; Santeliz, J & Karp, C. L. (2001). The germless theory of allergic disease: revisiting the hygiene hypothesis. *Nature Reviews Immunology* 1, 69–75; ISSN 1474-1733

Woolley, K.L; Gibson, P.G; Carty, K; Wilson, A.J; Twaddell, S.H & Woolley, M.J. (1996). Eosinophil apoptosis and the resolution of airway inflammation in asthma.

American Journal of Respiratory and Critical Care Medicine 154, 237–243; ISSN 1044-1549

Yamashita, M; Onodera, A & Nakayama T. (2007). Immune mechanism of allergic airway disease: regulation by transcriptions factors. *Critical Reviews in Immunology* 26. 539-546; ISSN 1040-8401

Zheng, S.G; Wang, J.H; Stohl, W; Kim, K.S; Gray, J.D & Horwitz, D.A. (2006). TGF-beta requires CTLA-4 early after T cell activation to induce FoxP3 and generate adaptive CD4+CD25+ regulatory cells. *The Journal of Immunology* 176, 3321–3329; ISSN 0022-1767

9

Asthma and Sensitization Pattern in Children

Ute Langen
Robert Koch-Institute,
Germany

1. Introduction

The prevalence of specific sensitization and its clinical relevance for the development of allergic diseases and asthma is one of the subjects currently being in the focus of scientific studies. In the field of asthma we find additionally several studies of occupational asthma with specific sensitization and of treatment efficacy and duration of omalizumab in asthma patients with high IgE levels, which will not be discussed in this chapter. Several other studies focus on general aspects of sensitization pattern or classification of specific sensitization corresponding to type or severity of asthma or globally the development of asthma in different populations. Based on a short literature review of such studies we will finally present own representative data of our German Health Interview and Examination Survey for Children and Adolescents (KiGGS).

In this presentation we will describe specific IgE levels to several common aeroallergens in asthmatic and nonasthmatic children, search for a possible correlation between the number of sensitizations and the development of asthma and correlations between age, gender, social and migration status and rural or urban residency of the children and their sensitization status. Finally we will try to identify high risk mono- and polysensitization for asthma and will compare typical combinations of sensitizations in children with and without asthma.

2. Asthma and specific sensitization in the literature

During the last years the scientific community seemed to feel more and more that asthma is a disease showing very different phenotypes with different courses of the disease and therapeutic outcomes and a different prognosis. So the disease has been described not only - as in former times - as eosinophilic or neutrophilic type asthma or intrinsic, extrinsic and mix type asthma but increasingly also as early onset and late onset asthma, childhood and adult onset asthma and several special asthma forms are subject of clinical studies as exercise induced asthma, seasonal asthma, variant asthma and so on. Together with this history also dependencies between specific allergic sensitization and asthma became a target of several studies.

The fact that asthma without any signs of allergy may occur is well known. Additionally, it has become clear that being measurably sensitized does not automatically mean to suffer from any allergic disease. Ten years ago in a population of nearly 800 school children in Italy, using a skin prick test, it was monitored (Crimi et al., 2001) that "about one third of the sensitized children were without symptoms" - meaning symptoms of asthma and/or rhinitis. So the question arose, how sensitization or special sensitization patterns may influence the development of allergic and atopic diseases like asthma.

Beforehand endeavour has been made to describe frequency and patterns of sensitization itself, for example in a population of more than 700 school children in Germany (Hader et al., 1990). 34.4 % of the studied children had been sensitized to one or more of the tested aeroallergens, 39.6 % of these monosensitized. The most common sensitization was that to grasspollen, followed by birch, than house-dust mite, cat and hazelpollen. Several patterns of mono- and polysensitization have been described.

Nowadays we have a wide overview of demographic distribution of sensitizations and its correlation to asthma. As one could expect, "residence of rural area is associated with a significant lower prevalence of allergic sensitization" seen in more than 400 school children 12-16 years old (Majkowska-Wojciechowska et al., 2007) and boys are significantly more often than girls sensitized to a wide range of allergens (Soto-Quiros et al., 1998) as they are more often affected by asthma. However, in Italy, polysensitization of children living in a rural area especially against pollen and mould led to comparable asthma prevalence as house dust mite sensitization in those living in urban regions (Verini et al., 2005). We will report about the special role of dust mite sensitization in asthma in the course of this review.

Reviewing studies using skin tests for defining sensitization, it has been clearly shown that "aeroallergen sensitization occurs in most patients with asthma" (Craig, 2010). It was concluded that in mild to moderate asthma about 95 % of patients show sensitization and in severe asthma still up to 90 %. Remembering the fact that up to 5 % of asthma patients show a neutrophilic asthma and nearly all of those patients develop a severe form of asthma and subtracting those patients from the selected patient groups this may mean that with the exception of neutrophilic asthma forms all other patients show a similar high percentage of sensitization independant from asthma severity grade. This review also showed that sensitization "pattern varies with ethnicity, location of residance, and onset of asthma, but not age".

The same author described two years earlier in a population of mild-to-moderate athma patients 14 % of these showing a sensitization only to 1 or 2 aeroallergens but 81 % showing a polysensitization to at least 3 aeroallergens (Craig et al., 2008). He was also able to demonstrate a correlation between sensitization and factors characterising asthma as exhaled nitric oxide measures as a sign of inflammation activity and lung function values.

Not only asthma severity grade correlates with sensitization but also the chance of asthma remission during childhood. In the data of ISAAC, the internatioal study of asthma and allergies in childhood and one of the most important international studies in this field, a cohort comparison of 7 - 8 year versus 11 - 12 year old school children showed that the "remission of asthma was 10 % yearly and inversely related to allergic sensitization" (Bjerg-Bäcklund et al., 2006).

The number of sensitizations against aeroallergens clearly correlates with the risk for asthma, as shown in a total of more than 3000 patients aged 10 to 50 years in Spain and Portugal (Valero Santiago et al. 2009).

Very interesting in this relation is the fact that asthma prevalence in children is enhanced by very different specific sensitizations. A study in a random population of more than 6000 children in New South Wales was able to show that high sensitization to house dust mites in coastal regions as well as high sensitization to alternaria in other regions correlated significantly with higher asthma prevalence compared with regions where sensitization levels are lower (Peat et al., 1995). Sensitization to house dust mite seems to be one of the most common sensitizations linked to asthma over the world, as for example also shown in children living in Florida, where 89.6 % of the asthmatic children showed a positive RAST result to Dermatophagoides pteronyssinus (Nelson et al., 1996). A similar prevalence was seen in Chinese asthmatic children by skin prick testing. 81.9 % showed a positive test to house dust mite (Leung et al., 2001). And also in Zimbabwe sensitization in RAST test to dust mites was the most common sensitization in atopic children (Kambarami et al., 1999).

Astonishingly another study in children living in high altitude (7200 feet) "in a mite-free environment with low levels of outdoor air pollution" saw a comparably high asthma prevalence rate of 6.3 % and high total IgE levels in asthmatic children (Sporik et al. 1995). The explanation of this finding was that 77 % of the studied households had a pet (cat or dog) and the predominant sensitization in children therefore was a sensitization to cat. That sensitization to cat allergen generally is a risk for childhood asthma was confirmed in a prospective birth cohort study in Germany (MAS 90), the German Multicenter Allergy Study (Lau et al., 2005).

In summary, indoor allergen sensitization seems to be closer connected to asthma than outdoor allergen sensitization. This was confirmed for two different ethnic groups living in the same environment of New York City (Rastogi et al. 2006). Similar environment led in both groups to similar sensitization and only indoor allergen sensitization was significantly associated not only with asthma prevalence but also with its severity. In contrary, different environmental circumstances lead not only to different sensitization prevalences and patterns, but also to different association levels with and different attributable fractions of asthma and other atopic diseases (Rona et al. 2008).

When the close correlation between childhood asthma and sensitization had become known, also efforts had been made to define correlations between adult onset asthma and sensitization. The result of a case-control study in Finland including only cases of adult onset asthma in patients 21 - 63 years of age was that specific "IgE antibodies to house dust mite and storage mite were significantly related to an incresased risk of asthma." The same correlation was found with IgE antibodies to aspergillus fumigatus and cladosporium herbarum (Jaakkola et al., 2006).

Nevertheless, one has to keep in mind sensitization being only one of several possible triggers for allergic asthma and these triggers probably showing dependencies among each other. An example was shown in children at high atopic risk, where the prevalence of asthma was higher for those children having suffered more from severe viral lower respiratory tract infections but only when they had also an early sensitization at the age 2 years or lower (Kusel et al., 2007).

From another perspective, specific sensitization only enhanced the risk of being asthmatic significantly for children with "a positive parental history of asthma or atopy" (Illi et al., 2001).

Also – as another example - the socioeconomic status influences sensitization in general, indoor sensitization and together with the latter the risk of asthma in the direction that sensitization is increased with lower socioeconomic status (Lewis et al., 2001). May anyone think sensitization against cockroach and animal to be understandable by social differences in residency environment and pet ownership, the significant increase in ragweed sensitization also will stay unexplainable by such obvious status dependant circumstances.

On the other hand, as we know as another result of the ISAAC study, the correlation between asthma and sensitization seems to be closer in developed countries with higher income (Weinmayr, 2006 2007).
Looking somewhat deeper into the description of sensitization in asthmatic patients, in asthmatic children prevalence rates of sensitization to cat were 40 %, to dog 34 %, to horse 28 %, to birch 23 % and to timothy 16 % and somewhat different to sensitization shown in other atopic diseases like rhinitis or eczema (Rönmark et al., 2003).
An association between different mono-sensitizations against pollen was seen in Sweden in a birth-cohort study with more than 2500 children, where especially birch pollen sensitization was closely correlated to allergic symptoms (Ghunaim et al., 2006).
Already several years ago the knowledge of correlations between sensitization and asthma had led to establishing a new asthma classification based on specific IgE antibodies among other parameters (Kumura 1994). In our time quite ambitious efforts have been made to redefine atopic phenotype and correlate the resultant patterns of sensitization with asthma and asthma outcome parameters even in a population-based birth cohort study (Simpson et al. 2010).

3. Asthma and sensitization pattern in a population-based study in German children and adolescents

Having performed the first population-based interview and examination survey in children and adolescents in Germany, we will seize the opportunity to look for correlations between sensitization and asthma in this population. As we will continue the study, later on we will have the chance to look for changes of sensitization in individuals over time and asthma development also.
For now we want to learn something about sensitization prevalence in German children and adolescents - as well in those with asthma as in nonasthmatic children - RAST classes of indentified sensitizations, demographically based differences in sensitizations and correlations of specific sensitizations with asthma.

3.1 The German health interview and examination survey for children and adolescents (KiGGS)

A total of 17641 children and adolescents from birth up to 17 years of age have been included in this survey, being studied in 167 study points throughout Germany between May 2003 and May 2006. The survey was composed of questionnaires filled in by the parents and parallel by children aged 11 years or older, a computer assisted personal interview (CAPI) performed by study physicians and physical examination and (laboratory) test parts.
A publication describing the study design and methods, patient enrollment and randomisation, response and representativeness can be found in BMC Public Health (Kurth et al., 2008). The response rate was 66.6 % and a non-response analysis based on "key socio-demographic and health-related characteristics for children and parents" was performed for about two thirds of the non-responders. The non-response analysis did not provide an indication of relevant differences in four health related variables compared to responders. Therefore the survey will provide us with as far as possible representative information about the health status of German children and adolescents.

3.2 Methods of assessing asthma and defining specific sensitization in KiGGS

During a Computer-assisted Personal Interview (CAPI) conducted by the studyteam physician parents had been asked wether their children ever had had a positive physicians diagnosis of asthma. Though the study results presented with some evidence that possibly more children suffered from asthma as being told to the parents - seen for example analysing the drug anamnesis regarding children having had specific asthma medication on prescription base without their parents having reported a physicians diagnosis of asthma as allready publicized (Langen & Knopf, 2007) - we think the accuracy of reported physicians diagnosis to be more reliable. So we will operate in this analysis with a positive answer to the question of physician diagnosed asthma as the decisive indicator for grouping participants in asthmatic and nonasthmatic children and adolescents.

In laboratory blood tests only the blood of children more than 2 years old and adolescents, had been tested for specific IgE-antibodies to 20 common allergens including 11 frequent inhalative indoor and outdoor allergens. The test system used was the ImmunoCAP® test of Phadia. The allergens involved included food allergens and the following groups and substances of inhalative allergens:

House dust mites:	Dermatophagoides pteronyssinus and dermatophagoides farinae
Animal epithelia:	Cat, horse and dog
Pollen:	Birch, mugwort, rye and timothy grass
Mould fungi:	Cladosporium herbarum and aspergillus fumigatus

In summary we will be able to present the data of 12911 children and adolescents from 3 years to 17 years of age having had a blood test for specific IgE antibodies and having their parents had answered the CAPI.

3.3 Statistical analysis of the KiGGS data

For this analysis SPSS (Statistical Package of the Social Sciences) Version 17 was used. The data have been weighted in the intention to adjust them for deviations between the sample group and German population statistics especially regarding "age structure and disproportionately higher sample size in Eastern vs. Western Germany" (Kurth, 2008). All analyses are based on "complex samples" procedures, so that estimated variations of the results became more realistic having in mind the complex sampling procedure of the study as in detail described in the above mentioned article.

3.4 Results and interpretation

In the entire study population, 4.7 % of the participants had a positive lifetime prevalence of asthma. At least one sensitization was identified in 40.8 % of the children aged 3 years or older and the adolescents.

As asthma and sensitization prevalence rise with increasing age, asthma prevalence in our population aged 3 years and older is measurably higher as in the entire population from birth to age 17. Also the prevalence in sensitization shows differences to the complete study population while we only analyzed the above described subgroup of children and adolescents.

3.4.1 Demographic data

In Table 1 we show demographic characteristics for asthmatic and nonasthmatic participants as well as for those without sensitization, being monosensitized or polysensitized. Statistically significant differences are shown in bold numbers.

	Asthmatic	Non-asthmatic	Not sensitized	Mono-sensitized	Polysensitized
Overall n=12911	5.5 % (5.0-6.0 %)	94.5 % (94.0-95.0 %)	62.8 % (61.6-64.0 %)	4.8 % (4.4-5.2 %)	32.4 % (31.3-33.6 %)
Age group					
3-6 years n=2936	**2.8** % (2.2-3.6 %)	97.2 % (96.4-97.8 %)	**77.9** % (76.1-79.6 %)	**3.6** % (2.9-4.5 %)	**18.5** % (16.8-20.3 %)
7-10 years n=3649	**4.7** % (4.0-5.6 %)	95.3 % (94.4-96.0 %)	**64.8** % (62.9-66.7 %)	5.0 % (4.3-5.9 %)	**30.2** % (28.5-32.0 %)
11-13 years n=2835	**7.1** % (6.0-8.3%)	92.9 % (92.1-94.1 %)	**57.5** % (54.8-60.2 %)	4.8 % (3.9-5.8 %)	**37.7** % (35.1-40.3 %)
14-17 years n=3468	6.8 % (5.9-7.9 %)	93.2 % (92.1-94.1%)	54.9 % (53.2-56.7 %)	**5.3** % (4.6-6.2 %)	39.8 % (38.0-41.6 %)
Sex					
Male n=6609	**6.3** % (5.7-6.9 %)	93.7 % (93.1-94.3%)	**58.5** % (57.0-60.0 %)	**4.0** % (3.6-4.6 %)	**37.5** % (36.1-38.9 %)
Female n=6279	**4.7** % (4.1-5.3 %)	95.3 % (94.7-95.9 %)	**67.4** % (66.0-68.8 %)	**5.5** % (4.9-6.2 %)	**27.0** % (25.7-28.5 %)
Parental allergy					
Yes n=5336	**7.2** % (6.5-7.9 %)	92.8 % (92.1-93.5%)	**55.3** % (53.7-56.9 %)	4.8 % (4.2-5.4 %)	**39.9** % (38.3-41.5 %)
No n=6977	**4.1** % (3.6-4.7 %)	95.9 % (95.3-96.4 %)	**68.7** % (67.2-70.2 %)	4.7 % (4.2-5.3 %)	**26.6** % (25.2-28.1 %)
Not known n=269	6.4 % (3.4-11.6 %)	93.6 % (88.4-96.6 %)	62.4 % (55.7-68.7 %)	7.0 % (4.3-11.1 %)	30.6 % (24.7-34.2 %)
Region					
North n=3276	6.2 % (5.3-7.4 %)	93.8 % (92.6-94.7 %)	**64.7** % (62.6-66.9 %)	5.4 % (4.7-6.2 %)	**29.8** % (27.8-32.0 %)
Middle n=5684	5.5 % (4.9-6.2 %)	94.5 % (93.8-95.1 %)	64.1 % (62.5-65.6 %)	4.3 % (3.7-5.0 %)	31.6 % (30.1-33.1 %)
South n=3920	5.0 % (4.3-5.9 %)	95.0 % (94.1-95.7 %)	**60.3** % (58.1-62.5 %)	4.8 % (4.2-5.4 %)	**34.9** % (32.8-37.0 %)
Migration status					
Yes n=1901	5.1 % (4.3-6.1 %)	94.9 % (93.9-95.7 %)	**65.8** % (63.6-67.9 %)	5.4 % (4.3-6.7 %)	**28.8** % (26.8-31.0%)
No n=10926	5.6 % (5.1-6.1 %)	94.4 % (93.9-94.9 %)	**62.2** % (60.9-63.5 %)	4.6 % (4.2-5.1 %)	**33.2** % (31.9-34.5 %)
Older siblings					
No n=3820	5.9 % (5.1-6.8 %)	94.1 % (93.2-94.9 %)	**60.9** % (58.8-62.9 %)	4.8 % (4.1-5.5 %)	**34.4** % (32.4-46.4 %)
One n=4395	5.3 % (4.6-6.1 %)	94.7 % (93.9-95.4 %)	63.7 % (61.8-65.5 %)	4.8 % (4.2-5.6 %)	31.5 % (29.8-33.3 %)
2 or more n=1461	4.2 % (3.2-5.5 %)	95.8 % (94.5-96.8 %)	**66.8** % (63.7-69.7 %)	3.8 % (2.9-5.0 %)	**29.4** % (26.6-32.4 %)

Table 1. Demographic characteristics of study population

We also analysed the population for differences regarding eastern or western region of Germany, rural or urban region, prematurity or underweight at birth, pets in household, preschool children's care outside the family (kindergarten etc.), sleeping behaviour, breast feeding and smoking behaviour and social status of the family. We have not been able to detect any additional statistically significant differences neither concerning asthma nor sensitization prevalence.

What we can clearly perceive is that sensitizations and asthma show a parallel continued rise from 3 years of age up to the age group of 11 - 13 years. Especially the polysensitizations make a major contribution to the increase in sensitization prevalence, whereas the rise in monosensitizations is significant between the agegroup of 3 - 6 and the agegroup of 14 - 17 years but numerically quite small.

Male children and adolescents suffer more often from asthma and sensitizations, both mono- and polysensitizations, than female. Such relationship between asthma and sex in children is described by the GINA (Global Initiative for Asthma) Report (GINA, 2009), while the causes for this difference are pictured as unknown. Nevertheless, the lung size, being smaller in male children and larger in male adults is mentioned as a possible reason for the different asthma prevalence. The importance of this argument may be supported by our data, as sensitizations to inhalative allergens remain more common in male adults than in female while asthma prevalence is decreasing. The fact that boys are more often sensitized than girls has been described in the literature - as mentioned in the review above - but the reasons for this gender based difference remain unclear.

Very well known in contrary is that children of atopic parents tend to more sensitizations and atopic diseases than those of healthy parents as is supported by our data.

Also living in the northern or southern part of Germany produces a significant difference regarding sensitizations. Significantly more study participants living in southern Germany suffer from polysensitizations. This finding may be caused by climatic differences as Germany borders in the North on the North and the Baltic Sea or by differences in the flora. Differences in asthma prevalence show descriptively the converse direction but did not reach significance.

Children belonging to a family with positive migration background show less polysensitizations than others, what may be explained by the known sensitization differences in differently developed countries with a more or less "westernized" lifestyle. Nevertheless, differences in asthma prevalence are barely detectable.

In the same way fitting into the so called hygiene hypothesis are the data showing children without older siblings suffering more from polysensitizations than children with two or more older siblings. This can be explained by the children with older siblings having had more contact with bacteria during early childhood leading in the maturing immune system to a decision more in favour of Th1 lymphocyte answer development which is needed for fighting infections than Th2 lymphocytes which contribute to allergic diseases. Nevertheless, the difference in asthma prevalence was not able to reach statistical significance although descriptively the correlation was similar.

3.4.2 Asthma and specific sensitizations to inhalative allergens

We have been able to scan the blood of nearly 13000 children and adolescents for specific IgE levels to certain common inhalative allergens. IgE is not detectable beneath a margin of 0.35 kU/l with the method used in this study and children not showing detectable IgE levels are defined as not sensitized as it is common in sensitization analyses. Also common understanding is to value a result between 0.35 and 0.69 kU/l as marginally positive and all results 0.7 or higher as positive. A clear correlation between the level of sensitization and clinical severity of symptoms has not been described.

Table 2 presents the results for the IgE levels in nonasthmatic and asthmatic study participants. It clearly shows up that sensitization prevalence for each single inhalative allergen shows statistically significant differences between the two groups. For better readability, variation has not been presented in the table. Significantly different prevalence rates between asthmatic and nonasthmatic subjects are presented in bold letters.

Additionally detectable is the fact that with the exemption of house dust mites and rye all other allergens show significantly different prevalence also regarding the lowest class between 0.35 and 0.69 kU/l. Our interpretation is that the relevance of such "marginally" positive results may be higher than estimated up to now.

Though we already knew that sensitization does not have to present automatically with clinical symptoms it remains interesting that we found also subjects sensitized with IgE levels of the highest class of 100 kU/l and more without asthma symptoms.

Unit: kU/l Nonasthmatic Asthmatic children	Not detectable <0.35	Low 0.35-0.69	Medium 0.70-3.49	High 3.50-17.49	Very high 17.5-49.99	Very high 50.0-99.99	Very high >=100
Derm. pteronyssinus	**80.7 %** **44.0 %**	3.3 % 3.7 %	**5.2 %** **9.5 %**	**4.4 %** **11.8 %**	**3.8 %** **12.4 %**	**1.6 %** **10.9 %**	**1.0 %** **7.8 %**
Derm. farinae	**80.7 %** **45.8 %**	3.4 % 3.1 %	**5.1 %** **9.3 %**	**4.5 %** **11.5 %**	**3.9 %** **12.9 %**	**1.7 %** **11.7 %**	**0.7 %** **5.8 %**
Cat	**93.1 %** **67.0 %**	**1.8 %** **4.6 %**	**3.2 %** **13.2 %**	**1.5 %** **7.1 %**	**0.3 %** **5.6 %**	**0.1 %** **2.0 %**	**0.0 %** **0.6 %**
Horse	**96.7 %** **75.6 %**	**1.1 %** **4.7 %**	**1.6 %** **10.7 %**	**0.4 %** **6.4 %**	**0.1 %** **2.0 %**	0.0 % 0.3 %	0.0 % 0.3 %
Dog	**91.9 %** **58.9 %**	**3.4 %** **12.4 %**	**4.0 %** **18.4 %**	**0.6 %** **7.5 %**	**0.1 %** **1.5 %**	**0.0 %** **0.7 %**	**0.0 %** **0.6 %**
Birch	**87.1 %** **58.7 %**	**2.3 %** **4.8 %**	**4.6 %** **10.3 %**	**3.4 %** **12.6 %**	**1.6 %** **7.6 %**	**0.6 %** **3.2 %**	**0.5 %** **2.9 %**
Mugwort	**89.9 %** **70.4 %**	**3.3 %** **8.9 %**	**5.0 %** **11.7 %**	**1.5 %** **7.5 %**	**0.3 %** **1.5 %**	0.0 % 0.0 %	0.0 % 0.0 %
Rye	**80.1 %** **47.2 %**	3.4 % 5.4 %	**5.8 %** **15.6 %**	**4.7 %** **12.1 %**	**3.1 %** **11.0 %**	**1.8 %** **5.2 %**	**1.1 %** **3.3 %**
Timothy	**78.6 %** **43.7 %**	**3.4 %** **5.5 %**	**5.9 %** **13.5 %**	**5.0 %** **13.5 %**	**2.9 %** **10.5 %**	**2.0 %** **6.9 %**	**2.2 %** **6.6 %**
Cladosporium herbarum	**98.7 %** **89.8 %**	**0.5 %** **1.7 %**	**0.6 %** **4.7 %**	**0.1 %** **2.8 %**	**0.0 %** **0.7 %**	0.0 % 0.3 %	0.0 % 0.0 %
Aspergillus fumigatus	**98.3 %** **86.8 %**	**0.8 %** **3.7 %**	**0.8 %** **6.6 %**	**0.1 %** **2.2 %**	**0.0 %** **0.4 %**	0.0 % 0.3 %	0.0 % 0.0 %

Table 2. Specific IgE to several inhalative allergens in asthmatic and nonasthmatic subjects

Nevertheless, the most subjects showing very high IgE levels equal or higher than 50 kU/l also suffered from asthma. Nearly 20 % of the asthmatic children and adolescents showed sensitizations to house dust mite in these both classes.

3.4.3 Number of sensitizations and asthma

When we saw the clear correlation between sensitizations to each of the tested inhalative allergens and asthma, the question arose, whether the development of asthma may also show a correlation with the number of sensitizations persons have developed during their life.

Figure 1 presents the correlation between asthma and the number of sensitizations we found in our study. We see that there seems to be a quite clear exponential relationship between the mentioned circumstances.

Only 2.1 % of the study participants without any sensitization suffered from asthma whereas 49.8 % of the participants showing sensitizations to each of the tested 11 inhalative allergens also have had an asthma anamnesis.

For those children and adolescents suffering from asthma but not showing sensitization to any of the inhalative allergens we made an additional analyses with the intention to indentify possible sensitizations to food allergens (egg white, milk protein, rice flour, peanut, soybean, carrot, potato, wheat flour or green apple) but were not able to find any correlation. Only a few single cases showed sensitizations to egg, milk or peanut, all other test results where negative.

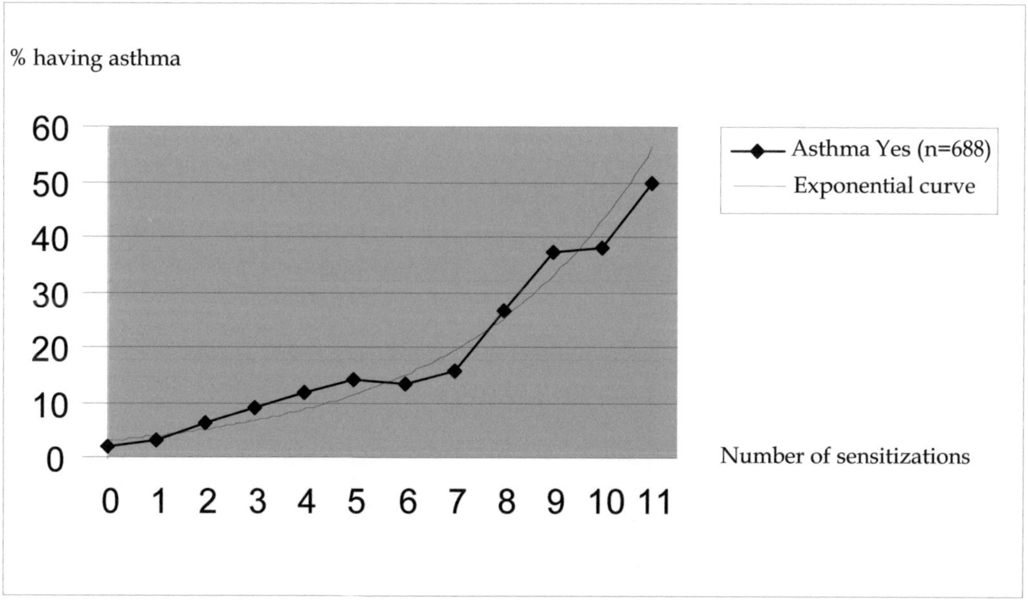

Fig. 1. Number of sensitizations to inhalative allergens and asthma

We also performed the same analyses for different age groups, sex, migration and social status as well as groups living in rural or urban regions of Germany. In each case we have been able to repeatedly find the same relationship - an exponentially sloping curve showing a positive correlation between the number of sensitizations and asthma. Additionally those curves are located very closely together so that the shown relationship seems to be somewhat like a constitutional or natural correlation.

3.4.4 Course of sensitizations with increasing age

With increasing age the prevalence of sensitizations is rising as well in children with as in those without asthma but in the former the rise starts on much higher values.

Table 3 shows in bold numbers statistically significant increases (those will be marked in all other tables in the same manner) of specific sensitizations with age in comparison with the youngest group or the last group having displayed significant differences already. Variations are presented, those in asthmatic children being much wider than the others as this group is much smaller as that of nonasthmatic children.

The first fact to detect is that in each case with only one exemption sensitization prevalence in asthmatic participants is statistically significant higher than that in nonasthmatic participants. Only in the age group 3 - 6 years sensitization to cladosporium herbarum does not reach significance between those two groups and this circumstance is explainable by the comparatively low prevalence of such sensitization in this age group.

Unit: kU/l Nonasthmatic Asthmatic children	3-6 years n=2936	7-10 years n=3649	11-13 years n=2835	14-17 years n=3468
Derm. pteronyssinus	**10.7** % (9.3-12.2) **32.3** % (22.5-44.2)	**15.8** % (14.4-17.4) 46.7 % (38.1-55.3)	**22.3** % (20.3-24.5) **59.0** % (50.2-67.3)	26.2 % (24.4-28.0) 65.4 % (58.5-71.7)
Derm. farinae	**10.7** % (9.4-12.1) **30.7** % (21.0-42.3)	**16.7** % (15.2-18.3) 45.5 % (37.1-54.1)	**21.8** % (19.8-23.9) **56.3** % (47.7-64.6)	25.5 % (23.8-27.3) 64.0 % (56.8-70.5)
Cat	**3.1** % (2.5-3.8) **16.9** % (9.6-28.1)	**6.7** % (5.8-7.6) 30.7 % (24.0-38.2)	7.3 % (6.0-8.8) **38.8** % (31.4-46.7)	**9.4** % (8.4-10.5) 34.6 % (28.0-41.9)
Horse	**1.4** % (1.0-1.9) 15.4 % (8.5-26.1)	**3.1** % (2.5-3.8) 20.8 % (14.4-29.0)	4.1 % (3.1-5.4) 24.4 % (18.1-32.0)	4.3 % (3.7-5.1) 28.9 % (22.9-35.7)
Dog	**3.1** % (2.5-3.9) **23.5** % (15.2-34.6)	**7.5** % (6.6-8.6) 31.1 % (23.4-40.0)	9.2 % (7.8-10.8) **45.4** % (37.4-53.6)	**11.3** %(10.2-12.4) 48.4 % (41.1-55.7)
Birch	**6.2** % (5.3-7.2) **21.1** % (12.8-32.7)	**12.3** % (11.1-13.6) 37.4 % (30.2-45.2)	15.2 % (13.2-17.4) **45.7** % (37.8-53.9)	**16.5** % (14.9-18.1) 46.0 % (39.2-52.9)
Mugwort	**3.4** % (2.7-4.3) **12.6** % (6.4-23.4)	**10.7** % (9.5-12.1) 21.2 % (15.2-28.7)	11.7 % (10.1-13.5) **32.7** % (25.8-40.4)	13.1 % (11.7-14.7) 36.6 % (30.5-43.1)
Rye	**9.5** % (8.2-11.0) **34.1** % (23.5-46.7)	**20.0** % (18.4-21.7) 40.4 % (33.0-48.3)	**24.2** % (21.8-26.8) **56.5** % (47.7-64.9)	24.0 % (22.1-26.1) 62.2 % (54.5-69.3)
Timothy	**11.3** % (9.9-12.9) **42.5** % (30.3-55.6)	**21.6** % (19.9-23.3) 42.5 % (34.6-50.8)	25.1 % (22.6-27.1) 60.2 % (51.8-68.0)	**25.5** % (23.7-27.6) **65.0** % (57.4-72.0)
Cladosporium herbarum	**0.7** % (0.4-1.1) **2.4** % (0.7-7.8)	1.3 % (1.0-1.8) 6.3 % (3.3-12.0)	1.2 % (0.8-1.7) 11.9 % (7.7-18.0)	**1.8** % (1.3-2.4) **13.1** % (9.1-18.7)
Aspergillus fumigatus	**0.8** % (0.6-1.3) 6.3 % (2.5-15.1)	1.6 % (1.2-2.1) 9.0 % (5.3-14.9)	**1.8** % (1.4-2.4) 17.3 % (12.0-24.3)	2.4 % (1.9-3.1) 14.6 % (10.5-20.0)

Table 3. Percentage of nonasthmatic and asthmatic participants of different age being specifically sensitized

Another fact we have to notice is the high prevalence of sensitizations in asthmatic children of very young age (3 - 6 years) to dermatophagoides pteronyssinus, dermatophagoides farinae, rye and timothy. The prevalence lies between more than 30 up to nearly 43 %. For the same allergens we see in the highest age group nearly two thirds of the asthmatic adolescents being sensitized. These findings support what was referred in the literature review - the most important role of house dust mite sensitization in asthma development.

A much minor role play sensitizations to moulds as shown in sensitizations to cladosporium herbarum and aspergillus fumigatus. The prevalence of sensitizations to pets and the not already mentioned pollen varies in between those described groups.

Sensitization rates in asthmatic children and adolescents rise significantly over time for each allergen with two exemptions: sensitizations to horse epithelia do not reach statistical significance although descriptively the rise seems quite clear, probably explained by the high variation of these results and the same holds true for sensitizations to aspergillus fumigatus where numbers may have become too small for showing significance in this somewhat less steep increase of sensitizations over time.

In nonasthmatic children as well as in asthmatic children we find the highest prevalence rate of sensitizations in the highest age group to the same allergens, both house dust mites, rye and timothy. So, from this point of view the kind of sensitization does not seem to influence the development of asthma in contrary to the number of sensitizations and - to some extent - the specific IgE level.

In the group of nonasthmatic children, increase over time did reach statistical significance for each tested inhalative allergen.

3.4.5 Demographic differences in sensitizations to inhalative allergens

Having learned boys to suffer more often from asthma as girls (in our study 5.5 % of the male children and adolescents have ever had a physician diagnosed asthma versus 3.9 of the female) and to be more often sensitized, as shown in table 1, we wanted to know whether sensitizations in boys and girls occur to different allergens.

The results are shown in table 4. All statistically significant differences between boys and girls did show up only in the group of nonasthmatic children and adolescents. Here we see differences in favour for the girls being less often sensitized for both house dust mites, cat and dog (but not horse), and all tested pollen but not to moulds.

Regarding the tested moulds, even here boys are descriptively more often sensitized but numbers all together are very small. Looking to the result for sensitization to horse epithelia girls are nearly as often sensitized as boys. This does not seem to be remarkable as horse riding in Germany has to be reckoned as a typical girl's hobby and only a small number of boys have horse contacts. So the greater sensitivity of boys for developing sensitizations seems to be counteracted by girls dealing more often with horses.

Again, the group of asthmatic children is clearly too small for differences in sensitizations between boys and girls becoming significant. With the exemption of horse epithelia sensitization, to all other allergens boys are descriptively more often sensitized than girls.

As mentioned above, with the development of polysensitization, the risk for asthma is increasing exponentially for boys and girls as well. Unfortunately not identifiable in the data is a sensitization pattern difference between boys and girls which could have explained the higher asthma prevalence in boys.

Unit: kU/l Nonasthmatic Asthmatic children	boys n=6609	girls n=6279
Derm. pteronyssinus	**22.3** % (21.1-23.6) 59.5 % (54.3-64.5)	**16.3** % (15.1-17.5) 51.1 % (44.5-57.6)
Derm. farinae	**22.5** % (21.3-23.7) 57.7 % (52.6-62.7)	**15.9** % (14.8-17.1) 49.3 % (42.6-55.9)
Cat	**8.3** % (7.5-9.1) 33.7 % (28.9-38.9)	**5.5** % (4.8-6.2) 32.0 % (26.6-37.9)
Horse	3.5 % (3.1-4.1) 24.0 % (19.7-29.1)	3.1 % (2.6-3.7) 24.9 % (20.0-30.5)
Dog	**9.8** % (8.9-10.7) 43.8 % (38.7-49.0)	**6.4** % (5.7-7.2) 37.2 % (31.7-43.1)
Birch	**15.0** % (13.8-16.3) 45.9 % (40.8-51.0)	**10.7** % (9.7-11.9) 34.9 % (29.4-40.9)
Mugwort	**11.9** % (10.7-13.6) 31.8 % (27.4-36.4)	**8.2** % (7.4-9.2) 26.4 % (21.2-32.4)
Rye	**23.7** % (22.2-25.4) 55.1 % (49.9-60.2)	**15.9** % (14.6-17.3) 49.6 % (42.9-56.3)
Timothy	**25.2** % (23.7-26.8) 60.0 % (54.7-65.1)	**17.4** % (16.0-18.8) 51.2 % (44.5-57.8)
Cladosporium herbarum	1.6 % (1.3-2.0) 11.3 % (8.1-15.5)	1.0 % (0.7-1.3) 8.5 % (5.4-13.3)
Aspergillus fumigatus	2.4 % (2.0-3.0) 15.4 % (11.8-19.9)	1.0 % (0.8-1.4) 10.2 % (6.7-15.1)

Table 4. Percentage of participants sensitized to inhalative allergens by sex

Regarding the social status of the families our participants live with, not many significant differences in sensitization status can be observed, as shown in table 5.

In nonasthmatic children with medium social status sensitizations to both house dust mites are significantly more common than in those with low social status. This may possibly be explainable by hygiene measures as vacuum cleaning, which may be – as other hygiene measures – more often practised in families with higher social status. In the literature, it has been shown that vacuum cleaning can enhance air levels of specific house dust allergens (Kalra et al., 1990, online 2003). In contrary, in asthmatic children that difference should not be able to play a major role as parents of those children should have been taught to use vacuum cleaners with small particle filters and especially parents with high social status are thought to follow those instructions closely.

Nonasthmatic children with medium social status are more often sensitized to horse epithelia than both, children with lower as well as those with higher social status, significantly more often compared to the children living in families with high social status. The reason of this difference seems to remain unclear. Horse riding may be a somewhat more expensive hobby so that children with low social status may not have as often contact to horses as other children, but this does not explain why children with high social status show significantly less often sensitizations to horse epithelia then those with medium social status.

Unit: kU/l Nonasthmatic Asthmatic children	Low social status n=3373	Medium social status n=5957	High social status n=3241
Dermatophagoides pteronyssinus	**17.5 %** (15.9-19.2) 54.3 % (46.9-61.6)	**20.5 %** (19.4-21.8) 55.9 % (49.6-62.0)	19.0 % (17.3-20.9) 57.7 % (49.6-65.3)
Dermatophagoides farinae	**16.8 %** (15.3-18.4) 51.4 % (43.5-59.2)	**20.2 %** (19.0-21.5) 53.8 % (47.7-59.8)	20.0 % (18.2-21.9) 57.7 % (49.5-65.5)
Cat	6.3 % (5.3-7.4) 25.9 % (20.1-32.8)	7.6 % (6.9-8.4) 36.0 % (30.2-42.3)	6.6 % (5.6-7.6) 34.7 % (28.2-41.9)
Horse	2.8 % (2.2-3.5) 19.5 % (14.3-26.0)	**4.1 %** (3.5-4.8) 25.6 % (20.4-31.7)	**2.6 %** (2.0-3.4) 28.7 % (22.2-36.3)
Dog	7.6 % (6.6-8.7) **35.4 %** (28.7-42.8)	9.0 % (8.1-9.9) 39.3 % (32.7-46.2)	7.3 % (6.3-8.4) **50.8 %** (43.8-57.7)
Birch	11.1 % (9.8-12.6) 31.7 % (24.7-39.6)	13.6 % (12.3-15.0) 44.2 % (38.1-50.4)	14.0 % (12.3-15.8) 47.4 % (38.8-56.1)
Mugwort	8.7 % (7.5-10.1) 25.0 % (18.6-32.7)	10.8 % (9.7-12.0) 29.8 % (24.9-35.3)	10.7 % (9.3-12.3) 34.4 % (27.1-42.4)
Rye	17.8 % (16.1-19.7) 46.2 % (37.8-54.9)	20.9 % (19.3-22.6) 55.4 % (49.2-61.5)	20.8 % (18.8-22.9) 56.4 % (48.4-64.2)
Timothy	19.6 % (17.8-21.5) 47.5 % (38.8-56.4)	22.3 % (20.7-24.1) 59.6 % (53.7-65.2)	22.0 % (20.1-24.2) 60.3 % (52.1-67.9)
Cladosporium herbarum	1.0 % (0.7-1.5) 14.1 % (9.3-20.9)	1.6 % (1.3-2.0) 8.3 % (5.2-12.9)	1.0 % (0.7-1.4) 8.9 % (5.4-14.2)
Aspergillus fumigatus	1.8 % (1.4-2.3) 12.9 % (8.3-19.5)	1.8 % (1.4-2.4) 13.8 % (9.9-19.0)	1.5 % (1.1-2.0) 12.5 % (8.4-18.2)

Table 5. Percentage of participants sensitized to inhalative allergens by social status

The only significant difference we can observe in asthmatic children is the very high degree of sensitizations to dog epithelia in children with high social status compared to those with low social status. Pet ownership and the development of asthma and other atopic diseases are very controversially discussed. Time point of pet contact, cat / dog ownership and other circumstances may be puzzle pieces of a picture not yet completely visible. Some studies seem to direct to early dog contacts being protective regarding a development of atopy (Gern et al., 2004). Having in mind, that dog ownership in Germany is more common in families with high social status (high income and house owner), as was shown in a situation bulletin to dog ownership in Germany by the German University of Göttingen (Ohr & Zeddies, 2006), we have to query a protective effect of dog ownership on asthma development. Cross-sectional studies showing a protective effect of dog ownership could be biased by atopic parents avoiding dog ownership leading to children more in danger of atopy development more often growing up in a household without dogs.

Descriptively but not statistically significant for all tested pollen sensitizations numbers rise from low over medium to high social status, what, if confirmed by other studies, could be explained by different free time behaviour. Children with lower social status are known to spend more time indoor than others, as confirmed by other analyses of the KiGGS study (Robert Koch Institut, 2008).

Independent of social status, in all three groups, again, number of asthma cases rises with rising number of sensitizations in an exponential manner.

Looking for children with or without migration background (table 6), we can observe more significant differences in sensitizations than in the above mentioned groups with different social status but only in nonasthmatic children.
To cat and horse but not dog children without migration background show more sensitizations. Unfortunately, we did not find data showing pet ownership behaviour in people living in Germany with migration background. Therefore we can not discuss pet ownership in relation to sensitization status. Sensitizations to horse epithelia nevertheless could be higher in children without migration background more due to income differences than cultural disparity.
Children without migration background are more often sensitized to all tested pollen than the other group of children. As it was previously shown in the KiGGS data, children with migration background spend much more time with indoor activities than children without such a background. Sensitization to pollen may be a consequence of outdoor activities.
No differences were seen regarding house dust mite and mould allergies. In children with migration background as in all other groups asthma prevalence rises with rising number of sensitizations.

Unit: kU/l Nonasthmatic Asthmatic children	With Migration background n=1906	Without Migration background n=10928
Dermatophagoides pteronyssinus	19,1 % (17.2-21.0) 67,2 % (56.6-76.2)	19,4 % (18.5-20.4) 54,0 % (49.3-58.6)
Dermatophagoides farinae	17,9 % (16.0-20.0) 64,7 % (54.5-73.6)	19,5 % (18.6-20.5) 52,4 % (47.8-56.9)
Cat	**5,0 %** (4.0-6.3) 30,6 % (22.0-40.8)	**7,3 %** (6.7-7.9) 33,5 % (29.6-37.6)
Horse	**2,0 %** (1.4-2.7) 16,2 % (9.9-25.0)	**3,6 %** (3.2-4.1) 26,0 % (22.1-30.3)
Dog	6,4 % (5.1-8.0) 38,8 % (28.9-49.6)	8,5 % (7.8-9.1) 41,6 % (37.4-45.9)
Birch	**8,7 %** (7.2-10.3) 36,0 % (27.2-46.0)	**13,8 %** (12.7-14.9) 42,4 % (38.3-46.6)
Mugwort	**7,5 %** (6.0-9.2) 22,5 % (15.0-32.4)	**10,7 %** (9.8-11.7) 30,9 % (27.1-35.0)
Rye	**15,9 %** (13.9-18.0) 57,8 % (47.4-67.5)	**20,8 %** (19.4-22.2) 52,0 % (47.2-56.7)
Timothy	**17,9 %** (15.9-20.0) 60,2 % (50.6-69.2)	**22,1 %** (20.8-23.5) 55,7 % (50.7-60.5)
Cladosporium herbarum	1,0 % (0.6-1.7) 7,3 % (2.9-17.3)	1,3 % (1.1-1.6) 10,7 % (8.1-14.0)
Aspergillus fumigatus	1,9 % (1.3-2.7) 13,6 % (6.9-24.9)	1,7 % (1.4-2.1) 13,2 % (10.4-16.4)

Table 6. Percentage of participants sensitized to inhalative allergens by migration status

Additionally we searched for differences in sensitizations between children living in more rural or urban regions of Germany. We have been able to identify only one single significant difference: in rural regions 12.7 % of the children without asthma where sensitized to mugwort, in small towns 10.4 % in medium towns 9.6 % and in large cities 8.5 %. The difference between the smallest and the biggest region class reaches significance. As, according to the hygiene hypothesis, sensitization occurs more easy in urban regions, these data in our view back up the hypothesis of outdoor activities leading to more sensitizations to outdoor allergens - independent of residence.
Descriptively, children with asthma show the same slope in sensitization prevalence to mugwort as children without asthma. Again, children in all regions show the above described exponential coherency between asthma and number of sensitizations.

3.4.6 Sensitization patterns in asthmatic children

In the intention to look for patterns of sensitizations we grouped sensitizations to house dust mites, animals, pollen and moulds respectively. In table 7 we demonstrate groups of children showing sensitizations to at least one allergen of one of the mentioned groups alone or to at least one allergen of the mentioned group and any other allergens and the prevalence of asthma in those groups compared to the overall prevalence.
If sensitizations to allergens of only one of the four groups show up, asthma prevalence is not enhanced with the exemption of sensitizations to animals. These more than double the asthma prevalence. In the underneath mentioned groups with combined sensitizations, asthma prevalence is enhanced in each group, what may result from the above described effect of multiple sensitizations exponentially leading to an increase of asthma.

Sensitization type	Asthma prevalence (%) n=690, 5.5 % (5.0-6.0)
only to house dust mites	5.9 % (4.5-7.7)
only to animals	**12.5 %** (7.7-19.8)
only to pollen	4.5 % (3.4-5.9)
only to moulds	5.4 % (0.7-30.4)
to house dust mites and other allergen(s)	**13.6 %** (12.1-15.3)
to animals and other allergen(s)	**19.8 %** (17.7-22.2)
to pollen and other allergen(s)	**12.7 %** (11.4-14.1)
to moulds an other allergen(s)	**27,2 %** (22.3-32.8)

Table 7. Percentage of sensitization types having asthma

Nevertheless, noticeably asthma prevalence is much higher in children with animal epithelia and other sensitizations as with house dust mite or pollen and other sensitizations and highest in the group of children and adolescents with mould and other sensitizations. So, in monosensitized children, sensitization to animals plays the major role and in polysensitizations animals and even more moulds.
After these insights we wanted to know exactly the sequence of mono- and polysensitizations regarding asthma prevalence and present the data in figure 2.

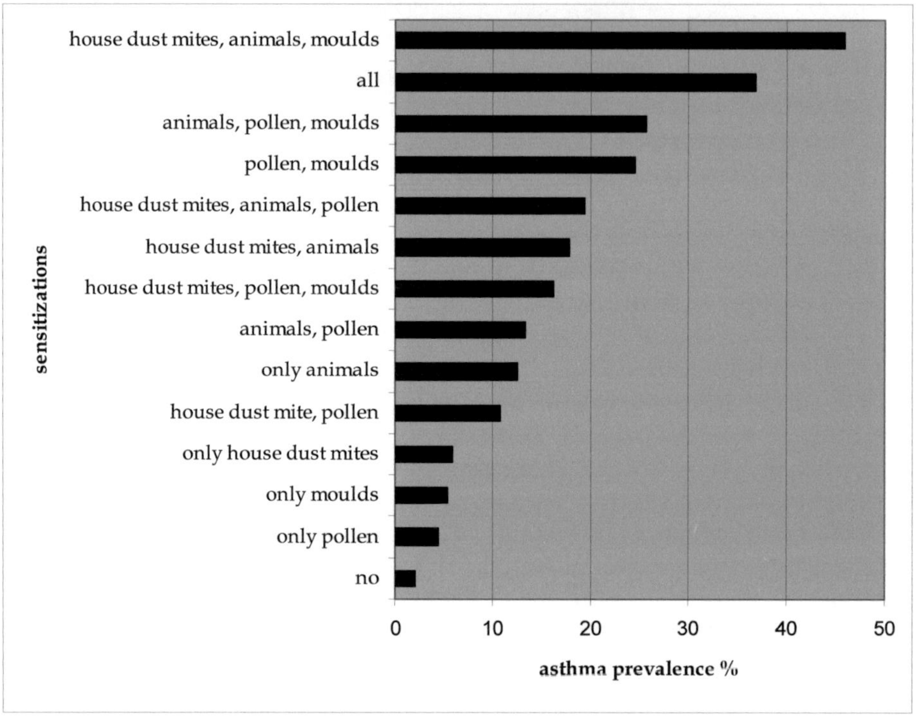

Fig. 2. Sensitization pattern and asthma prevalence

Combinations we did not find were that of animal and mould sensitizations and house dust mite and mould sensitizations.

Again, we have to keep in mind that increasing number of sensitizations lead to exponentially increasing asthma prevalence so that the shown figure must be strained by that effect. But - as an example - the combination of sensitizations to pollen and moulds seems to result in much higher asthma prevalence than the combination of sensitizations to pollen and animal epithelia, whereas the addition of a sensitization to animals to pollen and mould sensitizations does nearly not further enhance asthma prevalence.

Having a look into these data from another perspective we find that nearly a quarter of our asthmatic children and adolescents did not show any sensitization to the tested inhalative allergens (23.7 %). Never or infrequently (< 5 %) seen in the asthmatic children were sensitizations to mould only, pollen and mould, animals only, animals and mould, animals, pollen and mould, house dust mite and mould, house dust mite, pollen and mould, mould and animals as well as house dust mite, animals and mould. More frequently (5 - 10 %) we saw sensitizations to pollen only, animals and pollen and house dust mite only. Sensitizations to at least one allergen of each group were more frequent with 10.4 % of the asthmatic children concerned, sensitizations to house dust mite and pollen occurred in 10.9 % of the asthma cases and most frequent were sensitizations to house dust mites, pollen and animals in 22 % of asthmatic children.

In a cross-sectional study we are not able to detect the time sequence of acquired sensitizations. Alternatively we looked for dual combinations of sensitizations. Taking the assumption that sensitizations are livelong conditions, a dual combination could indirectly light the way of the beginning of multisensitizations and may show us, how sensitizations usually combine or start to build cluster.

In our data we found 1420 nonasthmatic and 86 asthmatic children with exactly two sensitizations (not grouped) as shown in figures 3 and 4 in absolute numbers.

Non-asthmatic	DermPt	DermFA	Cat	Horse	Dog	Birch	Mug-wort	Rye	Timothy	Clado	Asperg
DermPt											
DermFa	810										
Cat	4	2									
Horse	3		6								
Dog	1	3	24	2							
Birch	5	1	5		5						
Mugwort	3	4	1	1	2	10					
Rye	1	1				4	1				
Timothy	2	5	3	1	2	11	6	474			
Clado		1				1	1				
Asperg		4			1		1	1		7	
n=1420	829	21	39	4	10	26	9	475	0	7	

Fig. 3. Combinations of exactly two sensitizations in nonasthmatic children

Asthmatic	DermPt	DermFA	Cat	Horse	Dog	Birch	Mug-wort	Rye	Timothy	Clado	Asperg
DermPt											
DermFa	53										
Cat											
Horse			1								
Dog			3	1							
Birch											
Mugwort						1					
Rye											
Timothy			1			3		21			
Clado											
Asperg								1		1	
n=86	53	0	5	1	0	4	0	22	0	1	

Fig. 4. Combinations of exactly two sensitizations in asthmatic children

In the group of the nonasthmatic children we can observe that combinations of the two house dust mites are very common and also the combination between rye and timothy, two kinds of weed, so that these combinations are likely produced by cross reactivity. The same applies to the rarer combination of cat and dog sensitizations. The pattern in asthmatic

children is exactly the same, only the numbers are too small to show a peak at cat and dog sensitizations.
As a last step we then looked into the data of exactly two sensitizations in the above described sensitization groups and the results are shown in figure 5.

Non-asthmatic	House dust mite	Animals	Pollen	Moulds	Asthmatic	House dust mite	Animals	Pollen	Moulds
House dust mite					House dust mite				
Animals	125 (11.6 %)				Animals	23 (16.3 %)			
Pollen	607 (56.4 %)	292 (27.1 %)			Pollen	66 (46.8 %)	45 (31.9 %)		
Moulds	19 (1.8 %)	2 (0.2 %)	32 (3.0 %)		Moulds	0	0	7 (5.0 %)	
n=1077					N=141				

Fig. 5. Combinations of exactly two group sensitizations in children and adolescents

Again, it becomes clearly visible, that sensitization patterns of dual group sensitizations in our study do not differ between asthmatic and nonasthmatic children. The number of sensitizations influences asthma prevalence very much but patterns of sensitization to a much lesser degree - although the most differentiated analysis of the data shown in figure 2 seems to indicate some coherence between sensitization pattern and asthma.

3.5 Discussion and perspectives

We have been able to confirm data known from the literature on the grounds of a database as far as possible representative for German children and adolescents.
There is no mandatory coherency between sensitizations to inhalative allergens and asthma looking into individual developments. While in adults non allergic asthma forms concern a high percentage of asthmatic persons, in children it was thought that a broad majority suffers from allergic asthma. We identifyed 23.7 % of the asthmatic children not showing a sensitization to any of the tested inhalative allergens and additionally only a few of them showing sensitizations to food allergens. Though sensitizations to allergens not being included in our test are theoretically possible (included were the most common allergens being content of standard test series), possibly non allergic asthma forms in children may still be somewhat underestimated.
We also saw that sensitizations confirmed in the range of 0.35 - 0.69 kU/l and up to now regarded only as marginally positive are allready statistically significant more frequent in asthmatic children for all tested allergens with the exemption of the two house dust mites. Potentially such low sensitization results for animals, pollen and moulds should be noticed more attentively in clinical practise at least in children with a higher risk for the development of atopy.
In contrary, very high levels of sensitizations from 50.0 kU/l on have been seen nearly only in asthmatic children and only some single nonasthmatic individuals. Such high levels seem to be nearly an indicator for asthma development.
In contrast to the literatur identifying significantly less sensitizations in rural compared to urban regions, in Germany we were able to identify differences in sensitization patterns

between those regions but no overall differences regarding sensitization prevalence. Possibly life style differences between rural and urban regions in Germany are very low as we are a country with a pronounced "westernized lifestyle". A higher prevalence of sensitizations to pollen in rural regions already had been described for Italian children. We identified significantly higher sensitization prevalence in rural regions only for mugwort.

Sensitization prevalence being higher for boys compared to girls was already depicted. In connection with asthma it was an interesting fact that with increasing age sensitization prevalence in boys remains still higher than that in girls while asthma prevalence in boys declines. This could possibly back up the theory of lung size being an important factor in asthma prevalence differences in men and women being contrary to those in boys and girls.

Living in families with a lower social status was said to enhance the chance for having sensitizations. In our study, for most tested allergens the contrary held true. Especially regarding house dust mites, one of the most important factors for the development of asthma, higher social status was a risk factor for sensitizations. As far as causes are known, disproportionate hygiene behaviour could be one of the factors, what would fit in the widely respected hygiene hypothesis. We think that social habits like the use of desinfectants and odors in the househould and in public have to be questioned and that activities for prevention of allergies should be also directed to such behavioural factors.

The findings of polysensitization more often to cohere with asthma than monosensitization and the number of sensitizations to correlate with the risk for asthma were substanciated by our data. We have been able to show a clear exponential correlation between the number of sensitizations and asthma. This may be considered as an impulse to reconsider hyposensitization therapy in children at high risk for atopy. Maybe those children should undergo therapy the minute a second or third sensitization occurs regardless of symptoms of hayfever to prevent asthma development. As in the literature it was also shown that asthma remission relates inversely to sensitizations, this may make hyposensitization therapy also more fundamental in asthmatic children as it already is.

The special importance of house dust mite sensitizations was confirmed by our study, as was to be expected. Presumably based on cross reactivity sensitization to both tested house dust mites showed an overlap of nearly 100 % so that testing sensitizations to only one of the house dust mites would be in nearly every case able to confirm house dust mite allergy.

All in all we learned that the number of sensitizations was a much stronger element in asthma development than sensitization patterns. Nevertheless, it became clear that sensitizations to only animal epithelia more than double asthma prevalence compared to house dust mite, pollen or mould sensitizations only. In combined sensitization patterns containing animal sensitizations and by far more mould sensitizations are linked with enhanced asthma prevalence.

The KiGGS study will be carried forward and partly transformed into a longitudinal study. So we are looking forward to being better able to identify sensitizations or sensitization patterns really leading to asthma development. Additionally - as we will include in our study questions for hyposensitization therapy - we should be able to show whether early specific immunotherapy will be capable to prevent the development of polysensitizations and/or the development of asthma or influence asthma remission during adolescence.

Also the effectiveness of social measures such as proposed for example by the ABAP (an alliance for prevention of allergies initiated by the German Ministry for Health) could be followed up by this study.

4. References

Bjerg-Bäcklund, A., Bäcklund, AB., Perzanowski, MS., Platts-Mils, T., Sandström, T., Lundbäck, B., & Rönmark, E. (2006). Asthma during the primary school ages – prevalence, remission and the impact of allergic sensitization. *Allergy,* Vol. 61, No. 5, (May 2006), pp. 549-555, ISSN 0105-4538

Craig, TJ., King, TS., Lemanske, RF Jr., Wechsler, ME., Icitovic, N., Zimmerman, RR Jr., & Wasserman, S. (2008). Aeroallergen sensitization correlates with PC(20) and exhaled nitric oxide in subjects with mild-to-mederate asthma. *The Journal of allergy and clinical immunology,* Vol. 121, No. 3, (March 2008), pp. 671-677, ISSN 1097-6825

Craig, TJ. Aeroallergen sensitzization in asthma: prevalence and correlation with severity. *Allergy and asthma proceedings: the official journal of regional and state allergy societies,* Vol. 31, No. 2, (March 2010), pp. 96-102, ISSN 1539-6304

Crimi, P., Minale, P., Tazzer, C., Zanardi, S., & Ciprandi, G. (2001). Asthma and rhinitis in schoolchildren: the impact of allergic sensitization to aeroallergens. *Journal of Investigational Allergology and Clinical Immunology,* Vol. 11, No. 2, (2001), pp. 103-106, ISSN 1018-9068

Gern, JE., Reardon, C., Hoffjan, S., Nicolae, D., Li, Z., Roberg, KA., Neaville, WA., Carlson-Dakes, K,. Adler, K., Hamilton, R., Anderson, E., Gilbertson-White, S., Tisler, D., DaSilva, D., Anklam, K., Mikus, LD., Rosenthal, LA., Ober, C., Gangnon, R., & Lemanske, RF. Jr. (2004). Effects of dog ownership and genotype on immune development and atopy in infancy. *The Journal of allergy and clinical immunology,* Vol. 113, No. 2 (February 2004), pp. 307-314, ISSN 0091-6749

Ghunaim, N., Wickman, M., Almqvist, C., Söderström, L., Ahlstedt, S., & van Hage, M. (2006). Sensitization to different pollens and allergic disease in 4-year-old Swedish children. *Clinical and experimental allergy: journal of the British Society for Allergy and Clinical Immunology,* Vol. 36, No. 6, (June 2006), pp. 722-727, ISSN 09+54-7894

GINA (2009). GINA Report, Global Strategy for Asthma Management and Prevention, (2009), Available from http://www.ginasthma.com/Guidelineitem.asp??l1=2&l2=1&intId=1561

Hader, S., Kühr, J., Urbanek, R. (1990). Sensitization to 10 important air-borne allergens in school children. *Monatsschrift Kinderheilkunde: Organ der Deutschen Gesellschaft für Kinderheilkunde,* Vol. 138, No. 2, (February 1990), pp. 66-71, ISSN 0026-9298

Illi, S., von Mutius, E., Lau, S., Nickel, R., Niggemann, B., Sommerfeld, C., & Wahn, U. (2001). The pattern of atopic sensitization is associated with the development of asthma in childhood. *The Journal of allergy and clinical immunology,* Vol. 108, No. 5, (November 2001), pp. 709-714, ISSN 0091-6749

Jaakkola, MS., Ieromnimon, A., & Jaakkola, JJ. (2006). Are atopy and specific IgE to mites and moulds important for adult asthma? *The Journal of allergy and clinical immunology,* Vol. 117, No. 3, (March 2006), pp. 642-648, ISSN 0091-6749

Kalra, S., Owen, SJ., Hepworth J., & Woodcock, A. (1990, online 2003). Airborne house dust mite antigen after vacuum cleaning. *The Lancet,* Vol. 336, No. 8712, (August 1990, online 2003), p. 449, Available from http://www.sciencedirect.com/science/article/pii/0140673690920042

Kambarami, RA., Marechera, F., Sibanda, EN., Chitiyo, ME. (1999). Aero-allergen sensitisation patterns amongst atopic Zimbabwean children. *The Central African journal of medicine,* Vol. 45, No. 6, (June 1999), pp. 144-147, ISSN 0008-9176

Kumura, K. (2010). A new asthma classification based on its pathophysiology using IgE antibody (RAST) and lymphocyte activation as parameters. *Okayama Igakkai Zasshi,* Vol. 106, No. 9-10, (1994), pp. 1025-1033, ISSN 0030-1558

Kurth, BM. (2008). The challenge of comprehensively mapping children's health in a nation-wide health survey: Design of the German KiGGS-Study. *BMC Public Health,* Vol. 8, No. 196, (June 2008). URL: http://www.biomedcentral.com/1471-2458/8/196

Kusel, MMH., de Klerk, NH., Kebadze, T., Vohma, V., Holt, PG., Johnston, SL., & Sly, PD. (2007). Early-life respiratory viral infections, atopic sensitization, and risk of subsequent development of persistent asthma. *Journal of Allergy and Clinical Immunology,* Vol. 119, No. 5, (May 2007), pp. 1105-1110, ISSN 0091-6749

Langen, U., Knopf, H., (2007). Asthma bronchiale, obstruktive Bronchitis und ihre medikamentöse Therapie bei Kindern und Jugendlichen in Deutschland. *Pädiatrische Allergologie,* Vol. 10, No. 4, (April 2007), pp. 14-17, ISSN 1435-4233

Lau, S., Illi, S., Platts-Mills, TAE., Riposo, D., Nickel, R., Grueber, C., Niggemann, B., & Wahn, U. (2005). Longitudinal study on the relationship between cat allergen and endotoxin exposure, sensitization, cat-specific IgG and development of asthma in childhood - report of the German Multicentre Allergy Study (MAS 90). *Allergy (Oxford),* Vol. 60, No. 6, (June 2005), pp. 766-773, ISSN 0105-4538

Leung, TF., Li, AM., & Ha, G. (2000). Allergen sensitization in asthmatic children: consecutive case series. *Hong Kong medical journal,* Vol. 6, No. 4, (December 2000), pp. 355-360, ISSN 1024-2708

Lewis, SA., Weiss, ST., Platts-Mills, TA., Syring, M., & Gold, DR. (2001). Association of specific allergen sensitization with socioeconomic factors and allergic disease in a population of Boston women. *Journal of Allergy and Clinical Immunology,* Vol. 107, No. 4, (April 2001), pp. 615-622, ISSN 0091-6749

Majkowska-Wojciechowska, BM., Pelka, J., Korzon, L., Kozlowska, A., Kaczala, M., Jarzebska, M., Gwardys, T., & Kowalski, ML. (2007). Prevalence of allergy, patterns of allergic sensitization and allergy risk factors in rural and urban children. *Allergy (Oxford),* Vol. 62, No. 9, (September 2007), pp. 1044-1050, ISSN 0105-4538

Nelson, RP., Dinicolo, R., Fernandezcaldas, E., Seleznick, MJ., Lockey, RF., & Good, RA. (1996). Allergen-specific IgE levels and mite allergen exposure in children with acute asthma first seen in an emergency department and in nonasthmatic control subjects. *Journal of Allergy and Clinical Immunology,* Vol. 98, No. 2, (August 1996), pp. 258-263, ISSN 0091-6749.

Ohr, R., & Zeddies, G., (2006). Ökonomische Gesamtbetrachtung der Hundehaltung in Deutschland. Available from http://www.uni-goettingen.de/de/.../Abschlussbericht%20freigegeben%201.pdf

Peat, JK., Toelle, BG., Gray, EJ., Haby, MM., Belousova, E., Mellis, CM., & Wollcock, AJ. (1995). Prevalence and severity of childhood asthma and allergic sensitisation in seven climatic regions of New South Wales. *The Medical journal of Australia,* Vol. 163, No. 1, (July 1995), pp. 22-26, ISSN 0025-729X

Rastogi, D., Reddy, M., & Neugebauer, R. (2006). Comparison of patterns of allergen sensitization among inner-city Hispanic and African American children with asthma. *Annals of Allergy, Asthma and Immunology: official publication of the American College of Allergy, Asthma and Immunology,* Vol. 97, No. 5, (November 2006), pp. 636-642, ISSN 1081-1206

Robert Koch Institut & Statistisches Bundesamt (2008). *Beiträge zur Gesundheitsberichterstattung des Bundes. Lebensphasenspezifische Gesundheit von Kindern und Jugendlichen. Ergebnisse des Nationalen Kinder- und Jugendgesundheitssurveay (KiGGS).* Robert Koch-Institut, ISBN 978-3-89606-192-8, Berlin

Rönmark, E., Perzanowski, M., Platts-Mills, T., & Lundbäck, B. (2003). Different sensitization profile for asthma, rhinitis, and eczema among 7-8-year-old children: report from the Obstructive Lung Disease in Northern Sweden studies. *Pediatric Allergy and Immunology,* Vol. 14, No. 2, (April 2003), pp. 91-99, ISSN 0905-6157

Rona, RJ., Vargas, C., Vianna, EO., Bustos, H., Amigo, H., Mackenney, J., Barbieri, MA. (2008). Impact of specific sensitization on asthma and rhinits in young Brazilian and Chilean adults. *Clinical and experimental allergy: journal of the British Society for Allergy and Clinical Immunology,* Vol. 38, No. 11, (November 2008), pp. 1778-1786, ISSN 1365-2222

Simpson, A., Tan, VY., Winn, J., Svensén, M., Bishop, CM., Heckerman, DE., Buchan, I., Custovic, A. (2010). Beyond atopy: multiple patterns of sensitization in relation to asthma in a birth cohort study. *American journal of respiratory and critical care medicine,* Vol. 181, No. 11, (June 2010), pp. 1200-1206, ISSN 1535-4970

Soto-Quiros, M., Gutierrez, I., Calvo, N., Araya, C., Karlberg, J., Hanson, LÅ., & Belin, L. (2007). Allergen sensitization of asthmatic and nonasthmatic schoolchildren in Costa Rica. *Allergy (Copenhagen),* Vol. 53, No. 12, (December 1998), pp. 1141-1147, ISSN 0105-4538

Sporik, R., Ingram, JM., Price, W., Sussmann, JH., Honsinger, RW., & Platts-Mills, TA. (1995). Association of asthma with serum IgE and skin test reactivity to allergens among children living in high altitude. Tickling the dragon´s breath. *American journal of respiratory and critical care medicine,* Vol. 151, No. 5, (March 1995), pp. 1388-1392, ISSN 1073-449X

Valero Santiago, AL., Pereira, C., Loureiro, C., Martínez-Cócera, C., Murio, C., Rico, P., Palomino, R., & Dávila, I. (2009). Interrelationship between skin sensitization, rhinitis, and asthma in patients with allergic rhinitis: A study of Spain and Portugal. *Journal of Investigational Allergology and Clinical Immunology,* Vol. 19, No. 3, (2009), pp. 167-172. URL: http://www.jiaci.org/issues/vol19issue3/1.pdf

Verini, M., Nicodemo, A., Spagnuolo, C., Di Pillo, S., Morone, M., & Chiarelli, F. (2005). The effect of urban or rural environment on allergic sensitisation in children with asthma. *Italian Journal of Pediatrics,* Vol. 31, No. 5, (October 2005), pp. 329-334. URL: http://www.ijp.it/articoli/2005/vol-5-05/Verini.pdf

Weinmayr, G., Rzehak, P., Büchele, G., Björkstén, B., Brunekreef, B., Cookson, WOC., von Mutius, E., Strachan, DP., & Weiland, SK. (2006). International variation in prevalence of asthma symptoms and atopic sensitization: Results from phase II of the International Study of Asthma and Allergies in Childhood (ISAAC II). *Allergo Journal,* Vol. 15, No. 2, (March 2006), pp. 124-125, ISSN 0941-8849

Weinmayr, G., Weiland, SK., Bjorksten, B., Brunekreef, B., Buchele, G., Cookson, WOC., Garcia-Marcos, L., Gotua, M., Gratziou, C., van Hage, M., von Mutius, E., Riikjarv, MA., Rzehak, P., Stein, RT., Strachan, DP., Tsanakas, J., Wickens, K., & Wong, GW. (2007). Atopic sensitization and the international variation of asthma symptom prevalence in children. *American Journal of Respiratory and Critical Care Medicin,* Vol. 176, No. 6, (September 2007), pp. 565-574, ISSN 1073-449X

10

Wheezing Infant

Yukinori Yoshida, Tomoshige Matsumoto, Makoto Kameda,
Tomoki Nishikido, Isamu Takamatsu and Satoru Doi
Osaka Prefectural Hospital Organization,
Osaka Prefectural Medical Center for Respiratory and Allergic Diseases,
Japan

1. Introduction

Symptoms of Gastroesophageal Reflux Disease (GERD) are both esophageal and extraesophageal symptoms. The consensus statements on the definition of GERD in the pediatric population were reported that respiratory symptoms might be occurred by gastroesophageal acid reflux (Sherman et al.,2009). But, the definition of GERD used by gastroenterologists are much different from that used by allergists (Colombo, 2004).

Usually, the diagnosis of GERD is based on the reflux index (percentage of total recording time with a pH below 4) during 24-hour pH monitoring (pH monitoring) (Working group of the European society of pediatric gastroenterology and nutrition, 1992). But, this baseline of the reflux index was defined by gastroenterologists.In our previous study in asthmatic children with GERD, we showed that respiratory symptoms tended to worse not only at night but also in the daytime, and the index of the mean hourly number of acid refluxes (the mean number of acid reflux/h) which we defined parameters as the frequency of acid refluxes during upright position during pH monitoring was important for the diagnosis of GERD when associated with asthma (Yoshida et al., 2009).

In some previous reports, the frequency of GERD in children with respiratory symptoms was comparatively high (Saglani et al., 2006). But, at the present situation, it has not been cleared sufficiently when GERD should be considered in children with episodes of recurrent wheezing. In clinically, when episodes of recurrent wheezing are intractable regardless of doing medications, we suspect that GERD is associated with episodes of recurrent wheezing. So, in the present study, we investigated the difference of characteristics for diagnosis and treatment of GERD more appropriately in children with episodes of recurrent wheezing associated with GERD.

Proton pump inhibitors (PPIs) and histamine-2 receptor antagonists (H_2RAs) are widely used as acid suppression therapy of GERD (Scarupa et al.,2005). In recent years, not only H_2RAs but also PPIs were reported for treatment of GERD (Gustafsson et al.,1992; Harper et al., 1987; Khoshoo et al.,2003; Sopo et al.,2009; Stordal et al.,2005; The American lung association asthma clinical research center,2009). However, in Japan, we can only use the enteric-coated tablet-type PPIs. Therefore, PPIs are difficult to use for preschool children especially those under 5 years of age. So, we have no choice but to use the powdered-type H_2RAs in children under 5 years of age. In our country, the powdered-type H_2RAs we can use is famotidine. So, in the present study, we used famotidine as acid suppression therapy.

And, in our previous study, the mean number of acid reflux/h during the upright position exceeded 7 in all the children with GERD associated asthma (Yoshida, et al., 2009). So, in the present study, we diagnosed of GERD by the mean number of acid reflux/h which baseline was defined as exceeded 7 and response of acid suppression therapy.

2. Materials and methods

We performed pH monitoring between June 2007 and December 2008 in 52 preschool children with episodes of recurrent wheezing. All participant's chest radiograph were normal. They had no other respiratory disorders, for example, bronchiectasis, recurrent pneumonia, aspiration, intestinal lung disease and airway abnormality. And they had no neurological disorders, cardiac disease and gastrointestinal symptoms.

All patients received inhaled corticosteroid (ICS) for more than 3 months. The ICS used was fluticasone or hydrofluoroalkane-beclomethasone dipropionate more than 200 μg/day. But, their respiratory symptomatic days during one month were more than 5 days. Their respiratory symptoms were uncontrolled. So, we suspected that GERD was associated with their respiratory symptoms, and we performed the pH monitoring.

When the mean number of acid refluxes/h during upright position exceeded 7, by the result of pH monitoring, we started famotidine therapy (0.5mg/kg twice daily). And, we followed up the children who started famotidine therapy for one month. So, we counted respiratory symptomatic days for one month before and after starting the famotidine therapy. And we compared them before and after starting the famotidine therapy.

So, in the case that symptomatic days were decreased less than half days, we defined that framotidine therapy was effective. When famotidine therapy was effective, children formed the effective group. On the other hand, in the case that symptomatic days were not decreased less than half days, we defined that framotidine therapy was not effective. When famotidine therapy was not effective, children formed the no effective group. Then, we compared the patient's characteristics between the two groups. We investigated the patient's age, onset age of wheezing episodes, level of serum IgE, amount of ICS and results of pH monitoring as patient's characteristics. And we investigated modified asthma predictive index (mAPI) as the risk factors for the development of asthma (Panettieri et al., 2008).

The pH monitoring was performed using a Synectics Digitrapper MKIII (Synetics Medical Stockholm Sweden). The catheter had 4 probes that sensed acid reflux. The most upper probe (the first probe) was 20 cm above the bottom probe. The third probe of the catheter was placed 3-4 cm above the gastroesophageal junction, and its position was checked by chest radiography. We examined the mean number of acid refluxes/h during upright position and the reflux index at the third probe. The asthma medication was continued as usual during pH monitoring.

In our hospital, respiratory symptoms are recorded in a diary in order to acquire the precise clinical manifestation. At every patient's visit, each physician checked the diary.

3. Data analysis

Normal distributed data were presented as mean ± SD. Nonparametric data were expressed as median. The differences were assessed by the Mann-Whitney U-test. A p-vale <0.05 was considered to be statistically significant for all tests.

4. Results

Patient profiles were summarized in Table 1. 27 children showed the results that the mean number of acid reflux/h during upright position exceeded 7. In 18 of the 27 children, the reflux index exceeded 4%. In the remaining 25 children with the mean number of acid reflux/h during upright position being below 7, the reflux index was below 4%.

Gender	
- Male,n	35
- Female,n	17
Age,years*	3.1 (1.8)
Amount of ICS, µg/day*	219 (59.4)
Results of 24-hour pH monitoring	
- Reflux index,%*	6.2 (9.5)
- The mean number of acid reflux/h during upright position, times*	12.4 (13.6)
- The number of children with reflux index over 4 %, n	18
- The number of children with the mean number of acid reflux/h during upright position over seven, n	27

*Data are presented as mean (SD). n:number. ICS; inhaled corticosteroid

Table 1. Patient profiles (n=52)

19 of the 27 children profiles with the mean number of acid reflux/h during upright position being over 7 were summarized in Table 2. The remaining 8 children did not record respiratory symptoms in the diary or did not visit our hospital. Among the 19 children, 8 were included in the effective group and 11 were included in the no effective group.

Gender	
- Male,n	12
- Female,n	7
Age,year*	3.1 (1.33)
Amount of ICS, µg/day*	235 (236)
Results of 24-hour pH monitoring	
- The mean number of acid reflux/h during upright position, times*	19.5 (19.9)
- Reflux index,%*	9.0 (9.3)
The effective group	8
The no effective group	11

*Data are presented as mean (SD). n:number. ICS; inhaled corticosteroid

Table 2. Patient profiles with the mean number of acid reflux/h during upright position over 7 (n=19)

A comparison of patient's characteristics between the effective group and the no effective group was summarized in Table 3. The mean (SD) age was 2.4 (1.0) years old in the effective group, and 3.5 (1.3) years old in the no effective group ($p<0.05$). And, the mean (SD) onset

	Effective group n=8	No effective group n=11	p vale
Age,year	2.4(1.0)	3.5(1.3)	p<0.05
Onset age of episodes of wheezing, year	1.0(1.1)	3.0(1.0)	p<0.05
Serum IgE, IU/ml	209(201)	150(237)	n.s.
Amount of ICS, μg/day	237(106)	236(80)	n.s.
Results of 24-hour pH monitoring			
- reflux index,%	11.4(10.8)	7.6(9.8)	n.s.
- The mean number of acid reflux/h during upright position, times	20.9(9.5)	19.0(19.6)	n.s.
Respiratory symptomatic days			
- Before famotidine	16.0(7.2)	14.1(5.8)	n.s.
- After famotidine	5.6(5.4)	13.9(4.5)	p<0.05

Data are presented as mean(SD).

Table 3. Comparison of the effective group and the no effective group

age of wheezing was 1.0 (1.1) years old in the effective group, and 3.0 (1.0) years old in the no effective group (p<0.05). The mean (SD) respiratory symptomatic days before famotidine were 16.0 (7.2) in the effective group, and 14.1 (5.8) in the no effective group. The mean (SD) respiratory symptomatic days were 5.6 (5.4) in the effective group, and 13.9(4.5) in the no effective group (p<0.05). There was no significant difference between the two groups before famotidine tehapy. But, there was difference between the two groups after famotidine therapy. The changes of the respiratory symptomatic days between before and after famotidine therapy in each group were showed in figure 1. In the effective group, there was singinficant difference (p<0.05). There was no singinficant difference between the two groups about level of serum IgE, amount of ICS and the results of pH monitoring in Table 3. A comparison of modified asthma predictive index between the effective group the no effective group was summarized in Table 4. There was no singinficant difference about each index between the two groups.

Modified Asthma Prediction Index	Effective group (n=8)	No effective group (n=11)	p value
• Major criteria, n			
Parental history of asthma	3	5	n.s.
Physician-diagnosed atopic dermatitis	2	3	n.s.
Allergic sensitization to ≧ 1 aeroallergen	5	6	n.s.
• Minor criteria,n			
Allergic sensitization to milk, egg, or peanuts	3	3	n.s.
Wheezing unrelated to colds	8	11	n.s.
Blood eosinophils ≧ 4%	5	5	n.s.
The presence of 1 of the major criteria or 2 minor criteria,n	8 (100%)	11 (100%)	

Table 4. Comparison of Modified Asthma Prediction Index between the effective group and the no effective group

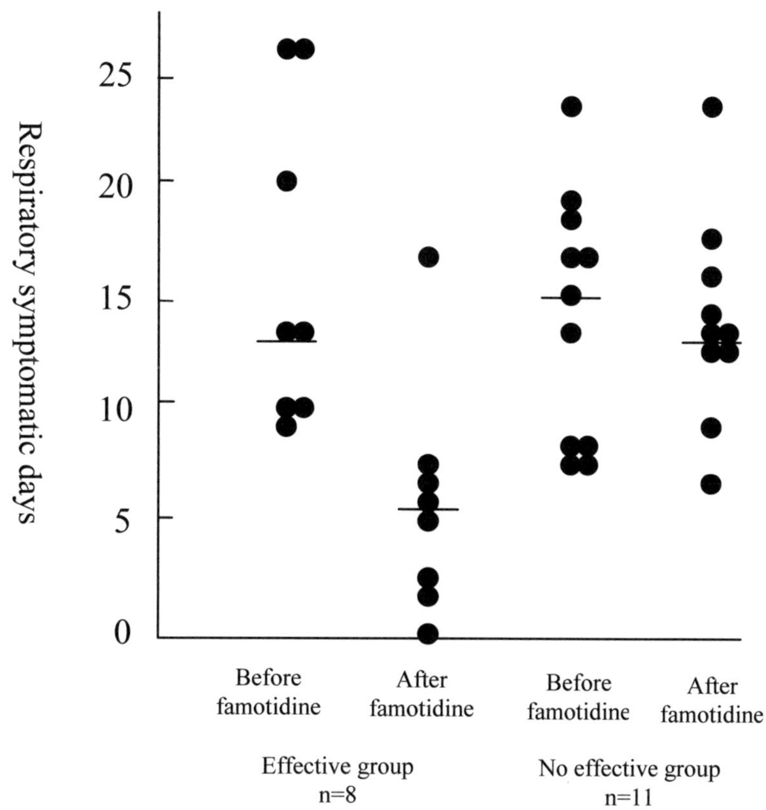

Fig. 1. The difference of the effective group and the no effective group of respiratory symptomatic days between before and after famotidine therapy

5. Discussion

The incidence of GERD was comparatively high in children with episodes of recurrent wheezing. The previous report had shown that the incidence of asthma in children with episodes of recurrent wheezing was 40.4%, and that of GERD was 23.4%. In particular, 57% children with asthma also had GERD (Saglani et al., 2006). But, the efficacy of acid suppression therapy was not cleared sufficiently for children with episodes of recurrent wheezing (Brand et al., 2008). For example, in the treatment of asthma, there was a report that PPIs did not improve asthma control (The American lung association asthma clinical research center, 2009). So, in the present study, we prescribed for famotidine based on result of pH monitoring in the lower age preschool children with episodes of recurrent wheezing, and compared between children with effective and ineffective of famotidine therapy. And, we showed that famotidine therapy could be more effective in the lower age preschool children with episodes of recurrent wheezing with associated GERD.

In the present study, 8 out of 19 (42%) children who received the famotidine therapy were included the effective group. And, in the effective group, the mean age and the onset age of first wheezing episode were significantly lower than that of the no effective group. Namely, in preschool children with episodes of recurrent wheezing associated with GERD, the lower age of and the lower onset age of first wheezing episodes were, the more effective famotidine therapy was. In clinically, a diagnosis of GERD is made by the efficacy of acid suppression therapy in addition to the results of pH monitoring. So, in the effective group, their respiratory symptoms could be defined that GERD was associated with episodes of recurrent wheezing. About relationship of gastroesophageal acid reflux (GER) and age, the other previous report had shown that GER occurs easily below one year of age (Nelson et al., 1997). From the present results and previous reports, we suggested that respiratory symptoms of lower age could be much associated with GERD witch symptoms were improved by famotidine in children with episodes of recurrent wheezing.

Some previous reports had shown the efficacy of PPIs for children with episodes of recurrent wheezing (Sopo et al., 2009; Stordal et al., 2005). PPIs were more effective than H_2RAs such as famotidine. But, PPIs available in Japan are difficult to use for preschool children. So, in the no effective group in the present study, there might be improved respiratory symptoms if PPIs were used. But, unfortunately, this problem could not be cleared in the present situation in Japan.

But, there are two treatment regimens of GERD. One treatment regimen witch is called the no effective therapy is to begin with H_2RAs. When symptoms are not improved by H_2RAs, then PPIs are used. The other medication witch is called step-down therapy is to begin with PPIs. But, in treatment of GERD, cost-effectiveness considerations must be needed when which medication is used (Hassall, 2008). In general, PPIs are superior to H_2RAs for erosive esophagitis (Vandenplas et al., 2009). So, PPIs were capable of being a cost-effective diagnostic test in adult (Ofman et al., 1999). But, in children, there was no study comparing these two medications (Hassall, 2008). In pediatric gastroesophageal reflux clinical practice guidelines, there needs special concern to prescription of PPIs in infants(Vandenplas et al., 2009). In previous report, PPIs were used over the age of 2 years old or those with moderate symptoms of GERD. But, under the age of 12 month, H_2RAs were better starting medication (Hassall, 2008; Vandenplas et al., 2009). So, in clinical cases, the medication is selected by considering age and severity of symptoms.

About symptoms of GERD, the presence of esophageal erosions or ulcers is one of the factors that determine the severity of GERD (Armstrong et al., 2005). But, the previous study showed that the presence of esophagitis did not always exist in children with refractory respiratory symptoms of GERD (Ravelli et al., 2006). So, the severity of GERD with episodes of recurrent wheezing could be defined "mild"

Another previous report showed that H_2RAs were safe and effective for the management of mild GERD symptoms (Vandenplas et al., 2009). So, we suggested that H_2RAs might be prescribed first for children with episodes of recurrent wheezing. H_2RAs include cimetidine, famotidine and ranitidine. There was no previous study about the effective of famotidine for respiratory symptoms. So, our present study is valuable.

Asthma is the most common cause in diseases with episodes of recurrent wheezing (Weinberger & Abu-Hasan, 2007). Recurrent wheezing during first 3 years is one of the established risk factor for the development of asthma in childhood (Panettieri et al., 2008). But, we must take careful of asthma like symptoms caused by other causes (Weinberger & Abu-Hasan, 2007). Diagnosis of asthma in preschool children with episodes of recurrent wheezing is difficult (Brand et al., 2008). The previous report had shown that the incidence of asthma in children with episodes of recurrent wheezing was 41%, and that of GERD was 23%, and that of predominantly infection was 13% (Saglani et al., 2006). One of the common diagnosis in the diseases of predominantly infection is protracted bacterial bronchitis (Gibson et al., 2010). Children with protracted bacterial bronchitis are sometimes erroneous

labeled as having severe asthma (Chang et al., 2008). So, the other previous report had shown that the differential diagnosis should be considered when young children with recurrent respiratory symptoms had a negative mAPI (Chipps, 2010).
The mAPI is a clinical index of asthma for 2 years of age and older (Panettieri et al., 2008). When the child has the presence of 1 the major criteria or 2 minor criteria in the mAPI, the recurrent respiratory symptoms of child might be developed persistent asthma (Chipps, 2010). So, we investigated mAPI whether there were differences about risk factor for asthma development between the effective group and the no effective group. As a result, there was no significant difference on each subject. And all children of each groups had the presence of 1 of the major criteria or 2 minor criteria. So, there was no significant difference about risk factor for asthma development according to the mAPI. But, in the no effective group, amount of ICS was increased within 3 months after famotidine therapy for controlling of respiratory symptoms. The mean (SD) amount of ICS was 308 (78) µg/day. (data not shown). We speculated that children in the no effective group had more progressive airway inflammation and had more risk for asthma development than children in the effective group. But, it is not cleared sufficiently in the present study.

6. Conclusion

It is not cleared sufficiently that we must consider what kind of preschool children with episodes of recurrent wheezing are prescribed for the acid suppression therapy. In our present study, in preschool children with episodes of recurrent wheezing associated with GERD, the lower age of and the lower onset age of first wheezing episodes were, the more effective famotidine therapy was. We suggest that lower age preschool children with episodes of recurrent wheezing whose symptoms are suspected associating with GERD from the result of pH monitoring might be prescribed acid suppression therapy actively.
And, famotidien is inferior to PPIs as the acid suppression therapy. But, we suggest that famotidine might be useful as primary medication for "mild" GERD which main symptom is recurrent wheezing.

7. Acknowledgment

We thank Dr. Ichiro Kawase who is director of our hospital for supervising of this study.

8. References

Armstrong, D et al. (2005). Canadian Consensus Conference on the management of gastroesophageal reflux disease in adults - update 2004. *Can J Gastroenterol.* Vol.19 (No.1): 15-35.

Brand, PL et al. (2008). Definition, assessment and treatment of wheezing disorders in preschool children: an evidence-based approach. *Eur Respir J.* Vol.32 (No.4): 1096-110.

Chang, AB et al. (2008). Chronic wet cough: Protracted bronchitis, chronic suppurative lung disease and bronchiectasis. *Pediatr Pulmonol.* Vol.43 (No.6); 519-531.

Chipps, BE. (2010) Evaluation of infants and children with refractory lower respiratory tract symptoms. *Ann Allergy Asthma Immunol.* Vol.104 (No.4): 279-83.

Colombo, JL. (2004). Gastroesophageal reflux and respiratory disorders. In: Behrman RE, Kliegman RM, Jenson HB (eds). *Nelson Textbook of Pediatrics.* 17th edn. Philadelphia: WB Sauders: 1430.

Gibson, PG et al. (2010). CIADA: Cough in Children and Adults: Diagnosis and Assesment. Australian cough gudelines summary statement. *Med J Aust.* Vol.192 (No.5): 265-271.

Gustafsson, PM et al. (1992). A trial of ranitidine in asthmatic children and adolescents with or without pathological gastro-oesophageal reflux. *Eur Respir J.* Vol.5 (No.2): 201-206.

Harper, PC et al. (1987). Antireflux treatment for asthma. Improvement in patients with associated gastroesophageal reflux. *Arch Intern Med.* Vol.147 (No.1):56-60.

Hassall E. (2008). Step-up and step-down approaches to treatment of gastroesophageal reflux disease in children. *Curr Gastroenterol Rep.* Vol.10 (No.3): 324-331.

Khoshoo, V et al. (2003). Role of gastroesophageal reflux in older children with persistent asthma. *Chest.* Vol.123 (No.4): 1008-1013.

Nelson, SP et al. (1997). Prevalence of symptoms of gastroesophageal reflux during infancy. A pediatric practice-based survey. Pediatric Practice Research Group. *Arch Pediatr Adolesc Med.* Vol.151 (No.6): 569-572.

Ofman, JJ et al. (1999). The cost-effectiveness of the omeprazole test in patients with noncardiac chest pain. *Am J Med.* Vol.107 (No.3):219-227.

Panettieri, RA Jr et al. (2008). Natural history of asthma: persistence versus progression-does the beginning predict the end?. *J Allergy Clin Immunol.* Vol.121 (No.3): 607-613.

Ravelli, AM et al. (2006). Pulmonary aspiration shown by scintigraphy in gastroesophageal reflux-related respiratory disease. *Chest.* Vol.130 (No.5): 1520-1526.

Saglani, S et al. (2006). Investigation of young children with severe recurrent wheeze: any clinical benefit? *Eur Respir J.* Vol.27 (No.1) :29-35.

Scarupa, MD et al.(2005). Gastroesophageal reflux disease in children with asthma: treatment implications. *Pediatr Drugs.* Vol. 7 (No.3): 177-186.

Sherman, PM et al.(2009).A global, evidence-based consensus on the definition of gastroesophageal reflux disease in the pediatric population. *Am J Gastroenterol* ,Vol.104 (No.5): 1278-1295.

Sopo, SM et al. (2009). Does treatment with proton pump inhibitors for gastroesophageal reflux disease (GERD) improve asthma symptoms in children with asthma and GERD? A systematic review. *J Investing Allergol Clin Immunol.* Vol.19 (No.1): 1-5.

Stordal, K et al. (2005). Acid suppression dose not change respiratory symptoms in children with asthma and gastroesophageal reflux disease. *Arch Dis Child.* Vol.90 (No.9): 956-960.

The American lung association asthma clinical research center. (2009). Efficacy of Esomeprazole for treatment of poorly controlled asthma. *N Engl J Med.* Vol.9;360 (No.15): 1487-1499.

Vandenplas, Y et al. (2009). Pediatric gastroesophageal reflux clinical practice guidelines: joint recommendations of the North American Society for Pediatric Gastroenterology, Hepatology, and Nutrition (NASPGHAN) and the European Society for Pediatric Gastroenterology, Hepatology, and Nutrition (ESPGHAN). *J Pediatr Gastroenterol Nutr* .Vol.49 (No.4): 498-547.

Weinberger, M. & Abu-Hasan, M. (2007). Pseudo-asthma: when cough, wheezing, and dyspnea are not asthma. *Pediatrics.* Vol.120 (No.4): 855-864.

Working group of the European society of pediatric gastroenterology and nutrition. (1992). A standardized protocol for the methodology of esophageal pH monitoring and interpretation of the data for the diagnosis of gastroesophageal reflux. *J Pediatr Gastroenterol Nutr.* Vol.14 (No.4): 467-471.

Yoshida, Y et al. (2009). Very short gastroesophageral acid reflux during the upright position could be associated with asthma in children. *Allergol Int.*Vol.58 (No.3): 395-401.

11

Comorbidities of Allergic Rhinitis

Doo Hee Han and Chae-Seo Rhee
Department of Otorhinolaryngology,
Seoul National University College of Medicine, Seoul,
Korea

1. Introduction

Allergic rhinitis (AR) is a symptomatic nose disorder induced after exposure to allergens via IgE-mediated hypersensitivity reactions, which are characterized by 4 cardinal symptoms: nasal obstruction, watery rhinorrhea, nasal itching and sneezing. For both children and adults, AR is more than just sneezing and nose itching. Complications of this disease are numerous and can have a significant impact, both physically and psychosocially. Major comorbidities in patients with AR include asthma, rhinosinusitis (RS), otitis media with effusion (OME), and sleep disturbance. The symptoms of AR can cause not only physical problems to the nose and lower airway, but also psychosocial problems including those in learning and cognitive processes and in missing work or school (Fig. 1). Thus, it is very important to understand other conditions caused by AR when managing this disorder.

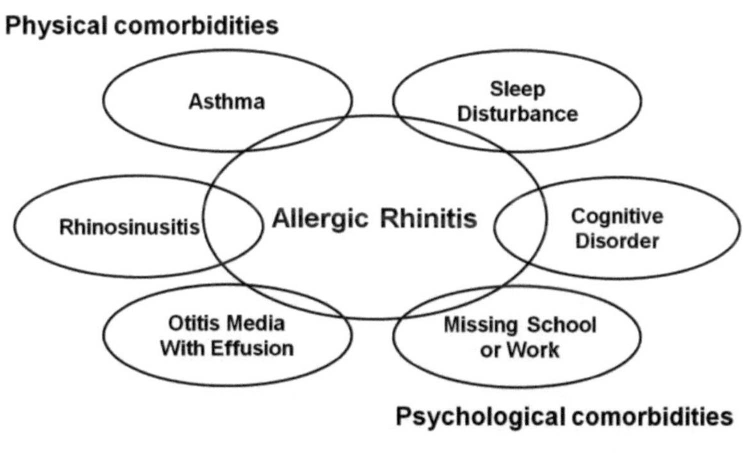

Fig. 1. Physical and psychological comorbidities of AR (Adapted from Spector, 1997)

The ongoing efforts of physicians to identify comorbidities of AR in the fields of allergy can be put to practical use in caring and protecting the community from the burden of disease as well as saving costs and offering preventive education. Moreover, providing information to the patients with AR is expected to have a direct and positive effect on their well being.
In this chapter, we will provide an overview of the comorbidities of AR that could cause both physical and psychosocial complications.

2. Physical comorbidities

2.1 AR and asthma

AR and asthma affect the upper and lower respiratory tract, respectively. Both are characterized by inflammation of the respiratory mucosa and involve similar inflammatory cells and mediators. Moreover AR and asthma have a considerable impact on quality of life, work and school productive, absenteeism, and individual and socioeconomic burden (Gaugris et al., 2006; Bachert et al., 2002; Bousquet et al., 2001). The socioeconomic burden via annual costs of treating AR and asthma, both direct costs such as hospitalization, medication and indirect costs such as time lost from work are substantial, and represent heavier burden in modern societies.

2.1.1 Association between AR and asthma

AR and asthma commonly coexist. Among asthmatic patients, approximately 85% also have AR. Conversely, up to 40% of AR patients have or will develop asthma (Bousquet et al., 2001; Guerra et al., 2002). There are many common anatomical and pathophysiological features between upper and lower airway disorders, primarily in histology and immunology. Examples of common anatomical features include ciliated columnar epithelial cells, mucinous glands, vasculature, and innervation (Baraniuk, 1997). Both AR and asthma are chronic inflammatory diseases of the upper and lower airways and their inflammatory mechanisms are characterized by inflammatory infiltrates made up of eosinophils, T cells, and mast cells that release several mediators, chemokines and cytokines, inducing local and systemic IgE synthesis, and activate a systemic link via the bone marrow.

AR has been shown to be a risk factor for asthma in children and adults (Leynaert et al., 2000). A longitudinal, population-based study confirmed an association between AR and adult-onset asthma (Shaaban et al., 2008). In another study, among 1,836 college freshman, those with AR were significantly more likely to have asthma by the 23-year follow-up than those without (Settipane et al., 1994).

In AR, one distinction is heavy vascularization of the nasal passages, which may lead to severe nasal obstruction. In asthma, the presence of smooth muscle from the trachea to the bronchioles can result in characteristic bronchoconstriction. Despite these differences, similarities exist. Notably, the anatomical structure and physiology of the airway mucosa are similar in both upper and lower airway (Bousquet et al., 2003).

Inflammation is a central component of both conditions. In AR, the inflammatory cascade is initiated by allergen deposition on the nasal mucosa and comprises early-phase and often late-phase responses. The antigen cross-links and activates IgE receptors, resulting in the degranulation of mast cells and the release of several mediators of inflammation, including histamine, prostaglandins, leukotrienes, and proteases, leading to sneezing, itching, rhinorrhea and congestion symptoms of AR. In asthma, antigen cross-linking and activation of IgE receptors may precipitate acute airway constriction.

AR may promote or exacerbate asthma through several physiological mechanisms that link 2 disorders. An early study investigating the integrated airway hypothesis suggested a nasobronchial reflex arc as a potential mechanism linking upper and lower airway disorders (Kaufman et al., 1970). Based on this hypothesis, nasal allergen challenge affects bronchial hyperresponsiveness through a reflex arc that involves trigeminal afferents and vagal efferents. In addition, other mechanisms include systemic release of mediators and cytokines, postnasal drip resulting irritation and oral breathing caused by nasal obstruction, which causes dry, cold air to penetrate into the bronchi and promote bronchial hyperresponsiveness (Meltzer, 2005) (Fig. 2).

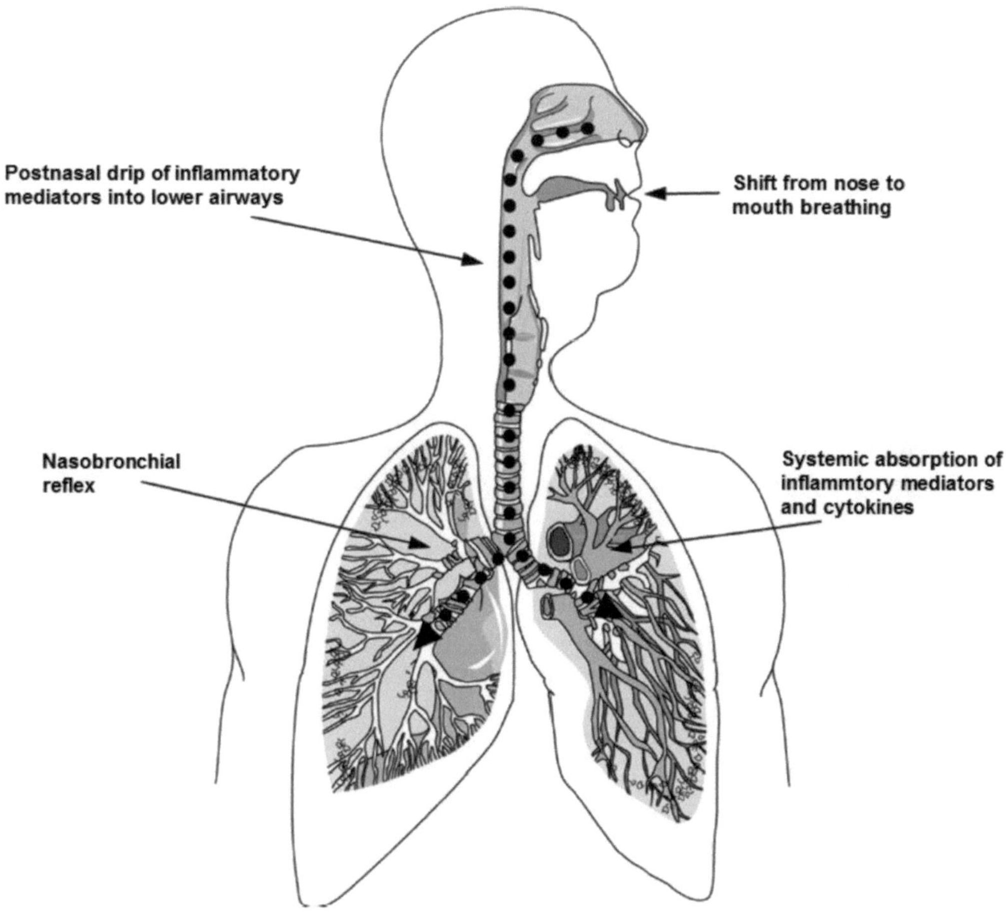

Fig. 2. Mechanisms of pathologic relationships between upper and lower airways (Adapted from Meltzer, 2005).

2.1.2 Asthma evaluation in AR

Allergic Rhinitis and its Impact on Asthma (ARIA) guidelines recommend that asthma patients be evaluated for AR and, conversely, that AR patients be evaluated for asthma (Bousquet et al., 2001). In a prospective study evaluating 375 adults with persistent moderate to severe AR and 115 controls, the authors concluded that patients with persistent moderate to severe AR without an asthma diagnosis should be evaluated for the lower airway with pulmonary function testing (Ciprandi et al., 2008). Similarly, ARIA 2008 updates recommend that persistent AR patients should be evaluated for asthma (Bousquet et al., 2008). In our previous study, 173 AR patients were evaluated for the lower airway with the methacholine bronchoprovocation test and we recommend lower airway evaluation for the selected patients with nasal polyps, moderate to severe symptoms, and high blood eosinophil count (>320 cells/μL) instead of a routine lower airway evaluation

(Ahn et al., 2010). In another study, persistent type of rhinitis and parental history of asthma were significant and independent risk factors for bronchial hyperresponsiveness in AR children (Choi et al., 2007).

2.1.3 Treatment of AR

Early, active treatment of AR may be appropriate to decrease the incidence and morbidity associated with asthma. In a retrospective US cohort study of medical records covering 1 year for 4,944 asthmatic patients, approximately 73% were treated for AR. Asthma-related events occurred more often in untreated patients than in treated patients (6.6% vs. 1.3%) (Crystal-Peters et al., 2002).

Controlling nasal symptoms with intranasal steroids improves asthma symptoms and nonspecific bronchial hyperresponsiveness (Watson et al., 1993). The authors reported that bronchial hyperresponsiveness to methacholine was significantly reduced in patients with perennial AR and asthma following treatment with intranasal steroids but not following intranasal placebo. More importantly, they also performed a radiolabeled deposition study of intranasal steroid administration and found that less than 2% was deposited in the chest area. These results suggest that treatment of inflammation in the upper airways indirectly improves asthma symptoms and decreases bronchial hyperresponsiveness, which is not a direct effect of the intranasally administered corticosteroid on the lower airways (Watson et al., 1993).

A 3-year retrospective cohort study conducted in 14 US centers evaluated whether treatment with intranasal corticosteroid (INS) in patients of 5 years or older with asthma was associated with a reduced risk of emergency room visits for asthma (Adams et al., 2002). Treatment of nasal conditions, particularly with INSs, appeared to prevent asthma exacerbations leading to emergency room visits.

2.2 AR and RS

AR and RS are increasingly being regarded as interrelated and part of a spectrum of upper airway inflammatory disease. AR also may be a contributing factor in 25% to 30% of patients with acute maxillary sinusitis and in as many as 60% to 80% of patients with chronic sinusitis (Spector, 1997). At the least, AR is associated with and probably a predisposing factor in the development of RS (Slavin, 1998). Both conditions are characterized by an inflammatory response leading to an altered milieu within the nose and paranasal sinuses, thus rendering normal host defenses weakened and susceptible to further inflammatory insult.

However, the role of allergy in the pathogenesis of RS has been under debate and controversy over the past several years.

2.2.1 Association between AR and RS

RS is an inflammation of the nose and paranasal sinuses, attributed to many potential factors. The term "rhinosinusitis" rather than "sinusitis" reflects more accurately close anatomical and pathophysiological relationship between rhinitis and chronic sinusitis, which are commonly comorbid. The typical pathophysiological scheme leading to the development of RS starts with some inciting agents (viral, bacterial, fungal, allergen) or predisposing factor (anatomical, immunological) leading to generalized mucosal edema and inflammation. In the development of RS, mucosal inflammation leads to ciliary dysfunction and mucus stasis, as well as edema of the sinus ostia. The stasis of secretions within the sinuses serves as a nidus for bacterial colonization and growth. These events coupled with the impairment of host defenses as a result of the inflammatory mediators released in response to the inciting agent, create a cycle of sustained inflammation that can chronically damage the nasal and paranasal sinus linings (Ahmad and Zacharek, 2008; Gwaltney et al., 1995) (Fig. 3).

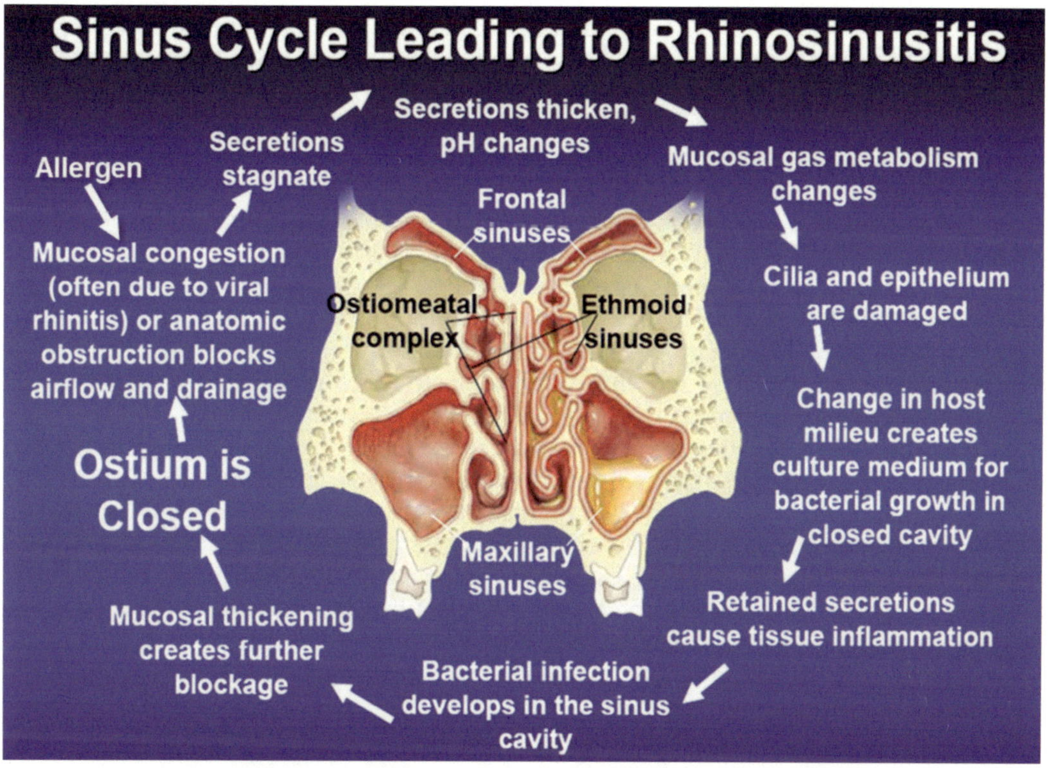

Fig. 3. Sinus cycle leading to RS (Adapted from Ahmad and Zacharek, 2008)

Adult chronic RS was defined as a group of disorders characterized by inflammation of the mucosa of the nose and paranasal sinuses of at least 12 weeks duration. In the past, chronic RS was characterized as a disease process caused by an anatomical obstruction of the sinus ostia, specifically ostiomeatal complex occlusion. The factors leading to this obstruction included viral infection aided by anatomical factors, leading to mucosal inflammation and edema, with thickening of mucus secretions and secondary bacterial infection. It has become clear that the pathogenic mechanisms are more complex than would be explained by a simple model and that there are other chronic inflammatory processes that contribute to the development of chronic RS. However, the exact mechanism by which allergy predisposes to the development of chronic RS has not been fully elucidated.

According to another model of the pathogenesis of RS, chronic RS is characterized by basement membrane thickening, subepithelial fibrosis and edema, goblet cell hyperplasia, and persistent inflammation (Christodoulopoulos et al., 2000). Like in asthma, remodeling of the mucosa occurs in response to this chronic and progressive inflammation. This model of pathogenesis also supports the notion of a unified airway with similar histopathological changes and immunological mechanism occurring as a result of inflammatory insult.

In a 1989 study, skin testing in 2 groups of young adults, one with acute maxillary sinusitis, and a matched group without sinusitis, revealed that the prevalence of positive allergen testing was greater in the group with RS (45% vs. 33%) (Savolainen, 1989). The author thus concluded that allergy did play a role in the development of acute RS, and that it was more common among atopic individuals. In another study, positive inhalant allergy testing was present in over 50% of the 120 patients undergoing endoscopic sinus surgery, which led him to conclude that allergy may be a predisposing cause of chronic sinusitis (Kennedy, 1992).

The contribution of allergy in the pathophysiology of both acute and chronic RS has been supported by studies examining the role of the ethmoid sinuses in terms of immunological, histopathological and postsurgical changes. The ethmoid mucosa affected by RS demonstrates an increased CD4/CD8 ratio and increase in the number of eosinophils and mast cells as well as extracellular matrix deposition, basement membrane disruption, and denudation of the epithelium (Christodoulopoulos et al., 2000). These findings are similar to the effect of allergy on other parts of the respiratory tract. In another study attempting to correlate tissue histopathology in chronic RS with immune mechanisms in allergic disease, the conclusions were that the proposed method for quantifying tissue eosinophilia in sinus mucosa was reliable and valid and that a relatively strong correlation existed between CT scan stage and tissue eosinophilia in chronic RS (Bhattacharyya et al., 2001).

Several studies examining the relationship between allergen exposure or provocation and RS exacerbation have also suggested a common mechanism in AR and RS (Pelikan and Pelikan-Filipek, 1990; Conner et al., 1989; Slavin, 1998). The investigators demonstrated an increase in metabolic activity of the maxillary sinus mucosa in chronic RS patients during ragweed season, using single-photon emission CT scanning (Slavin, 1998).

Evidence of a common pathophysiological mechanism between AR and RS is convincing. Although a clear causal mechanism leading from AR to the development of RS remains to be elucidated, an increasing number of studies have found the possibility and evidence of this link.

2.3 AR and OME

OME is one of the most commonly encountered diseases in children, affecting approximately 90% of children at some time before school age (Tos, 1984). OME is characterized by an accumulation of fluid in the middle ear behind an intact tympanic membrane in the absence of signs and symptoms of acute infection. If we look at the natural history of OME, many cases are self-limited and resolve spontaneously (Williamson et al., 1994). But, OME is the most frequent cause of hearing loss in children (Thomas et al., 2006; Shekelle et al., 2002).

An epidemiologic link between OME and AR has been demonstrated in many trials (Alles et al., 2001; Tomonaga et al., 1988). Prevalence of AR among patients with chronic or recurrent OME is higher than that seen in the same age group in the general population.

2.3.1 Pathophysiology of OME and AR

The etiology of OME is multifactorial. It may be related to bacterial infection, poor clearance due to Eustachian tube (E-tube) dysfunction, local inflammatory reactions and possibly atopy (Thomas et al., 2006; Luong and Roland, 2008).

Data from several animal studies have suggested a link between nasal allergic inflammation and E-tube dysfunction. For example, an intranasal pollen antigen challenge significantly compromised E-tube function in 23 passively sensitized juvenile rhesus monkeys (Doyle et al., 1984). A nasal allergen challenge in rats resulted in E-tube inflammation, negative pressure and hindrance of mucociliary clearance (Ebert et al., 2007). Another previous study showed negative middle ear pressure following nasal allergen challenge in subjects with AR and hypothesized the involvement of both immunological and mechanical mechanisms (O'Connor et al., 1984). E-tube dysfunction developed during allergy season in 60% of children with seasonal AR and correlated with AR symptom severity (Osur et al., 1989).

Because the E-tube lining is contiguous with the nasopharynx, allergic disorders such as AR may cause inflammation and swelling in this region resulting in E-tube obstruction in the same manner as in the nasal mucosa (Alles et al., 2001; Luong and Roland, 2008; Fireman, 1988) (Fig. 4). Furthermore, it has been found that a reduction in the size of the lumen in an inflamed E-tube could impede mucociliary function, thus delaying clearance of acute infective middle ear effusion, leading to recurrent OME (Alles et al., 2001).

Several studies analyzing middle ear mucosa and effusions in atopic patients with OME have demonstrated that the composition of the inflammatory substrate in acute otitis media is similar to the type I late-phase allergic response seen in other areas of the respiratory tract, such as in AR, chronic RS, and asthma (Nguyen et al., 2004; Sobol et al., 2002; Hurst, 1996). The middle ear effusions of atopic patients with OME showed significantly higher levels of eosinophils, T lymphocytes, and IL-4 mRNA+ cells ($p<0.01$) and significantly lower levels of neutrophils and IFN-γ mRNA+ cells ($p<0.01$) compared to non-atopic patients with OME (Nguyen et al., 2004). Similarly, in another study, a higher percentage of eosinophils and T lymphocytes, and a higher percentage of cells expressing IL-4 and IL-5 were found among atopic patients with OME (Sobol et al., 2002).

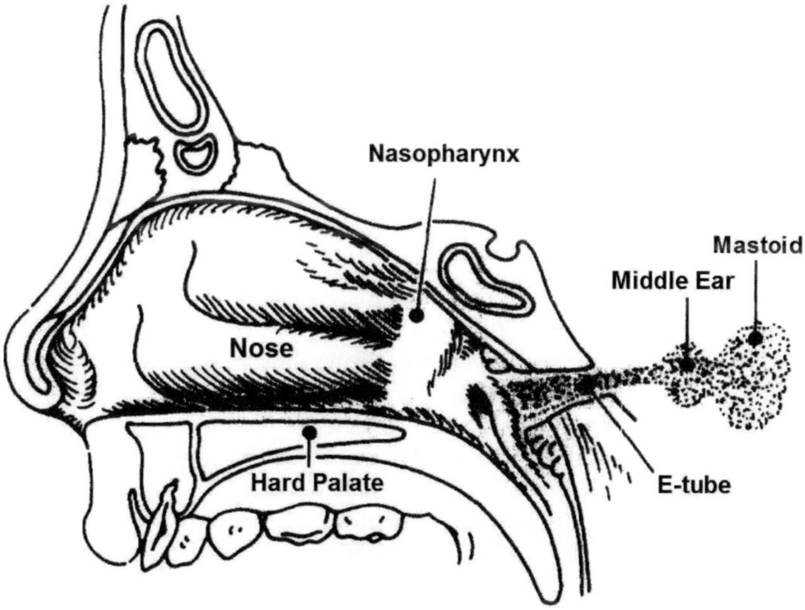

Fig. 4. Schematic diagram showing anatomical relationship of E-tube between the nasopharynx and middle ear (Adapted from Fireman, 1988)

2.3.2 Treatment of OME

Because of the pathophysiological associations of AR with OME, treatments focusing on allergic inflammation may be helpful in the management of OME (Caffarelli et al., 1998; Fireman, 1988).

A meta-analysis of 16 randomized controlled trials demonstrated no significant benefit from antihistamines, decongestants, or combined antihistamines and decongestants versus placebo for treatment of OME (Griffin et al., 2006). However, in a meta-analysis of 6 randomized clinical trials, oral steroids administered for 7-14 days increased the rate of complete effusion resolution versus no steroid (Rosenfeld et al., 1991). A Cochrane database review yielded very similar results, demonstrating a quicker resolution of OME in the short term (≤2 wk) with oral steroids alone or in combination with antibiotics (Thomas et al., 2006). However, there are likely to be safety concerns surrounding oral corticosteroids, such as behavioral changes, increased appetite, weight gain, and adrenal and growth suppression. On the contrary, INS has limited systemic absorption, these drugs offer safety advantages over oral corticosteroids and would be expected to exert their anti-inflammatory effects more locally in the nose, nasopharynx, and E-tube (Tracy et al., 1998). In this study, the authors compared the effects of prophylactic antibiotic alone or in combination with either intranasal beclomethasone or placebo on middle ear pressure, otoscopic examination, and symptom scores in 61 children with persistent middle ear effusion greater than 3 months. Subjects with the beclomethasone plus antibiotic group improved more rapidly in middle ear pressure and otoscopic examination than those with the antibiotic alone or placebo groups during the initial 8 wk. At 12 wk, only the combination treatment showed significant improvement in bilateral ear pressures. In addition, symptom resolution was significantly greater at 12 wk with antibiotic plus beclomethasone group than with the antibiotic alone group. However, there were no differences in outcomes between atopic and nonatopic subjects (Tracy et al., 1998). In another previous study, patients with OME treated with mometasone furoate nasal spray experienced significantly higher rates of resolution of OME at 6 wk compared with untreated controls (42.2% vs. 14.5%; $p<0.001$) (Cengel and Akyol, 2006).

In conclusion, atopic status should be evaluated in recurrent or chronic OME patients who had no response to antibiotic therapy and INS could be used as an adjunct to treatment of OME patients with AR. However, further studies are needed to elucidate whether atopic status or rhinitis itself may influence the development of OME.

2.4 AR and sleep disturbance

The effect of AR on sleep can impair a patient's quality of life (Canonica et al., 2007; Schatz, 2007). A nationwide controlled cross-sectional study showed that patients with AR have more difficulties in falling asleep, take more sleeping drugs, suffer from nocturnal awakenings, and feel that they do not get sufficient sleep when compared to healthy controls (Leger et al., 2006). Children with AR can experience micro-arousal during their sleep and irregular breathing.

A prospective study of 39 children with habitual snoring revealed that 14 subjects (36%) showed sensitivity to allergens (McColley et al., 1997), which is higher than expected for the general pediatric population. Based on subjective criteria, sleep apnea syndrome has also been found to be more prevalent in AR than in controls (Leger et al., 2006). The reasons for poor sleep in AR are not clearly understood, but may be related, at least in part, to nasal congestion (Meltzer, 2004). Several studies have shown the relationships between AR and nasal obstruction and abnormal breathing during sleep, snoring and sleep apnea (Scharf and Cohen, 1998; Young et al., 1997).

The impact of the severity of rhinitis on quality of life including sleep, daily activities, and work performance was shown to be stronger than the duration of rhinitis (Bousquet et al., 2006). Another study showed that the severity of rhinitis, but not its frequency, was significant factors for severe insomnia, hypersomnia, respiratory arrest, apnea, sleepiness, and regular use of sedatives (Leger et al., 2006). Recently, we are conducting multi-center cohort study on the complication of rhinitis in Korean children. All patients were classified into 4 categories (intermittent mild, intermittent moderate to severe, persistent mild and persistent moderate to severe) using ARIA classification, and Korean version of Obstructive Sleep Apnea 18 (KOSA-18) questionnaire were performed. High KOSA-18 scores mean more sleep disturbance. In our cohort study, the preliminary results (n=999) showed that sleep disturbance was more frequent according to the ARIA classification (Fig. 5) and there were no differences between atopic and nonatopic patients (48.7±17.5 vs. 51.1±19.7, p=0.120) (unpublished data).

In these groups, after the treatment of rhinitis, KOSA-18 scores at 6 months were lower than those of baseline; sleep disturbance were improved after the 6-month follow-up (Fig. 6).

AR appears to increase the risk of obstructive sleep apnea syndrome (OSAS) in children. Adequate treatment of AR can reduce the severity of OSAS and prevent the emergence of an elongated face, which predisposes patients to OSAS. It may also reduce the severity of coexisting OSAS.

3. Psychosocial comorbidities

3.1 AR and cognitive disorder

AR leads to psychosocial complications such as cognitive impairment and learning problems as well as physical complications. Young people, with and without treatment, were given the task, during the ongoing pollen season, to learn about agriculture in desert environments. The results showed that individuals receiving placebo or sedative antihistamines performed significantly worse than healthy controls (Vuurman et al., 1993). In another study, patients allergic to ragweed have impaired cognitive learning during the pollen season and some also had memory impairment (Marshall et al., 2000). It was also shown that patients with AR symptoms take a longer time to make decisions and have a slower psychomotor rate than healthy control subjects.

However, it is under debate whether AR itself does or does not lead to learning problems among allergic students. Resultant symptoms, such as sleep deprivation and general malaise can affect concentration and learning. Consequently, this theory argues that cognitive difficulties are a secondary result of sleep problems.

The consequences of AR effect on learning and other cognitive functions in relation to school performance have been established. A case-control study was conducted on 1,834 students sitting for the national examinations in mathematics, English and science (Walker et al., 2007). Those who had allergic symptoms during the examination period had a 40% higher risk of achieving lower grades than students who did not have symptoms.

Children with AR may fall behind in classes. Sniffling, rubbing and blowing the nose are more common among children with AR than those without. These behaviors make children self-conscious and peers may be annoyed by them, leading to teasing and a further increase in their stress levels (Meltzer, 2001) and may cause behavioral disorders. Thus, adequate treatment of AR should be needed, especially in school children.

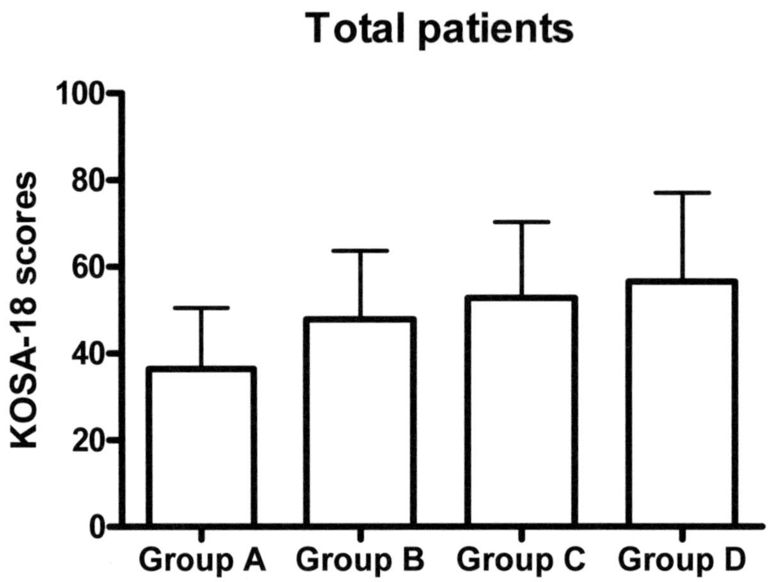

(a) Total patients

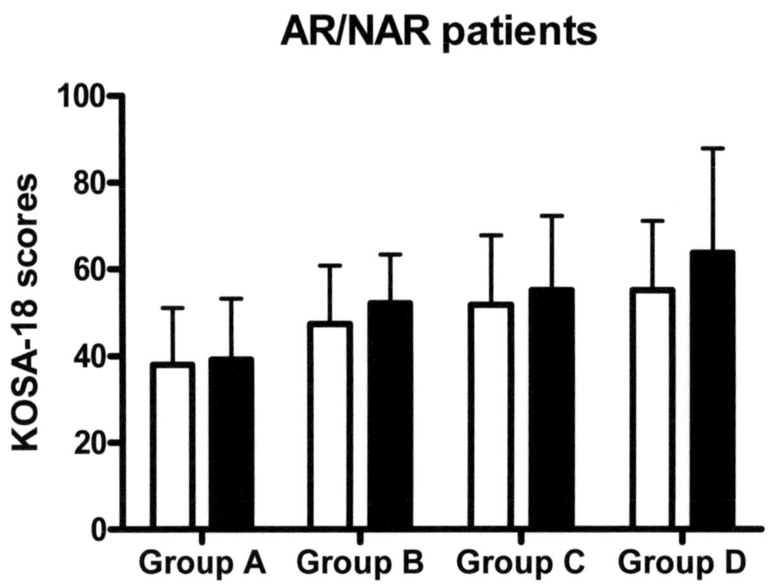

(b) AR/NAR patients

Fig. 5. Mean differences of KOSA-18 scores according to ARIA classification among (a) total patients and (b) allergic rhinitis (AR)/non allergic rhinitis (NAR) patients. All the data showed statistical significances ($p<0.001$, adjusted to age). Group A: intermittent mild, Group B: intermittent moderate to severe, Group C: persistent mild, Group D: persistent moderate to severe. □: AR patients, ■: NAR patients

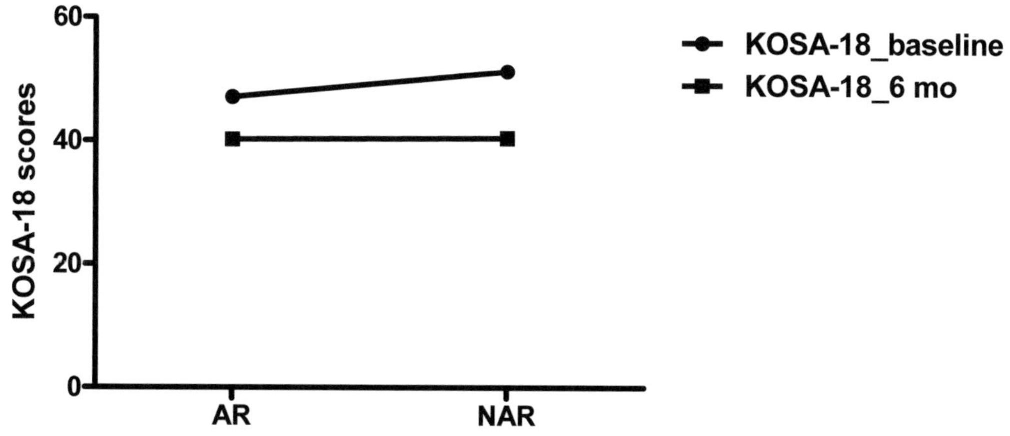

(a) KOSA-18 scores changes between AR/NAR patients

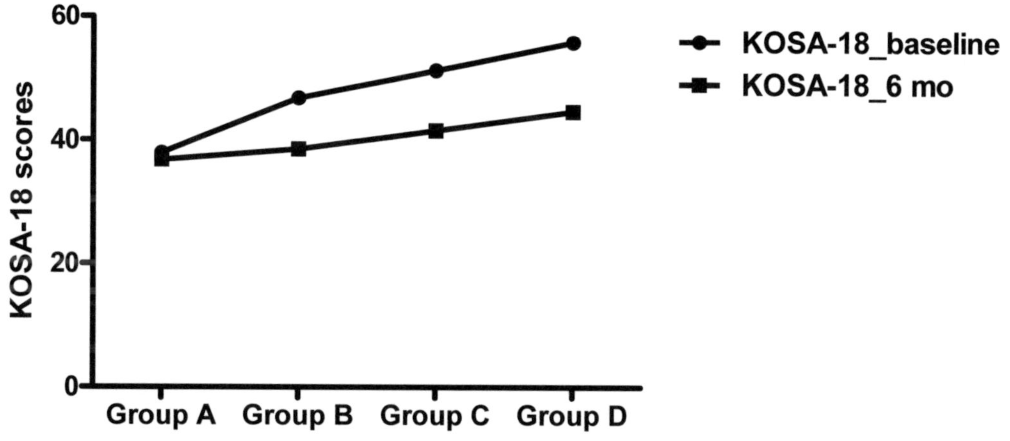

(b) KOSA-18 scores changes according to ARIA classification

Fig. 6. Mean differences of KOSA-18 scores after the treatment of rhinitis (a) between AR/NAR patients and (b) according to ARIA classification. Group A: intermittent mild, Group B: intermittent moderate to severe, Group C: persistent mild, Group D: persistent moderate to severe.

3.2 AR and missing school or work

AR has considerable negative effects on both school-aged children and adult workers. Especially in school-aged children, it can not only affect sleep and cognitive function, but also cause school absenteeism and presenteeism. Untreated AR in childhood could cause sleep disturbances and daytime sleepiness, absenteeism and presenteeism (inattention, distraction, lack of concentration), irritability and mood disorders (Jauregui et al., 2009). In terms of adult workers, a previous study in the US evaluated economic impact of workplace productivity losses due to AR (Lamb et al., 2006). A total of 8,267 US employees at 47 employer locations volunteered to participate in health/wellness screenings. AR was the most prevalent; 55% of employees reported AR symptoms for an average of 52.5 days, were absent 3.6 days per year. The mean total productivity losses (absenteeism+presenteeism) were 593 US dollars for AR, 518 dollars for high stress, 277 dollars for migraine, 273 dollars for depression, 269 dollars for arthritis/rheumatism, 248 dollars for anxiety disorder, 181 dollars for respiratory infections, 105 dollars for hypertension, 95 dollars for diabetes, 85 dollars for asthma, and 40 dollars for coronary heart disease. Thus, the authors suggested that allergies are major contributors to the total cost of health-related absenteeism and presenteeism.

4. Conclusion

AR has a considerable effect on one's quality of life and can have significant consequences if left untreated. The consequences are more far-reaching than expected. Because all the possible comorbidities of AR have significant consequences to the community, it is fair to say that physicians and patients should pay close attention to prevent the occurrence of comorbidities. Furthermore, the adequate treatment of AR could prevent physical and psychosocial complications.

5. References

Adams RJ, Fuhlbrigge AL, Finkelstein JA, Weiss ST. Intranasal steroids and the risk of emergency department visits for asthma. *J Allergy Clin Immunol* 2002;109:636-42.

Ahmad N, Zacharek MA. Allergic rhinitis and rhinosinusitis. *Otolaryngol Clin North Am* 2008;41:267-81, v.

Ahn Y, An SY, Won TB et al. Nasal polyps: An independent risk factor for bronchial hyperresponsiveness in patients with allergic rhinitis. *Am J Rhinol Allergy* 2010;24:359-63.

Alles R, Parikh A, Hawk L, Darby Y, Romero JN, Scadding G. The prevalence of atopic disorders in children with chronic otitis media with effusion. *Pediatr Allergy Immunol* 2001;12:102-6.

Bachert C, van Cauwenberge P, Khaltaev N. Allergic rhinitis and its impact on asthma. In collaboration with the World Health Organization. Executive summary of the workshop report. 7-10 December 1999, Geneva, Switzerland. *Allergy* 2002;57:841-55.

Baraniuk JN. Pathogenesis of allergic rhinitis. *J Allergy Clin Immunol* 1997;99:S763-72.

Bhattacharyya N, Vyas DK, Fechner FP, Gliklich RE, Metson R. Tissue eosinophilia in chronic sinusitis: quantification techniques. *Arch Otolaryngol Head Neck Surg* 2001;127:1102-5.

Bousquet J, Van Cauwenberge P, Khaltaev N. Allergic rhinitis and its impact on asthma. *J Allergy Clin Immunol* 2001;108:S147-334.

Bousquet J, Vignola AM, Demoly P. Links between rhinitis and asthma. *Allergy* 2003;58:691-706.

Bousquet J, Neukirch F, Bousquet PJ et al. Severity and impairment of allergic rhinitis in patients consulting in primary care. *J Allergy Clin Immunol* 2006;117:158-62.

Bousquet J, Khaltaev N, Cruz AA et al. Allergic Rhinitis and its Impact on Asthma (ARIA) 2008 update (in collaboration with the World Health Organization, GA(2)LEN and AllerGen). *Allergy* 2008;63 Suppl 86:8-160.

Caffarelli C, Savini E, Giordano S, Gianlupi G, Cavagni G. Atopy in children with otitis media with effusion. *Clin Exp Allergy* 1998;28:591-6.

Canonica GW, Bousquet J, Mullol J, Scadding GK, Virchow JC. A survey of the burden of allergic rhinitis in Europe. *Allergy* 2007;62 Suppl 85:17-25.

Cengel S, Akyol MU. The role of topical nasal steroids in the treatment of children with otitis media with effusion and/or adenoid hypertrophy. *Int J Pediatr Otorhinolaryngol* 2006;70:639-45.

Choi SH, Yoo Y, Yu J, Rhee CS, Min YG, Koh YY. Bronchial hyperresponsiveness in young children with allergic rhinitis and its risk factors. *Allergy* 2007;62:1051-6.

Christodoulopoulos P, Cameron L, Durham S, Hamid Q. Molecular pathology of allergic disease. II: Upper airway disease. *J Allergy Clin Immunol* 2000;105:211-23.

Ciprandi G, Cirillo I, Pistorio A, La Grutta S, Tosca M. Impact of allergic rhinitis on asthma: effects on bronchodilation testing. *Ann Allergy Asthma Immunol* 2008;101:42-6.

Conner BL, Roach ES, Laster W, Georgitis JW. Magnetic resonance imaging of the paranasal sinuses: frequency and type of abnormalities. *Ann Allergy* 1989;62:457-60.

Crystal-Peters J, Neslusan C, Crown WH, Torres A. Treating allergic rhinitis in patients with comorbid asthma: the risk of asthma-related hospitalizations and emergency department visits. *J Allergy Clin Immunol* 2002;109:57-62.

Doyle WJ, Friedman R, Fireman P, Bluestone CD. Eustachian tube obstruction after provocative nasal antigen challenge. *Arch Otolaryngol* 1984;110:508-11.

Ebert CS, Jr., Rose AS, Blanks DA et al. Immune modulatory oligonucleotides in prevention of nasal allergen-induced Eustachian tube dysfunction in rats. *Otolaryngol Head Neck Surg* 2007;137:250-5.

Fireman P. Otitis media and nasal disease: a role for allergy. *J Allergy Clin Immunol* 1988;82:917-26.

Gaugris S, Sazonov-Kocevar V, Thomas M. Burden of concomitant allergic rhinitis in adults with asthma. *J Asthma* 2006;43:1-7.

Griffin GH, Flynn C, Bailey RE, Schultz JK. Antihistamines and/or decongestants for otitis media with effusion (OME) in children. *Cochrane Database Syst Rev* 2006:CD003423.

Guerra S, Sherrill DL, Martinez FD, Barbee RA. Rhinitis as an independent risk factor for adult-onset asthma. *J Allergy Clin Immunol* 2002;109:419-25.

Gwaltney JM, Jr., Jones JG, Kennedy DW. Medical management of sinusitis: educational goals and management guidelines. The International Conference on sinus Disease. *Ann Otol Rhinol Laryngol Suppl* 1995;167:22-30.

Hurst DS. Association of otitis media with effusion and allergy as demonstrated by intradermal skin testing and eosinophil cationic protein levels in both middle ear effusions and mucosal biopsies. *Laryngoscope* 1996;106:1128-37.

Jauregui I, Mullol J, Davila I et al. Allergic rhinitis and school performance. *J Investig Allergol Clin Immunol* 2009;19 Suppl 1:32-9.

Kaufman J, Chen JC, Wright GW. The effect of trigeminal resection on reflex bronchoconstriction after nasal and nasopharyngeal irritation in man. *Am Rev Respir Dis* 1970;101:768-9.

Kennedy DW. Prognostic factors, outcomes and staging in ethmoid sinus surgery. *Laryngoscope* 1992;102:1-18.

Lamb CE, Ratner PH, Johnson CE et al. Economic impact of workplace productivity losses due to allergic rhinitis compared with select medical conditions in the United States from an employer perspective. *Curr Med Res Opin* 2006;22:1203-10.

Leger D, Annesi-Maesano I, Carat F et al. Allergic rhinitis and its consequences on quality of sleep: An unexplored area. *Arch Intern Med* 2006;166:1744-8.

Leynaert B, Neukirch F, Demoly P, Bousquet J. Epidemiologic evidence for asthma and rhinitis comorbidity. *J Allergy Clin Immunol* 2000;106:S201-5.

Luong A, Roland PS. The link between allergic rhinitis and chronic otitis media with effusion in atopic patients. *Otolaryngol Clin North Am* 2008;41:311-23, vi.

Marshall PS, O'Hara C, Steinberg P. Effects of seasonal allergic rhinitis on selected cognitive abilities. *Ann Allergy Asthma Immunol* 2000;84:403-10.

McColley SA, Carroll JL, Curtis S, Loughlin GM, Sampson HA. High prevalence of allergic sensitization in children with habitual snoring and obstructive sleep apnea. *Chest* 1997;111:170-3.

Meltzer EO. Quality of life in adults and children with allergic rhinitis. *J Allergy Clin Immunol* 2001;108:S45-53.

Meltzer EO. Introduction: Stuffy is also related to Sleepy and Grumpy--the link between rhinitis and sleep-disordered breathing. *J Allergy Clin Immunol* 2004;114:S133-4.

Meltzer EO. The relationships of rhinitis and asthma. *Allergy Asthma Proc* 2005;26:336-40.

Nguyen LH, Manoukian JJ, Sobol SE et al. Similar allergic inflammation in the middle ear and the upper airway: evidence linking otitis media with effusion to the united airways concept. *J Allergy Clin Immunol* 2004;114:1110-5.

O'Connor RD, Ort H, Leong AB, Cook DA, Street D, Hamburger RN. Tympanometric changes following nasal antigen challenge in children with allergic rhinitis. *Ann Allergy* 1984;53:468-71.

Osur SL, Volovitz B, Dickson S, Enck DC, Bernstein JM. Eustachian tube dysfunction in children with ragweed hayfever during natural pollen exposure. *Allergy Proc* 1989;10:133-9.

Pelikan Z, Pelikan-Filipek M. Role of nasal allergy in chronic maxillary sinusitis--diagnostic value of nasal challenge with allergen. *J Allergy Clin Immunol* 1990;86:484-91.

Rosenfeld RM, Mandel EM, Bluestone CD. Systemic steroids for otitis media with effusion in children. *Arch Otolaryngol Head Neck Surg* 1991;117:984-9.

Savolainen S. Allergy in patients with acute maxillary sinusitis. *Allergy* 1989;44:116-22.

Scharf MB, Cohen AP. Diagnostic and treatment implications of nasal obstruction in snoring and obstructive sleep apnea. *Ann Allergy Asthma Immunol* 1998;81:279-87; quiz 87-90.

Schatz M. A survey of the burden of allergic rhinitis in the USA. *Allergy* 2007;62 Suppl 85:9-16.

Settipane RJ, Hagy GW, Settipane GA. Long-term risk factors for developing asthma and allergic rhinitis: a 23-year follow-up study of college students. *Allergy Proc* 1994;15:21-5.

Shaaban R, Zureik M, Soussan D et al. Rhinitis and onset of asthma: a longitudinal population-based study. *Lancet* 2008;372:1049-57.

Shekelle P, Takata G, Chan LS et al. Diagnosis, natural history, and late effects of otitis media with effusion. *Evid Rep Technol Assess (Summ)* 2002:1-5.

Slavin RG. Complications of allergic rhinitis: implications for sinusitis and asthma. *J Allergy Clin Immunol* 1998;101:S357-60.

Sobol SE, Taha R, Schloss MD et al. T(H)2 cytokine expression in atopic children with otitis media with effusion. *J Allergy Clin Immunol* 2002;110:125-30.

Spector SL. Overview of comorbid associations of allergic rhinitis. *J Allergy Clin Immunol* 1997;99:S773-80.

Thomas CL, Simpson S, Butler CC, van der Voort JH. Oral or topical nasal steroids for hearing loss associated with otitis media with effusion in children. *Cochrane Database Syst Rev* 2006;3:CD001935.

Tomonaga K, Kurono Y, Mogi G. The role of nasal allergy in otitis media with effusion. A clinical study. *Acta Otolaryngol Suppl* 1988;458:41-7.

Tos M. Epidemiology and natural history of secretory otitis. *Am J Otol* 1984;5:459-62.

Tracy JM, Demain JG, Hoffman KM, Goetz DW. Intranasal beclomethasone as an adjunct to treatment of chronic middle ear effusion. *Ann Allergy Asthma Immunol* 1998;80:198-206.

Vuurman EF, van Veggel LM, Uiterwijk MM, Leutner D, O'Hanlon JF. Seasonal allergic rhinitis and antihistamine effects on children's learning. *Ann Allergy* 1993;71: 121-6.

Walker S, Khan-Wasti S, Fletcher M, Cullinan P, Harris J, Sheikh A. Seasonal allergic rhinitis is associated with a detrimental effect on examination performance in United Kingdom teenagers: case-control study. *J Allergy Clin Immunol* 2007;120:381-7.

Watson WT, Becker AB, Simons FE. Treatment of allergic rhinitis with intranasal corticosteroids in patients with mild asthma: effect on lower airway responsiveness. *J Allergy Clin Immunol* 1993;91:97-101.

Williamson IG, Dunleavey J, Bain J, Robinson D. The natural history of otitis media with effusion--a three-year study of the incidence and prevalence of abnormal tympanograms in four South West Hampshire infant and first schools. *J Laryngol Otol* 1994;108:930-4.

Young T, Finn L, Kim H. Nasal obstruction as a risk factor for sleep-disordered breathing. The University of Wisconsin Sleep and Respiratory Research Group. *J Allergy Clin Immunol* 1997;99:S757-62.

12

Allergy and Benign Lesions of the Vocal Cord Mucosa

Alenka Kravos
University Clinical Centre Maribor, Slovenia

1. Introduction

Hoarseness is a result of the vocal cords not working properly and it can be detected by hearing. Basic and higher harmonic tones are associated with severe hoarseness, as well as noises replacing the harmonic noise. Hoarseness can also appear as a result of organic changes of the vocal cords (also caused by allergic mucosal changes) or functional disorders.

The most common organic changes of the vocal cords are polyps, nodules and Reinke's oedema (1). Under a microscope they share many common characteristics of mucosal changes and indicate pathological changes in the superficial layer of the lamina propria, in the so-called Reinke's space (2). The main changes include: fluid oedema, elevated interstitial and exudative proteins, dilated or hypertrophic vein walls. The aetiology of the benign changes is, however, slightly different although the changes in the lamina propria are quite similar. The most common cause is trauma (phonotrauma), exposure to unfavourable microclimate conditions, smoking, voice overuse or incorrect vocal technique, hormonal changes, and allergy (3).

Reinke's oedema is a swelling of vocal cords that mostly occurs bilaterally. It is a chronic benign condition. On examination a transparent, sometimes a pink swelling is seen along the length and on the upper side of the vocal cord. As long as the swelling remains small, the vocal cords can vibrate normally. However, as the oedema grows and therefore changes the biomechanics of the larynx, the functional impairment of the phonation appears, vocal cords do not vibrate appropriately and the voice becomes low-pitched and hoarse.

Histologically, the mucosa is covered by a layer of normal and hyperplastic epithelium. By enlargement of the swelling, it may become atrophic. Persisting etiologic factors can cause the epithelium to thicken or become hypetrophic. Simple hyperplasia is the most common form of the epithelial changes due to hypertrophy (1).

A polyp is a mucosal thickness usually found at the front midpoint of the vocal cord. It is most commonly thought to be caused by vocal overuse or incorrect vocal technique. It is very similar to the Reinke's oedema, except that the polyp is localised.

Of all the benign oedematous vocal cord lesions, nodules are the smallest and by aetiology similar to polyps. The oedema is modified as in Reinke's oedema or polyps.

2. Allergy and Reinke's edema

There is a lack of research on aetiologic factors such as allergies, allergic inflammation, and hormonal changes. We became suspicious of their influence over oedematous changes of the mucosa only on the basis of our clinical experience. Pathohistological examination did not reveal any pathognomonic changes of the mucosa neither during an allergy nor during hormonal changes. The changes of the lamina propria in Reinke's oedema, polyps and nodules are nearly the same: oedema with interstitial proteins (collagen, elastane), fibroblasts, intercellular substance (glycoproteins and proteoglycans), dilated vessels, thickened basal membrane. The number of inflammatory cells in the lamina propria in the tissue samples of patients with and without allergy was the same: individual monocytes are visible (4).
Reinke's oedema patients are not more allergy-prone compared to normal population. A study carried out among ENT outpatient clinic patients with Reinke's oedema showed that the frequency of allergy was 20%, which complies with the number of allergies among normal population (5).

3. Hypersensitivity skin tests and Reinke's edema

On the basis of history we determined how many patients with Reinke's edema (N=80) suspected on possible hypersensitiveness. Only in five cases patients noticed changes in their voice in contact with a certain substance or in certain circumstances. In the study group there were 16 patients with clinical signs of allergy and positive allergy skin tests, and in the control group (N=80) there were 19 subjects with proven allergy type I.; this did not present a statistically significant difference (χ_c = 0,59 ; p = 0,57). 16 subjects were hypersensitive to inhalatory allergens, three among them also to food allergens (flour, eggs, fruit). Hypersensitivity to mite was the most frequently established.

4. Allergic rhinitis ena Reinke's edema

Among the patients with Reinke's edema on vocal folds (N=80) there were 28 subjects with chronic hyperplastic rhinitis (35,0%). In 11 patients with Reinke's edema and hyperplastic rhinitis allergy was proven by skin tests. In the control group there were 9 such patients with allergic rhinitis and positive skin tests. The difference in the prevalence of allergic hyperplastic rhinitis between the groups was not statistically significant (χ_c=0,06, p= 0,863).
We also compared the prevalence of allergy between the patients with RE and rhinitis, and the patients with Reinke's edema without rhinitis. Allergy skin tests were positive in the group with rhinitis and RE in 11 cases, and in the group with Reinke's edema without rhinitis in 5 subjects, what presented a statistically significant difference (χ_c= 13,29, p=0,001).

5. Thyroid disease and Reinke's edema

In the study group there were 13 patients who claimed thyroid diseases in the history: 9 subjects had enlarged thyroid gland in euthyroid state, and 4 subjects had hypothyroidism. In the control group two subjects had difficulties with the thyroid gland (one hypothyroidism, the other hyperthyroidism).

The prevalence of other risk factors for the occurrence of Reinke's edema in the study and control groups is represented in Table 1.

Etiological factor	Study group n=80	Control group n=80	P
Smoking	69	10	0.001
Thyroid diseases	13	2	0.003
Gastroesophageal reflux	38	20	0.003
Microclimate conditions	25	12	0.015
Unsuitable speaking and voice technique	21	7	0.04

Table 1. Prevalence of some risk factors for the occurrence of RE on vocal folds in the study and control groups

6. Discussion

According to the results of our study we suppose that allergy is one of the factors contributing to the occurrence of RE on vocal cords, but it is by no means a crucial one. We have established that other risk factors (smoking, unsuitable speaking habits and vocal load at work, gastroesophageal reflux, thyroid diseases) are much more frequent (5).

Allergy type I was confirmed on the basis of history, clinical examination and skin tests in 20% of patients from the study group with RE and in 23.8% of subjects from the control group; this is similar to the prevalence of allergy in general. Among general population the prevalence of allergy type I is about 20% (6). In the case that allergy type I is an important factor in the etiology of RE, an infiltration of eosinophils in the vocal cord mucosa is expected. Actually, there were no eosinophils found in the removed vocal fold mucosa in any of 10 patients who had previous surgery on vocal folds because of RE. Similar data were also reported by Hočevar-Boltežar et al. who on the basis of history and clinical data presumed the allergy as an etiologic factor in the patients with RE and other epithelial hyperplastic lesions on vocal cords, however histopathological picture of vocal cord mucosa did not confirm it (7).

In studying allergy as an etiological factor for the occurrence of epithelial hyperplastic lesions on vocal cords, we suppose that immediate hypersensitivity type I, according to Gel and Coombs, does not play a significant role, because there are other types of hypersensitivity that are much more important. Immediate hypersensitivity is easier to study because the tests are fast, easy and reliable tests for determining it. However, medical literature describes that the most notable type of allergy causing laryngeal mucosa lesions is allergy type III but this one is difficult to prove. Sometimes we can rely only on anamnestic data which present the basis for the performance of a tolerance test - a patient is exposed to a particular allergen.

It is possible that allergy type I is relevant for the occurrence of RE only in connection with the other risk factors. Despite the fact that allergy is not more frequent in the patients with RE than in the population in general, we have to consider it and decide for allergy skin tests if there is anamnestically and clinically set suspicion to allergy. This is important primarily in the patients with RE and hyperplastic rhinitis. Regarding the results of our study, allergy was the cause of rhinitis almost in 40% of patients with RE and hyperplastic rhinitis. On the basis of test results the patient will find out which allergens should be avoided.

In the patients with RE, we have found a relatively frequent occurrence of hyperplastic rhinitis (35% of the study group). It is possible that apart from allergy type I there are also other factors - above all unfavourable microclimate conditions in workplace - affecting the occurrence of rhinitis.

All authors investigating the etiology of RE agree that smoking is the main risk factor for the occurrence of RE (3). In our study, there were significantly more smokers in the study group than in the control group. Smoking was the only risk factor merely in 8 patients with RE on vocal folds, in all the others it was one of two or more simultaneously acting factors. There were also some previous researches emphasizing the importance of simultaneous acting of several risk factors (8).

In the study group we expected a greater percentage of those who incorrectly of excessively strain vocal folds while speaking. This factor was only on the fourth place among the most important etiologic causes for RE. Voice strain or incorrect speaking technique is performed by abnormal activity of the muscles participating in speaking. The fluid accumulates in the RS because of microtraumas of vocal folds' vessels, caused by greater mechanical forces during vocal folds' vibration. The mechanical stress makes the vessels more permeable because their walls degenerate faster. At indirect laryngoscopy, adduction of ventricular folds during phonation is often noticed. Their contraction pushes intersticial fluid down into the vocal fold and enlarges the edema in RS (9). Learning correct speaking and voice technique is the most important step in the treatment of RE, besides giving up smoking. It is especially important after the vocal folds' surgery for RE..

Due to limited technical possibilities in our study, we determined GER on the basis of history, and estimation of typical changes in the larynx and pharynx at indirect laryngoscopy performed with the rigid laryngoscope. The findings of the esophagogastroscopy which was carried out in less than one quarter of the patients before the inclusion in the study confirmed the diagnosis. In our study GER was significantly more often present in the study group than in the control group. Therefore, we presume that GER is an important factor in the etiology of RE on vocal folds but not the only one and not a crucial one. GER has never occurred as the only etiologic factor. It was always accompanied by at least one more risk factor for the occurrence of RE. GER causes inflammation of laryngeal mucosa, so the vessels become more fragile. Thick mucus accumulated in the posterior part of the larynx forces patients to clear their throats. Coughing represents a huge mechanical strain of vocal folds and results in their damage.

Until now, not much has been determined about the role of thyroid hormones in the occurrence of RE. The main cause for RE is most probably hypotyroidism. In 1992, Benfary performed a thorough study on assessing the thyroid function by measuring seven different parameters after indirectly stimulating the thyroid gland with TRH (thyrotropin-releasing hormone). As much as 78% of patients had pathological tests which indicated subclinical hypothyroidism (10). In our study we stated statistically significant difference between the study group and the control group regarding thyroid gland problems. The majority of subjects with thyroid gland problems had normal serum levels of TSH and thyroid hormones. During the research period only 3 subjects had increased level of TSH. According

to the findings of the endocrinologist two subjects needed treatment. Our scarce experience with the relation between hypotyroidism and RE indicate that a wider spectrum of tests (for example, thyroid stimulation test, determination of thyroid antibodies) is necessary in the estimation of thyroid function.
Laryngeal lesions in subjects working in unfavourable microclimate conditions in chemical industry were studied. Some chronic inflammatory changes on laryngeal mucosa were found also in the workers without any subjective laryngeal problems. It was supposed that the damages of the laryngeal mucosa occurred because of the irritation of chemicals or harmful concentration of inhaled dust (11). More recent studies presumed that the possible cause of laryngeal inflammation could also be an allergic reaction to chemicals and dust (12). Therefore, the laryngeal inflammation can be the consequence of immunological and non-immunological reaction to the unfavourable microclimate at work. In our study we determined only how unpleasant microclimate in workplace influences the occurrence of vocal fold swelling without getting in details. The results have shown that the subjects from the study group were significantly more often exposed to unfavourable microclimate conditions than the subjects from the control group. Patients stated constant flow of cold air in workplace as the most frequent unpleasant factor. This factor has not been stated by studies already mentioned; they even very rarely mentioned temperature changes in workplace. According to the frequency of appearance, the unpleasant microclimate factors are arranged in the following order: dust, industrial chemicals, detergents, cold air due to refrigerating chamber or air-conditioning systems, welding gases, lathe dust, cement dust, hair-dressing chemicals, and hot water steam. On the basis of our researche we claim that microclimate conditions in workplace have a significant influence on the occurrence of the vocal fold swelling. The inflammation that occurs as a consequence of their irritating effect, changes vessel walls in vocal folds. The changed vessels get more permeable after the action of mechanical forces occurring during phonation. Because almost one third of the patients with RE from our study was exposed to harmful substances or abnormal temperature in workplace, it would be useful to expand the research with the cooperation of other experts from this field. Patients with the recurrence of RE on vocal folds were also significantly more frequently exposed to unfavourable microclimate than the patients who had the first occurrence of RE.

7. Conclusion

On the basis of the results of the study we have found out that in the majority of patients with RE at least two risk factors were present simultaneously, sometimes even more. Every otorhinolaryngologist treating a patient with RE has to be aware of the interconnectedness of all the factors. He/she should think about all six factors described and exclude or confirm them with selected diagnostic procedures. The treatment has to be etiological, otherwise vocal fold swelling can also reoccur after the surgical treatment. We wish to stress that in all patients with the recurrence of RE we found at least two risk factors which undoubtedly brought up the recurrence of the disease.

8. References

[1] KambičV, Gale N. Epithelial hyperplastic lesions of the larynx. Amsterdam Elsevier 1995: 9-28.

[2] Kambič V, Gale N, Radšel Z. Die anatomische merkmale des Reike - Raumes und die Aethio-Pathogenese des Reinke-Oedems. Laryngo Rhino Otol 1989; 68: 231-5.
[3] Fuchs B. Zur pathogenese und klinik des Reinke-oedems. HNO 1989; 37: 490-5.
[4] Kahane JC. Connective tissue changes in the larynx and its effect on voice. J Voice 1987; 1: 27-30.
[5] Kravos A, Boltežar Hočevar I, Čizmarevič B, Župevc A. The role of allergy in the etiology of Reinke9s edema on vocal folds. Wien Klin Wochenschr 2010; 122 Suppl 2: 44-8.
[6] Corey JP, Gungor A, Karnell M. Allergy for the laryngologist. Otolaryngol Clin North Am 1998; 31: 189-205.
[7] Hočevar-Boltežar I, Radšel Z, Žargi M. The role of allergy in the etiopathogenesis of laryngeal mucosal lesions. Acta Otolaryngol (Stockh) 1997; Suppl 527: 134-7.
[8] Wirchow R. The basement membrane in diseases of the vocal cords: electron microscopy and immunomorphologic findings. Laryngorhinootologie 1994; 73: 642-6.
[9] Coombs RRA, Gel PGH. The classification of allergic reactions. Malbry RL, Faoa F. Otolaryngic Allergy. Otolaryngol Clin North Am 1992; 25: 159-60.
[10] Benfari G, Carluccio F, Murgiano S, Lentini A. Thyroid gland stimulation test in Reinke's edema. A study of 28 patients. An Otolaryngolog Ibero Am 1992; 19: 485-91.
[11] Raabe J, Paschler W. Das Reinke-eodem. Eine untersuchung zu fragen der aetiologie, der prognose und der wirksamkeit terapeutischer interventionen. Laryngo Rhino Otol 1999; 78: 97-101.
[12] Tee RD. Allergens in workplace. In: Kay AB. Basic clinical allergy. Bailere Tindal, London 1987: 865-901.

13

Drug Hypersensitivity

María L. Sanz[1], Cristobalina Mayorga[2],
Ruben Martínez-Aranguren[1] and Pedro M. Gamboa[3]
[1]*Departamento de Alergología e Inmunología Clínica, Clínica Universidad de Navarra,*
[2]*Unidad de Investigación, Hospital Carlos Haya, Malaga,*
[3]*Servicio de Alergia, Hospital Basurto, Bilbao,*
Spain

1. Introduction

The in vitro diagnosis of allergic reactions to drugs is of particular interest to clinicians, as neither the clinical history nor the in vivo tests are fully conclusive. In addition, these tests may often be associated with risk, as occurs with the drug provocation test. Various different in vitro tests are available for the evaluation of drug hypersensitivity depending on the immunological mechanism involved, either IgE mediated or T cell mediated.

For IgE-mediated reactions, the determination of serum-specific IgE, antigen-specific histamine release and sulphidoleukotriene production after in vitro stimulation of effector cells, as well as analysis of the activation markers of these cells (the basophil activation test), provide greater diagnostic precision.

Serum-specific IgE assays are still the most common in vitro method for evaluating immediate reactions. However, either there is no great commercial availability of fixed drugs for this study, with the exception of antibiotics (penicillin G and V, ampicillin, amoxicillin and cefaclor), a few muscle relaxants and certain substances, like insulins and ACTH. The most validated immunoassay, ImmunoCAP (Phadia, Uppsala, Sweden), has been widely used to evaluate immediate reactions to beta-lactams, mainly penicillins, with a specificity approaching 90% and a sensitivity of up to 50% (Blanca et al., 2001; Sanz et al., 2002a)

The in vitro study of the cell response in non-immediate reactions mainly assesses the T-cell response. A cellular response involving drug-related T-cell activity may be assessed in vitro by means of both the lymphocyte transformation test (LTT) (Pichler & Tilch, 2004) and the flow cytometric lymphocyte activation test, based on upregulation of the activation marker CD69 (Beeler et al., 2008). The combination of these tests with an assay of the production of drug-specific cytokines (e.g., IFN-g, IL-2, IL-5, IL-8 and IL-12) can increase the sensitivity and specificity to 48% and 82%, respectively (Romano et al., 2011; Rozieres et al., 2009a).

2. Cellular tests for the diagnosis of immediate type drug hypersensitivity reactions

2.1 The Basophil activation test

The in vitro diagnosis of drug allergies has advanced much over recent years, mainly due to the incorporation of new technologies, such as flow cytometry, which permits the analysis of various types of cells, even when they are poorly represented in peripheral blood, as is the case with basophils. These cells are a useful model for the study of IgE-mediated reactions, as they are effectors of the reactions (Schleimer et al., 1985).

Basophils are able to release the content of their granules (either preformed mediators, like histamine, or formed de novo, like sulphidoleukotrienes) after antigen-specific activation. In addition, after this process they express, or overexpress, activation molecules on their membranes (Fig. 1).

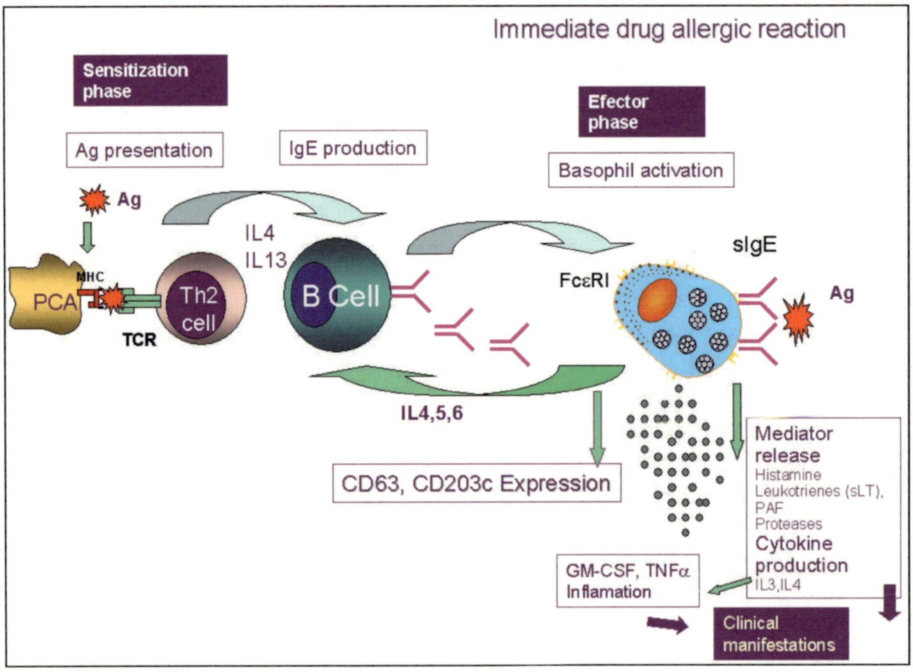

Fig. 1. Immune response in Immediate drug allergic reaction.

The basophil activation test (BAT) is based on the identification of basophils by labelling with monoclonal antibodies against different molecules, such as the IgE receptor, anti-CD 123 (IL-3 receptor) and fluorochrome-labelled anti-HLA-DR or anti-CCR3. This strategy, coupled with the identification of cell activation markers, such as CD63 or CD 203c, enables the comparison of cell activation before and after in vitro antigen-specific stimulation (Sanz et al., 2002b). Parallel to this process there is production of mediators, such as sulphidoleukotrienes that can be quantified simultaneously.

The CD63 molecule is a tetraspan, 53 kDa granular protein that is expressed not only on basophil granules but also on monocytes, macrophages and platelets. The expression of this marker correlates with degranulation and histamine release, which makes it an ideal marker of basophil activation (De Weck et al., 2008).

For in vitro stimulation with allergen, the peripheral blood cells are incubated with the suspected allergen for 15-40 minutes at 37ºC (Fig. 2).

After stopping the reaction, the cells are labelled with anti-CD63-PE and anti-IgE-FITC monoclonal antibodies. Two controls are used: a negative control in which the cells are incubated with the stimulation buffer used in the assay and that often contains IL-3 (negative control alias basal stimulation); as a positive control, an anti-IgE or an anti-IgE receptor antibody can be used (Sanz et al., 2008) (Fig. 3). The results are analised through flow cytometry (Fig. 4).

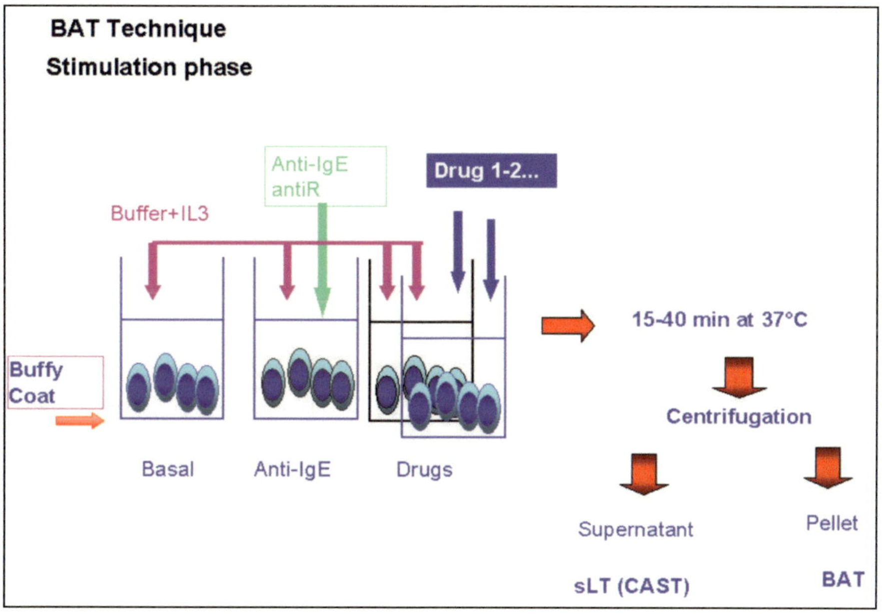

Fig. 2. Basophil activation test. Stimulation phase.

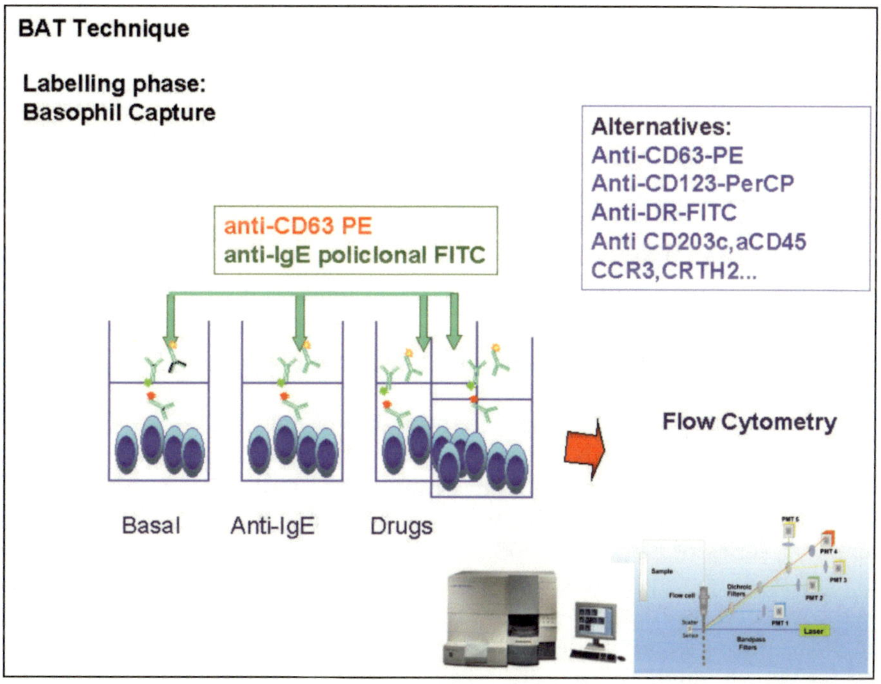

Fig. 3. Basophil activation test. Labelling phase.

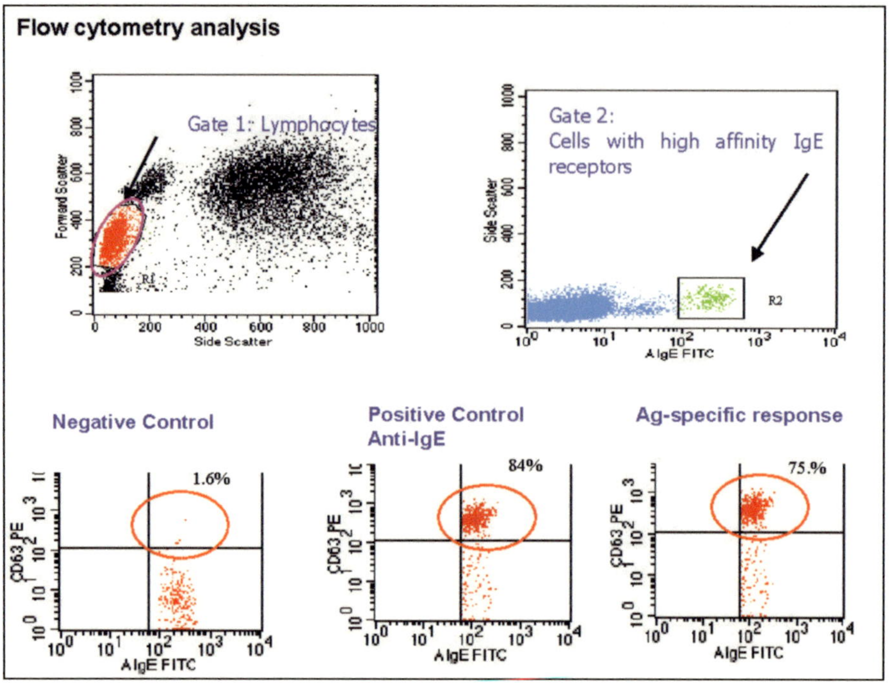

Fig. 4. Flow cytometry analysis.

Numerous studies over recent years have shown the usefulness of this technique for the in vitro diagnosis of allergic diseases (Ebo et al., 2006a, 2004a; Kleine-Tebbe et al., 2006) involving different allergens, such as inhalants (Paris-Köhler et al., 2000; Sanz et al., 2001; Saporta et al., 2001), hymenoptera venoms (Sabbah et al., 1998; Sainte-Laudy et al., 2000), or latex (Ebo et al., 2002; Sanz et al., 2003). For the diagnosis of allergy to drugs like muscle relaxants (Abuaf et al., 1999; Monneret et al., 2002), betalactam antibiotics (Sanz et al., 2001b, 2002a; Torres et al., 2004), pyrazolones (Sabbah et al., 1997; Sanz et al., 2005) and non steroidal anti-inflammatory drugs (NSAIDs) (Gamboa et al., 2004) BAT has opened up an important diagnostic pathway, either on its own or combined with other techniques (de Weck et al., 2008b; Gamboa et al., 2003a), allowing avoidance of challenge tests in an important number of cases (Hausmann et al., 2009; Romano et al., 2011; Sanz et al., 2009).

2.1.1 Basophil activation test and sulphidoleukotriene production in immediate type allergic reactions to beta-lactams

We studied the reliability of BAT, the determination of specific IgE by CAP (CAP-FEIA, Phadia, Uppsala, Sweden) and the production of leukotrienes after antigen-specific stimulation using the Cellular Antigen Stimulation Test (CAST ELISA (Bühlmann Laboratories, Allschwill, Switzerland) for the in vitro diagnosis of immediate allergy to betalactams in a series of 81 patients (58 patients with positive and 23 with negative skin tests) and in 30 healthy controls (Gamboa et al., 2004b; Sanz et al., 2001b, 2002a). Our results, as well as those found by Torres et al (Torres et al., 2004), showed that the sensitivity of BAT in the diagnosis of immediate hypersensitivity reactions to beta-lactams was 50%, and the specificity 93.3%, although there were certain differences depending on the technique applied (e.g., use of total blood or isolated cells) (de Weck et al., 2008a).

In our study (Sanz et al., 2002a) the best predictive values were obtained with BAT, in comparison with immunoassay or CAST. The positive predictive value of BAT was 18.9% and the negative predictive value 97.7%, with amoxicillin being the antibiotic with the highest predictive values. The joint use of CAP (Phadia) and BAT allowed identification of 65.2% of the betalactam allergic patients, with a specificity of 83.3% (Sanz et al., 2008).

In betalactam allergic patients with negative skin tests BAT was positive in 39.1%, CAST was positive in 22.7% with a specificity of 83.3%, and CAP showed a sensitivity of 21.7% with a specificity of 83.3%. The association of all three techniques allowed diagnosis in 60.9% of the patients of this group, with a specificity of 70% (Gamboa et al., 2004b).

Torres et al (Torres et al., 2004) studied the reliability of BAT in 70 patients with immediate allergic reactions. Like us, these authors found a greater positivity to amoxicillin (28.6%), followed by benzylpenicillin (BP) (21.7%), penicilloyl polylysine (PPL) (20%), ampicillin (12.5%) and MDM (2.2%).

They, too, reported a BAT sensitivity for cephalosporins of 77.7%. These results have since been confirmed in a multicentre study involving 181 betalactam allergic patients and 80 controls. This study concluded that the association of this technique with the determination of the production of antigen-specific sulphidoleukotrienes increases the sensitivity to 62% (de Weck et al., 2008b).

A certain lack of association exists between clinical and BAT cross-reactivity, which restricts the usefulness of this method for predicting cross-reactive responses in beta-lactam reactions. With BAT it is possible to find positive results when BP is used as the hapten in patients who are selective responders to amoxicillin (Torres et al., 2004).

2.1.2 BAT in IgE-mediated hypersensitivity reactions to quinolones

IgE-mediated hypersensitivity reactions to quinolones are a particularly difficult situation for the clinician as skin testing may induce false positive results. A recent report confirms that BAT is a useful method for diagnosing patients with confirmed immediate allergic reactions to quinolones (Aranda et al., 2011). In this study, involving 38 patients, the Sepharose-RIA technique was positive in 12 cases (31.57%), BAT in 27 (71.05%) and the combination of both tests showed positive results in 28 (73.68%). The drug most frequently involved in the reaction was moxifloxacin (63.2%), followed by ciprofloxacin (28.9%). The authors conclude that the BAT is a useful method for diagnosing patients, especially in those with severe reactions where drug provocation testing may increase the risk.

2.1.3 Basophil activation test in muscle relaxant allergic reactions

Muscle relaxants are an important group of drugs involved in 60% of adverse reactions during anaesthesia. Relevant studies have found that BAT sensitivity and specificity for muscle relaxants varied from 36% to 92% and 93% to 100%, respectively (Sudheer et al., 2005). Most of these studies reported a high specificity and a sensitivity above 50%, reaching 91% (Abuaf et al., 1999; Kvedariene et al., 2006; Laxenaire et al., 1999; Monneret et al., 2002; Moss, 1995; Stellato et al., 1991).

This sensitivity is lower (36%) when the marker CD203c is used (Sudheer et al., 2005). However, results are discordant; Kvedarine et al. (Kvedariene et al., 2006) observed in 47 patients a sensitivity of 36% and a specificity of 93% performing BAT (CD63 in whole blood). On the other hand, Ebo et al. (Ebo et al., 2006b) reported the sensitivity of a similar BAT technique to be 91.7% and the specificity 100% for rocuronium in a study including 14 patients with an anaphylactic reaction to drugs and with a positive skin test to rocuronium. However, the sensitivity apparently increases up to 80% when BAT is performed shortly after the clinical reaction (Kvedariene et al., 2006); this technique allows evaluation of the cross-reactivity between different muscle relaxants (Ebo et al., 2006b).

Leysen et al (Leysen et al., 2011) recently reported that BAT is complementary to skin testing in the assessment of cross-reactivity between rocuronium and vecuronium. In patients with negative skin tests and positive sIgE results, BAT helps in interpreting the clinical significance of a positive sIgE result.

These authors found a cross-reactivity with vecuronium in 69% of 104 curarized patients with a history of profound hypotension and severe bronchospasm immediately after induction of anaesthesia

2.1.4 Basophil activation test as a diagnostic tool for immediate radiocontrast media (RCM) hypersensitivity

A study involving 26 patients with immediate RCM reactions and 43 specimens from healthy volunteers found that the specificity of BAT ranged from 88.4% to 100%, with a sensitivity around 50% (most of the patients in this study experienced only mild skin symptoms) (Pinnobphun et al., 2011). The authors demonstrated the potential of BAT as a diagnostic tool for immediate RCM hypersensitivity, particularly as a confirmation test, with significantly higher activated basophil percentages in BAT in patients with a history of immediate RCM reactions than in normal controls. The time between the RCM reaction and the BAT in their study was rather long (1–4 years), and this time lag may have lowered BAT reactivity.

2.1.5 Basophil activation test in IgE-mediated selective reactions to NSAIDs

Until now only two articles have been published on selective NSAID reactors, patients reacting exclusively to only one NSAID family through an IgE-mediated mechanism and tolerating other NSAID groups (Gamboa et al., 2003a; Gómez et al., 2009). The first study comprised 26 patients with exclusive IgE-mediated allergy to methamizole. BAT sensitivity was 42.3% and specificity 100%. Upon adding the leukotriene release test, the sensitivity increased to 52% in the overall patient group, with a specificity of 92% (Gamboa et al., 2003a). In the second study, involving 51 patients with immediate reactions also to methamizole, the sensitivity was 54.9% but with a lower specificity, 85.71% (Gómez et al., 2009). The differences in the sensitivities and specificities may have been due to differences in the time interval between the in vitro test being performed and the reaction (16.9 versus 8 months, respectively), and the number of cases with anaphylaxis (57.5% versus 74.5%). Importantly, the BAT was positive in 38.5% of patients with negative skin tests but even more importantly, the BAT was positive in 75% of patients with anaphylaxis and negative skin tests. (Gómez et al., 2009).

BAT is the only in vitro technique currently available which allows the evaluation, with sufficiently high sensitivity and specificity values, of patients with selective IgE-mediated reactions to methamizole without the use of drug provocation tests and their associated dangers for patients. Negative BAT testing is associated with the delay to the test after the occurrence of the reaction.

2.1.6 Basophil activation test in NSAID hypersensitivity reactions

The mechanism involved in these type of reactions is not well known although it is clear that it is a non immunological mechanism.

In this first study (Gamboa et al., 2004a) in 60 patients with this syndrome the use of only 2 drugs (aspirin and diclofenac) allowed a diagnosis to be reached in 58% of these patients, with a specificity of 90%. In similar studies carried out in 43 patients with NSAID hypersensitivity (Rodríguez-Trabado et al., 2008), BAT achieved a sensitivity of 43% with a specificity of 100%. Subsequently, the European Network for Drug Allergy began a multi-centre study to validate the real usefulness of this technique (de Weck et al., 2010). However, a notable heterogeneous response in the results from each participating group in both sensitivity and specificity was observed that can be attributed to two main factors: different clinical characteristics in the study patients and technical variation between the different groups. The specificity value was notably better in those groups that used buffy coat than in those using plasma leukocytes. The lower values in sensitivity and specificity found by others increase the need for further studies. In this paper (de Weck et al., 2010), we further analyzed basophil activation in vitro in apparently normal individuals tolerating the administration of NSAIDs, in particular the specificity of these reactions and the role of technical conditions, such as the cell isolation technique. Different clinical and technical conditions may give rise to discordant results relating to NSAID hypersensitivity reactions (de Weck et al., 2009).

2.1.7 Basophil activation test in various drug-allergic reactions

Other drugs are also of interest since evaluation of allergy to drugs that cannot be studied by other in vitro techniques is interesting. BAT has proven useful for the in vitro diagnosis of such allergy-causing drugs as corticosteroids (Lehmann Ott, 2008), heparins (Caballero & Fernández-Benítez, 2003; Ebo et al., 2004b), omeprazole (Gamboa et al., 2003b), cyclosporine (Ebo et al., 2001), Gelofusine (Apostolou et al., 2006), dexchlorpheniramine (Caceres Calle & Fernández-Benítez, 2004), chlorhexidine (Ebo et al., 2006c), iodinated povidone (Le Pabic et al., 2003), hyaluronidase (Ebo et al., 2005), or bovine serum albumin (Orta et al., 2003).

2.1.8 The sensitivity of BAT for evaluating immediate allergic reactions to drugs may decrease over time

The diagnostic capacity of BAT has been shown to fall as the time increases between the clinical reaction and the test, both for allergic reactions to betalactams (where the sensitivity of BAT decreases to 12.5% one year after the reaction) (Blanca et al., 1999), and for reactions to muscle relaxants, where the sensitivity fell from 85.7% to 47.6% 4-8 years after the reaction (Abuaf et al., 1999) as well as for allergy to dipyrone, where 60% of the patients had a negative BAT 6 months after the reaction (Gómez et al., 2009), or expressed another way, if the tests are carried out within 6 months from the initial drug reaction, the efficacy of the BAT increases to 56% (Gamboa et al., 2003a). Thus, it is generally recommended to perform BAT at least two weeks after the allergic reaction but within no more than 6 months (Rodríguez Trabado et al., 2006), given that negativization of BAT does not correlate with tolerance to the drug (Antúnez et al, 2006).

In summary, BAT is a useful technique for the diagnosis of allergy to drugs, though additional validation studies are warranted.

3. Cellular tests in the diagnosis of non-immediate type drug hypersensitivity reactions

Although it has been shown that delayed reactions to drugs are mediated by effector T lymphocytes (Fernández et al, 2010) with a Th1 profile, based on the transcription factors involved and with cytokine and chemokine production (Cornejo-Garcia et al., 2007; Fernández et al., 2009; Mullen et al., 2001; Rengarajan et al., 2000), an important number of heterogeneous clinical manifestations nevertheless indicate that different mechanisms with different cell subsets and mediators may be involved (Posadas et al., 2002) (Fig. 5).

3.1 Lymphocyte transformation test

Among the in vitro tests proposed for delayed hypersensitivity reactions to drugs, the lymphocyte transformation test (LTT) was one of the earliest. However, for some years now its role in the evaluation of these reactions has been questioned. This is owing to the existence of studies reporting series with a low number of cases where many drugs were involved and the clinical entities experienced by the patients were very heterogeneous (Mayorga et al., 2006; Luque et al., 2001). However, promising results together with the need for an in vitro test are now revitalizing its use.

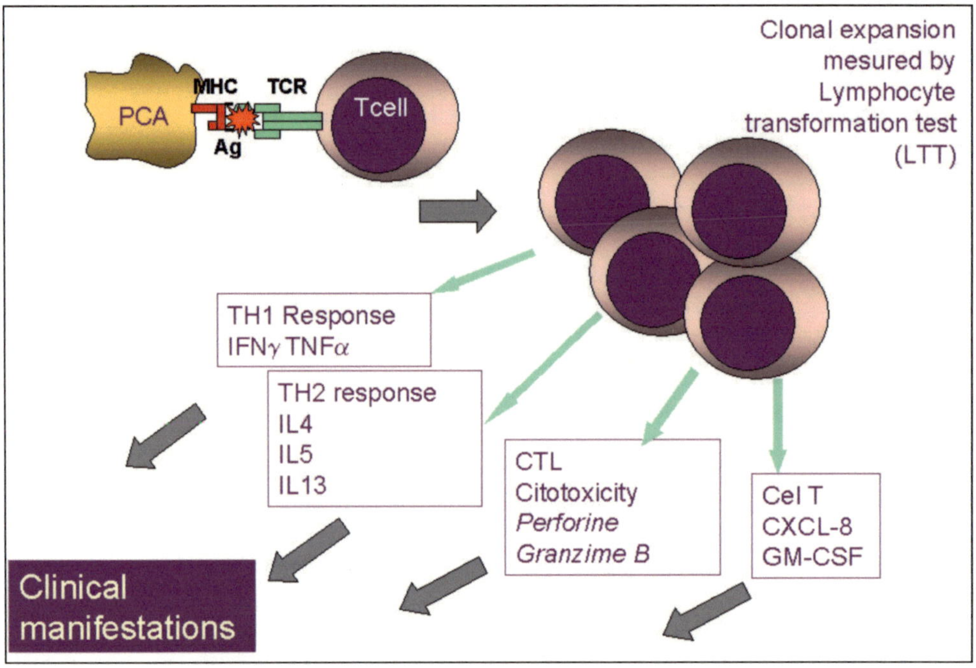

Fig. 5. Non immediate drug allergic reactions. Different profiles of T response.

The LTT enables identification of the drug involved and cross-reactivities, but it is important to take into account that a negative LTT does not always indicate the absence of a delayed reaction to the drug.

Different studies have shown the good sensitivity and specificity of the LTT, with heterogeneity in the drugs and clinical entities (Luque et al., 2001; Naisbitt et al., 2003a, 2003b; Nyfeler & Pichler, 1997; Schnyder & Pichler 2000). The most frequent drugs studied are beta-lactam antibiotics and anti-epileptics, particularly carbamazepine (Hertl et al., 1993; Luque et al., 2001; Mauri-Hellweg et al., 1995; Nyfeler & Pichler, 1997; Tapia et al., 2004; Yawalkar et al., 2000). These studies have shown an overall sensitivity of 60-70% for LTT (Lerch et al., 2007; Luque et al., 2001; Mauri-Hellweg et al., 1995; Pichler & Tilch, 2004). In the case of beta-lactams, for immediate and non immediate reactions, the sensitivity was 64.5% and 57.9%, respectively and the specificity was 92.8% (Luque et al., 2001; Pichler & Tilch, 2004). In a retrospective analysis of patients with adverse drug reactions, the LTT sensitivity was seen to depend also on the drug involved in the reaction (Nyfeler & Pichler, 1997; Roujeau et al., 1985) and the sensitivity might significantly improve when LTT is performed at the optimal time (Kano et al., 2007). This timing could vary depending on the clinical manifestations, since it has been shown that LTT should be performed within one week for patients with MPE and SJS/TEN whereas 5-8 weeks is optimal for patients with DRESS (Kano et al., 2007).

Recently, a modification of the LTT with inclusion of monocyte derived dendritic cells as antigen presenting cells has shown promising results, with higher sensitivity and specificity in delayed reactions to amoxicillin, heparins, glucocorticosteroids and contrast media, as well as providing the possibility of detecting a response over a longer period of time, preserving sensitivity to the culprit drug (Lopez S et al., 2009, 2010; Nyfeler & Pichler, 1997; Rodríguez-Pena et al., 2006).

3.2 ELISPOT

The Elispot assay is based on the detection of a cytokine caught by an immobilized antibody and revealed by a secondary antibody (Czerkinsky et al., 1988). With this method it is possible to detect different cytokines as well as cytotoxic markers released by antigen or drug stimulated cells (Beeler et al., 2006, 2008; Rozieres et al., 2009a; Zawodniak et al., 2010). This test has a high sensitivity, and is able to detect fewer than 25 secreting cells per million PBMC (Schmittel et al., 1997, 2001). The results are expressed as spot forming cells obtained from the rate between the cytokine secretion produced in the presence of the drug compared to the absence of stimulus. The Elispot assay has detected lymphocytes secreting cytokines such as IFN-γ, IL-5, IL-13 from allergic patients in the presence of the culprit drug. Recently, this test has been used to determine the release of the granule content (granzymes and perforin) by cytotoxic cells after activation with the culprit drug (Zawodniak et al, 2010). The test showed a high sensitivity and specificity, although in some cases no correlation with LTT results was found, probably because cytotoxicity-based tests measure effector cell function, which is distinct from proliferative response.

The secretion of cytokines (IFN-γ) or cytotoxic granules (Granzyme B) has been detected in vitro in response to the culprit drug in allergic patients but not in tolerant subjects (Rozieres et al., 2009a; Zawodniak et al., 2010), demonstrating that the Elispot can be a complementary method to evaluate delayed reactions to drugs.

3.3 Monitoring delayed reaction to drugs

Another approach for the in vitro evaluation of delayed reactions to drugs is the follow-up of the immunopathological response by performing serial determinations in peripheral blood and the affected skin, from the acute phase to basal conditions (Mayorga et al., 2006). This enables an idea of the underlying process to be built up, not only in the development and progress of the reaction but also related to the degree of response to treatment (Mayorga et al., 2003). These reactions involve not only different cell populations but also activation markers, signalling molecules, cytokines, chemokines and transcription factors. These are all assessed and it is important to determine the changes in the different markers rather than their quantification *per se*.

Among the available methods the most widely used are flow cytometry and mRNA gene expression by real time PCR. These methodologies provide important information about the immunological mechanisms involved, since different clinical manifestations like urticaria, MPE, DRESS, AGEP, FDE or TEN are produced by different cell subsets contributing to each particular entity. Different authors have shown that $CD4^+$ T lymphocytes are mainly involved in MPE, DRESS, and AGEP (Fernandez et al., 2009; 1995; Hertl et al., 1993; Mauri-Hellweg et al., 1995; Pichler, 2003; Schnyder et al., 2000; Shiora & Muzukawa, 2007; Torres et al., 2006, 2009; Whittam et al., 2000; Zedlitz et al., 2002), whereas $CD8^+$ T lymphocytes are the effector cells in FDE and TEN (Alanko et al., 1987; Chung et al., 2008; Nassif et al., 2002, 2004a). Although other studies indicate that both $CD4^+$ and $CD8^+$ T lymphocytes may be involved in TEN (Torres et al., 2006) and $CD8^+$ T cells have been found in the epidermis of non bullous lesions including MPE (Rozieres et al., 2009b).
These cells become activated and express high levels of CD25, CD69, CD71 and HLA-DR (Leyva et al., 2000; Mayorga et al., 2003; Nishio et al., 2007; Shiohara & Mizukawa, 2007; Torres et al., 2008). Apart from activation, different chemokine and chemokine receptors involved in cell recruitment to the affected organ, mainly the skin, can also be analyzed. Thus, an increase in the expression of cutaneous lymphocyte-associated antigen (CLA), a skin homing receptor in delayed reactions to drugs, correlates with disease severity (Blanca et al., 2000; Mullen et al., 2001; Torres et al., 2006). In a study in patients with drug-induced MPE, an increase in the expression of Th1 chemokines (CXCL9 and CXCL10) and their specific receptor CXCR3, as well as in the expression of the cutaneous homing chemokines (CCL17, CCL20, and CCL27) and their receptors (CCR4, CCR6, CCR10), with high production of TNF-α and IFN-γ, was found at the acute phase of the reaction (Fernandez et al., 2008). In MPE or DRESS an increase has also been found in IL-5 and chemokines such as RANTES and eotaxins, which explains the involvement of eosinophils expressing CCR3 (Hertl et al., 1993). In AGEP, another severe delayed drug-induced reaction, lymphocytes have a dual role as cytotoxic agents and inducing migration of neutrophils to the skin by producing IL-8 (Britschgi & Pichler, 2002; Hertl et al., 1993; Padial et al., 2004; Yawalkar et al., 2000). At the acute phase of TEN, T cells are recruited to the skin, producing cytotoxic markers such as perforin and granzyme B (Fernandez et al., 2010; Mayorga et al., 2003; Pichler, 2003; Posadas et al., 2002; Torres et al., 2006; Zawodniak et al., 2010), and they express high levels of CCR10 and their chemokine CCL27 (Tapia et al., 2004).
As mentioned, this monitoring is useful in order to understand not only the underlying mechanisms but also to assess the response to treatment. This latter was analyzed during the follow-up of TEN, where the administration of gamma globulin was associated with a rapid decrease in the cytotoxic markers (Mayorga et al., 2003).
A Th1 pattern with expression of IFN-γ, IL-12, and TNF-α and down-regulation of IL-4 has been found in delayed reactions to drugs (Cornejo-Garcia et al., 2007; Posadas et al., 2000). The polarizations also extend to the expression of transcription factors, such as T-bet in Th1 and inhibition of c-maf and GATA3 in Th2 (Cornejo-Garcia et al., 2007).

3.4 Trafficking between different organs

Since the skin is the organ most frequently affected in delayed reactions to drugs, it is possible to assess the parallel course in the two compartments, the skin (in both biopsies and blister fluid cells) and the peripheral blood. At the very early stage of the reaction, there is an increase in the blister fluid of CLA+ cells which later appear in peripheral blood, probably due to recirculation from the skin (Leyva et al., 2000; Mayorga et al., 2003). These cells also show a Th1 profile, with high production of perforin and granzyme B that correlates with the reaction and its severity (Nassif et al., 2004a; 2004b).

In patients with MPE (Fernandez et al., 2008) an increase in the expression of Th1 chemokines, including CXCL9 and CXCL10, as well as cutaneous homing chemokines such as CCL17, CCL20, and CCL27, was found only in the skin. In this study they also found a high production of TNF-α and IFN-γ as well as the presence of Th1 cytotoxic T lymphocytes in the skin. However, in the peripheral blood T lymphocytes expressing only the chemokine receptors CXCR3, CCR4, CCR6, and CCR10 were found. These data indicate that during the reaction there is recruitment of Th1 cytotoxic T lymphocytes to the skin induced by different chemokines produced by cutaneous cells (Fernandez et al., 2008).

4. Acknowledgments

MLS, PMG and CM are supported by grant RD07/0064 from the Spanish Research Network on Adverse Reactions to Allergens and Drugs (RIRAAF: Red de Investigation de Reacciones Adversas a Alérgenos y Fármacos) of the Carlos III Health Institute.

5. References

Abuaf N., Rajoely B., Ghazouani E., Levy D.A., Pecquet C., Chabane H. & Leynadier F. (1999). Validation of flow cytometry assay detecting in vitro basophil activation for the diagnosis of muscle relaxant allergy. *J Allergy Clin Immunol;* 1999; 104: 411-8.

Alanko T., Stubb S. & Reitamo S. (1987). Topical provocation of fixed drug eruption. *Br J Dermatol;* 1987, 116: 561-567.

Antúnez C., Fernández T., Blanca-Lopez N., Torres M.J., Mayorga C., Canto G., Fernández J., Moya M.C. & Blanca M. (2006) IgE antibodies to betalactams: relationship between the triggering hapten and the specificity of the immune response. *Allergy;* 61:940-6.

Apostolou E., Deckert K., Puy R., Sandrini A., de Leon M.P., Douglass J.A., Rolland J.M. & O'hehir R.E. (2006) Anaphylaxis to Gelofusine confirmed by in vitro basophil activation test: a case series. *Anaesthesia;* 61:264- 268.

Aranda A., Mayorga C., Ariza A., Doña I., Rosado A., Blanca-Lopez N., Andreu I. & Torres MJ. (2011). In vitro evaluation of IgE-mediated hypersensitivity reactions to quinolones. *Allergy;* 66(2):247-54.

Beeler A., Engler O., Gerber B.O. & Pichler WJ. (2006). Long-lasting reactivity and high frequency of drug-specific T cells after severe systemic drug hypersensitivity reactions. *J Allergy Clin Immunol;* 117:455-462.

Beeler A., Zaccaria L., Kawabata T., Gerber B.O. & Pichler W.J. (2008) CD69 upregulation on T cells as an in vitro marker for delayed-type drug hypersensitivity. *Allergy;* 63:181-8.

Blanca M., Torres M.J., García J.J., Romano A., Mayorga C., de Ramon E., Vega J.M., Miranda A. & Juarez C. (1999). Natural evolution of skin test sensitivity in patients allergic to beta-lactams. *J Allergy Clin Immunol;* 103:918-924.

Blanca M., Posadas S., Torres M.J., Leyva L., Mayorga C., Gonzalez L., Juarez C., Fernandez J. & Santamaria L.F. (2000) Expression of the skin-homing receptor in peripheral blood lymphocytes from subjects with nonimmediate cutaneous allergic drug reactions. *Allergy*; 55:998-1004.

Blanca M., Mayorga C., Torres M.J., Reche M., Moya M.C., Rodriguez J.L., Romano A. & Juarez C. (2001). Clinical evaluation of Pharmacia CAP System RAST FEIA amoxicilloyl and benzylpenicilloyl in patients with penicillin allergy. *Allergy*; 56: 862–870.

Britschgi M., Steiner U.C., Schmid S., Depta J.P., Senti G., Bircher A., Burkhart C., Yawalkar N. & Pichler W.J. (2001). T- cell involvement in drug-induced acute generalized exanthematous pustulosis. *J Clin Invest*;107(11):1433–41.

Britschgi M. & Pichler W.J. (2002). Acute generalized exanthematous pustulosis, a clue to neutrophil-mediated inflammatory processes orchestrated by T cells. *Curr Opin Allergy Clin Immunol*; 2:325-331.

Caballero M.R. & Fernandez-Benitez M. (2003). Allergy to heparin: a new in vitro diagnostic technique. *Allergol Immunopathol*; 31:324-328.

Caceres Calle O, Fernandez-Benitez M. (2004). Allergy to dexchlorpheniramine. Study of a case. *Allergol Immunopathol*; 32: 306-309.

Chung W.H., Hung S.I., Yang J.Y., Su S.C., Huang S.P., Wei C.Y., Chin S.W., Chiou C.C., Chu S.C., Ho H.C., Yang C.H., Lu C.F., Wu J.Y., Liao Y.D., Chen Y.T. (2008). Granulysin is a key mediator for disseminated keratinocyte death in Stevens-Johnson syndrome and toxic epidermal necrolysis. *Nat Med*; 14:1343-1350.

Cornejo-Garcia J.A., Fernandez T.D., Torres M.J., Carballo M., Hernan I., Antunez C., Blanca M. & Mayorga C. (2007). Differential cytokine and transcription factor expression in patients with allergic reactions to drugs. *Allergy*.;62(12):1429-38.

Czerkinsky C., Moldoveanu Z., Mestecky J., Nilsson L.A. & Ouchterlony O. (1988). A novel two colour ELISPOT assay. I. Simultaneous detection of distinct types of antibody-secreting cells. *J Immunol Methods*;115:31-37.

De Weck A.L., Sanz M.L., Gamboa P.M., Aberer W., Bienvenu J., Blanca M., Demoly P., Ebo D.G., Mayorga L., Monneret G. & Sainte-Laudy J. (2008). Diagnostic tests based on human basophils: more potentials and perspectives than pitfalls. *Int Arch Allergy Immunol*; 146: 177-89.

De Weck A.L., Sanz M.L., Gamboa P.M., Aberer W., Bienvenu J., Blanca M., Demoly P., Ebo D.G., Mayorga L., Monneret G., Sainte Laudy J. (2008). Diagnostic tests based on human basophils: more potentials and perspectives than pitfalls. II. Technical issues. *J Investig Allergol Clin Immunol*; 18: 143-55.

De Weck A.L., Sanz M.L., Gamboa P.M., Aberer W., Blanca M., Correia S., Erdman S., Jermann J.M., Kanny G., Kowalski M., Mayorga L., Medrala W., Merk A., Sturm G.J., Sainte-Laudy J., Schneider M.S., Sczczeklik A., Weber J.M. & Wedi A. (2009). Nonsteroidal anti-inflammatory drug hypersensitivity syndrome. A multicenter study. I. Clinical findings and in vitro diagnosis. *J Investig Allergol Clin Immunol*;19(5):355-69.

De Weck A.L., Sanz M.L., Gamboa P.M., Jermann J.M., Kowalski M., Medrala W., Sainte-Laudy J., Schneider M.S., Weber J.M. & Wolanczyk-Medrala A. (2010). Nonsteroidal anti-inflammatory drug hypersensitivity syndrome: a multicenter study. II. Basophil activation by nonsteroidal anti-inflammatory drugs and its impact on pathogenesis. *J Investig Allergol Clin Immunol*;20(1):39-57.

Ebo D.G., Piel G.C., Conraads V. & Stevens W.J. (2001). IgE-mediated anaphylaxis after first intravenous infusion of cyclosporine. *Ann Allergy Asthma Immunol*; 87:243-245.

Ebo D.G., Lechkar B., Schuerwegh A.J., Bridts C.H., De Clerck L.S., Stevens W.J. (2002). Validation of a two-color flow cytometric assay detecting in vitro basophil activation for the diagnosis of IgE mediated natural rubber latex allergy. *Allergy*; 57: 706-12.

Ebo D.G., Haine S.E., Hagendorens M.M., Bridts C.H., Conraads V.M., Vorlat A., Vrints C.J., De Clerck L.S. & Stevens W.J. (2004). Hypersensitivity to nadroparin calcium: case report and review of the literature. *Clin Drug Investig*; 24:421-426.

Ebo D.G., Hagendorens M.M., Bridts C.H., Schuerwegh A.J., De Clerk L.D. & Stevens W.J. (2004). In vitro allergy diagnosis: should we follow the flow? *Clin Exp Allergy*; 34: 332-9.

Ebo D.G., Goossens S., Opsomer F., Bridts C.H. & Stevens W.J. Flow-assisted diagnosis of anaphylaxis to hyaluronidase. (2005). *Allergy*; 60:1333-1334.

Ebo D.G., Sainte-Laudy J., Bridts C.H., Mertens C.H., Hagendorens M.M., Schuerwegh A.J., De Clerck L.S. & Stevens W.J. (2006). Assisted allergy diagnosis: current applications and future perspectives. *Allergy*; 61: 1028-39.

Ebo D.G., Bridts C.H., Hagendorens M.M., Mertens C.H., De Clerck L.S. & Stevens W.J. (2006). Flow-assisted diagnostic management of anaphylaxis from rocuronium bromide. *Allergy*; 61: 935–9.

Ebo D.G., Bridts C.H. & Stevens W.J. IgE-mediated anaphylaxis from chlorhexidine: diagnostic possibilities. (2006). *Contact Dermatitis*; 55:301-302.

Fernandez T.D., Mayorga C., Torres M.J., Cornejo-Garcia J.A., López S., Chaves P., Rondon C. & Blanca M. (2008). Cytokine and chemokine expression in the skin from patients with maculopapular exanthema to drugs. *Allergy*; 63:712-719.

Fernández T.D., Canto G. & Blanca M. Molecular mechanisms of maculopapular exanthema. Curr Opin Infect Dis. 2009 Jun;22(3):272-8.

Fernandez T.D., Torres M.J., Lopez S., Antunez C., Gomez E., Del Prado M.F., Canto G., Blanca M. & Mayorga C. (2010). Role of effector cells ($CCR7^{-}CD27^{-}$) and effector-memory cells ($CCR7^{-}CD27^{+}$) in drug-induced maculopapular exanthema. *Int J Immunopathol Pharmacol*;23:437-447.

Gamboa P.M., Sanz M.L., Caballero M.R., Antépara I., Urrutia I., Jáuregui I., González G., Diéguez I. & De Weck A.L. (2003). Use of CD63 expression as a marker of in vitro basophil activation and leukotriene determination in metamizol allergic patients. *Allergy* 2003; 58: 312-7.

Gamboa P.M., Sanz M.L., Urrutia I., Jáuregui I., Antépara I., Diéguez I. & De Weck A.L. (2003). CD63 expression by flow cytometry in the in vitro diagnosis of allergy to omeprazole. *Allergy*; 58:538-539.

Gamboa P, Sanz ML, Caballero MR, Urrutia I, Antépara I, Esparza R, de Weck AL. (2004). The flow-cytometric determination of basophil activation induced by aspirin and other non-steroidal antiinflammatory drugs (NSAIDs) is useful for in vitro diagnosis of the NSAID hypersensitivity syndrome. *Clin Exp Allergy*; 34: 1448-57.

Gamboa P.M., García-Avilés M.C., Urrutia I., Antépara I., Esparza R. & Sanz M.L. (2004). Basophil activation and sulfidoleukotriene production in patients with immediate allergy to betalactam antibiotics and negative skin tests. *J Investig Allergol Clin Immunol*;14(4):278-83.

Gómez E., Blanca-Lopez N., Torres M.J., Requena G., Rondon C., Canto G., Blanca M. & Mayorga C. (2009). IgE- mediated immediate allergic reactions to dipyrone: value of basophil activation test in the identification of patients. *Clin Exp Allergy*;39(8):1217-24.

Hausmann O.V., Gentinetta T., Bridts C.H. & Ebo D.G. (2009). The Basophil Activation Test in Immediate-Type Drug Allergy. *Immunol Allergy Clin North Am*; 29 :555-566.

Hertl M., Geisel J., Boecker C. & Merk H.F. (1993). Selective generation of CD81 T-cell clones from the peripheral blood of patients with cutaneous reactions to beta-lactam antibiotics. *Br J Dermatol* ;128(6):619–26.

Kano Y., Hirahara K., Mitsuyama Y., Takahashi R. & Shiohara T. (2007). Utility of the lymphocyte transformation test in the diagnosis of drug sensitivity: dependence on its timing and the type of drug eruption. *Allergy*;62:1439-1444.

Kleine-Tebbe J., Erdmann S., Knol E.F., Macglashan D.W. Jr, Poulsen K.L. & Gibbs BF. (2006). Diagnostic tests based on human basophils: potentials, pitfalls and perspectives. *Int Arch Allergy Immunol;* 141: 79-90.

Kvedariene V., Kamey S., Ryckwaert Y., Rongier M., Bousquet J., Demoly P. & Arnoux B. (2006). Diagnosis of neuromuscular blocking agent hypersensitivity reactions using cytofluorimetric analysis of basophils. *Allergy;* 61:311–315.

Laxenaire M.C., and the perioperative anaphylactic reactions study group. (1999). Epidemiology of anesthetic anaphylactoid reactions. Fourth multicentric survey. *Ann. Fr Anesth Reanim*; 18:796–809.

Lehmann S. & Ott II. (2008). Glucocorticoid hypersensitivity as a rare but potentially fatal side effect of paediatric asthma treatment: a case report. *J Med Case Report;* 2:186.

Le Pabic F., Sainte-Laudy J., Blanchard N. & Moneret-Vautrin D.A. (2003). First case of anaphylaxis to iodinated povidone. *Allergy*; 58:826-827.

Lerch M., Keller M., Britschgi M., Kanny G., Tache V., Schmid D.A., Beeler A., Gerber B.O., Luethi M., Bircher A.J., Christiansen C. & Pichler W.J. (2007). Cross-reactivity patterns of T cells specific for iodinated contrast media. *J Allergy Clin Immunol*;119(6):1529–36.

Leyva L., Torres M.J., Posadas S., Blanca M., Besso G., O'Valle F., del Moral R.G., Santamaría L.F. & Juárez C. (2000). Anticonvulsant-induced toxic epidermal necrolysis: monitoring the immunologic response. *J Allergy Clin Immunol*; 105:157-165

Leysen J., Bridts C.H., De Clerck L.S., Vercauteren M., Lambert J., Weyler J.J., Stevens W.J. & Ebo D.G. (2011). Allergy to rocuronium: from clinical suspicion to correct Diagnosis. *Allergy*; DOI:10.1111/j.1398-9995.2011.02569

Lopez S., Torres M.J., Rodríguez-Pena R., Blanca-Lopez N., Fernandez T.D., Antunez C., Canto G., de Luque V. & Mayorga C. (2009). Lymphocyte proliferation response in patients with delayed hypersensitivity reactions to heparins. *Br J Dermatol;* 160:259-65.

Lopez S., Torres M.J., Antunez C., Rodríguez-Pena R., Canto G., Blanca M. & Mayorga C. (2010). Specific immunological response to budesonide in a patient with delayed-type hypersensitivity reaction. *J Invest Dermatol;* 130(3):895-7.

Luque I., Leyva L., José Torres M., Rosal M., Mayorga C., Segura J.M., Blanca M. & Juárez C. (2001). In vitro T-cell responses to beta-lactam drugs in immediate and nonimmediate allergic reactions. *Allergy;* 56:611-8.

Mauri-Hellweg D., Bettens F., Mauri D., Brander C., Hunziker T. & Pichler W.J. (1995). Activation of drug-specific CD41 and CD81 T cells in individuals allergic to sulfonamides, phenytoin, and carbamazepine. *J Immunol;* 155(1):462- 72.
Mayorga C., Torres M.J., Corzo J.L., Sanchez-Sabate E., Alvarez J., Vera A., Posadas S., Jurado A. & Blanca M. (2003). Improvement of toxic epidermal necrolysis after the early administration of a single high dose of intravenous immunoglobulin. *Ann Allergy Asthma Immunol;* 91:86–91.
Mayorga C., Pena R.R., Blanca-López N., López S., Martin E. & Torres M.J. (2006). Monitoring the acute phase response in non-immediate allergic drug reactions. *Curr Opin Allergy Clin Immunol;*6:249-57.
Monneret G., Benoit Y., Debard A.L., Gutowski M.C., Topenot I. & Bienvenu J. (2002). Monitoring of basophil activation using CD63 and CCR3 in allergy to muscle relaxant drugs. *Clin Immunol;* 102 :192-9.
Moss J. (1995). Muscle relaxants and histamine release. *Acta Anaesthesiol Scand;* 39(S106):7-12.
Orta M., Ordoqui E., Aranzábal A., Fernández C., Bartolomé B. & Sanz M.L. (2003). Anaphylactic reaction after artificial insemination. *Ann Allergy Asthma Immunol;* 90:446-451.
Mullen A.C., High F.A., Hutchins A.S., Lee H.W., Villarino A.V., Livingston D.M., Kung A.L., Cereb N., Yao T.P., Yang S.Y. & Reiner S.L. (2001). Role of T-bet in commitment of Th1cells before IL-12-dependent selection. *Science;* 292:1907–1910.
Naisbitt D.J., Farrell J., Wong G., Depta J.P., Dodd C.C., Hopkins J.E., Gibney C.A., Chadwick D.W., Pichler W.J., Pirmohamed M., & Park B.K. (2003). Characterization of Skin Homing Lamotrigine-specific T-cells from hypersensitive patients. *J Allergy Clin Immunol;* 111:1393–1403.
Naisbitt D.J., Britschgi M., Wong G., Farrell J., Depta J.P., Chadwick D.W., Pichler W.J., Pirmohamed M. & Park B.K. (2003). Hypersensitivity reactions to carbamazepine: characterization of the specificity, phenotype, and cytokine profile of drug-specific T-cell clones. *Mol Pharmacol;* 63:732–741.
Nassif A., Bensussan A., Dorothée G., Mami-Chouaib F., Bachot N., Bagot M., Boumsell L., Roujeau J.C. Drug specific cytotoxic T-cells in the skin lesions of a patient with toxic epidermal necrolysis. *J Invest Dermatol* 2002; 118:728- 733.
Nassif A., Bensussan A., Boumsell L., Deniaud A., Moslehi H., Wolkenstein P., Bagot M., & Roujeau J.C. Toxic epidermal necrolysis: effector cells are drug-specific cytotoxic T cells. *J Allergy Clin Immunol* 2004; 114:1209-1215.
Nassif A., Moslehi H., Le Gouvello S., Bagot M., Lyonnet L., Michel L., Boumsell L., Bensussan A. & Roujeau J.C. (2004). Evaluation of the potential role of cytokines in Toxic Epidermal Necrolysis. *J Invest Dermatol;* 123:850-855.
Nishio D., Izu K., Kabashima K. & Tokura Y. (2007). T cell populations propagating in the peripheral blood of patients with drug eruptions. *J Dermatol Sci;* 48:25-33.
Nyfeler B. & Pichler W.J. (1997). The lymphocyte transformation test for the diagnosis of drug allergy: sensitivity and specificity. *Clin Exp Allergy;* 27:175–181.
Padial M.A., Alvarez-Ferreira J., Tapia B., Blanco R., Mañas C., Blanca M. & Bellón T. (2004). Acute generalized exanthematous pustulosis associated with pseudoephedrine. *Br J Dermatol* ;150:139-142.

Pâris-Köhler A., Demoly P., Persi L., Lebel B., Bousquet J. & Arnoux B. (2000). In vitro diagnosis of cypress pollen allergy by using cytofluorometric analysis of basophils (Basotest). *J Allergy Clin Immunol;* 105: 339-45.

Pichler W.J. (2003). Delayed drug hypersensitivity reactions. *Ann Intern Med;* 139:683-693.

Pichler W.J. & Tilch J. (2004). The lymphocyte transformation test in the diagnosis of drug hypersensitivity. *Allergy;* 59:809-20.

Pinnobphun P., Buranapraditkun S., Kampitak T., Hirankarn N. & Klaewsongkram J. (2011). The diagnostic value of basophil activation test in patients with an immediate hypersensitivity reaction to radiocontrast media. *Ann Allergy Asthma Immunol;*106(5):387-93.

Posadas S.J., Leyva L., Torres M.J., Rodriguez J.L., Bravo I., Rosal M., Fernandez J., Juarez C. & Blanca M. (2000). Subjects with allergic reactions to drugs show polarized patterns of cytokine expression depending on the chronology of the clinical reaction. *J Allergy Clin Immunol;* 106:769-776.

Posadas S.J., Padial A., Torres M.J., Mayorga C., Leyva L., Sanchez E., Alvarez J., Romano A., Juarez C. & Blanca M. (2002). Delayed reactions to drugs show a Th1 profile and levels of perforin, granzyme B and Fas-L related to disease severity. *J Allergy Clin Immunol;* 109:155–161.

Rengarajan J., Szabo S.J. & Glimcher LH. (2000). Transcriptional regulation of Th1/Th2 polarization. *Immunol Today;* 21:479–483.

Rodriguez-Pena R., Lopez S., Mayorga C., Antunez C., Fernandez T.D., Torres M.J. & Blanca M. (2006). Potential involvement of dendritic cells in delayed-type hypersensitivity reactions to beta-lactams. *J Allergy Clin Immunol;* 118:949-56.

Rodríguez Trabado A., Cámara Hijón C., Porcel Carreño S.L., Rodríguez Martín E., Fletes Peral C., Pereira Navarro G., Jiménez Timón S., Hernández Arbeiza F.J. & Fernández Pereira L. (2006). Anaphylaxis caused by cloxacillin: diagnosis with seriated analysis by way of basophil activation test. *Allergy Asthma Proc;* 27:269-72.

Rodríguez-Trabado A., Cámara-Hijón C., Ramos-Cantariño A., Porcel-Carreño S.L., Jiménez-Timón S., Pereira-Navarro G., Hernández-Arbeiza F.J. & Fernández-Pereira L. 2008. Basophil activation test for the in vitro diagnosis of nonsteroidal anti-inflammatory drug hypersensitivity. *Allergy Asthma Proc;* 29:241-9.

Romano A., Torres M.J., Castells M. & Sanz M.L. (2011). Diagnosis and management of drug hypersensitivity reactions. *J Allergy Clin Immunol;*127:S67-73.

Romano A., Torres M.J., Castells M., Sanz M.L. & Blanca M. (2011). Diagnosis and management of drug hypersensitivity reactions. *J Allergy Clin Immunol;*127:67-73.

Roujeau J.C., Albengres E. & Moritz S. (1985). Lymphocyte transformation test in drug induced toxic epidermal necrolysis. *Int Arch Allergy Appl Immunol;*78:22–4.

Rozieres A., Vocanson M., Nosbaum A., Cuerq C., Rouzaire P. & Ben Saïd B. (2009). Role of T cells in non-immediate allergic drug reaction. *Current Op Allergy Clin Immunol;*9(4):305-10.

Rozieres A., Hennino A., Rodet K., Gutowski M.-C., Gunera-Saad N., Berard F., Cozon G., Bienvenu J. & Nicolas J.-F. (1997). Detection and quantification of drug-specific T cells in penicillin allergy. *Allergy;* 64: 534–542.

Sabbah A., Sainte-Laudy J., Drouet M., Lauret M.G. & Loiry M. (1997). Anaphylactic or anaphylactoid reactions to paracetamol. Report of 3 cases. *Allerg Immunol (Paris);* 29: 60-2.

Sabbah A., Plassais R., Grenapin S., Drouet M., Lauret M.G., Loiry M. & Sainte-Laudy J. (1998). Testing basophil activation by flow cytometry in the diagnosis of allergy to hymenopteran venom. *Allerg Immunol (Paris);* 30: 44- 8.

Sainte-Laudy J., Sabbah A., Drouet M., Lauret M.G. & Loiri M. (2000). Diagnosis of venom allergy by flow cytometry. Correlation with clinical history, skin tests, specific IgE, histamine and leukotriene C4 release. *Clin Exp Allergy;* ; 30: 1166-71

Sanz M.L., Sánchez G., Gamboa P.M., Vila L., Uasuf C., Chazot M., Diéguez I. & De Weck A.L. (2001). Ag-induced basophil activation: CD63 cell expression detected by flow cytometry in patients allergic to Dermatophagoides pteronyssinus and Lolium perenne. *Clin Exp Allergy;* 31: 1007-13.

Sanz M.L., De Weck A.L., Uasuf C., Gamboa P.M. & Chazot M. (2001). Use of flow cytometry to assess basophil activation in patients allergic to betalactam antibiotics. Correlation between Flow cytometric Alergen Stimulation Test (FAST) and other in vivo and in vitro tests. *Int Arch Allergy Immunol,* 124: 307-8.

Sanz M.L., Gamboa P.M., Antépara I., Uasuf C., Vila L., Garcia-Avilés C., Chazot M., & De Weck AL. (2002). Flow- cytometric basophil activation test by detection of CD63 expression in patients with immedate type reactions to Betalactam antibiotics. *Clin Exp Allergy;* 32: 277-86.

Sanz M.L., Maselli J.P., Gamboa P.M., Oehling A., Diéguez I. & de Weck A.L. (2002). Diagnosis and management of drug hypersensitivity. *J Invest Allergol Clin Immunol;* 12:143-54.

Sanz M.L., Gamboa P.M., García-Avilés C., Vila L., Diéguez I., Antépara I., de Weck A.L. (2003). Flow-cytometric cellular allergen stimulation test in latex allergy. *Int Arch Allergy Immunol;* 130: 33-9.

Sanz M.L., Gamboa P.M. & De Weck A.L. (2005). A new combined test with flowcytometric basophil activation and determination of sulfidoleukotrienes is useful for in vitro diagnosis of hypersensitivity to aspirin and other nonsteroidal anti- inflammatory drugs. *Int Arch Allergy Immunol;* 136: 58-72.

Sanz M.L., Gamboa P.M. & De Weck A.L. (2008). Cellular test in the diagnosis of drug hypersensitivity. *Curr Pharml Des,* 14: 2803-2808.

Sanz M.L., Gamboa P.M. & Mayorga C. (2009). Basophil activation tests in the evaluation of immediate drug hypersensitivity. Curr Opin Allergy Clin Immunol; 9: 298-304

Saporta M., Kamei S., Persi L., Bousquet J. & Arnoux B. (2001). Basophil activation during pollen season in patients monosensitized to grass pollens. *Allergy;* 56: 442-5

Schleimer R.P., Fox C.C., Togias A., Norman P. & Lichtenstein LM. (1985). Role of human basophils and mast cells in the pathogenesis of allergic diseases. *J Allergy Clin Immunol;* 76, 369-74.

Schmittel A., Keilholz U. & Scheibenbogen C. (1997). Evaluation of the interferon-gamma ELISPOT-assay for quantification of peptide specific T lymphocytes from peripheral blood. *J Immunol Methods;*210:167-174.

Schmittel A., Keilholz U., Bauer S., Kuhne U., Stevanovic S., Thiel E. & Scheibenbogen C. (2001). Application of the IFN- gamma ELISPOT assay to quantify T cell responses against proteins. *J Immunol Methods;*247:17-24.

Schnyder B., Burkhart C., Schnyder-Frutig K., von Greyerz S., Naisbitt D.J., Pirmohamed M., Park B.K. & Pichler W.J. . (2000). Recognition of sulfamethoxazole and its reactive metabolites by drug-specific CD4+ T cells from allergic individuals. *J Immunol;* 164:6647-6654.

Schnyder B. & Pichler W.J. (2000). Skin and laboratory tests in amoxicillin- and penicillin-induced morbilliform skin eruption. *Clin Exp Allergy;* 30: 590–595.

Shiohara T. & Mizukawa Y. (2007). Fixed drug eruption: a disease mediated by self-inflicted responses of intraepidermal T cells. *Eur J Dermatol;*17(3):201-8.

Sudheer P.S., Hall J.E., Read G.F., Rowbottom A.W. & Williams PE. (2005). Flow cytometric investigation of peri- anaesthetic anaphylaxis using CD63 and CD203c. *Anaesthesia;* 60:251–256.

Stellato C., de Paulis A., Cirillo R., Mastronardi P., Mazzarella B. & Marone G. (1991). Heterogeneity of human mast cells and basophils in response to muscle relaxants. *Anesthesiology;* 74:1078-86.

Tapia B., Padial A., Sanchez-Sabate E., Alvarez-Ferreira J., Morel E., Blanca M. & Bellon T. (2004). Involvement of CCL27- CCR10 interactions in drug-induced cutaneous reactions. *J Allergy Clin Immunol* ;114:335-340.

Torres M.J., Padial A, Mayorga C., Fernandez T., Sanchez-Sebate E., Cornejo-Garcia J.A., Antúnez C. & Blanca M. (2004). The diagnostic interpretation of basophil activation test in immediate allergic reactions to betalactams. *Clin Exp Allergy;* 34: 1768-75.

Torres M.J., Mayorga C., Fernández T.D., Cornejo-García J.A., Antúnez C., Valenzuela M., Del Prado M.F., Rodriguez- Pena R. & Blanca M. (2006). T cell assessment in allergic drug reactions during the acute phase according to the time of occurrence. *Int J Immunopathol Pharmacol;* 19(1):119-30.

Torres M.J., Mayorga C., Cornejo-Garcia J.A., Lopez S., Chaves P., Rondon C., Fernandez T. & Blanca M. (2008). Monitoring non-immediate allergic reactions to iodine contrast media. *Clin Exp Immunol;* 152:233-238.

Torres M.J., Mayorga C. & Blanca M. (2009). Nonimmediate allergic reactions induced by drugs: Pathogenesis and diagnostic tests. *J Investig Allergol Clin Immunol;* 19: 80-90.

Whittam L.R., Wakelin S.H. & Barker JNWN. (2000). Generalized pustular psoriasis or drug-induced pustuloderma? The use of patch testing. *Clin Exp Dermatol;* 25: 122-124.

Yawalkar N., Shrikhande M., Hari Y., Nievergelt H., Braathen L.R. & Pichler WJ. (2000). Evidence for a role of IL-5 and eotaxin in activating and recruitment of eosinophils in drug-induced cutaneous eruptions. *J Allergy Clin Immunol;* 106:1171-6.

Zawodniak A., Lochmatter P., Yerly D., Kawabata T., Lerch M., Yawalkar N. & Pichler WJ. (2010). In vitro detection of cytotoxic T and NK cells in peripheral blood of patients with various drug-induced skin diseases. *Allergy;*65:376- 384.

Zedlitz S., Linzbach L., Kaufmann R. & Boehncke W.H. (2002). Reproducible identification of the causative drug of a fixed drug eruption by oral provocation and lesional patch testing. *Contact Dermatitis;* 46: 352-353.

14

Diagnosis and Management of Cows' Milk Protein Allergy in Infants

Elisabeth De Greef, Gigi Veereman-Wauters, Thierry Devreker, Bruno Hauser and Yvan Vandenplas
Pediatric Gastroenterology, Hepatology and Nutrition, University Children's Hospital Brussels, Free University Brussels, Belgium

1. Introduction

Cow's milk protein allergy (CMPA) is defined as an immunological reaction to one or more milk proteins(1). A variety of symptoms can be suggestive for CMPA. CMPA is suspected clinically in 5-15% of infants (2), while most estimates of prevalence of CMPA vary from only 2 to 5 % (1). Confusion regarding CMPA prevalence is often due to differences in study population, and a lack of defined diagnostic criteria for CMPA. The importance of defined diagnostic criteria needs to be emphasised. It precludes infants from an unnecessary diet (3) and avoids delay in diagnosis, which can lead to malnutrition (4).
The intention of this manuscript is to help diagnose and manage CMPA. Most of the recommendations are based on recently published guidelines on CMPA diagnosis and management (3, 5-9).

2. Manifestations

CMPA may develop in breastfed (BF) and in cow's milk formula (CMF) fed infants and usually occurs within the first weeks after cow's milk introduction. The presentation is variable; no symptom is pathognomonic. Manifestations mainly occur at the level of the digestive tract (50-60%), the skin (50-60%) and the respiratory tract (20-30%) (2). They vary from mild-moderate to severe (Table 1).
There are two clinical types of CMPA: the immediate and the delayed type. The immediate type presents shortly after ingestion of cow's milk protein (CMP) (urticaria, angio-oedema, vomiting or an acute flare of atopic dermatitis) and is present in slightly more than half of the patients with CMPA(10). They are more likely to have positive skin prick test (SPT) (wheel size $\geq$3 mm) or positive serum specific Immunoglobulin e (IgE) (10). The amount of cow's milk necessary to elicit an immediate reaction varies from one drop to more than 150 ml, which shows that some patients tolerate a considerable amount of milk before manifestations develop (11). Delayed reactions such as atopic dermatitis or gastrointestinal manifestations like proctocolitis or enteropathy, usually present after hours or days.
Immunologically, CMPA can be IgE or non-IgE mediated (12). IgE mediated reactions are clinically more often of the immediate type and can be confirmed with SPT or serum specific

IgE. Non-IgE mediated reactions are due to a cellular immune response or to a mixed immune response in which IgE and immune cells play a role. This type of reaction is more difficult to prove by specific testing.

SEVERE MANIFESTATIONS	
Organ Involved	**Manifestation**
Gastro-intestinal tract	Failure to thrive
	Iron deficiency anemia
	Enteropathy
Skin	Exudative/Severe atopic dermatitis
Respiratory tract	Larynx oedema
General	Anaphylaxis
MODERATE-MILD MANIFESTATIONS	
Organ involved	**Manifestations**
Gastrointestinal tract	Regurgitations and vomiting
	Diarrhea
	Constipation
	Colitis
	Colic/Abdominal pain
Skin	atopic dermatitis
	Angio-Oedema
	Urticaria
	Swollen lips
Respiratory tract	Rhinitis
	Conjunctivitis
	Wheezing
General	Irritability

Table 1. Clinical Manifestations suggesting CMPA.

3. Diagnosis

None of the diagnostic tests available in routine clinical situations prove or exclude CMPA completely (11). A thorough history, including family history of atopy, and a careful clinical examination are therefore the key elements in the diagnostic process. Clinicians may perform SPT (preferable with fresh cows' milk or whole CMP extracts), determination of specific IgE, or patch tests, but they merely indicate sensitisation to the substrate and are not necessarily proof of an allergic reaction. The rate of outgrowing CMPA varies between 30-79% in IgE mediated CMPA (13); consecutive IgE measurements can be indicative in this process (14). If serum specific IgE and/or SPT at time of diagnosis are negative, tolerance is obtained at a younger age and the risk of severe acute reaction is small. On the contrary, persistant high IgE titers increase the risk of developing other atopic conditions like asthma, rhino-conjunctivitis and atopic dermatitis. Patch testing, still a topic of on-going research, can aid in the diagnosis of non-IgE mediated reactions.

3.1 Diagnostic challenge procedures

The double-blind placebo-controlled challenge is considered the gold standard in CMPA diagnosis, but in practice only an open challenge is often performed.(3) The patient with suspected CMPA will follow a cow's milk free diet for 2-4 weeks. Formula fed infants get an extensively hydrolyzed formula (eHF) and breastfeeding mothers follow a cow's milk free diet. If CMPA is present, clinical manifestations will disappear. Cow's milk protein is reintroduced progressively thereafter and clinical symptoms are monitored. The risk of an open challenge is an overestimation of the diagnosis.(15) A double-blind placebo-controlled challenge will blind the parent and the doctor as for the introduction of cow's milk protein and is the only objective measure to make the diagnosis. Unfortunately, it is expensive, requires extensive preparation, is time consuming and is difficult to perform.(16)

Medical supervision during a challenge is necessary because the severity of symptoms cannot be predicted (17, 18). When additional allergy testing (serum specific IgE, SPT) is negative, life threatening manifestations are extremely rare and a non-hospital setting with medical supervision is often sufficient (19), but in patients with a history of severe reactions or high IgE levels, a hospital setting with an established protocol is indicated. In case of an unequivocal history of recent anaphylactic reaction to cow's milk, a challenge is debatable.

When CMPA is confirmed, the infant should be maintained on an elimination diet until the infant is between 9-12 months or at least for 6 months, whichever occurs first. A new challenge is then performed. Children who do not develop allergy-related manifestations during challenge and up to one week thereafter can resume their normal diet.

If the patient with CMPA is on amino acid formula (AAF) because of ongoing allergic manifestations under an eHF, the debate whether to challenge with an eHF or standard infant formula is still ongoing. After the initial phase, allergic symptoms may not recur on an eHF challenge and the formula can be used as a less expensive and more palatable treatment. (20) Whereas in the same patient recurrence of symptoms after a challenge with normal cow's milk formula might be more likely.

3.2 Differential diagnosis

The list of potential differential diagnoses for CMPA is long including repetitive viral infections and transient lactose intolerance. Concurrent conditions can also be present: troublesome regurgitation occurs in 20 % of all infants, with or without CMPA. On the other hand, gastro-oesophageal reflux has been mentioned as a possible manifestation of CMPA. (21) CMPA has also been related to infantile colic; CMPA contributes to colic in about 10% of colicky infants (22).

Although in some young infants, a correlation between atopic dermatitis and CMPA is suggested, many cases of atopic dermatitis are not related. The younger the infant and/or the more severe the atopic dermatitis, the stronger the association appears to be (23).

Reactions to other foods - especially egg and soy, wheat, fish and peanut - occur frequently and often in combination with CMPA (24). Therefore, complementary feeding and, preferentially, all supplementary feeding should be avoided during the diagnostic elimination diet.

4. Management of CMPA

The principles for the management of CMPA differ in breastfed and formula fed infants.

4.1 Management of CMPA in exclusively breastfed infants (Figure 1)

Breastfeeding is the gold standard feeding in infant nutrition and is recommended exclusively at least for the first four months of life.(25) Only about 0.5% of exclusively breast-fed infants show a reproducible clinical reaction to CMP, mostly mild to moderate.(2) Life-threatening symptoms due to CMPA in breast-fed infants are extremely rare, but severe cases with protein losing enteropathy and atopic dermatitis have been described. (24) Any other underlying disease should be looked for in severe cases.

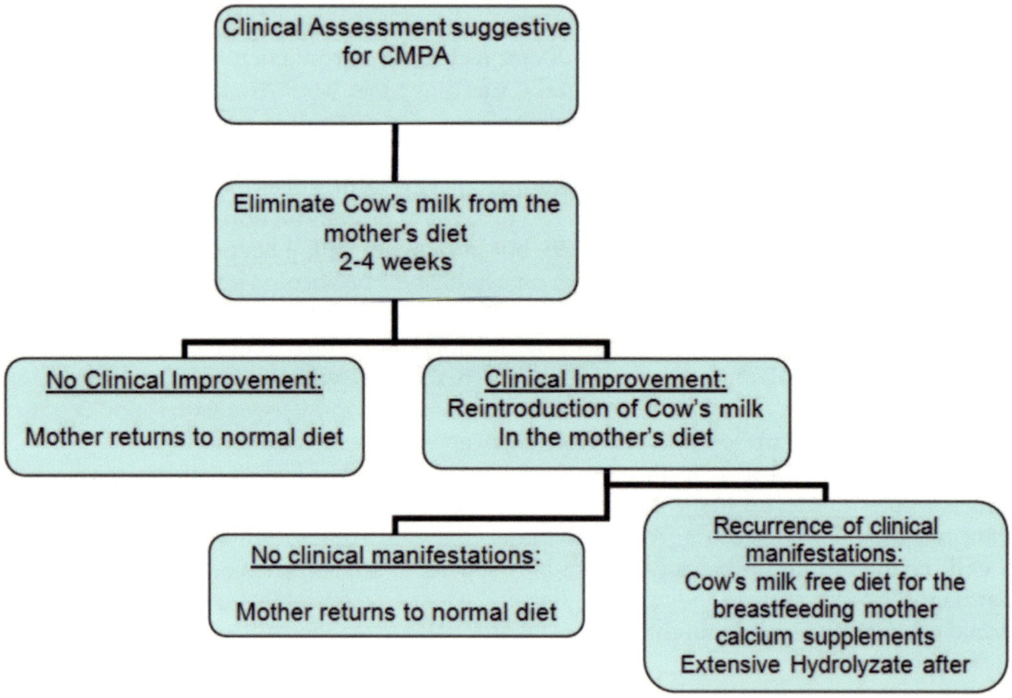

Fig. 1. Decision tree for the diagnosis and treatment of CMPA in Breastfed infants with mild to moderate symptoms

Due to the many benefits of breastfeeding, clinicians should advise to continue, even if the infant has CMPA. A cow's milk elimination diet for the mother is then indicated. The maintenance of a strict avoidance of CMP is mandatory if supplementary feeding is being given to the infant. (23) The elimination diet for breastfeeding mother and child should be continued for a minimum of two (to four) weeks. In cases of atopic dermatitis, symptoms may not have disappeared after two to four weeks, in which case, clinical experience suggests that other food proteins, such as egg, peanut, fish and wheat may as well sensitise an infant through its mother's milk. If so, elimination diet should be adapted accordingly. Advice of a dietician is often required in order to help the mother to keep a nutritionally balanced diet; an adequate calcium intake (1000 mg per day) needs special attention.

If symptoms disappear, cows' milk should be reintroduced in the mother's diet after 2 to 4 weeks. If symptoms relapse, the milk should be eliminated from the mother's diet as long as she is breastfeeding. When the mother wants to wean, the infant should receive an extensive hydrolysed formula (eHF). When the elimination diet fails to improve the symptoms or when the patient remains asymptomatic on reintroduction of specific food proteins, the mother should resume her normal diet.

4.2 Management of CMPA in formula-fed infants (Figure 2)

4.2.1 Mild- moderate manifestations

In formula-fed infants with mild to moderate symptoms related to CMPA, a "therapeutic formula" is the first choice. According to consensus in literature, a therapeutic formula is a formula tolerated by at least 90% (with 95% confidence) of CMPA infants (26, 27). Many eHF's based on whey, casein or another protein source comply to those criteria as well as amino acid based formulae (AAF). During a diagnostic elimination diet, all other food intake should be stopped to avoid misinterpretation of manifestations due to other allergens. The CMP-free diet should be maintained for at least 6 months. To maintain a balanced therapeutic diet, help of a dietician is often needed.

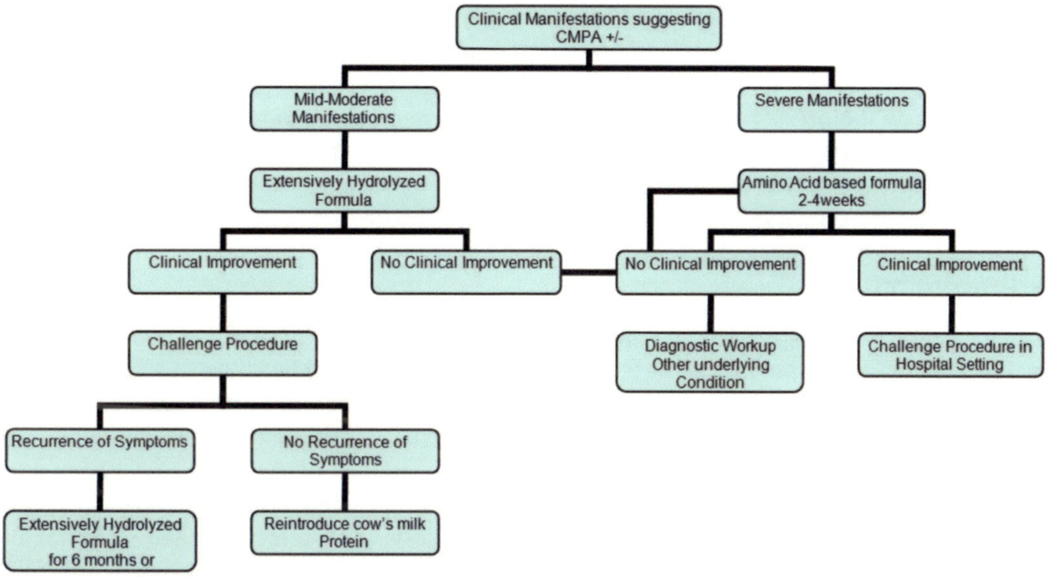

Fig. 2. Decision tree for diagnosis and treatment of formula fed infants with suspected CMPA

Because of high cross-reactivity (up to 80%) and nutritional inadequacy, the use of most animal milk is precluded (28-30). Rice based hydrolysates, available in certain countries, may offer an alternative approach in the treatment of CMPA. (31-33) However, any protein hydrolysate, independent of its origin, has a certain residual allergenicity. Residual symptoms on eHF is often due to a non IgE related mechanisms (20). Failure on eHF may be up to 10% in CMPA children in tertiary care centres (20). There are no data available from primary health care centres.

Although eHF is the treatment of choice in formula fed CMPA infants, AAF can sometimes be indicated if symptoms persist beyond 2-4 weeks on eHF. AAF has the advantage of no residual protein allergenicity, since AAF is a pure chemically made formula, not derived from cow's milk (or any native protein) containing isolated amino-acids instead of peptides. If symptoms persist on an AAF, the CMPA diagnosis should be questioned.

4.3 Severe manifestations

Formula-fed infants with severe CMPA should be given AFF, "the most effective" elimination diet. There is no specific evidence for the use of AAF in severe symptoms, but the risk to aggravate further weight loss and nutritional deficiencies is hereby minimised. Patients with life-threatening, particularly respiratory symptoms or anaphylaxis need immediate referral to the nearest emergency department.

4.4 Soy formula in CMPA

The discussion on the use of soy-based infant formula is difficult, since scientific societies have different recommendations. There is a broad consensus on the following statements: The incidence of soy allergy in soy formula-fed infants is comparable to that of CMPA in cows' milk formula-fed babies (34). Cross reactivity to soy has been reported in 10 to 35% of infants with CMPA, regardless whether they were positive or negative for specific IgE for CMP (10) . In particular, infants with multiple food allergies and eosinophilic enterocolitis also react to soy protein (35). Therefore, different specialist groups have different standpoints on the use of Soy formula for CMPA, but is generally not recommended before the age of 6 months (26, 34, 36, 37). Soy could be considered as an alternative, the possible cross reactivity in mind, in cultures where the hydrolyzation process with pork-derived enzymes is considered a problem and beyond the age of 6 months.

5. Prevention

Genetic predisposition, environmental factors and the influence of allergen exposure early in life may play a role in the development of allergy (38). There are no data on the development of CMPA in atopic versus non-atopic families. A comprehensive history (including family history of atopy) and careful physical examination are therefore an important part of diagnosis.
Irrespective of the atopic heredity, exclusive breastfeeding remains the best nutrition for all infants up to the age of 4-6 months, even as prevention of CMPA. If breastfeeding is not an option, hydrolysed formulas with proven efficacy are recommended in high risk infants (39) combined with the avoidance of solid food and cow's milk for the same period. (25)

6. Conclusion

CMPA can present in BF and FF infants. The manifestations are non pathognomonic and a comprehensive history and thorough clinical examination form the basis of the diagnosis. Confirmation with SPT, serum specific IgE or patch testing, unfortunately lack specificity and a double blind placebo controlled food challenge, remains the gold standard.
Although several groups have published recommendations (3, 6, 40), the ongoing debate on CMPA management is still dependent on the primary outcome measure chosen: most

efficient or cheapest solution. BF remains the best and cheapest option to feed healthy infants, even in CMPA. When BF is not an option, eHF in CMPA is recommended as by European consensus.

7. Acknowledgement

EDG, TD, BH and YVDP wrote paper. YVDP had primary responsibility for final content. All authors have read and approved the final manuscript.

8. References

[1] Hill DJ, Firer MA, Shelton MJ, Hosking CS. Manifestations of milk allergy in infancy: clinical and immunologic findings. The Journal of pediatrics. 1986 Aug;109:270-6.
[2] Host A. Frequency of cow's milk allergy in childhood. Ann Allergy Asthma Immunol. 2002 Dec;89:33-7.
[3] Vandenplas Y, Koletzko S, Isolauri E, Hill D, Oranje AP, Brueton M, Staiano A, Dupont C. Guidelines for the diagnosis and management of cow's milk protein allergy in infants. Archives of disease in childhood. 2007 Oct;92:902-8.
[4] Viera MC MM, Spolidoro JVN, Toporovski MS, Cardoso AL, 1raujo GTB, Nudelman V, Fonseca MCM. A survey on clinical presentation and nutritional status of infants with suspected cow'milk allergy. BMC Pediatrics. 2010;10:25.
[5] Fiocchi A, Schunemann HJ, Brozek J, Restani P, Beyer K, Troncone R, Martelli A, Terracciano L, Bahna SL, et al. Diagnosis and Rationale for Action Against Cow's Milk Allergy (DRACMA): a summary report. The Journal of allergy and clinical immunology. 2010 Dec;126:1119-28 e12.
[6] Allen KJ, Davidson GP, Day AS, Hill DJ, Kemp AS, Peake JE, Prescott SL, Shugg A, Sinn JK, Heine RG. Management of cow's milk protein allergy in infants and young children: an expert panel perspective. Journal of paediatrics and child health. 2009 Sep;45:481-6.
[7] Kneepkens CM, Meijer Y. Clinical practice. Diagnosis and treatment of cow's milk allergy. European journal of pediatrics. 2009 Aug;168:891-6.
[8] Fiocchi A, Brozek J, Schunemann H, Bahna SL, von Berg A, Beyer K, Bozzola M, Bradsher J, Compalati E, et al. World Allergy Organization (WAO) Diagnosis and Rationale for Action against Cow's Milk Allergy (DRACMA) Guidelines. Pediatr Allergy Immunol. 2010 Jul;21 Suppl 21:1-125.
[9] Boyce JA, Assa'ad A, Burks AW, Jones SM, Sampson HA, Wood RA, Plaut M, Cooper SF, Fenton MJ. Guidelines for the Diagnosis and Management of Food Allergy in the United States: summary of the NIAID-sponsored expert panel report. Journal of the American Dietetic Association. Jan;111:17-27.
[10] Klemola T, Vanto T, Juntunen-Backman K, Kalimo K, Korpela R, Varjonen E. Allergy to soy formula and to extensively hydrolyzed whey formula in infants with cow's milk allergy: a prospective, randomized study with a follow-up to the age of 2 years. The Journal of pediatrics. 2002 Feb;140:219-24.

[11] Vanto T, Juntunen-Backman K, Kalimo K, Klemola T, Koivikko A, Koskinen P, Syvanen P, Valovirta E, Varjonen E. The patch test, skin prick test, and serum milk-specific IgE as diagnostic tools in cow's milk allergy in infants. Allergy. 1999 Aug;54:837-42.
[12] Sicherer SH, Noone SA, Koerner CB, Christie L, Burks AW, Sampson HA. Hypoallergenicity and efficacy of an amino acid-based formula in children with cow's milk and multiple food hypersensitivities. The Journal of pediatrics. 2001 May;138:688-93.
[13] Wood RA. The natural history of food allergy. Pediatrics. 2003 Jun;111:1631-7.
[14] Shek LP, Soderstrom L, Ahlstedt S, Beyer K, Sampson HA. Determination of food specific IgE levels over time can predict the development of tolerance in cow's milk and hen's egg allergy. The Journal of allergy and clinical immunology. 2004 Aug;114:387-91.
[15] Venter C, Pereira B, Voigt K, Grundy J, Clayton CB, Gant C, Higgins B, Dean T. Comparison of open and double-blind placebo-controlled food challenges in diagnosis of food hypersensitivity amongst children. J Hum Nutr Diet. 2007 Dec;20:565-79.
[16] Bindslev-Jensen C, Ballmer-Weber BK, Bengtsson U, Blanco C, Ebner C, Hourihane J, Knulst AC, Moneret-Vautrin DA, Nekam K, et al. Standardization of food challenges in patients with immediate reactions to foods--position paper from the European Academy of Allergology and Clinical Immunology. Allergy. 2004 Jul;59:690-7.
[17] Barbi E, Gerarduzzi T, Longo G, Ventura A. Fatal allergy as a possible consequence of long-term elimination diet. Allergy. 2004 Jun;59:668-9.
[18] Flinterman AE, Knulst AC, Meijer Y, Bruijnzeel-Koomen CA, Pasmans SG. Acute allergic reactions in children with AEDS after prolonged cow's milk elimination diets. Allergy. 2006 Mar;61:370-4.
[19] Bock SA, Sampson HA, Atkins FM, Zeiger RS, Lehrer S, Sachs M, Bush RK, Metcalfe DD. Double-blind, placebo-controlled food challenge (DBPCFC) as an office procedure: a manual. The Journal of allergy and clinical immunology. 1988 Dec;82:986-97.
[20] Vanderhoof JA, Murray ND, Kaufman SS, Mack DR, Antonson DL, Corkins MR, Perry D, Kruger R. Intolerance to protein hydrolysate infant formulas: an underrecognized cause of gastrointestinal symptoms in infants. The Journal of pediatrics. 1997 Nov;131:741-4.
[21] Hill DJ, Heine RG, Cameron DJ, Catto-Smith AG, Chow CW, Francis DE, Hosking CS. Role of food protein intolerance in infants with persistent distress attributed to reflux esophagitis. The Journal of pediatrics. 2000 May;136:641-7.
[22] Jakobsson I, Lindberg T. Cow's milk proteins cause infantile colic in breast-fed infants: a double-blind crossover study. Pediatrics. 1983 Feb;71:268-71.
[23] Isolauri E, Tahvanainen A, Peltola T, Arvola T. Breast-feeding of allergic infants. The Journal of pediatrics. 1999 Jan;134:27-32.
[24] Saarinen UM, Kajosaari M. Breastfeeding as prophylaxis against atopic disease: prospective follow-up study until 17 years old. Lancet. 1995 Oct 21;346:1065-9.

[25] Host A, Halken S, Muraro A, Dreborg S, Niggemann B, Aalberse R, Arshad SH, von Berg A, Carlsen KH, et al. Dietary prevention of allergic diseases in infants and small children. Pediatr Allergy Immunol. 2008 Feb;19:1-4.
[26] American Academy of Pediatrics. Committee on Nutrition. Hypoallergenic infant formulas. Pediatrics. 2000 Aug;106:346-9.
[27] Giampietro PG, Kjellman NI, Oldaeus G, Wouters-Wesseling W, Businco L. Hypoallergenicity of an extensively hydrolyzed whey formula. Pediatr Allergy Immunol. 2001 Apr;12:83-6.
[28] Restani P, Gaiaschi A, Plebani A, Beretta B, Cavagni G, Fiocchi A, Poiesi C, Velona T, Ugazio AG, Galli CL. Cross-reactivity between milk proteins from different animal species. Clin Exp Allergy. 1999 Jul;29:997-1004.
[29] Restani P, Beretta B, Fiocchi A, Ballabio C, Galli CL. Cross-reactivity between mammalian proteins. Ann Allergy Asthma Immunol. 2002 Dec;89:11-5.
[30] Spuergin P, Walter M, Schiltz E, Deichmann K, Forster J, Mueller H. Allergenicity of alpha-caseins from cow, sheep, and goat. Allergy. 1997 Mar;52:293-8.
[31] Terracciano L, Isoardi P, Arrigoni S, Zoja A, Martelli A. Use of hydrolysates in the treatment of cow's milk allergy. Ann Allergy Asthma Immunol. 2002 Dec;89:86-90.
[32] Savino F, Castagno E, Monti G, Serraino P, Peltran A, Oggero R, Fanaro S, Vigi V, Silvestro L. Z-score of weight for age of infants with atopic dermatitis and cow's milk allergy fed with a rice-hydrolysate formula during the first two years of life. Acta Paediatr Suppl. 2005 Oct;94:115-9.
[33] Reche M, Pascual C, Fiandor A, Polanco I, Rivero-Urgell M, Chifre R, Johnston S, Martin-Esteban M. The effect of a partially hydrolysed formula based on rice protein in the treatment of infants with cow's milk protein allergy. Pediatr Allergy Immunol. Jun;21:577-85.
[34] ESPGHAN Committee on Nutrition; Agostoni C AI, Goulet O, Koletzko B, Michaelsen KF, Puntis J, Rieu D, Rigo J, Shamir R, Szajewska H, Turck D. Soy protein infant formulae and follow-on formulae: a commentary by the ESPGHAN Committee on Nutrition. J Pediatr Gastroenterol Nutr 2006;42:352-61.
[35] Nowak-Wegrzyn A, Sampson HA, Wood RA, Sicherer SH. Food protein-induced enterocolitis syndrome caused by solid food proteins. Pediatrics. 2003 Apr;111:829-35.
[36] Bocquet A, Bresson JL, Briend A, Chouraqui JP, Darmaun D, Dupont C, Frelut ML, Ghisolfi J, Goulet O, et al. [Infant formulas and soy protein-based formulas: current data]. Arch Pediatr. 2001 Nov;8:1226-33.
[37] Bhatia J, Greer F. Use of soy protein-based formulas in infant feeding. Pediatrics. 2008 May;121:1062-8.
[38] Wahn U. Aspects of nutritional management of food allergy. Pediatr Allergy Immunol. 2001;12 Suppl 14:75-7.
[39] Osborn DA, Sinn J. Formulas containing hydrolysed protein for prevention of allergy and food intolerance in infants. Cochrane database of systematic reviews (Online). 2006:CD003664.

[40] Kemp AS, Hill DJ, Allen KJ, Anderson K, Davidson GP, Day AS, Heine RG, Peake JE, Prescott SL, et al. Guidelines for the use of infant formulas to treat cows milk protein allergy: an Australian consensus panel opinion. The Medical journal of Australia. 2008 Jan 21;188:109-12.

15

Natural Rubber Latex Allergy

Ana Maria Sell and Jeane Eliete Laguila Visentainer
Universidade Estadual de Maringá,
Brazil

1. Introduction

Natural rubber latex (NRL) is a milky fluid from the *Hevea brasiliensis* (Hev b) tree, which functions as a protective sealant (Ownby, 2002). Because of its excellent elastic properties, it is widely used in the manufacture of medical devices and in a variety of everyday articles such as gloves, condoms, balloons, baby nipples, syringe plungers, and vial stoppers. As many as 40 000 types of consumer products may contain NRL (Perkin et al., 2000). The use of rubber for surgical gloves was first made in 1984 by Richard Cook and who popularized the use of rubber gloves in surgery was William Hasted (Dyck, 2000).

NRL allergy is a common occupational disease. The induction of latex allergy commonly occurs after exposure of skin or mucous membrane to natural rubber latex. It is usually a contact dermatitis or delayed allergy (type IV), and reaction mediated by IgE (type I) or immediate hypersensitivity. Latex allergy symptoms can be mild or severe and manifest as contact urticaria, rhinoconjunctivitis, asthma, and mucosal swelling; systemic reactions consist of generalized urticaria and anaphylactic shock (Hamann et al., 1998; Agarwal & Gawkrodger, 2002; Cao et al., 2010; Cleenewerck, 2010).

It affects people who are frequently exposed to products made of natural rubber latex, such as health care workers HCWs (5 to 17%); and groups at high risk included spina bifida cystica patients (to almost 65%), latex industry workers, specific food-allergy patients, and patients with a history of atopy or multiple surgical procedures (Nettis et al., 2002; Turjanmaa et al., 2002; Sullivan, 2005; Sukekava & Sell, 2007; Armentia et al., 2010; Bains et al., 2010; Radauer et al., 2011).

Knowledge about latex allergy is important for three reasons: firstly, it is potentially fatal if the patient is not properly managed; secondly, it is common in healthcare workers (HCWs) as an occupational disease; and thirdly, its incidence has been increasing due to increased use of latex gloves as a barrier against viral infections (Agarwal & Gawkrodger, 2002). Also, latex has cross reactivity to banana, avocado, kiwi and other foods.

Undiagnosed latex allergy is potentially very serious for patients and is increasingly recognized as a significant contributor to morbidity and mortality during medical and surgical procedures, and anaphylactic shock has been documented (Kosti & Lambrianidis, 2002; Sonofuchi et al., 2010).

At present, latex avoidance is the only available treatment and is the key to preventing allergic reactions in latex-sensitized individuals.

This chapter will present the etiology, epidemiology, and pathogenesis of natural rubber latex allergy.

2. Latex allergens

Latex products are ubiquitous in our environment and its use and choice is attributed to its biomechanical performance characteristics, which include strength, elasticity, tear resistance, and superior barriers qualities.

Raw latex is a milky sap harvested from the rubber tree *(Hevea brasiliensis)* and it is subsequently vulcanized into elastic rubber with which we are all familiar. This milky substance is the cytoplasm of the cells of the lactiferous system of the tree. The vast majority of *Hevea brasiliensis* cultivation occurs in Malaysia, Indonesia and Thailand. After harvest by sap collection, NRL is ammoniated to prevent bacterial contamination and coagulation, resulting in the hydrolysis to latex proteins. Prior to use in manufacturing, the latex is formulated by the addition of multiple chemicals: accelerators, antioxidants, and secondary preservatives. Thus human exposure is a mixture of residual chemicals and hydrolyzed latex peptides. The proteins components have been responsible for type I latex-specific allergy and the accelerators and antioxidants are agents of type IV allergic reactions (contact dermatitis). Not until Charles Goodyear developed the process of vulcanization to stabilize rubber and prevent it from easily melting or freezing, did the rubber industry become important (Dyck, 2000).

The essential structural functional unit in processed latex is an aqueous elastomer emulsion containing mainly cis-1,4-polyisoprene (30%-40%) and water (55%-65%), which is coated with a layer of protein, lipid, and phospholipids. The protein content of rubber tree sap is approximately 15mg/ml and includes more than 240 polypeptides, and 60 of these react to latex-specific IgE. Latex proteins can be divided into: water-soluble proteins, starch-bound proteins, and latex-bound proteins. Of the multiple proteins found in latex, certain specific proteins have been identified as being the major concern in causing IgE-mediated allergic reactions. Fourteen proteins have been identified, characterized, and officially accepted as allergenic components (Sussman & Beezold, 1994; Lee et al., 2010; Ott et al., 2010).

The WHO_International Union of Immunological Societies Allergen Nomenclature Committee (www.allergens.org) listed 14 NRL Hev b allergens (Hev b 1-14) characterized at the molecular level. It has included Hev b 1, rubber elongation factor (Chen et al., 1997); Hev b 2, b-1,3-glucanase (Yagami et al., 2002); Hev b 3, small rubber particle protein - a 24-kDa protein (Wagner et al., 1999); Hev b 4, a component of the microhelix protein complex – lecithinase homologue; Hev b 6, prohevein/hevein precursor; Hev b 7; patatin-like protein; and Hev b 13, esterase (Beirnstein et al., 2003); Hev b 5, acidic protein – proline-rich protein (Slater et al., 1996); Hev b 8, profiling (Nieto et al., 2002); Hev b 9, enolase (Wagner et al., 2000); Hev b 10, manganese superoxide dismutase (Rihs et al., 2001); Hev b 12, non-specific lipid transfer protein 1 (Beezhold et al., 2003); and Hev b 11, class I chitinase, and Hev b 14, hevamine, that no allergenicity has been described yet. The epitopes identified as IgE-binding areas have been defined (Pedraza-Escalona et al., 2009; Rougé et al., 2010). Natural rubber latex (NRL) allergenic proteins are listed in Table 1.

It has been suggested that Hev b 1 and Hev b 3 are major allergens in children with spina bifida and urological congenital anomalies (Baur et al., 1995; Yeang et al., 1996; Chen et al., 1997). Berstein et al. (2003) identified Hev b 2, 5, 6.01 and Hev b 13 as the major *in vivo* allergens among HCWs with allergy to NRL, confirmed by percutaneous sensitivity to nonammoniated latex (NAL). These differences of epitopes reactivity can be explained by the different allergen profiles on internal and external surfaces of natural rubber latex gloves (Peixinho et al., 2008).

Biochemical name	Allergen name	WM		Allerginicity reference
Rubber elongation factor	Hev b 1	14	mainly associated with spina bifida patients	Chen et al., 1997
b-1,3-glucanase	Hev b 2	34	linked more to adult latex-allergy patients	Yagami et al., 2002
Small rubber particle protein	Hev b 3	24	mainly associated with spina bifida patients	Wagner et al., 1999
Lecithinase homologue	Hev b 4	53-55		Beirnstein et al., 2003
Acidic protein	Hev b 5	16	linked more to adult latex-allergy patients	Slater et al., 1996
Hevein precursor	Hev b 6	20	linked more to adult latex-allergy patients	Beirnstein et al., 2003
Patatin-like protein	Hev b 7	42		Beirnstein et al., 2003
Profilin	Hev b 8	15		Nieto et al., 2002
Enolase	Hev b 9	51		Wagner et al., 2000
Superoxide dismutase (Mn)	Hev b 10	26		Rihs et al., 2001
Class I chitinase	Hev b 11	30	no allergenicity described	
Non-specific lipid transfer protein 1	Hev b 12	9		Beezhold et al., 2003
Esterase	Hev b 13	42	linked more to adult latex-allergy patients	Beirnstein et al., 2003
Hevamine	Hev b 14	30	no allergenicity described	

Table 1. Natural rubber latex (NRL) allergenic proteins

3. Hypersensitivity reactions

Specific immune responses are normally stimulated when an individual is exposed to a foreign antigen and this process is called immunization. Immune responses are specific for different structural components of the most complex proteins and polysaccharides antigens. The portions of such antigens are specifically recognized by distinct lymphocytes are called epitopes. This fine specificity exists because T and B lymphocytes express membrane receptors that distinguish subtle difference between distinct antigens. *Naïve* lymphocytes are continually released from the primary lymphoid organs into the periphery (secondary lymphoid organs). Antigen-binding can lead to activation of a T or B cell. All of the progeny cells derived from any single *naïve* lymphocytes that constitute a clone.

Responses to most immunogens can begin only after the immunogen has been captured, processed, and presented by an APC (antigen-processing cell) to CD4 T cells (T_H0). The reason of this is that T cells only recognize immunogens that are bound to major histocompatiblity complex (MHC) proteins on the surfaces of other cells. There are two different classes of MHC proteins. Class I MHC proteins are expressed virtually by all somatic cell types and are used to present substances to CD8 T cells, most of which are cytotoxic T cells. Class II MHC proteins, on the other hand, are expressed only by macrophages and a few other cells types and are necessary for antigen presentation to CD4 T cells - the subset that includes most helper cells. Since helper-cell activation is necessary for virtually all responses, the class II-bearing APCs plays a pivotal role in controlling such responses.

Exogenous immunogens can be captured in a variety of ways. After captured by APCs become enclosed within membrane-lined vesicles in the cytoplasm and, within these vesicles, undergo a series of alterations called antigen processing and a limited number of the resulting peptides associated non-covalently with class II MHC proteins and transported to APC surface, where they can be detected by CD4 T cells. This process is called antigen presentation. At specific antigen recognition the sequences of events induced in lymphocytes initiate the activation phase. First, the lymphocyte proliferate, leading to expansion of the clones of antigen-specific lymphocytes and amplification of the protective response. Second, lymphocytes differentiate to cells that functions are to eliminate foreign antigens: thus, B cells transform to plasma cells that secret specific antibody that binds to soluble antigen; and some T cells (CD4 or T helper) differentiate into cells that activate phagocytes to kill intracellular antigens, and other T cells (CD8) that directly lyses cells that are producing foreign antigens such as viral proteins. The effector phase is the stage that activated performs the functions that lead to elimination of the antigens: inflammatory response is amplified after recruitment of specific and nonspecific effectors cells (lymphocytes, macrophages, basophiles, mast cells) and their soluble components production (lymphokines, monokines, complement, kinines, arachidonic acid derivates, and mast cells- basophile products).

The immune response serves to protect the individual from foreign antigens with a well-controlled immune and inflammatory response. However damage to host tissues and diseases can result from dysfunction of any component of the host defense system, like hypersensitivity or allergy.

The allergy results when an exposure to the allergens induces an immune response, referred to as "sensitization" rather than immunization. Once sensitization occurs, an individual will be not symptomatic until there is a new exposure to the same allergen. Then the reaction of allergen with specific antibody or sensitized effector T lymphocyte induces an inflammatory response, producing the symptoms and signs of the allergic reaction.

The reactions characteristic of type I hypersensitivity are dependent on the specific triggering of IgE-sensitized mast cell by allergen. The sensitization occurs when foreign antigens or allergens enter in the host, are processed and presented to APC to the T helper 2 (T_H2) cells. T_H2 cells secrete cytokines (interleukins: IL-4, IL-5 and IL-6) that induces B cells proliferation and favour to production of an allergens specific-IgE response. IgE binds, via Fc_ε receptors, to mast cells and basophiles thus sensitizing them. When allergen subsequently reaches the sensitized mast cells it cross-links surphace-bound IgE and increases intracellular calcium that triggers the release of pre-formed mediators, such as histamine and proteases, and newly synthesized, lipid-derived mediators such as leukotrienes and prostaglandins. These autacoids produce the clinical symptoms of allergy (asthma, eczema, and anaphylaxis).

Type IV (delayed) hypersensitivity reactions involve cell-mediated immune reactions rather than humoral response. The sensitization occurs when Langerhans cells process foreign antigens and present them to T helper 1 (T_H1) cells. The T cells responsibly for the delayed response have been specifically sensitized by a previous encounter, and act recruiting other cell types to the site of the reaction. Contact hypersensitivity is characterized by an eczematous reaction at the point of the contact with an allergen.

4. Latex sensitization

Sensitization and development of latex allergy arise from exposure to products containing residual latex proteins and chemical additives in latex products. Latex proteins are potent allergens capable of inducing fatal anaphylaxis.

Sensitization of latex allergy can occur through the skin, by inhalation or by internal exposure (mucous membranes of the mouth, vagina or rectum). Medical devices (anesthetic masks, condom catheters, ileostomy bags, balloon catheters used for enemas and latex gloves) can induce sensitization and then subsequently cause an allergy to develop on re-exposure. The addiction of cornstarch powder of gloves, in 1947, to prevent sticking and give a smoother fit, has been shown to increase the leaching of latex proteins and exposure latex proteins on the surface. Powder from latex gloves serves as vector of the dangerous proteins that then trigger an allergic response. Cornstarch also promotes aerosolization of the latex proteins when gloves are removed, and its release powder into the air and latex proteins are inhaled by all individuals in the room. Rubber is extensively distributed in the environment and we are in contact with it virtually all the time.

Latex absorption through the skin is postulated as the major route of sensitization in health care workers by the soluble proteins. Friction, pressure, heat, and perspiration are among the nonspecific factors that influence the occurrence, severity, and sites of involvement of hypersensitivity and cutaneous manifestations.

5. Pathogenesis and clinical manifestations

Clinical manifestations include irritant contact dermatitis, allergic contact dermatitis (type IV), and immediate hypersensitivity reaction mediated by IgE (type I) (Table 2). It can affect the skin, eyes and lungs (Nutter, 1979; Hamann et al., 1998; Mebra & Hunter, 1998; Agarwal & Gawkrodger, 2002; Cao et al., 2010; Cleenewerck, 2010).

5.1 Irritant contact dermatitis

Irritant contact dermatitis (ICD) is not an allergic reaction. It occurs when an exogenous substance without previous sensitization causes direct damage to the skin. Usually it is the result of contact with glove additives. Chapped skin from hand washing can be responsible for this symptom. Early manifestations of this type of reaction include itchy (most common symptoms), but morphological features (dry, crusted lesions) are similar in allergic dermatitis, especially on fingers webs and under rings. Greater degrees of irritation result in burning, red or swollen tissues. Vesiculation is a late manifestation, but rarely occurs. ICD has a diagnosis for exclusion, and patch testing is negative. Management includes careful hand washing techniques, use of skin emollients, and an effective routine.

5.2 Type IV hypersensitivity - Delayed reactions

Delayed (type IV) allergy or contact dermatitis to rubber gloves is primarily caused by accelerators added to speed up rubber vulcanization, including carbamates, thiurams, 2-mercaptobenzothiszole, and 1,3-diphenylguanidina. It may also cause by antioxidants that prevent rubber deterioration, such as black rubber mix chemicals (*p*-phenylenediamines (Cao et al., 2010). It typically manifests within 24 to 48 hours after contact with the allergen. It is localized to the skin or mucous membrane. The patient presents a diffuse or patchy eczema on the dorsal surface of the hands, wrists, and distal forearms. Latter the reaction can become generalized, and chronic exposure leads to hyperkeratosis and lichenification, and at times either hyper- or hypopigmentation. The scalp and palms have a greater resistance to contact allergic and irritant reactions than other skin areas. The eyelids, penis, and scrotum often show erythema and edema rather than vesiculation. Patch testing is positive in these patients. The development of a type IV hypersensitivity allergic response may occur after years of contact with the substance.

5.3 Type I hypersensitivity - Immediate reactions

Type I reactions to latex involve specific immunoglobulin IgE and mediators of anaphylaxis. It is caused by latex proteins that direct sensitize the patients, and reactions occur within 1-30 minutes. There may be a wide spectrum of clinical presentations. The route of latex antigen presentation will usually dictate the clinical manifestations. The skin manifestations include itching, swelling, localized pruritus and urticaria (direct contact). Respiratory involvement consists of sneezing, wheezing and rhinitis; and the eyes may water, itch and conjunctivitis (aerosol exposure or facial contact – latex proteins are adsorbed on gloves powder that becomes airborne and can be directly inhaled). A mucosal route of exposure to latex allergens is often associated with anaphylactic reactions. The clinical manifestations may be serious and give rise to a generalized shock-like reaction: systemic reactions such as broncospasm, hypotension, cardiorespiratory collapse, and shock can occur with more substantial exposure and in extremely sensitive individuals.

Contact urticaria is the most common early manifestation of rubber allergy, particularly in latex-sensitive health care workers. Symptoms appear within 10-15 min after donning gloves. No residual coloration occurs after resolution of the urticaria.

Anaphylactic shock is potentially fatal and anaphylactic response to latex exposure occurs most commonly intraoperatively. However, anaphylactic reactions have been encountered during gloving, exposure to dental dams, condom use, and even after indirect exposition by contact with individual who use latex gloves. The response appears minutes after the administration the allergen, manifesting as a respiratory distress, followed by vascular collapse and shock. Cutaneous symptoms, pruritus and urticaria, often occur with or without angioedema. Gastrointestinal manifestations involved nausea, vomiting, crampy abdominal pain, and diarrhea.

Non-Immunological and Immunological Reactions	Symptoms	Etiology	Allergens
Irritant Contact Dermatitis	Irritant contact dermatitis	Non-immunological	Gloves additives
Type I hypersensitivity Immediate reactions	Contact urticaria, asthma, rhinithis, angioedema, generalized anaphylaxis	IgE antibody produced by B cells	Latex proteins
Type IV hypersensitivity Delayed reactions	Contact dermatitis	T cells sensitized to antigens	Chemicals used in manufacture of latex

Table 2. Pathogenesis and clinical manifestations to the allergy of latex

6. Incidence of latex allergy

Latex allergy is now an important medical, occupational, medico-legal and financial problem, and it is essential that policies are developed to reduce it.

The diffusion of the "universal precautions", promoted in 1987 by the Center for Disease Control and Prevention, dramatically increased the use of latex glove in health care workers (HCWs) to reduce the risk of infection, for protection against the HIV and HBV. The increased demand caused an increased production of gloves, and a different chemical treatment of rubber trees which lowered the glove quality, that means high levels of antigens and high powder content. This situation causes an increase of allergic frequency (type I and type IV) and irritant reactions to latex gloves in health care workers.

The prevalence of latex allergy in the general population was estimated at 0.7%-1% in the most reports, but some reports now show numbers up to 6%. A high prevalence of latex hypersensitivity is observed in certain occupational and other high-risk groups with frequent exposure to NRL products, including health care workers (ranges from 2.8% to 17%), operating room personal (15-20%), rubber industry workers (near 10%), spina bifida cystica patients (to almost 65%), atopic individuals (7%), and those who have had multiple surgical operations (6.5%), patients with congenital urologic abnormalities, and those with a coexisting food allergy, most often related to certain fruits. The risk is associated with the peoples who are frequently exposed to products made of natural rubber latex such as in different regions, age, sex and ethnic groups.

6.1 General population

Although data is difficult to obtain, estimates now indicate that 1% to 6% of the general population has some sensitivity or allergy to latex. In 1994, Ownby et al. measured latex-specific IgE in the serum from 1000 blood donors and 6.5% were positive. Prevalence of positive samples was not associated to race or age.

6.2 Risk groups

6.2.1 Health care workers

The major source of workplace exposure has been powered natural rubber latex gloves used mainly by HCW. It has been a problem especially for HCW working in surgical areas or in places where there is more use of latex gloves, in function of the high levels of airbone latex particles in these areas. The prevalence of immediate latex allergy increased with increasing duration of latex exposure. Studies have reported a prevalence of latex sensitization of from 2.8 to 17% of the hospital workpopulation.

The first scientific work describing dermatitis from rubber gloves was published in 1933 (Downing, 1933). Nutter (1979) was the first investigator to describe contact urticaria to rubber gloves: the condition occurred in a house-wife with atopic dermatitis, and during the exacerbation of her hand eczema she noted intensive itching for her hands which occurred 5 min after donning a pair of rubber gloves. The urticaria was confirmed by a patch test using a small piece of rubber gloves and with a skin prick test. One year later, Förström described the first case of contact urticaria from latex surgical gloves in a nurse with history of atopic dermatitis and allergic rhinitis.

In 1987, Turjanmaa was the first to evaluate the frequency of latex gloves allergy among health care workers. A total of 512 hospital employees were screened by using a latex gloves scratch-chamber test and subsequent prick test for individuals who are positive in screening. Twenty-three (4.5%) had positive scratch-chamber test, and the prick test was positive in 15 of these 23 patients. Most of them had a personal history of atopy, asthma, allergic rhinitis, and atopic eczema. Latex gloves allergy was significantly more frequent in personal of operative room.

Arellano et al. (1992) were the first to report the prevalence of latex sensitization among physicians using latex gloves in a North American Hospital setting. Using a latex skin prick test they determined the sensitization in 9.9% of the North American physicians.

Since 1987, the number of HCW with positive test results for NRL has been increased. In 1994, Charous et al. reviewed medical histories of symptomatic workers with occupational exposure to latex and they evidenced that the number of patients reporting onset of latex-induced contact dermatitis had remained relatively constant, whereas the number of the patients with contact dermatitis and systemic reactions had markedly increased.

Some reports about prevalence of latex allergy in HCW in different countries are presented. At an Italy Hospital, a high prevalence of rubber glove-induced dermatoses among the employees were evidenced: about of 24% the health care workers, who used or had used latex gloves at work, reported glove-induced symptoms, namely, cutaneous symptoms in all the cases. Non-cutaneous symptoms appeared in 8.1%. Positive patch tests to rubber-related allergens were exhibited at 10.5% of symptomatic employees (Nettis et al., 2002).

The prevalence of latex allergy among HCWs in Russia, and adjacent eastern European countries was available and considerably less than reported in Western Europe and the United States. Skin test to latex was positive in 5.4% of HCWs and 1.9% were classified as latex-allergic based on positive skin tests to latex associated with allergy symptoms with exposure. Some of them had experienced anaphylactic reactions to latex. The low prevalence of latex allergy suggests that lessened exposure to natural latex powdered gloves in HCWs in Russia (Nolte et al., 2002).

To assess the allergic risk induced by latex gloves in HCWs, a meta-analysis was carried out under the auspices of the French National Regulatory Authority. Latex allergy was found in 4.32% (range, 4.01% to 4.63%) of HCWs and in 1.37% (range, 0.43% to 2.31%) of the general population. Latex-positive skin prick test responses ranged from 2.1% to 3.7% in the general population and from 6.9% to 7.8% for the HCWs (Bousquet et al, 2006).

To determine the main factors associated with latex allergy and to quantify levels of airborne latex particles in different areas of Spanish hospital, a cross-sectional study was conducted by Diéguez et al. (2007). More allergic patients were found in the surgery department, intensive care unit, and vascular radiology unit.

In Taiwan, natural rubber latex is the most important occupational allergen among medical workers. To evaluate immediate latex allergy and contact dermatitis, 1253 medical workers were interviewed using a screening questionnaire and skin prick testing with commercial latex extract was performed. The prevalence of contact hand dermatitis from latex gloves was 35%. Twelve percent had positive latex skin prick test, suggesting that they had been sensitized to latex proteins. Seventy nine subjects (6%) had immediate allergic reactions to latex products (Lin et al., 2008).

The prevalence of hypersensitivity to natural rubber latex and potential food cross reactions in operation room personnel in Shiraz hospitals revealed a significant correlation between those with positive skin tests to latex with atopia, urticaria, and food hypersensitivity. About 18% of operating room personnel showed positive latex skin tests. The prevalence did not vary by sex, age, education, surgical and non-surgical gloves users, or history of contact dermatitis (Nabavizadeh et al., 2009).

Dates from Asia countries with regard to latex allergy are scarce. Amarasekera et al. (2010) determined the prevalence and risk factors among healthcare workers in a hospital in Sri Lanka. Symptoms suggestive of latex allergy were reported in 16% of the subjects. A considerable proportion (11.4%) of workers had been suffering from latex allergy for more than 5 years.

Oral health care professionals have been shown to be at risk for developing a type I allergy to natural rubber latex (NRL). The prevalence of this allergy in dental hygienists has been evaluated. Hamann et al. (2005) investigated by screened positive for a type I allergy to NRL (SPT-positive) 582 participants to 2000-2002 American Dental Hygienists' Association (ADHA) national meetings. Risk factors and symptom assessments were questioned and were based on a self-reported health history. About 5% screened positive for a type I allergy to NRL (SPT-positive). They observed that the NRL allergy was significantly more likely to report an allergy to cross-reacting foods, plants, moulds, and pollens, and to report reactions to rubber products. Sukekava & Sell (2007) determined the incidence of latex gloves allergy among dental care workers. Latex gloves reaction occurred in 19% of them, and 5% reported allergic reactions to other latex products; 2.5% reported symptoms suggesting contact dermatitis and anaphylaxis hypersensitivities, 1.5% reported contact dermatitis, and 1% reported anaphylaxis symptoms when wearing them.

6.2.2 Latex industry workers

Latex industry workers have an increased prevalence of chronic respiratory symptoms and reduced lung function. In 1988, Bascom et al. described a spectrum of respiratory illness associated with eosinophilia that occurred in a group of rubber workers exposed to fumes from a synthetic rubber-based curing operation. Two years latter, 81 latex industry workers were evaluated, and 7 had spirometric changes consistent with asthma, and two of them had positive skin prick test to latex. To known the relation of rubber tree dust exposure to respiratory and skin symptoms, asthma and lung function in regard to wood dust from the rubber tree, a cross-sectional study was carried out among 103 workers in a rubber tree furniture factory and 76 office workers in four factories in Thailand. Factory workers showed increased risk of wheezing, nasal symptoms and asthma compared to office workers. There was a dose-dependent increase in wheeze and skin symptoms in regard to dust level. Significantly increased risks of nasal symptoms and asthma were detected in the low exposure category (Sripaiboonkij et al., 2009).

6.2.3 Patients with spina bifida cystica

Patients with spina bifida cystica form a population at highest risk of latex allergy. Management of infants with spina bifida cystica involves different procedures that include immediate operative skin closure of an open or thin walled defect, ventriculoperitoneal shunting of hydrocephalus, bracing of the lower extremities, and other surgical procedures to address sensory deficits, bowel and bladder dysfunction, pain elimination, orthopedic problems, and minimize or prevent associated neurologic defects. The major risk factors for latex sensitization in spina bifida cystica children include atopy, familiarity propensity for allergy, and very early exposure with mucosal absorption of allergen related to number of surgical procedures. Kelly et al. (1991) pointed out in their studies that spina bifida pediatric patients have 500 times greater a risk of latex-related anaphylaxis during operative procedures than of the general pediatric population: eight of the 10 pediatric patients experiencing anaphylaxis during surgery. Prevalence of latex sensitivity among the spina bifida cystica pediatric population was among 40 to 65%. The recommendation is that children with spina bifida avoid contact with NRL products from birth.

7. Cases reports of latex-induced anaphylactic reactions

The prevalence of latex allergy is increasing in general population and surgical patient individuals. Several anaphylactic events during some surgical procedures are still rare; however they are associated with increased morbidity and mortality. Undiagnosed latex allergy is potentially very serious for patients. The risk factors for latex skin sensitization were: a previous history of atopy and asthma; history of surgery; pre-existing hand dermatitis; work-related symptoms; and positive skin tests to common inhalant and certain foods. Avoidance of exposure to the allergen is essential to minimizing preoperative complications in patients suspect to be at risk.

In 2003, Verdolin et al. described an accidental diagnosis of latex allergy after urological surgery under spinal anesthesia when patient presented clinical manifestation of anaphylactic shock: confusion, dyspnea, generalized pruritus and erythema, bronchospasm, arterial hypotension, and tachycardia. In Japan, Ueda et al. (2008) reported an anaphylactic reaction to latex forty-three minutes subsequent to spinal anesthesia in a 46-year-old man with a history of atopic dermatitis and bronchial asthma underwent surgery for an inguinal hernia. Sonofuchi et al. (2010) reported anaphylactic shock after introduction of the general anesthesia in the patient who had latex allergy. Machado et al. (2011) described a case of severe latex induced anaphylactic reaction in a patient with a diagnostic suspicion of appendicitis who underwent an emergency surgery under spinal anesthesia. The symptoms occurred approximately 30 minutes after beginning the surgery.

One of the groups that are at risk for anaphylactic reactions to latex during surgical and medical procedures is represented by the obstetric and gynecologic population. A case was reported when an anaphylactic reaction to latex occurred in a pregnant woman patient who underwent a caesarean section that the diagnosis of latex allergy was missed. Following day the woman underwent a surgical re-exploration complicated by fatal cardiovascular arrest. At post-mortem examination, pulmonary mast cells in the bronchial walls and capillary septa were identified, and a great number of degranulating mast cells with tryptase-positive material outside the cells was documented and the latex-specific IgE test showed a high title. Latex-induced fatal anaphylactic shock was recorded as the cause of death. This case highlights some of the practical difficulties in the initial diagnosis and subsequent investigation of fatal anaphylactic reaction during anesthesia. Anaphylaxis is often misdiagnosed because many other pathologic conditions may present identical clinical manifestations, so anaphylactic shock must be differentiated from other causes of circulatory collapse. Although latex allergy usually has a delayed onset after the start of the surgery and most often a slow onset too, it should be always suspected if circulatory collapse and respiratory failure occur during surgery, even if the patient does not belong to a risk group; in the presence of identified risk factors for latex allergy a well-founded suspicion must be stronger, leading to an immediate discontinuation of the potential trigger (Turillazzi et al., 2008).

8. Immunological cross-reactivity between latex and other products

8.1 Food cross-reactivity

Latex allergy has been reported to be associated with allergy to certain foods. Approximately 30-50% of individuals who are allergic to natural rubber latex (NRL) show an associated hypersensitivity to some plant-derived foods, especially freshly consumed fruits. This association of latex allergy and allergy to plant-derived foods is called latex-fruit syndrome. An increasing number of plant sources have been associated with this syndrome. The most frequently involved are banana, avocado, kiwi, and chestnut, although several others may also be included as peach, grape, pineapple, nuts, figs, passion fruit, celery, citrus fruits, chestnut, peach, tomato, potato and bell pepper. Some studies have found out immunological and clinical cross-reactivity.

The hypothesis is that allergen cross-reactivity is due to IgE antibodies that recognize structurally similar epitopes on different proteins that are phylogenetically closely related or represent evolutionarily conserved structures. Several types of proteins have been identified to be involved in the latex-fruit syndrome. Two of these are higher plant defense proteins. Class I chitinases containing an N-terminal hevein-like domain cross-react with hevein (Hev b 6.02). A beta-1,3-glucanase was identified as an important latex allergen which shows cross-reactivity with proteins of bell pepper and banana. Nine distinct IgE-binding epitopes were identified along the entire amino acid sequence of the major latex allergen Hev b 2 (beta-1,3-glucanase), and a smaller number of IgE-binding epitopic areas was identified on the banana beta-1,3- glucanase, which exhibits a very similar overall conformation and charge distribution. Plant defense-related proteins are relatively conserved in the course of evolution and can supply cross-reactive epitopes. It is important to note that various stresses can stimulate the expression of these proteins, which implies that allergens increase in plants under stressful conditions like severe growing situations and exposure to some kinds of chemicals. Another important NRL allergen, Hev b 7, is a patatin-like protein that shows cross-reactivity with its analogous protein in potato (Wagner and Breiteneder, 2002; Barre et al., 2009).

Axelsson e cols. were one of the first researches to described an association between latex allergy and fruit. They describe a 12-year-old girl who developed rhinoconjuntivitis and itching in the throat after eating stone fruits. Subsequently, she developed angioedema after inflating a rubber balloon (Woods et al., 1997). Recently, anaphylactic shock was related in a woman underwent a cardiac catheter examination, and a Swan-Ganz catheter was inserted. She declared no past history of latex allergy, but did have a banana allergy. Skin prick test showed a positive reaction to an extract of latex gloves an extract of the balloon of a Swan-Ganz catheter (Sekiya et al., 2011). It is necessary to pay attention to not only latex allergy but also fruit allergies with cross-reactivity to latex.

Up to 2 out of 3 spina bifida patients with natural rubber latex (NRL) antibodies have crossreacting IgE-antibody against tropical fruit, due to structural homologies between several NRL antigens and allergenic fruit proteins. To investigate whether the patients were first sensitized against NRL or fruit, Cremer et al. (2011) investigated sera of 96 patients for specific IgE antibody against NRL, banana and kiwi as examples for cross reacting fruit. Only two patients developed antibody against fruit without being sensitized against NRL. In most cases the sensitization against fruit follows the NRL sensitization. There is no need to recommend spina bifida patients without NRL sensitization to primarily avoid tropical fruit.

Allergen cross-reactivity between tobacco and other species of Solanaceae family (tomato, potato, aubergine, and egg plant) have been reported. Armentia et al. (2010) have recently studied IgE response to tobacco in asthmatic patients sensitized to Lolium perenne (Perennial rye grass pollen), and have found that 30% of the tobacco responsive patients also have latex sensitization. They concluded that exist cross-reactivity between latex and tobacco allergens, and smoker patients with IgE response to tobacco may be a risk population for latex sensitization.

8.2 Gutta-percha and gutta-balata

In general dental practice, there is over than 30 products containing latex rubber. The practitioner should be cautions when threatening patients with a history or allergy to latex products. Gutta-percha and gutta-balata, used in endodontic treatment, are derived from the *Paliquium gutta* and *Mimusops globsa* trees, respectively, that are in the same botanical family of the rubber tree *Hevea brasiliensis*. For this reason immunological cross-reactivity between gutta-percha, gutta-balata and NRL were investigated (Costa et al., 2001): no detectable cross-reactivity was observed with any of the raw or clinically used gutta-percha products. In contrast, gutta-balata released proteins that were cross-reactive with latex. Because gutta-balata is sometimes added to commercial gutta percha products, caution should be taken if these products are used in endodontic care of latex-allergic individuals.

Many cases of anaphylaxis reactions occurrence in patient sensitive to latex during endodontic treatment has been reported. Boxer et al. (1994) described a latex-allergic dental hygienist who experienced immediate lip and gingival swelling and diffuse urticaria after the insertion of gutta-percha points into her maxillary molar by a general dentist. Immediately after removal of the gutta-percha, relief of the oral discomfort was noted, and the urticaria resolved several hours thereafter.

9. Genetic predisposition

The intensity of latex exposure, the route of sensitization, the genetically determined susceptibility, or the combination of all may have significant influence on pathogenesis of type I reaction to latex allergens. Although exposure to NRL products is necessary for sensitization, it is not sufficient.

The field of genome-based medicine, which attempts to identify genetic ffactors some individuals have, which may protect them or created problems when they undergo medical intervention, is rapidly evolving and affecting all fields of medical practice. Allergic diseases are dependent on the specific triggering of IgE-sensitized mast cell and their activation resulting in an inflammatory response. Immunological specific mechanism is genetically controlled and some individuals are more susceptible to allergic manifestations. Any steps of immunological and inflammatory reactions could be involved and are target of investigations. Polymorphism in over 30 genes localized on 15 different chromosomes has been associated with human allergy. Although the importance of these genetic components in the development of allergic diseases, susceptibility genes have been difficult to identify given the multigenic nature of this effect. The genetic/ immunologic risk factors of diseases susceptibility, that had been most studied, are the classic and non-classic alleles of the Major Histocompatibility Complex (MHC), and promoter genes of cytokine polymorphisms.

The Major Histocompatibility Complex (MHC), located on chromosome 6p21, is the most polymorphic genetic system in mammalians, and has been studied with regard to a wide variety of diseases of distinct etiology. The fundamental role of the different molecules within the MHC is antigen processing and presentation to the T-cell receptor (TCR), which is crucial for the cell interactions in immune response. In humans, while the classic class I *loci*, HLA-A, -B, and -C, bind peptides of intra-cellular origin and present them to CD8 T cells, the classic class II *loci*, HLA-DR, -DQ, and -DP, primarily bind peptides of extra-cellular origin and present them to CD4 T cells, resulting in cytokine production that drives an antibody production.

Focusing specifically on NRL allergy, Rihs et al. (2002) demonstrated the association between the specific IgE response to the major latex allergen hevein (Hev b 6.02) in HCW with latex allergy and latex-sensitized patients with spina bifida, and HLA class II alleles of DQB1 and DRB1, DRB3, DRB4, and DRB5. The class II HLA-DQB1*03:02 (DQ8) allele and HLA-DQB1*03:02 (DQ8)-DRB1*04(DR4) haplotype were significantly involved in the hevein-specific IgE immune response in HCW with latex allergy. NRL-sensitized patients with spina bifida showed an increase HLA-DQB1*03:02 frequency, but this result was not significant.

Two genes that have been of interest with regard to NRL allergy are *IL13* and *IL18*. IL-13, along with IL-4, is critical for the promotion of allergic response. IL-13 plays an important role in mediating airway hyperresponsiveness in asthma. Binding of IL-4 and IL-13 to the α chain of the IL-4 receptor activates germline transcription of the ε heavy-chain gene locus and isotype switching of B cells to IgE production. IL-18 can stimulate interferon production or enhance cytokines and IgE production. SNPs in these genes have been postulated to influence physiologic functions that are important in development of atopy (Monitto et al., 2010). Genetic predisposition to natural rubber latex allergy in the health care workers was available, and has been shown to be associated with promoter polymorphisms in *IL13* and *IL18* genes when compared with nonatopic controls (Brown et al., 2005). This association was not seen when these patients were genotyped for SNPs in other immunomodulatory genes, including *IL4*, tumor necrosis factor- α and -β, CC chemokine receptor 2 and 5, and toll-like receptor 4. In patients born with spina bifda and or genitourinary abnormalities the association of promoter polymorphisms in *IL13* and *IL18* genes was not observed (Monitto et al., 2010).

10. Diagnosis of latex allergy

To manage latex allergy appropriately, prompt and correct diagnosis is essential, and both *in vivo* and *in vitro* assays have been included. There are two elements to consider in latex allergy diagnosis: history and qualitative and quantitative tests.

10.1 History

The diagnosis of latex requires a thorough and accurate medical history. Screening patients is the first step for minimizing the risk of a latex allergic reaction. It is necessary to have a high index of suspicion, especially for patients in high risk occupations or with medical histories that induce repeated exposure to latex. Patients at special risk are those individuals with frequent or prolonged exposure to latex products. The following points must be considered: history of atopy (general allergies); food allergies (especially bananas, kiwi, avocados, chesnut, fig, tomato); history of allergic reactions to latex (including hives, swelling, eye/nose symptoms, asthma, and anaphylaxis); and undiagnosed reactions or complications during anesthesia, surgery, or dental work.

The medical clinical history about manifestations is often similar among individuals affected by latex allergy. Onset is often insidious with dermatitis of the hands, which patients attribute to frequent hand washing and irritation. After a short period of time (less than a year) erythema, papulovesiculation, induration, and pruritis emerge within 1-3 hours after onset of gloves use. Among HCW, one may often elicit a history of respiratory symptoms, which is pronounced while at work. For patients presenting contact dermatitis or urticaria, the physician should ask about localization and time of onset of the eruption, morphology, nature of progression, and recurrence or periodicity (Woods et al., 1997).

10.2 Diagnostic testing

Latex allergy can be diagnosed by skin prick testing, latex-specific serum immunoglobulin E testing, glove provocation testing, and patch testing. Both *in vivo* and *in vitro* testing methods have been used to diagnose latex allergy with varying degrees of success.

10.2.1 Skin prick testing (SPT)

The cutaneous test or skin prick tests with latex extracts are commonly used in the diagnostic approach to natural rubber latex allergy. For this, a minute quantity of the allergen is introduced into the dermis to cause a reaction with IgE antibodies fixed to cutaneous mast cells for release of mediators, producing a visible wheal and erythema. After 20 minutes the reactions are graded and recorded. The skin of the back or upper arms can be used. It should be done by trained allergists in a hospital setting with adequate resuscitation and medical support services. Reports of anaphylaxis during SPT for latex allergy emphasize the need to safe testing methods for diagnosis. This test has the advantage of being sensitive, rapid, and cost-effective. Reactivity in SPT is related to the potency of the SPT solution used: as a rule solutions with higher protein and antigen contents gave better results. Commercial extracts are used with good specificity and sensivity. Ammoniated and non-ammoniated latex extracts and Hev b 1, 2, 3, 4, 6.01, 7.01, and 13 allergens and recombinant Hev b 5 (rHev b 5) allergens are commonly used for this purpose. Serial dilutions extracts and NRL allergens were employed in skin testing. It is important to consider that sensitivity and specificity of different commercially available skin prick tests could vary (Bernardini et al., 2008b; van Kampen et al., 2010).

10.2.2 *In vitro* assays for latex-specific IgE

Quantitative measurement of allergen-specific IgE antibodies in serum requires special methods to detect the extremely minute quantities (pictograms per milliliter) found in allergic patients. Sensitive and specific commercial *in vitro* serological assays that have been developed for the diagnosis of IgE-mediated latex allergy include a radioallergosorbent assay - RAST, and enzyme-immunoassay method - ELISA. These occur in a 2-phase (solid/liquid) system using an insolubilized allergen that is incubated first in the test serum to react with latex specific IgE and then in radio, fluoro or enzyme- labeled heterologous anti-human IgE isotype. These tests require purified preparations of allergens (Hev b 1, Hev b 3, Hev b 5 - rHev b 5, Hev b 6.02, Hev b 8, and Hev b 13) and anti-human IgE. The differences in preparations of latex allergen and the existence of possible cross-reacting antibodies contribute to variance in accuracy of these tests. In atopic individuals, especially in patients with allergies to fruits or vegetables, these serological tests can produce false-positive results. The diagnostic sensitivity and specificity of the latex-specific IgE serology can be less when compared with skin tests (Smith et al., 2007).

10.2.3 Microarray technology

Microarray technology has recently been introduced being a reliable tool for diagnosing latex allergy (Ebo et al., 2010; Ott et al., 2010). A positive specific IgE (sIgE) result for latex does not always mirror the clinical situation and is frequently found in individuals without overt latex allergy. The diagnosis of latex allergy could be established by the combination of recombinant latex components present on the microarray (Hev b 1, Hev b 3, Hev b 5 and Hev b 6.02). The reaction can be performed with different platforms, the ImmunoCAP ISAC microarray and traditional singleplexed ImmunoCAP. Microarray can improve the diagnosis of IgE-mediated latex allergy by discriminating between genuine allergy and sensitization.

10.2.4 Provocation test

Occasionally, it is desirable to test the target (cutaneous, respiratory, or gastrointestinal) tissue responsiveness to the allergen under controlled conditions. Cutaneous provocation tests have been used in patients with suspect latex allergy: they wore a latex glove on one hand and a vinyl glove on the other hand for 15 minutes. Sensitivity is 90%, but some studies have indicated it may be more dangerous than skin testing in very allergic individuals. In the nasal provocation test, changes in nasal airways resistance and visible signs of congestion and rhinorrhea are observed after exposure to quantitative allergen challenge. To examine the responses in patients with positive SPT to nasal provocation test, Unsel et al. (2009) found that nasal provocation test has a sensitivity of 96%, specificity of 100%, negative predictive value of 98% and positive predictive value of 100%.

10.2.5 Path testing

Path testing is helpful in differentiating irritant contact dermatitis from allergic contact dermatitis mediated by type IV hypersensitivity reactions. It's a definitive test for diagnosis of patients with type IV hypersensitivity to latex products using a standard battery of rubber additives. The series of rubber allergen were applied on normal skin, usually on the patient's back or arms, under a small semi occlusive dressing. It is left in place for 24-48 hours. The results are first read in 30 minutes after removing patches, and again 24 or 48 h. The positive reaction can be accepted as the cause of the present eruption. Accelerators evoke positive patch tests in 82% patients with occupationally induced contact dermatitis associated with glove use. The allergens that most commonly yielded positive reactions have been carbamates, 4,4-dithiodimorpholine, thiurams mix, 2-mercaptobenzothiazole, and 1,3-diphenylguanidine (Woods et al., 1997; Bendewald et al., 2010; Cao et al., 2010).

11. Management and treatment

At present, latex avoidance is the only available treatment and has been the key to preventing allergic reactions in latex-sensitized individuals. For patients, avoidance of exposure to the allergen is essential to minimizing perioperative complications (Heitz &

Bader, 2010). In 1998, the Food and Drug Administration (FDA) started to require the labeling of medical devices made from rubber latex; since that time substantial progress had been made in identifying latex-free alternatives.

Avoidance of exposure to allergen is essential to minimizing complications in patients suspected to be at risk. The patient must be aware of the long list of medical and consumer products containing latex. Because there is cross reactivity between latex and fruit antigens, patients should be careful when first consuming these fruits after diagnosis. Procedures performed on latex-sensitive patients should be performed in latex-safe environment. A latex-safe environment is one in which no latex gloves are used; in addition, there must be no latex accessories (masks, rebreathing, cannulas, catheters, adhesives, tourniquets, anesthesia equipment) that come in direct contact with the patients. Prophylactic premedication is used by many centers for surgical patients with high risk of latex allergy. The use must be begin 24 h before surgery. In cases of minor reactions, such as contact dermatitis, the gloves should be removed immediately. For severe cases involving pruritus and erythema, therapy with H_1 antagonists should be initiated; H_2 blockers also can be used. In cases of severe systemic anaphylaxis, initial attention should focus on pulmonary and cardiovascular manifestations of the reaction, because these are the major causes of death.

The health care workers with latex allergy must be protected from adverse reaction to latex. Sensitization to latex antigens is commonly encountered in HCW wearing latex gloves with high latex allergen concentrations and in workers wearing powdered latex surgical gloves. HCW who have contact dermatitis to latex products can avoid it by changing to a different brand of gloves like vinyl and other synthetic gloves. Workers with a documented type I latex allergy must be protected from serious systemic reactions. Basically this involves latex avoidance. Low-protein, in powder-free gloves, decreases the sensitization potential of the latex and avoids some of the granuloma associated with the powder. Latex proteins are adsorbed by glove powder and may be airbone and the use of powder-free gloves can sometimes reduce the aerosol levels. In a review of claims data from 1997 to 2005 about the switch to powder-free latex gloves, Malerich et al. (2008) concluded that it was associated with a significant decrease in workers' compensation for latex-related illness. The cost of gloves increased but was partially offset by a decrease in workers' compensation payments and operating room expenses.

Future strategies must focus not only on the reduction of allergens during latex manufacture and development of suitable non-latex gloves, but also the immunotherapy including desensitization of latex allergic individuals and development of candidate vaccine (Belleri & Crippa, 2008; Bernardini et al., 2008a; Rolland & O'Hehir, 2008; Nettis et al., 2010).

In allergy desensitization treatment, the immune response itself can be altered. In practice, true desensitization is rare: specific IgE- mediated allergy is significantly lessened but not eliminated, even after many years of treatment. Immunological changes during desensitization therapy for IgE- mediated disease consist of increased IgG antibody levels and decreased IgE production. IgG are called "blocking antibody". Sublingual immunotherapy (SLIT) with natural rubber latex (NRL) has recently been proposed and was safe and effective; no SLIT-related side effects had been observed. Bernardini et al. (2008a) used commercial latex SLIT in pediatric patients and observed the effect for three years. A significant reduction of the glove-use score was observed after 1, 2, and 3 years of treatment with SLIT. Baseline wheal areas of skin prick test and baseline values of serum specific IgE were significantly reduced. They concluded that three years of latex SLIT is safe, and it consolidates the efficacy of treatment in pediatric patients. In addition, current

subcutaneous immunotherapy schedules have been tested for treatment of latex allergy with evidence of efficacy, but the risks of adverse events have been high.
For such potent allergens as latex, hypoallergenic but T cell-reactive preparations are required for clinical use. For this, it is essential to identify allergenic components of latex products with generation of monoclonal antibodies and recombinant allergens, allowing sequence determination and mapping of T cell and B cell epitopes. Potential hypoallergenic latex preparations identified include modified non-IgE-reactive allergen molecules and short T cell epitope peptides. Together, these reagents and data should facilitate improved diagnostics and investigation of novel-specific therapeutics. The co-administration of adjunct therapies, such as anti-IgE or corticosteroids, and appropriate adjuvant for induction of regulatory T cell response offer promise for clinically effective, and development of safe latex-specific candidate vaccines.

12. Conclusion

Latex products have had many useful roles in the medical fields. Unfortunately the allergic responses to latex have become causes of both morbidity and mortality. Avoidance of exposure to allergen is essential to minimizing complications in patients suspected to be at risk, butthere is lack of information concerning latex allergen content of medical equipment leading to an increased risk to sensitized patients. Occupational health need to be a guideline and should be prepared for any emergency. Patients with well documented latex hypersensitivity can undergo surgical procedures with proper panning and care. Further strategies must be focused not only on the reduction of allergens during latex manufacture and development of suitable non-latex gloves, but also on the immunotherapy and development of vaccine.

13. References

Amarasekera, M., Rathnamalala, N., Samaraweera, S. & Jinadasa, M. (2010). Prevalence of latex allergy among healthcare workers. *Int J Occup Med Environ Health.*, Vol.23, No.4, (May-Jun 2010), pp.391-396, ISSN 1232-1087

Arellano, R., Bradley, J. & Sussman, G. (1992). Prevalence of the latex sensitization among hospital physicians occupationally exposed to latex gloves. *Anesthesiology*, Vol.77, No.5, (Nov 1992), pp.905-908, ISSN 0003-2999

Agarwal, S. & Gawkrodger, D.J. (2002). Latex allergy: a health care problem of epidemic proportions. *Eur J Dermatol.*, Vol.12, No.4, (Jul-Aug 2002), pp.311-315, ISSN 1167-1122

Armentia, A., Dueñas-Laita, A., Bartolomé, B., Martín-Gil, F.J., San Miguel, A. & Castrodeza, J.J. (2010). Clinical significance of cross-reactivity between tobacco and latex. *Allergol Immunopathol.*,Vol.38, No.4, (Jul-Aug 2010), pp.187-196, ISSN 0301-0546

Ausili, E., Tabacco, F., Focarelli, B., Nucera, E., Patriarca, G. & Rendeli, C. (2007). Prevalence of latex allergy in spina bifida: genetic and environmental risk factors. *Eur Rev Med Pharmacol Sci.*, Vol.11, No.3, (May-Jun 2007), pp.149-153, ISSN 1128-3602

Bains, S.N., Hamilton, R.G., Abouhassan, S., Lang, D., Han, Y., & Hsieh, F.H. (2010). Identification of clinically relevant cross-sensitization between *Soliadgo virgaurea* (Goldenrod) and *Hevea brasiliensis* (Natural Rubber Latex). *J Investig Allergol Clin Immunol.*, Vol.20, No.4, pp.331-339, ISSN 1018-9068

Barre, A., Culerrier, R., Granier, C., Selman, L., Peumans, W.J., Van Damme, E.J., Bienvenu, F., Bienvenu, J. & Rougé, P. (2009). Mapping of IgE-binding epitopes on the major latex allergen Hev b 2 and the cross-reacting 1,3beta-glucanase fruit allergens as a molecular basis for the latex-fruit syndrome. *Mol Immunol.*, Vol.46, No.8-9, (May 2009), pp.1595-1604, ISSN 0161-5890

Bascom, R., Fisher J.F., Thomas, R.J., Yang, W.N., Baser, M.E. & Baker, J.H. (1988). Eosinophilia, respiratory symtoms, and pulmonary infiltrates in rubber workers. *Chest.* Vol.93, No.1, (Jan 1988), pp.154-158, ISSN 0012-3692

Baur, X., Chen, Z,. Rozynek, P., Duser, M. & Raulf-Heimsoth, M. (1995). Cross-reacting IgE antibodies recognizing latex allergens, including Hev b, as well as papain. *Allergy,* Vol. 50, No.7, (Jul 1995), pp. 604-609, ISSN 0105-4538

Belleri, L. & Crippa, M. (2008). Old and new types of sanitary gloves: what has improved? *Med Lav.,*Vol. 99, No.2, (Mar-Apr 2008), pp.80-84, ISSN 0025-7818

Bendewald, M.J., Farmer, S.A. & Davis, M.D. (2010). An 8-year retrospective review of patch testing with rubber allergens: the Mayo Clinic experience. *Dermatitis,*Vol.21, No.1, (Feb 2010), pp.33-40, ISSN 1710-3568

Bernardini, R., Pecora, S., Milani, M. & Burastero, S.E. (2008a). Natural rubber latex allergy in children: clinical and immunological effects of 3-years sublingual immunotherapy. *Eur Ann Allergy Clin Immunol.*, Vol.40, No.4, (Dec 2008), pp.142-147, ISSN 1764-1489

Bernardini, R., Pucci, N., Azzari, C., Novembre, E., De Martino, M. & Milani, M. (2008b). Sensitivity and specificity of different skin prick tests with latex extracts in pediatric patients with suspected natural rubber latex allergy-a cohort study. *Pediatr Allergy Immunol.*, Vol.19, No.4, (Jun 2008), pp.315-318, ISSN 0905-6157

Bernstein, D.I., Biagini, R.E., Karnani, R., Hamilton, R., Murphy, K., Bernstein, C., Arif S.A., Berendts, B. & Yeang, H.Y. (2003). *In vivo* sensitization to purified *Hevea brasiliensis* proteins in health care workers sensitized to natural rubber latex. *J Allergy Clin Immunol.,* Vol.111, No.3, (Mar 2003), pp.610-616, ISSN 0091-6749

Beezhold, D.H., Hickey, V.L., Kostyal, D.A., Puhl, H., Zuidmeer, L., van Ree, R., Sussman, GL. (2003). Lipid transfer protein from Hevea brasiliensis (Hev b 12), a cross-reactive latex protein. *Ann Allergy Asthma Immunol.* Vol.90, No.4, (Apr 2003), pp.439-445, ISSN 1081-1206

Bousquet, J., Flahault, A., Vandenplas, O., Ameille, J., Duron, J.J., Pecquet, C., Chevrie, K. & Annesi-Maesano, I. (2006). Natural rubber latex allergy among health care workers: a systematic review of the evidence. *J Allergy Clin Immunol.,* Vol.118, No.2, (Aug 2006), pp.447-454, ISSN 0091-6749

Boxer, M.B., Grammer, L.C., Orfan, N. (1994). Gutta-percha allergy in a health care worker with latex allergy. *J Allergy Clin Immunol.*, Vol.93, No.5, (May 1994), pp.943-944, ISSN 0091-6749

Brown, R.H., Hamilton, R.G., Mintz, M., Jedicka, A.E., Scott, A.L. & Kleeberger S.R. (2005). Genetic predisposition to latex allergy. Role of Interleukin 13 and Interleukin 18. *Anesthesiology,* Vol.102, No.3, (Mar 2005), pp.496-502, ISSN 0003-2999

Cao, L.Y., Taylor, J.S., Sood, A., Murray, D. & Siegel, P.D. (2010). Alergic contact dermatitis to synthetic rubber gloves: changing trends in patch test reactions to accelerators. *Arch Dermatol.*, Vol.146, No.9, (Sep 2010), pp.1001-1007, ISSN 0003-987X

Charous, B.L., Hamilton, R.G. & Yonginger, J.W. (1994). Occupational latex exposure: characteristics of contact and systemic reactions in 47 Works. *J Allergy Clin Immunol.*, Vol.94, No.1, (Jul 1994), pp.12-18, ISSN 0091-6749

Chen, Z., Cremer R, Posch, A., Raulf-Heimsoth, M., Rihs, H., Baur, X. (1997). On the allergenicity of Hev b 1 among health care workers and patients with spina bifida allergic to natural rubber latex. *J Allergy Clin Immunol.*, Vol.100, No.5, (Nov 1997), pp.684-693, ISSN 0091-6749

Cleenewerck, M.B. (2010). Update on medical surgical gloves. *Eur J Dermatol.*, Vol.20, No.4, (Jul-Aug 2010), pp. 434-442, ISSN 1167-1122

Costa, G.E., Johnson, J.D. & Hamilton, R.G. (2001). Cross-reactivity studies of guttapercha, gutta-balata, and natural rubber latex (*Hevea brasiliensis*). *J Endod.*, Vol. 27, No.9, (Sep 2001), pp.584-587, ISSN 0099-2399

Cremer, R. & Mennicken O. (2011). Longitudinal study on specific IgE against natural rubber latex, banana and kiwi in patients with spina bifida. *Klin Padiatr.*, (Apr 2011). [Epub ahead of print], ISSN 1439-3824

Diéguez, M.C., Pulido, Z., de la Hoz, B., Blanco, R., Cerecedo, I., Fernández-Caldas, E. & Swanson, M. (2007). Latex allergy in healthcare workers: an epidemiological study in a Spanish hospital. *Allergy Asthma Proc.*, Vol.28, No.5, (Sep-Oct 2007), pp.564-570, ISSN 1088-5412

Downing, J. (1993). Dermatitis from rubber gloves. *N Engl J Med.*, Vol.208, (Jan 1993), pp.196-198, ISSN 0028-4793

Dyck, R.J. (2000). Historical development of latex allergy. *AORN J.*, Vol.72, No.1, (Jul 2000), pp.27-40, ISSN 0001-2092

Ebo, D.G., Hagendorens, M.M., De Knop, K.J.,Verweij, M.M., Bridts, C.H., De Clerck, L.S. & Stevens, W.J. (2010). Component-resolved diagnosis from latex allergy by microarray. *Clin Exp Allergy*, Vol.40, No.2, (Feb 2010), pp.348-358, ISSN 0954-7894

Förström, L. (1980). Contact urticaria from latex surgical gloves. *Contact Dermatitis*, Vol.6, No.1, (Jan 1980), pp.33-34, ISSN 0105-1873

Hamann, C.P., Rodgers, P.A. & Sullivan, K.M. (2005). Prevalence of type I natural rubber latex allergy among dental hygienists. *J Dent Hyg.*, Vol.79, No.2, (Apr 205), pp.7, ISSN 1043-254X

Hamann, C.P., Turjanmaa, K., Rietschel, R., Siew, C., Owensby, D., Gruning,er S.E. & Sullivan K.M. (1998). Natural Rubber Latex Hypersensitivity: Incidence and Prevalence of Type I Allergy in the Dental Professional. *JADA*, Vol.129, No.1, (Jan 1998), pp.43-54, ISSN 0002-8177

Heitz, J.W. & Bader, S.O. (2010). An evidence-based approach to medication preparation for the surgical patient at risk for latex allergy: is it time to stop being stopper poppers? *J Clin Anesth.*, Vol.22, No.6, (Sep 2010), pp.477-83, ISSN 0952-8180

Kelly, K.J., Setlock, M. & Davis, J.P. (1991). Anaphylactic reactions during general anesthesia among pediatric patients. *MMWR*, Vol.40, No.26, (Jul 1991), pp.437-443, ISSN 0149-2195

Kosti, E. & Lambrianidis, T. (2002). Endodontic treatment in cases of allergic reaction to rubber dam. *J. Endod.*, Vol.28, No.11, (Nov 2002), pp.787-789, ISSN 0099-2399

Lin, C.T., Hung, D.Z., Chen, D.Y., Wu, H.J., Lan, J.L. & Chen, Y.H. (2008). A hospital-based screening study of latex allergy and latex sensitization among medical workers in Taiwan. *J Microbiol Immunol Infect.*, Vol.41, No.6, (Dec 2008), pp.499-506, ISSN 1684-1182

Machado, J.A., da Cunha, R.C., de Oliveira, B.H. & da Silva, J. (2011). Latex-induced anaphylactic reaction in a patient undergoing open appendectomy. Case report. *Rev Bras Anestesiol.*, Vol.61, No. 3, (May-Jun 2011), pp.360-366, ISSN 0034-7094

Malerich, P.G., Wilson, M.L. & Mowad, C.M. (2008). The effect of a transition to powder-free latex gloves on workers' compensation claims for latex-related illness. *Dermatitis*, Vol.19, No.6, (Nov-Dec 2008), pp.316-318, ISSN 1710-3568

Mebra, P. & Hunter, M.J. (1998). Latex allergy: a review of considerations for the oral and maxillofacial surgeon. *J Oral Maxillofac Surg.*, Vol.56, No.12, (Dec 1998), pp.1426-1430, ISSN 0278-2391

Monitto, C.L., Hamilton, R.G., Levey, E., Jedlicka, A.E., Dziedzic, A., Gearhart, J.P., Boyadjiev, S.A. & Brown, R.H. (2010). Genetic predisposition to natural rubber latex allergy differs between health care workers and high-risk patients. *Anesth Analg.*, Vol.110, No.5, (May 2010), pp.1310-1317, ISSN 0003-2999

Nabavizadeh, S.H., Anushiravani, A. & Amin, R. (2009). Natural rubber latex hypersensitiveity with skin prick test in operating room personnel. *Iran J Allergy Asthma Immunol.*, Vol.8, No.4, (Dec 2009), pp.219-20, ISSN 1735-1502

Nettis, E., Di Leo, E., Calogiuri, G., Milani, M., Donne, PD., Ferrannini, A. & Vacca, A. (2010). The safety of a novel sublingual rush induction phase for latex desensitization. *Curr Med Res Opin.*, Vol.26, No.8, (Aug 2010), pp.1855-1859, ISSN 0300-7995

Nettis, E., Assennato, G., Ferrannini, A. & Tursi, A. (2002). Type I allergy to natural rubber latex and type IV allergy to rubber chemicals in health care workers with glove-related skin symptoms. *Clin Exp Allergy*, Vol.32, No.3, (Mar 2002), pp.441-447, ISSN 0954-7894

Nieto, A., Mazón, A., Boquete, M., Carballada, F., Asturias, J.A., Martínez, J., Martínez, A. (2002). Assessment of profilin as an allergen for latex-sensitized patients. *Allergy*, Vol.57, No.9, (Sep 2002), pp.776-784, ISSN 0105-453

Nolte, H., Babakhin, A., Babanin, A., Bakhutashvili, V., Beloglazov, V., Bezruchenko, O., Blaziene, A., Chuchalin, A., Drannik, G., Endre, L., Khaitov, R., Khanferyan, R., Kowal, K., Kowalski, M., Markov, A., Petrov, R., Puchlik, B., Rosovenko, A., Sepiashvili R., Stepka, K., Titov, L., Tsybulkina, V., Yashina, L., Zakirova, I. & DuBuske, L.M. (2002). Prevalence of skin teste reactions to natural rubber latex in hospital personnel in Russia and Eastern Europe. *Annals of Allergy, Asthma & Immunology*, Vol.89. No.5, (Nov 2002), pp.452-456, ISSN 1081-1206

Nutter, A.F. (1979). Contact urticaria to rubber. *Br J Dermatol.*, Vol.101, No.5, (Nov 1979), pp.597-598, ISSN 0007-0963

Ott, H., Schröder, C., Raulf-Heimsoth, M., Mahler, V., Ocklenburg, C., Merk, H.F. & Baron, J.M. (2010). Microarrays of Recombinant *Hevea brasiliensis* Proteins: A novel tool for the component-resolved diagnosis of natural rubber latex allergy. *J Investig Allergol Clin Immunol.*, Vol.20, No.2, pp.129-138, ISSN 1018-9068

Ownby, D.R., Ownby, H.E., McCullough, J.A. & Shafer, A.W. (1994). The prevalence of anti-latex antibodies in 1000 volunteer blood donors. *J Allergy Clin Immunol.*, Vol.97, No.6, (Jun 1994), pp.1188-1192, ISSN 0091-6749

Ownby, D.R. (2002). A history of latex allergy. *J Allergy Clin Immunol.*, Vol.110, (Aug 2002), pp.S27-32, ISSN 0091-6749

Pedraza-Escalona, M., Becerril-Luján, B., Agundis, C., Domínguez-Ramírez, L., Pereyra, A. Riaño-Umbarila, L. & Rodríguez-Romero, A. (2009). Analysis of B-cell epitopes from the allergen Hev b 6.02 revealed by using blocking antibodies. *Mol Immunol.*, Vol.46, No.4, (Feb 2009), pp.668-676, ISSN 0161-5890

Peixinho, C., Tavares-Ratado, P., Tomás, M.R., Taborda-Barata, L. & Tomaz, C.T. (2008). Latex allergy: new insights to explain different sensitization profiles in different risk groups. *Br J Dermatol.*, Vol.159, No.1, (Jul 2008), pp.132-136, ISSN 0007-0963

Perkin, J.E. (2000). The latex and food allergy connection. *J Am Diet Assoc.*, Vol.100, No. 11, (Nov 2000), p.1381-1384, ISSN 0002-8223

Radauer, C., Adhami, F., Fürtler, I., Wagner, S., Allwardt, D., Scala, E., Ebner, C., Hafner, C., Hemmer, W., Mari, A. & Breiteneder, H. (2011). Latex-allergic patients sensitized to the major allergen hevein and hevein-like domains of class I chitinases show no increased frequency of latex-associated plant food allergy. *Mol Immunol.*, Vol.48, No.4, (Jan 2011), pp.600–609, ISSN 0161-5890

Rihs, H.P., Chen, Z., Rozynek, P., Cremer, R. (2001). Allergenicity of rHev b 10 (manganese-superoxide dismutase). *Allergy*, Vol.56, No.1, (Jan 2001), pp.85-86, ISSN 0105-4538

Rihs, H-P., Chen, Z., Ruëff, F., Cremer, R., Raulf-Heimsoth, M., Baur, X., Moneret-Valtrin, D.A. & Brüning, T. (2002). HLA-DQ8 and the HLA-DQ8-DR4 haplotype are positively associated with the hevein-specific IgE immune response in health care workers with latex allergy. *J Allergy Clin Immunol.*, Vol.110, No.3, (Sep 2002), pp.507-514, ISSN 0091-6749

Rolland, J.M. & O'Hehir, R.E. (2008). Latex allergy: a model for therapy. *Clin Exp Allergy*, Vol.38, No.6, (Jun 2008), pp.898-912, ISSN 0954-7894

Rougé, P., Culerrier, R., Campistron, M., Granier, C., Bienvenu, F., Bienvenu, J., Didier, A. & Barre, A. (2010). Allergenicity of Hev b 13, a major esterase allergen in natural rubber latex (*Hevea brasiliensis*) allergy, does not only depend on its carbohydrate moiety. *Mol Immunol.*, Vol.47, No.4, (Jan 2010), pp.871-7, ISSN 0161-5890

Sekiya, K., Watai, K., Taniguchi, M., Mitsui, C., Fukutomi, Y., Tanimoto, H., Kawaura, N., Akiyama, K. (2011). Latex Anaphylaxis caused by a Swan-Ganz catheter. *Intern Med.*, Vol.50, No.4, (Feb 2011), pp.355-357, ISSN 18410987

Slater, J.E., Vedvick, T., Arthur-Smith, A., Trybul, D.E. Kekwick, R.G.O. (1996). Identification, Cloning, and Sequence of a Major Allergen (Hev b 5) from Natural Rubber Latex (*Hevea brasiliensis*). *The Journal of Biological Chemistry*, Vol.271, No.41, (October 1996), pp. 25394–25399, ISSN 0021-9258

Smith, A.M., Amin, H.S., Biagini, R.E., Hamilton, R.G., Arif, S.A., Yeang, H.Y. & Bernstein, D.I. (2007). Percutaneous reactivity to natural rubber latex proteins persists in health-care workers following avoidance of natural rubber latex. *Clin Exp Allergy*, Vol.37, No.9, (Sep 2007), pp.1349-56, ISSN 0954-7894

Sonofuchi, K., Watanabe, K., Onuma, T., Kaneko, T., Ohmizo, H., Furuta, S., Endo, K. & Morota, T. (2010). A case of anaphylactic shock by multiple causes. *Masui-The Japanese Journal of anesthesiology*, Vol.59, No.8, (Aug 2010), pp.1032-1035, ISSN 0021-4892

Sripaiboonkij, P., Phanprasit, W. & Jaakkola, M.S. (2009). Respiratory and skin effects of exposure to wood dust from the rubber tree *Hevea brasiliensis*. *Occup Environ Med.*, Vol.66, No.7, (Jul 2009), pp.442-447, ISSN 1351-0711

Sukekava, F. & Sell, A.M. (2007). Rubber latex gloves hypersensitivities in dental workers. *Acta Sci. Health Sci.*, Vol.29, No.1, (Jan-Jun, 2007), pp.39-44, ISSN 1679-9291.

Sussman, G.L. & Beezold, D.H. (1994). Latex allergy- a clinical perspective. *J Long-Term Effects Med Implants*, Vol.4, No.2-3, (Jul 1994), pp.95-110, ISSN 1050-6934

Turillazzi, E., Greco, P., Neri, M., Pomara, C. Riezzo, I. & Fineschi, V. (2008). Anaphylactic latex reaction during anesthesia: the silent culprit in a fatal case. *Forensic Sci Int.*, Vol.179, No.1, (Jul 2008), pp.5-8, ISSN 0379-0738

Turjanmaa, K., Kanto, M. Kautiainen, H., Reunala, T., Palosuo, T. (2002). Long-term outcome of 160 adult patients with natural rubber latex allergy. *J Allergy Clin Immunol.*, Vol.110, (Aug 2002), pp.S70-4, ISSN 0091-6749

Turjanmaa, K. (1987). Incidence of immediate alergy to latex gloves in hospital personnel. *Contact Dermatitis*, Vol.17, No.5, (Nov 1987), p.270-275, ISSN 0105-1873

Ueda, N., Kitamura, R., Wakamori, T., Nakamura, K., Konishi, K. (2008). Anaphylactic reaction to latex during spinal anesthesia: a case report. *Masui-The Japanese Journal of anesthesiology*, Vol.57, No.5, (May 2008), pp.637-639, ISSN 0021-4892

Unsel, M., Mete, N., Ardeniz, O., Göksel, S., Ersoy, R., Sin, A., Gulbahar, O. & Kokuludag, A. (2009). The importance of nasal provocation test in the diagnosis of natural rubber latex allergy. *Allergy*, Vol.64, No.6, (Jun 2009), pp.862-867, ISSN 0105-4538

van Kampen, V., Raulf-Heimsoth, M., Sander, I. & Merget, R. (2010). Diagnostics of occupational type I allergies-comparison of skin prick test solutions from different manufacturers for selected occupational allergens. *Pneumologie.*, Vol.64, No.5, (May 2010), pp.271-277, ISSN 0033-4073

Verdolin, B.A., Villlas Boas, W.V. & Gomez, R.S. (2003). Latex Allergy: accidental diagnosis after urological procedure. Case Report. *Rev. Bras. Anestesiol.*, Vol.53, No.4, (Aug 2003), pp.496-500, ISSN 0034-7094

Wagner, S. & Breiteneder, H. (2002). The latex-fruit syndrome. *Biochem Soc Trans.*, Vol.30, No.6, (Nov 2002), pp.935-940, ISSN 0300-5127

Wagner, B., Krebitz., M, Buck, D., Niggemann, B., Yeang, H.Y., Han, K.H., Scheiner, O. & Breiteneder H. (1999). Cloning, expression, and characterization of recombinant Hev b 3, a *Hevea brasiliensis* protein associated with latex allergy in patients with spina bifida. *J Allergy Clin Immunol.*, Vol.104, No.5, (Nov 1999), pp.1084-1092, ISSN 0091-6749

Wagner, S., Breiteneder, H., Simon-Nobbe, B., Susani, M., Krebitz, M., Niggemann, B., Brehler, R., Scheiner, O., Hoffmann-Sommergruber, K. (2000). Hev b 9, an enolase and a new cross-reactive allergen from hevea latex and molds. Purification, characterization, cloning and expression. *Eur J Biochem.*, Vol.267, No.24, (Dec 2000), pp.7006-7014, ISSN 0014-2956

Woods, J.A., Lambert, S., Platts-Mills, T.A.E., Drake, D.B. & Edlich, R. (1997). Natural rubber latex allergy: spectrum, diagnostic approach, and therapy. *The Journal of Emergency Medicine*, Vol.15, No.1, (Jan-Feb 1997), p.71-85, ISSN 0736-4679

Yagami, T., Osuna, H., Kouno, M., Haishima, Y., Nakamura, A., Ikezawa, Z. (2002). Significance of carbohydrate epitopes in a latex allergen with beta-1,3-glucanase activity. *Int Arch Allergy Immunol.*, Vol.129, No.1, (Sep 2002), pp.27-37, ISSN 1018-2438

Yeang, H.Y., Cheong, K.F., Sunderasan, E., Hamzah, S., Chew, N.P., Hamid, S. Hamilton R.G., Cardosa, M.J. (1996). The 14.6 kD (Hev b3) rubber particle proteins are recognized by IgE from spina bifida patients with allergy. *J Allergy Clin Immunol.*, Vol.98, No.3, (Sep 1996), pp.628-639, ISSN 0091-6749

Part 3

Specific Aspects of Allergic Diseases

16

Psychological Factors in Asthma and Psychoeducational Interventions

Lia Fernandes
Department of Psychiatry and Mental Health, Faculty of Medicine, University of Oporto, Psychiatry Service of S. João Hospital, Oporto, Portugal

1. Introduction

This subject is of interest as asthma has increased over the last two decades. Despite therapeutic advances, morbidity and mortality are increasing (Global Initiative for Asthma [GINA], 2010), particularly due to the development of western standards of living, where psychological factors have regained notability (Busse et al., 2000). This brings about a worsening in psychological factors and quality of life which entails high socioeconomic costs (direct and indirect) (Sulivan 1996; Suissa 2000).

Since the most remote times of medical history (Maimonides 1990, Alexander 1940, Dunbar 1948), it has been possible to determine a connection between asthma and emotional factors. In this study, besides the epidemiological aspects and the determinant psychopathological issues of this illness, some of the main psychological factors that influence and are influenced by this complex illness are reviewed in a multidimensional systemic vision (Gregerson, 2000; Jasnoski et al., 1994; Dirks et al., 1978).

Parallel to the importance given to biological factors, social and physical variables have also been enhanced, as have conditionings brought about by stress, which intervene and condition psychoneuroimmunohormonal mechanisms in the evolution of the illness (Goodwin & Eaton, 2003).

In the most severe cases of asthma, psychological factors such as depression, anxiety, stress, psychopathology, psychiatric expression of asthma and side effects of medication will be implicated. In this context, the coping mechanisms involved, as well as different life events and other psychosocial conditions are of the utmost importance. The transformation of these people's lives inevitably involves their families, making problem solving difficult, and determining the outcome and the treatment of this pathology (Scott et al., 2007; Fernandes et al., 2010; Thomas et al., 2011; Di Marco et al., 2011).

On the other hand, less adapted behaviours become related to minor compliance in the care of asthma, which leads to the worsening of the symptoms of asthma, causing self-perpetuation mechanisms, with chronically inflammatory processes, pulmonary remodelling and irreversibility in the size of the airways (Rietveld, 2000; Fonseca et al., 2004).

Therapeutically, in people with moderate to severe asthma, besides the usual, preventive and pharmacological approaches, it is essential to turn to psychoeducational and

multifamily programmes, in order to increase the control of the illness, and allow more efficient treatment (Yorke et al., 2007; Smith et al., 2007).
It is in this multisystemic context only by deepening the reciprocal relationships among psychological and biological, family and social factors can one find answers for the enormous complexity of the asthmatic illness. As a corollary of this, the confirmation that only a sufficiently widespread intervention that simultaneously combines the premises previously formulated, will allow an increased therapeutic effectiveness (Fernandes, 2009).
This conceptual transformation into a multifactorial model influences also methodologically the psychosomatic research (Gregerson, 1995). The focus of this approach is based not so much on the causes (as in the linear model) but above all, in intervention and treatment (Mathison, 1993; Stout & Creer, 1997).
Illustrating this, two studies will be presented. The first one, Psychological and Psychosocial Factors in Asthma, will study the influence of the psychological (anxiety, depression, psychopathology) and psychosocial variables of asthmatics with the clinical variables (symptoms, spirometry, inflammatory marker, severity and duration) and morbidity (quality of life, control of asthma, medication, use of health care and absenteeism). In the second study, Psychoeducational and Multifamily Interventions in asthma will presented the effectiveness of these interventions in this illness.

2. Clinical review

Asthma is a chronic inflammatory disease of the airways, which has a great impact on the quality of life of these patients.
In Portugal, as in the majority of western countries, asthma is increasing, which brings about high socioeconomic costs and an increase in mortality and morbidity (GINA, 2010).
For a long time the involvement of psychosocial factors in this disease has been known. Among different respiratory illnesses asthma presents the most profound links between psychological, social, biological and physiological factors. This is why it is considered the prototype of psychosomatic diseases (Isenberg et al., 1992; Lehrer et al., 1993; Mackenzie, 1886).
Much has been achieved since the 1960s, with the psychoanalytic approach to asthma in children, viewed as crying repression (French & Alexander, 1941).
Great progress has been made in the field of medical knowledge namely concerning the neuroimunohormonal mechanisms involved in the etiopathogenesis of this disease. There is increasing evidence that the immune system is not working autonomously. In spite of this it will be connected with many psychophysiological processes under the regulatory modulation of the brain (Ader & Cohen, 1985). This branch of study we call psychoneuroimmunology. In this way it makes sense that we speak in the long term about changes that can stabilize resistance to the disease. This individual stability could be organized in each patient's personality structure, which could confront the different challenges and stress events of daily life (Goldstein & Dekker, 2001).
However the precise physiological mechanisms involved are very complex, needing more profound research. The psychological disorders seem to produce systemic effects in the immune system function, in metabolic and hormonal processes and in the peripheral and central nervous system, in interactional and reciprocal mechanisms instead of being focused on one organ, as was commonly thought for a long time (Kang et al., 1997; Cohen et al., 1991; Rietveld & Everaerd, 2000; Di Marco et al., 2011).

Nowadays in a more realistic perspective, it is considered that negative emotions (fear, panic, anger, anxiety and depression) are linked in a fluctuating process of bronchoconstriction of the airways, based on a mechanism of worsening crises of asthma (Hollaender & Florin, 1983; Silverglade et al., 1994; Lehrer, 1998; ten Brinke et al., 2001).

In an indispensable holistic vision of this disease the psychological aspects become inseparable from the remaining symptoms when it is a question of making a diagnosis or prognosis or treating asthma (Lehrer et al., 2002).

It is well known that these patients' behaviour strongly influences the course of the illness and the treatment, determining the exposure to allergic factors, in the perception and assessment of the symptoms, in the search for adequate medical care and compliance with the therapeutic plan, being strongly predictive for the frequency and severity of the worsening of the disease (Levy, 1994; van der Berg et al., 1997; Miller & Hotses, 1995; Devriese et al., 2000).

Determinants of this behaviour are indubitable the psychopathology and familiar disorganization which is reflected in the worsening of the disease, in a decrease in quality of life as well as in the increasing health care costs involved. In some more extreme conditions these factors increase risk to life (Nouwen et al., 1999).

Near-fatal asthma deserves scrutiny due to the severity of these events and because of its impact on subsequent asthma morbidity and healthcare costs. The first studies emphasized the role of psychological variables (Campbell et al., 1994; Strunk et al., 1999; Innes et al., 1998; Di Marco et al., 2011).

Furthermore, special attention has to be devoted to the subgroup of severe asthma which is difficult and complex - implying avoidance of multiple environmental stimuli, with a variety of medications for controlling chronic inflammation or acute broncho-dilatation, with complex planning and high costs (Boulet et al., 1991; Woller et al., 1993; Kelloway et al., 2000).

Besides that, knowing that asthma is not a behavioural disease, there is evidence that some changes in some asthmatic groups can condition the evolution of the disease. On the other hand there is also evidence that asthma has a role in the development of some psychiatric diseases (Lehrer et al., 2002; Scott et al., 2007).

Some negative emotions, particularly panic and depression, even not severe enough to be classified as psychiatric disorders, can produce respiratory effects and lead to worsening of asthma, directly by psychophysiological effects or indirectly by neglecting self-management of the illness. Conversely, these emotional disorders can also be worsened by asthma itself (Nouwen et al., 1999; ten Brinke et al., 2001; Lehrer et al., 2004).

A prospective Swiss community-based longitudinal cohort study (Hasler et al., 2005) reported that having a diagnosis of asthma may result in the subsequent development of panic in some patients with an odds ratio of 4.5. On the other hand, the same study also reported that the presence of panic disorder predicted subsequent asthma with an odds ratio of 6.3, suggesting that psychological dysfunction may precede the development of asthma.

A UK primary care survey published in 2007 (Cooper et al., 2007), reported higher anxiety and depression scores in adults with asthma than the general community, and a prevalence of panic disorder of 16% in those with asthma.

There are other psychological factors with a similar relationship to asthma worsening, which deserve a deeper study, particularly personality characteristics and their relation to the perception of asthma symptoms. The state of the art test pinpoints for endorphin activity on the basis of this respiratory sensitivity (Rietveld et al., 2000).

In a recent study (Fernandes et al., 2005) the predominance of neurotic characteristics in asthmatic patients was confirmed. They also presented lower extroversion, openness to experience, agreeableness and conscientiousness when compared to the general population. These characteristics were linked to the severity and duration of the disease.

On the other hand, an increasing consensus is becoming established concerning the emotional triggers of asthma, focusing on psychophysiological mechanisms. This is demonstrated in recent studies where in response to emotional states there is a bronchoconstriction as well as registered cardiovascular and electrodermal modifications. Particularly in asthma the respiratory reaction in the airways is well known, when psychologically induced, including the variations in airways narrowing, which characterize the typical fluctuations of the disease (Lehrer et al., 2003, 2004).

Nowadays bronchoconstriction in asthma is defined by direct sympathetic nervous system action or indirect parasympathetic nervous system action by a rebound effect (Manto, 1969; Isenberg et al., 1992; Lehrer et al., 1997), under some specific psychological states (sadness, stress, etc.), or by an inflammatory reaction. Although it remains less well-investigated, it is the last characteristic component in the pathology of asthma, i.e., blood vessel proliferations with increased airways wall thickness, as well as mucus hypersecrection (Lehrer et al., 1998).

In some patients, stress in particular is the essential trigger for asthma attacks. Anxiety symptoms in asthmatics have been revealed as strong predictors of respiratory illness in those patients. Besides that, anxiety and depression seem to be much more prevalent in the asthmatic population than in the normal one (Rietveld et al., 2000; Thomas et al., 2011).

Different surveys using different methodologies and instruments indicate that anxiety and depression disorders are up to six times more common in people with asthma than in the general population (Goodwin & Eaton, 2003; Lavoie et al., 2006).

In a recent study (Fernandes et al., 2010) the high prevalence of anxiety in asthmatic patients as well as its associations with worse subjective asthma outcomes and increased used of medications/healthcare services was confirmed.

Anxiety and depression are also particularly reported with severe and difficult to control asthma (Heaney et al., 2005) and impaired emotional coping mechanisms (Lavoie et al., 2010).

Both psychological manifestations inherent in the asthmatic process itself and other clinical situations that can be asthma like, or present some aspects of this illness, have in core genesis a common mechanism: psychosomatic structure (Horton et al., 1978).

Some of that asthma like illnesses have present in their origin above all a psychological mechanism. These kinds of clinical expressions can vary from somatoform disorder to factitious or conversion disorder. In any case it is mainly a functional disturbance, with a physiological minor component (Luparello et al., 1968).

From an investigational perspective there has been a huge change in the techniques used. In the majority of the research, scientists look for physical data when trying to understand this complex system, where psychological factors and emotions are involved.

In this context, some respiratory changes are measured and studied, in some experiments with emotional content in films (Levenson, 1979), in contrast with saline solution inhalation, both by the action of suggestion (Luparello, 1968; McFadden et al., 1969; Neild & Cameron, 1985).

In spite of this, all researchers are using a model, which follows a linear mechanism of thinking. According to some authors (Ford, 1987; Ford & Urban, 1998), who mostly reflected on psychosomatic methodology research, this paradigm is considered completely inappropriate since we involve the behavioural component. In none of these studies, for

example, was the individual and unique experience of each patient taken into account, neither were their past nor their future hopes, considered as a part of the study context.
In fact, any biological, physical or chemical system works like a complex system in which the inherent proprieties are not totally explained, by each constituent part (Gallagher & Appenzeller, 1999). This kind of approach has given rise to some findings in the chemical field (Whitesides & Ismagilov, 1999) in biological signal systems (Weng et al., 1999) and the nervous system (Koch & Laurent, 1999).
Alternatively a new model was suggested, with particular relevance to human being studies. In this, as underlined by Borkovec (1997), the involved processes are linked in a nonlinear dynamic, just as with attention, thinking, images, memory, emotion, physiology and behaviour, all in a permanent interaction, and answering to interpersonal and environmental changes, with a background of biological and developmental history.
In an attempt to adapt this model to the investigation of emotional phenomena in asthma, it will probably be as difficult as to adapt it to the chemical field (Whitesides & Ismagilov, 1999). This becomes even more difficult if we take into consideration that asthma is particularly sensitive to the initial conditions with small variations, having a great number of independent components, which interact in multiple pathways, through which all of these mechanisms could be involved. These conditions raise a multiplicity of potential respiratory patterns.
Through this kind of alternative approach, we will be able to allow a draw study project based above all on the reality of the phenomena investigated. This will bring us close to the necessary conditions to finally get solid evidence in the clarification of the complexity of all of these mechanisms involved with stress and emotions in the present disease. Not only will we get solutions for centuries of old mysteries but it will be possible to have new approaches in the treatment of asthma (Gallagher & Appenzeller, 1999; Koch & Laurent, 1999).
It is in this new contextualization that the importance of psychoeducational programs in asthma is growing. The preliminary data about this intervention gives emphasis to educational, communicational and self-efficacy aspects (Yorke et al., 2007; Fernandes, 2009).
There are already some series of randomized multicenter educational programmes for asthma (Taitel et al., 1995; Kotses et al., 1995; Wilson et al., 1996; Bruzzese et al., 2001). The focus of these programmes is in the clarification of the importance of specific components of the illness. In spite of this, feedback to patients with an assessment of these educational programmes is lacking, as well as an adaptation into short interventions that can work in clinical practice or even in a multifamily context (McFarlane et al., 1995; Devine, 1996; Fernandes, 2009).
Furthermore, it will be important to establish this kind of intervention in more specific groups, such as children with more vulnerability in asthmatic crises, people in high risk groups where stress clearly triggers the worsening of the disease (Bernard-Bonnin et al., 1995; Smith et al., 2005).
There is also some relevance of specific programmes for tobacco reduction, with use of psychotherapy, particularly in the cognitive and family therapy fields. These studies took a privileged focus on the control and treatment in daily life, of this complex chronic disease (Irvine et al., 1999; Silagy, 1999; Gustafsson & Cederblad, 1986; Lask & Matthew, 1979; Sun et al., 2010).
Another important aspect is the identification of some specific characteristics of these patients (in terms of severity, personality and even psychological aspects) in subpopulations that most benefit from these education programmes. Eventually the longitudinal assessment in different contexts will be fundamental.

In conclusion, from a research perspective, a distinct kind of approach will be necessary, based on a reality of these phenomena studied, that allows association mechanisms to be established among multiple factors involved, leading to a more modern methodology in a systemic framework, that puts emphasis on the multifactorial model (Fernandes, 2009).

3. Study 1: Psychological and psychosocial factors

3.1 Objectives

The present study aims to study the influence of psychological factors (state and trait anxiety, anger, depression, psychopathology) and psychosocial variables of asthma with clinical characteristics (spirometry, inflammatory marker, severity and duration) and morbidity criteria (quality of life, control of asthma, medication, use of health care services and absenteeism).

The second aim is to study the integration of these data into the cultural diversity of the present population, from a demographic perspective.

3.2 Methods

In this transversal study, 299 outpatients of the Immunoallergology department of the S. João Hospital, of both sexes, were recruited with asthma diagnosis, between the ages of 17 and 75 years.

With the 217 patients that participated, a psychiatric clinical interview was carried out, and psychiatric clinical cases were excluded, by the General Health Questionnaire - GHQ-28 (Goldberg & Hillier, 1979), as well as alcohol and drug abuse cases. Inclusion criteria were previous medical diagnosis of asthma and specific criteria (anti-asthmatic therapy, tests of unspecified bronchial hyper-reactivity and bronchodilation, inflammatory marker, spirometry).

Thus, 195 patients were studied according to the duration of the illness, symptoms, morbidity criteria (use of health care, medication and absenteeism), spirometry (FEV1, PEF), test of bronchial hyper-reactivity (PD20 metacolina), inflammatory markers (FENO), severity of asthma (GINA, 2010) and atopy and rhinitis.

They were evaluated according to the following scales: Self Anxiety Scale - SAS (Zung, 1971), State-Trait Anxiety Inventory - STAIY (Spielberger, 1983), State-Trait Anger Expression Inventory - STAXI (Spielberger, 1988), Beck Depression Inventory - BDI (Beck et al., 1961), Hopkins Symptom Distress Checklist 90-Revised - SCL90R (Derogatis & Savitz, 1999), Ways of Coping with Asthma in Everyday Life - WCAEL (Aalto et al., 2002), Mini Asthma Quality of Life Questionnaire - MiniAQLQ (Juniper et al., 1999a) and Asthma Control Questionnaire - ACQ (Juniper et al., 1999b).

Patient informed consent was obtained and the study was approved by the hospital Ethics Committee.

3.3 Results

In this sample (n=195), most of the patients were female (76.4%), with ages ranging from 17 to 75 years. The mean (sd) age was 38(14.5) years. Most of the patients have low education (70.2%). There was a predominance of low and very low classes (72.4%), according to the Graffar social classification (Graffar, 1956).

The mean duration of the disease was 19.8(14.0) years. The severity of the illness was distributed in the following way: Intermittent (8.2%), Mild persistent (12.8%), Moderate persistent (12.8%) and Severe persistent (66.2%).

The respiratory values found were: spirometry FEV1 83.5(22.4) (min.19%, max.120%), inflammatory marker FENO P50 28 (min.4, max.222). Most of these patients concomitantly have atopy (80.9%) and rhinitis (60.3%).

Total = 195		
Age (years) mean (sd)	38.0	(14.6)
Gender n(%)		
Male	46	(23.6)
Female	149	(76.4)
Education n(%)		
≤ 9	137	(70.2)
10-11	37	(19.0)
> 12	21	(10.8)
Socio-economic classification n(%)		
High and very high	16	(8.2)
Median	38	(19.5)
Low	59	(30.3)
Very low	82	(42.1)
Asthma duration (years) mean (sd)	19.8	(14.0)
Asthma severity n (%)		
Intermittent	16	(8.2)
Mild persistent	25	(12.8)
Moderate persistent	25	(12.8)
Severe persistent	129	(66.2)

Table 1. Demographic and clinical characteristics of sample

From a psychological point of view, the asthmatics of the sample were individuals with a high level of anxiety state (70%): 13.3% had scores suggesting anxiety and 56.4% suffered from high-anxiety (Ponciano et al., 1982).

Considering the anxiety trait, assessed by STAIY, there was a mean (sd) value of 40.82 (12.18). On this scale, state-anxiety had a mean (sd) of 44.8 (13.16).

In this sample, the mean values of contained and manifested anger (mean 15.94, sd 4.05; mean 13.31, sd 12.0) were much higher than the mean standard results found in the normative Portuguese population (Martins, 1995).

Additionally the analysis of the degree of depression, assessed by BDI, allowed us to conclude that in the majority of the sample (72%) depression was absent. Only 6.2% of these patients revealed symptoms of severe and 22% mild/moderate depression.

Psychopathology assessed in the different list of symptoms of Hopkins-Review SCL-90-R, had in general normal values, with the exception for somatization (mean 1.4, dp 0.8) and anxiety (mean 1.06, dp 0.68), higher than the mean values standardized for the Portuguese population.

In the present sample, the most important coping mechanism found was hiding asthma, with a mean (dp) value of 13.08 (2.21), followed by worry with the disease, with a mean (dp) value of 9 (2.12), corroborated by the global score (mean 82, dp 7.63).

The mean (sd) values for quality of life, according to the MiniAQLQ were 4.9 (1.3), with a minimum of 2 and a maximum of 7.

For asthma control, assessed by ACQ (with 0 FEV1), P50 (min.0 /max. 5.2), the mean (sd) was 1.5 (1.2).
In the present study we verified a correlation between sex (higher in women) and anxiety ($p<0.001$), as well as depression ($p=0.000$) and psychopathology ($p=0.001$).
There was a positive correlation between age and anxiety state ($p=0.006$) and trait ($p=0.037$), depression ($p=0.001$), psychopathology ($p=0.025$), as well as coping mechanism ($p<0.001$).
A worsening in breathing was noted (spirometry values) only with psychopathology - obsession ($p=0.05$).
On the other hand, these psychological variables (anxiety $p\leq0.001$, psychopathology - somatization $p=0.001$) were related to the decrease in the inflammatory marker, indicating higher health care use and an increase in medication intake (mainly preventative).
Above all anxiety state was related to more hospitalization ($p=0.007$) as well as non-scheduled consultations ($p=0.008$) and routine ones ($p=0.001$).
Anxiety and depression also increased absenteeism ($p=0.011$; $p=0.017$).
These psychological variables also increased with the severity ($p\leq0.001$; $p\leq0.001$) and with the duration of the disease ($p=0.002$; $p=0.023$). However, psychopathology only increased with severity ($p=0.002$).
Another result found, was that anxiety ($r=0.638$; $p\leq0.001$), anger ($r=-0.343$; ≤0.001) and depression ($r=-0.527$; $p\leq0.001$) worsened the quality of life (Figure 1 and 2).

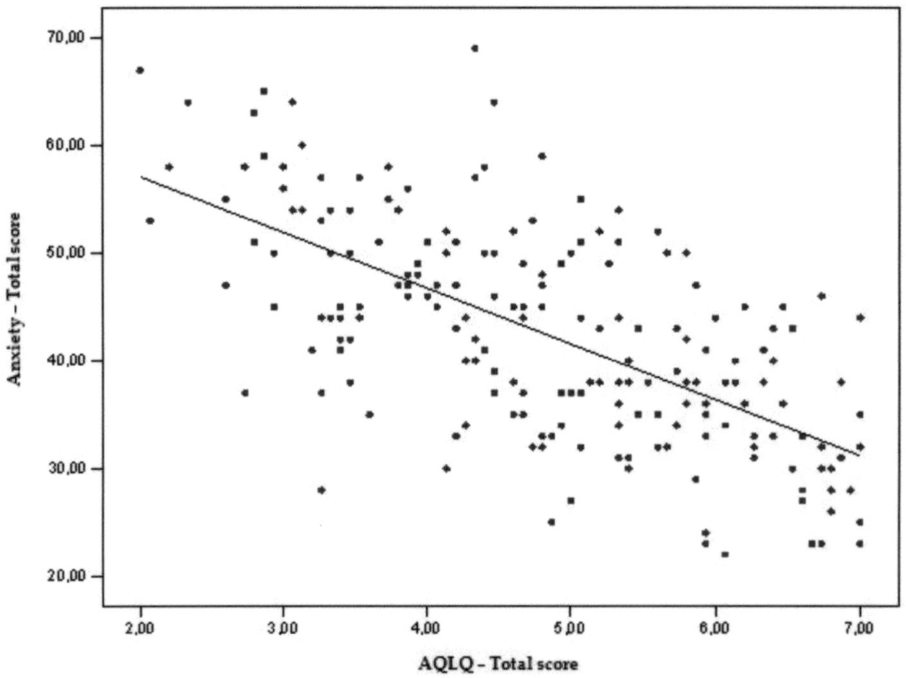

Fig. 1. Correlation between anxiety and quality of life

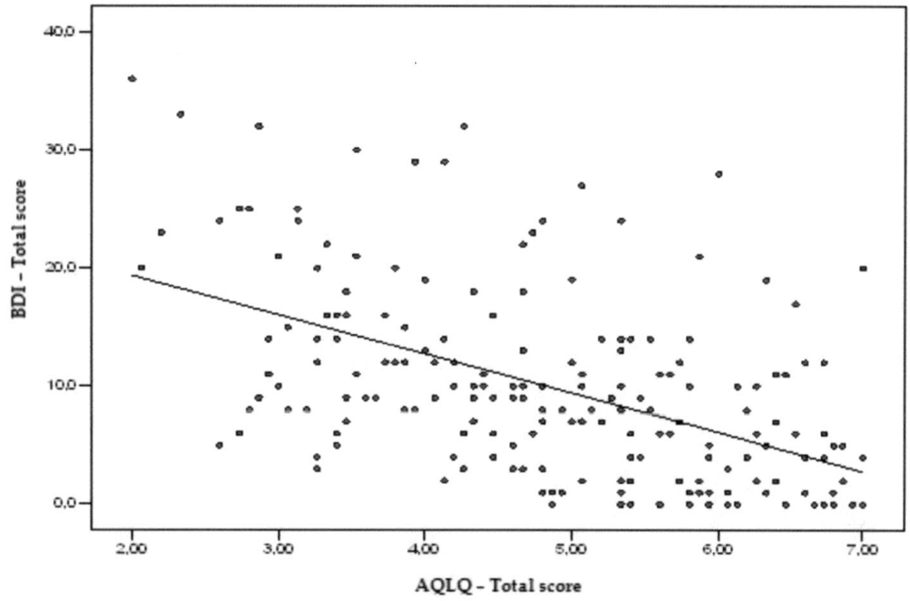

Fig. 2. Correlation between depression and quality of life

The control of asthma was correlated with anxiety state (r=0.554; p≤0.001) and trait (r=0.357; p=0.000), as well as anger (r=0.221; p=0.016) (Figure 3). Another clinical variable was also associated with control of asthma, which is depression (r=0.656; p≤0.001) (Figure 4).

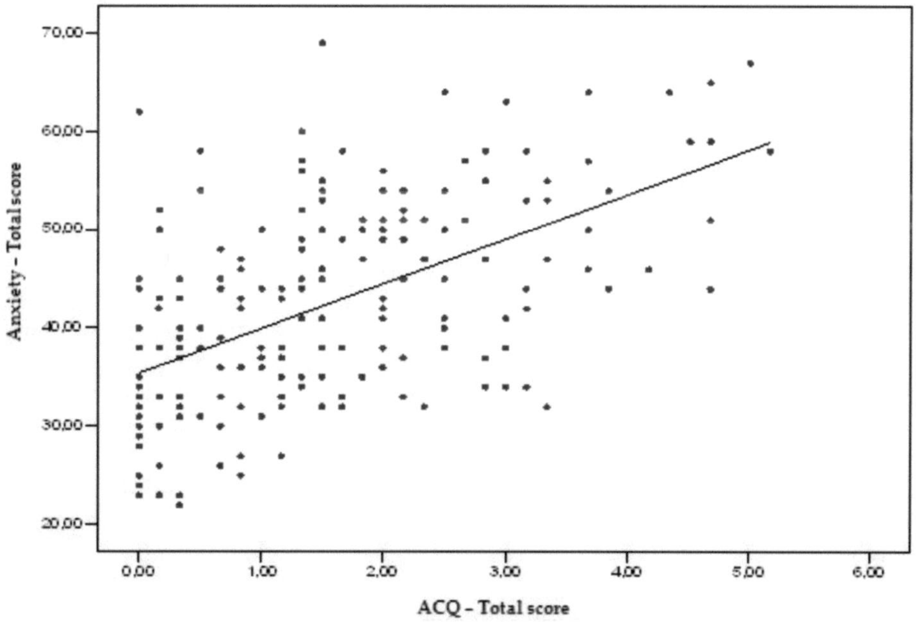

Fig. 3. Correlation between anxiety and asthma control

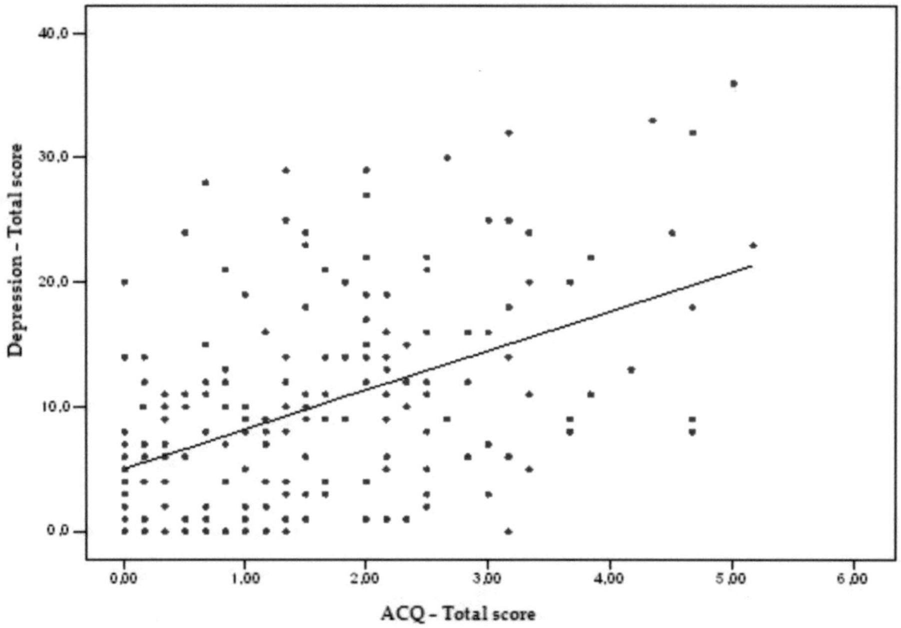

Fig. 4. Correlation between depression and asthma control

Increase in age implied better disease adaptation ($p \leq 0.001$). The severity of asthma sustained lower total coping mechanisms (p=0.021), as well as positive reappraisal (p=0.009), assessed by WCAEL.
Of special note, the coping mechanism restricted lifestyle (p=0.021) increased with duration of the disease. The positive reappraisal had a negative correlation with the duration of the disease (p=0.028).
Absenteeism was also directly related to restricted lifestyle and reverse with seeking information, the two coping mechanisms.
The coping mechanism worry with asthma decreased the quality of life (r=-0.239; p=0.044). The most mobilizing mechanism for looking for medical care: consultation (p=0.014) was restricted lifestyle. An opposite implication for denial (p=0.015) mechanism was found, and leading to less intake of corticosteroids.

3.4 Discussion and conclusion

According to the standard values for the Portuguese population (Ponciano et al., 1982), this group has a clear predominance of anxiety in 70% of the sample, as defined in the literature (Vila et al., 2000; Goodwin & Eaton, 2003). This is reinforced by the high levels of anger-in as well as anger-out, that almost all duplicated in this sample (when compared to the normal values of general population), which may be related to more physiological activation, as found for the studies with hypertension (Spielberger & London, 1990).
In contrast we found lower psychopathology levels, particularly depression, probably explained by the selection criteria of the present sample and because the influence of the well-known low compliance in this kind of study of these particular patients.
Anxiety, depression, psychopathology and coping increased with age. However, only anxiety was correlated with low socioeconomic level, as corroborated in other studies (Rumbak et al., 1993).

In the present sample a high correlation with sex, especially for women was found with anxiety, depression and psychopathology, which is in accordance in the previous studies (Eysenck, 1969; Dalton et al., 1975; Mayer-Cross et al., 1969; Thomas et al., 2011).

Anxiety, anger and depression correlated with the duration of asthma episodes and their acuteness (in the GINA classification), which is in agreement with former studies (Mrazeck et al., 1998; Sandberg et al., 2000; ten Brinke et al., 2001; Barton et al., 2005; Wainwright et al., 2007; Dahlem et al., 2009), associating the early onset of asthma with a negative impact on psychological adaptation to the disease, which implies the development of more clinical anxiety and depression.

The use of healthcare services by asthmatic patients as well medication (especially relief and preventive ones) was also directly linked with anxiety. Particularly, anxiety is predicted due to hospitalizations (Dirks et al., 1978, 1981; Kinsman et al., 1982) and their duration (Put et al., 1999).

These results agree with others, who argue that high anxiety leads to poor discrimination between anxiety symptoms and breathing symptoms, thus leading to an overuse of medical care (Spinhoven et al., 1997; Cluley & Cochrane, 2001). There was also a significant relationship between a great number of hospital admissions and higher scores of anxiety, which strengthens the conclusions of previous studies, where anxiety is predictive of more hospital admissions (Bender et al., 2006; Prueter & Norra, 2005) and longer duration.

There was a relationship between exhaled nitric oxide (FENO) and anxiety and somatization. This marker for airway inflammation had a negative correlation with anxiety. In other words, as the levels of anxiety increase, there is evidence of a decrease in inflammation. A possible interpretation of this inverse association may be found in the characteristics of high anxiety of this sample, calling for the use of greater medical care (ten Brinke et al., 2001b). In turn physicians may be influenced by the increased expression of symptoms by the patients. As a consequence more anti-inflammatory treatment is prescribed as patients are identified as more acutely ill (Hibbert & Pilsbury, 1988; Hornsveld & Garssen, 1996). The inflammatory marker decreases because it is particularly sensitive to changes in medication, specifically corticosteroids (Chetta et al., 1998). However, the changes are not reflected in other, less sensitive markers of this disease, namely, lung-function (FEV and PEF), for which no significant relationship with anxiety was found. This lack of association between lung function and anxiety has been previously reported (Thomas et al., 2001).

This tendency toward increasing anxiety was seen for the greater degrees of asthma severity. This agrees with studies in which anxiety in asthmatics is seen as a risk factor for increase in asthma morbidity and mortality (Wright et al., 1998; Forsythe et al., 2004). A similar correlation was found for psychopathology which is corroborated by other studies (Chetta et al., 1998), namely when this is linked with near-fatal asthma attacks (Yellowees et al., 1988; Boulet et al., 1991; Garden et al., 1993; Campbell et al., 1995a; McQuaid et al., 2001). This severity was also correlated positively with depression, in accordance with other studies (Strunk et al., 195; Picado et al., 1989; Campbell et al., 1995a; Martin et al., 1995). This relation between depression and severity asthma is particularly relevant in the case of recent bereavement (Levitan, 1985), as well as death by asthma with hopelessness and despair in the days before the relative's death (Miller et al., 1989).

By using STAI-Y, the average values for the anxiety trait (i.e., a measure for an individual's tendency for anxiety) were higher than those found in other studies for the Portuguese population (Santos & Silva, 1997; Silva & Campos, 1998) and that have been used as standard references. These characteristics agree with some other previous studies (Boulet et al., 1991; Chetta et al., 1998) which argue that there is a strong link between anxiety trait and asthma, as well as a greater manifestation of the symptoms of this ailment (Kinsman et al., 1973; Dirks et al., 1978; Friedman & Booth-Kewley, 1987; Yellowlees & Kalucy, 1990). More recently Rimington et al (2001) further supports this notion and states that as anxiety increases (state and trait) a poorer quality of life is evidenced, and Baumeister et al (2005) makes similar observations between higher anxiety and less asthma control (Thomas et al., 2011).

The present study also recognized worse control of the disease with anger and depression, as found in other studies (Cluley & Cochrane, 2001; Thomas et al., 2011). Is well known that patients classified as non-adherent (those taking less 70% of the prescription) presented high anxiety and depression levels (Zigmond et al., 1983; Thomas et al., 2011).

Corroborating former studies (Dirks et al., 1978; Staudenmayer et al., 1979; Dirks & Kinsman, 1981; Baron et al., 1986; Put et al., 1999), the data from this study suggest that the most anxious patients are more vigilant over their symptoms, use more medication and more often turn to healthcare services for help. With this behaviour they would suffer from great psychological stress with their disease in the short term (higher values of anxiety, with less quality of life associated with asthma), but in the long run it may result in better control over the illness. Thus, this anxiety which is specifically related to asthma can be beneficial, by making the individual aware of the bodily symptoms related to asthma, through a process of focusing attention. However, excessively high levels of anxiety may lead to super-perception of asthma symptoms, with the patient thus becoming more disorganized in behavioural terms, with negative consequences upon the development of the ailment. In this way we may understand the association observed: as the state of anxiety increases, asthma control becomes worse.

The most important coping mechanism in this study was hiding asthma, considered as a passive one. This mechanism as well as avoidance and denial were linked with less mobilized strategies in chronic diseases (Felton et al., 1984; Santavirta, 1997; Osowiecki & Compas, 1999). In other studies, asthma denial has been recognized as an important risk factor for asthma attacks, and more emergency treatment (Dirks et al., 1978; Miller, 1987; Steiner et al., 1987; Yellowlees & Ruffin, 1989; Lavoie et al., 2010). The coping mechanism in general (total scores) and particularly the positive reappraisal were also correlated with greater severity of asthma.

Another important mechanism found in this sample was worry about the disease, which is considered as the most emotionally involving, correlated with poor quality of life. This is in accordance with the worst adjustment to the disease, related to emotional involvement (Bombardier et al., 1990; Landreville & Veniza, 1994; Scharloo et al., 1998).

Related also with poor quality of life are depressive symptoms (Goethe et al., 2001), which seem to measure negative feelings as well as neuroticism (Koivumaa-Honkanen et al., 2000), and this is corroborated in the present study.

With these results we are witnessing a multiple confluence of biological, environmental, psychological and social factors in asthma, as well as in its evolution, treatment and prognosis, understandable in the complexity of systemic and multiple interaction of all these factors, which influence and are simultaneously influenced by the disease.

The behavioral disorders found are translated by clinical and morbidity criteria, leading to higher use of healthcare and medication, and absenteeism, with poorer disease control and quality of life.

In this way, the need for better and more accurate assessment emerge, not at a symptomatic level but also discriminating different types of anxiety, depression, associated psychopathology that determine the diagnosis and development of this disease.
In future studies a cluster selection of individuals will be required who combine physical and psychological characteristics, above all with severe or unstable asthma, with more adequate clinical interventions. This is taking into account that even if we cannot change personalities, we can at least modify behaviour, with efficacy in healthy habits and attitudes, namely concerning compliance to treatment.

4. Study 2: Psychoeducational and multifamily interventions in asthma

4.1 Objectives

This study aims to analyse the effects of psychoeducational and multifamily interventions in asthma, in biological variables (spirometry and inflammatory marker), morbidity criteria (health care use, absenteeism, medication, quality of life and control of disease) and psychological outcomes (anxiety, depression and coping mechanisms).

4.2 Methods

We conducted a five-month prospective study, randomized with simple occultation, with two intervention groups and a control group, according to the criteria defined and presented in the previous study, where 195 patients were studied. Of these, the ones with moderate or severe persistent asthma were selected.
This Random Control Trial was carried out in the Allergy & Immunology outpatients' department of the University Hospital S. João in Oporto.
The randomization resulted in the balanced inclusion of 141 patients, divided into three groups (according to levels of anxiety and depression). The studied sample, in two observations, was the following: Psychoeducational Group (PG) intervention and usual pharmacological treatment (n=38), Multifamily Group (MG) intervention and usual pharmacological treatment (n=29), Control group (CG) with only usual pharmacological treatment (n=44) (Figure 5).

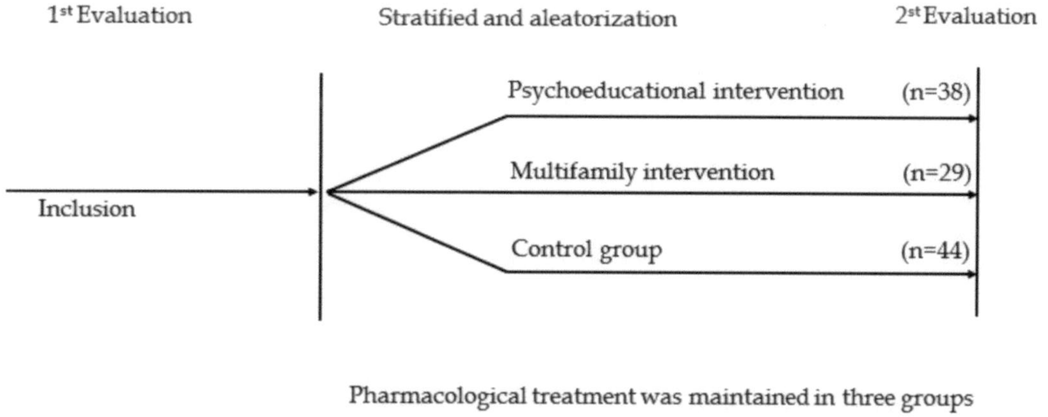

Fig. 5. Clinical study design

For comparison with the evaluation made in the second study, the following scales of evaluation were used: Self Anxiety Scale - SAS (Zung, 1971), State-Trait Anxiety Inventory - STAIY (Spielberger, 1983), Beck Depression Inventory - BDI (Beck et al., 1961), Ways of Coping with Asthma in Everyday Life - WCAEL (Aalto et al., 2002), Mini Asthma Quality of Life Questionnaire - MiniAQLQ (Juniper et al., 1999a) and Asthma Control Questionnaire - ACQ (Juniper et al., 1999b).

They were still compared according to their asthma symptoms, spirometry, inflammatory marker and morbidity criteria.

All psychological and clinical measures were assessed twice, before and after interventions.

Only adding information and knowledge became incomplete (Costa & MacCrane, 1987; Clark et al., 2002). With these interventions the aim is not to modify personalities, but change behaviour and attitudes (Costa & MacCrane, 1986).

In this context, the general principles of two interventions included both transmission of information, promoting behaviour change and improvement of self-efficacy. This implies a bidirectional process with interactions between health professionals and asthmatic patients and families. There are some objectives in this communication, mainly in answer to different issues, erasing false constructs, reduction of anxiety due to illness and promoting healthy habits and attitudes

Specifically for the **Psychoeducational programme**, the present intervention was focused on results in three levels of learning: knowledge transmission, education for instrumental attitudes and finally integration of the former. This empowered the patients by increasing self-efficacy and improvement in problem-solving of asthma. These sessions were not only didactic but also interactive.

The **Multifamily programme** was based on three distinct components: educational (sharing of experiences between families and patients, mediation by psychotherapists), social network (cross over difficult situations) and problem-solving (extending solutions, training strategies to deal with illness). This intervention was structured as a "group within a group", based on the Multifamily Discussion Group of Gonzalez and Steinglass (Gonzalez et al., 1986, Gonzalez & Steinglass, 2002; Steinglass, 1998).

4.3 Results

The intervention groups and control group had balanced demographic, psychological and clinical characteristics (Table 2).

Considering the total sample of asthmatics (n=141), the majority was female (78.7%), with a mean age (sd) of 39.3 (14.2). There was also a predominance of lower socio-economic classes (75.1%). The mean duration of the disease was 21.5 (14.8) years and most of the patients had severe persistent asthma (76.6%).

There was an improvement in both intervention programmes, in psychological variables. Depression only achieved statistical significance in the PG ($p \leq 0.05$), but anxiety state was significant in all groups (MG $p<0.01$; PG $p<0.01$), as well as anxiety trait (MG $p<0.001$; PG $p<0.01$) (Table 3).

In the MG, there was a relevant decrease in the coping mechanism of worry with asthma ($p=0.000$).

In both programs there was an improvement in the quality of life (MG $p<0.05$; PG $p<0.01$), increasing in 0.8U in PG and 0.5U in MG, taking into consideration effective results since 0.5U, according Juniper´s references (Juniper et al., 1999a).

	Multifamily (n=46)	Psychoeducacional (n=47)	Control (n=48)
Age (years) mean (sd)	40.2(16.3)	37.8(14.1)	40.0(12.3)
Gender n(%)			
Male	7(15.2)	8(17.0)	15(31.3)
Female	39(84.8)	39(83.0)	33(68.8)
Socio-economic classification n(%)			
High and very high	3(6.5)	3(6.4)	5(10.4)
Median	6(13.0)	11(23.4)	7(14.6)
Low	12(26.1)	10(21.3)	14(29.2)
Very low	25(54.3)	23(48.9)	22(45.8)
Disease duration (years) mean (sd)	24.4(15.0)	20.4(14.6)	19.7(14.8)
Asthma severity n(%)			
Moderate persistent	9(19.6)	8(17.0)	16(33.4)
Severe persistent	37(80.4)	39(83.0)	32(66.7)

Table 2. Demographic and clinical characteristics of sample

	MULTIFAMILY (*n=29*)			PSYCOEDUCACIONAL (*n=38*)		
	1º Av.	*2ª Av.*		*1º Av.*	*2ª Av.*	
Anxiety state[1]	11.2 (3.3)	9.8 (3.7)	Imp **	11.4 (3.0)	9.4 (2.6)	Imp **
Anxiety trait[2]	49.5 (12.4)	38.8 (11.4)	Imp ***	45.8 (11.8)	41.2 (10.7)	Imp **
Depression[3]	12.3 (9.1)	11.9 (10.2)	Imp. NS	10.7 (6.9)	8.0 (8.3)	Imp *
Quality of life[4]	4.5 (1.3)	5.0 (1.4)	Imp. *	4.3 (1.2)	5.1 (1.3)	Imp **
Asthma control[5]	2.0 (1.1)	1.5 (1.4)	Imp *	1.9 (1.1)	1.5 (1.3)	Imp *

Note: $p<0.001$ ***; $p<0.01$**; $p<0.05$*; NS - non-significant, imp. - improved; [1]SAS; [2]STAI-Y; [3]BDI; [4]MiniAQLQ; [5]ACQ

Table 3. Psychological and clinical outcomes in experimental groups

There was also an increase in the control of asthma in both groups (MG $p<0.05$; PG $p<0.05$). In morbidity criteria, there was a reduction in the use of corticotherapy ($p=0.01$) in the MG, and in hospitalization ($p=0.000$) in the PG. There was an improvement in spirometry: FEV1 (MG $p<0.05$, PG $p<0.05$) and PEF (MG $p<0.05$, PG $p<0.01$).

4.4 Discussion and conclusion

The intention of this pioneer study in Portugal was to contribute to the characterization of the clinical situation of asthmatic patients in a hospital context, as well as the importance of group interventions (mainly educational and communicational) carried out in the context of a multidisciplinary programme (Fernandes, 2009).

Rejecting the linear model of etiological causality, the multisystemic model is strengthened with this psychoeducational intervention, in which all factors influence and are influenced by the illness.

In moderate/severe asthma, besides the usual preventive and pharmacological approaches, it is essential to turn to a widespread intervention: psychoeducational and multifamily programmes, with a multidisciplinary team, to increase the control of the illness and allow therapeutic effectiveness (Wamboldt et al., 1995; Devine, 1996; Steinglass et al., 2002; Yorke et al., 2007)

The innovative therapeutic interventions (Psychoeducational and Multifamily) revealed promising results, as demonstrated in the present study. Namely in both interventional groups, there were good results, with statistically significant improvement in quality of life, asthma control, psychological variables (anxiety state and trait, depression and coping mechanisms) and clinical parameters (spirometry).

With the present intervention we try to demonstrate that behavioural changes brought about, improvement in the psychological parameters, as well as in the clinical parameters.

The present results encourage further studies, with larger samples and longitudinal interventions, in order to evaluate the stability of the positive effects found.

An accurate selection for a therapeutic approach is also necessary to cater for specific characteristics of these patients, more orientated for control and self-efficacy in psychoeducational or solution focused/emotional confrontation for more psychotherapeutic intervention.

Only in this way, can we pursue a holistic comprehension of the complexity of these physiopathological processes involved in asthma, with a more integrated and efficient treatment.

5. Acknowledgements

The author wish to thank J. Fonseca, S. Martins, M. Ribeiro, L. Delgado, A. Costa Pereira and M. Vaz.

6. References

Aalto, A.M.; Härkäpää, K.; Aro, A.R. & Rissanen, P. (2002). Ways of coping with asthma in everyday life validation of the asthma specific coping scale. *Journal of Psychosomatic Research*, Vol. 53, pp. 1061-1069.

Ader, R. & Cohen, N. (1985). CNS-immune system interaction conditioning phenomena. *Behavioral and Brain Sciences*, Vol. 8, pp- 379-394.

Baron, C., Lamarre, A., Veilleux, P., Ducharme, G., Spiet, S. & Lapierre, J.G. (1986). Psycho maintenance of childhood asthma: a study of 34 children. Journal of Asthma, Vol. 23, pp. 69-79.

Barton, C.A., McKenzie, D.P., Walters, E.H. & Abramson, M. (2005). Interactions between psychosocial problems and management of asthma: who is at risk of dying? *J Asthma*, Vol. 42, pp. 249-56.

Baumeister, H. (2005). [Bronchial asthma and mental disorders -- a systematic review of empirical studies]. *Psychother Psychosom Med Psychol*, May, Vol. 55, No. 5, pp. 247-55.

Beck, A.T., Ward, C.H., Mendelson, M., Mock, J. & Erbaugh, J. (1961). An Inventory for Measuring Depression. *Arch Gen Psychiat*, Vol. 4, pp. 561-571.

Bender, B.G. (2006). Risk taking, depression, adherence, and symptom control in adolescents and young adults with asthma. *Am J Respir Crit Care Med*, Vol. 173, No. 9, pp. 953-7

Bernard-Bonnin, A.C., Stachenko, S., Bonin, D., Charette, C. & Rousseau, E. (1995). Self-management teaching programs and morbidity of pediatric asthma: a meta-analysis. *Journal of Allergy and Clinical Immunology*, Vol. 95, pp. 34-41.

Bombardier, C.H., D'Amico, C. & Jordan, J.S. (1990). The relationship of appraisal and coping to chronic illness adjustment. *Behav Res Ther*, Vol. 28, pp. 297-304.

Borkovec, T.D. On the need for a basic science approach to psychotherapy research. *Psych Sci*, Vol. 8, pp. 145-147.

Boulet, L.P., Deschesnes, F., Turcotte, H. & Gignac, F. (1991). Near-fatal asthma: Clinical and physiologic features, perception of bronchoconstriction, and psychologic profile. *J Allergy Clin Immunol*, Vol. 88, No. 6, pp. 838-846.

Bruzzese, J.M., Markman, L.B., Appel, D. & Webber, M. (2001). An evaluation of Open Airways for Schools: using college students as intructors. *Journal of Asthma*, Vol. 38, pp. 337-342.

Busse, W.B. (2000). A 47-year-old woman with severe asthma. Clinical crossroads. *JAMA*, Vol. 284, pp. 2225-2233.

Campbell, D.A., McLennan, G., Coates, J.R., Frith, P.A., Gluyas, P.A., Latimer, K.M., Luke, C.G., Martin, A.J., Roder, D.M. & Ruffin, R.E. (1994). A comparison of asthma deaths and near-fatal asthma attacks in South Australia. *Eur Respir J*, Vol. 7, pp. 490–497.

Campbell, D.A., Yellowlees, P., McLennan, G., Coates, J.R., Frith, P.A., Gluyas, P.A., Latimer, K.M., Luke, C.G., Martin, A.J. & Ruffin, R.E. (1995a). Psychiatric and medical features of near fatal asthma. *Thorax*, Vol. 50, pp. 254-259.

Chetta, A., Gerra, G., Foresi, A., Zaimovic, A., Del Donno, M., Chittolini, B., Malorgio, R., Castagnaro, A. & Olivieri, D. (1998). Personality profiles and breathlessness perception in outpatients with different grading of asthma. *Am J Respir Crit Care Med*, Vol. 157, pp. 116-22.

Clark, N.M. & Partridge, M.R. (2002). Strengthening asthma education to enhance disease control. *Chest*, Vol. 121, pp. 1661-1669.

Cluley, S. & Cochrane, G.M. (2001). Psychological disorder in asthma is associated with poor control and poor adherence to inhaled steroids. *Respir Med*, Vol. 95, pp. 37- 9.

Cohen, S., Tyreli, D.A. & Smith, A.P. (1991). Psychological stress in humans and susceptibility to the common cold. *New England Journal of Medicine*, Vol. 325, pp. 606-612.

Cooper, C.L., Parry, D.G., Saul, C., Morice, A.H., Hutchcroft, B.J., Moore, J. & Esmonde, L. (2007). Anxiety and panic fear in adults with asthma: prevalence in primary care. BMC Fam Prat, Vol. 8, pp. 62.

Costa, P.T. & McCrae, R. (1986). Personality stability and its implications for clinical psychology. *Clinical Psychology Review*, Vol. 6, pp. 407-423.

Costa, P.T. & McCrae, R. (1987). Neuroticism, somatic complaints and disease: Is the bark worse than the bite? *Journal of Personality*, Vol. 55, No. 2, pp. 299-316.

Dahlem, N.K., Kinsman, R.A. & Horton, D.J. (2009). Panic-fear in asthma: requests for asneeded medication in relation to pulmonary function measurements. *J Allergy Clin Immunol*, Vol. 60, pp. 295-300.

Derogatis, L.R. & Savitz, K.L. (1999). The SCL-90-R, brief symptom inventory, and matching clinical rating scales. In: Maruish (Ed), *The use of psychological testing for treatment planning and outcomes assessment*. Mahwah, NJ. Erlbaum, pp. 679-724.

Devine, E.C. (1996). Meta-analysis of the effects of psychoeducational care in adults with asthma. *Research in Nursing and Health*, Vol. 19, pp. 367-376.

Devriese, S., Winters, W., Stegen, K., van Diest, I., Veulemans, H., Nemery, B., Eelen, P., Van de Woestijne, K. & Van den Bergh, O. (2000). Generalization of acquired somatic symptoms in response to odors: A Pavlovian perspective on multiple chemical sensitivity. *Psychosomatic Medicine*, Vol. 62, pp. 751-759.

Di Marco, F., Santus, P. & Centanni, S. (2011). Anxiety and depression in asthma. *Curr Opin Pulm Med*, Vol. 17, No. 1, pp. 39-44.

Dirks, J.F. & Kinsman, R.A. (1981). Clinical prediction of medical rehospitalization: psychological assessment with the battery of asthma illness behavior. *J Pers Assessment*, Vol. 45, pp. 608-613.

Dirks, J.F., Kinsman, R.A., Horton, D.J., Fross, K.H. & Jones, N.F. (1978). Panic-fear in asthma: rehospitalization following intensive long-term treatment. *Psychosom Med*, Vol. 40, pp. 5-13

Eysenck, H.J. (1969). Research findings with the MPI. In: Eysenck, H.J. & Eysenck, S.B.C., Personality Structure and Measurement. London: Routledge & Kegan Paul.

Felton, B.J., Revenson, T.A. & Hinrichsen, G.A. (1984). Stress and coping in explenation of psychosocial adjustment among chronically ill adults. *Soc Sci Med*, Vol. 18, pp. 889-98.

Fernandes, L. (2009). Dos Factores Biopsicológicos às Intervenções Multifamiliares e Psicoeducacionais na Asma. Edição Bial.

Fernandes, L., Fernandes, M., Cruz, R., Gonçalves, R., Martins, S., Rodrigues, J., Almeida, J., Pinto, A. & Vieira, A. (2005). Caracterização da personalidade dos doentes asmáticos. *Revista Portuguesa de Pneumologia*, Jan-Fev, *Vol.*11, No. 1, pp. 7-34.

Fernandes, L., Fonseca, J., Martins, S., Delgado, L., Pereira, A.C., Vaz, M. & Branco, G. (2010). Association of anxiety with asthma: subjective and objective outcome measures. *Psychosomatics*, Jan, Vol. 51, No. 1, pp. 39-46.

Fonseca, J.A., Fernandes, L., Delgado, L., Costa-Pereira, A., Sousa, M., Martins, S., Gomes, S., Moreira, A., Vaz, M. & Castel-Branco, G. (2004). Asthmatic patients with anxiety:

more symptoms and medication but a better adherence and less Exhaled Nitric Oxide. *Journal Investigational Allergology Clinical Immunology*, Vol. 14, (suppl 1).

Ford, D.H. & Urban, H.B. (1998). Contemporary models of psychotherapy. A comparative Analysis (2nd ed). New York: John Wiley.

Ford, D.H. (1987). Humans as self –construction living systems. A developmental perspective on behavior, personality, and health. New York: Erlbaum.

Forsythe, P., Ebeling, C., Gordon, J.R., Befus, A.D. & Vliagoftis, H. (2004). Opposing effects of short- and long-term stress on airway inflammation. *Am J Respir Crit Care Med*, Vol. 169, pp. 220-6.

French, T.M. & Alexander, F. (1941). Psychogenic factors in bronchial asthma. *Psychosom Med Monographs*, Vol. 4, pp. 1941.

Friedman, H.S. & Booth-Kewley, S. (1987). The "disease-prone personality". A meta-analytic view of the construct. *American Psychologist*, Vol. 42, No. 6, pp. 539-555.

Gallagher, R. & Appenzeller, T. (1999). Beyond reductionism. *Science*, Vol. 284, pp. 79.

Garden, G.M. (1993). Psychiatric and social aspects of brittle asthma. *Thorax*, Vol. 48, pp. 501-505.

GINA - Global Initiative for Asthma (2010). *Global Strategy for Asthma Management and Prevention. National Institutes of Health.* National Heart, Lung, and Blood Institute. Available at: www.ginasthma.org.

Goethe, J.W., Maljanian, R., Wolf, S., Hernandez, P. & Cabrera, Y. (2001). The impact of depressive symptoms on the functional status of inner-city patients with asthma. *Ann Allergy Asthma Immunol*, Vol. 87, pp. 205-210.

Goldberg, D.P. & Hillier, V.F. (1979). A Scaled Version of the General Health Questionnaire. *Psychological Medicine*, Vol. 9, pp. 139-145.

Goldstein, D.S. & Dekker, M. (2001). *The autonomic nervous system in health and disease.* Informa Healthcare.

Gonzalez, S., & Steinglass, P. (2002). Application of Multifamily Groups in Chronic Medical Disorders. In: McFarlane, W. *Multifamily Groups in the Treatment of Severe Psychiatric Disorders*. New York: The Guilford Press.

Gonzalez, S., Steinglass, P., & Reiss, D. (1986). *Family- centred interventions for the chronically disabled: The 8-session multiple-family group programme: Treatment manual.* Washington, DC: George Washington University Rehabilitation Research and Training Center.

Goodwin, R.D. & Eaton, W.W. (2003). Asthma and the risk of panic attacks among adults in the community. *Psychological Medicine*, Vol. 33, pp. 879-885.

Graffar, M. (1956). Une méthode de classification sociale d'échantillons de population. *Courier, Vol.* 6, pp. 455-459.

Gregerson, M.B. (2000). The curious 2000-year case of asthma. *Psychosom Med*, Vol. 62, pp. 816-827.

Gustafsson, P.A. & Cederblad, M. (1986). Family therapy in the treatment of severe childhood asthma. *Journal of Psychosomatic Research*, Vol. 30, pp. 369-374.

Hasler, G., Gergen, P.J., Kleinbaum, D.G. & Ajdacic, V. (2005). Asthma and Panic in Young Adults. A 20-Year Prospective Community Study. *American Journal of Respiratory and Critical Care Medicine*, Vol. 171, pp. 1224-1230.

Heaney, L.G., Conway, E., Kelly, C. & Gamble, J. (2005). Prevalence of psychiatric morbidity in a difficult asthma population: relationship to asthma outcome. *Respir Med*, Vol. 99, pp. 1152–1159.

Hibbert, G.A. & Pilsbury, D. (1988). Demonstration and treatment of hyperventilation causing asthma. *Br J Psychiatry*, Vol. 153, pp. 687-9.

Hollaender, J. & Florin, I. (1983). Expressed emotion and airway conductance in children with bronchial asthma. *Journal of Psychosomatic Research*, Vol. 27, pp. 307-311.

Hornsveld, H.K. & Garssen, B. (1996). Double-blind placebo-controlled study of thehyperventilation provocation test and the validity of the hyperventilation syndrome. *Lancet*, Vol. 384, pp. 158.

Horton, D.J., Suda, W.L., Kinsman, R.A., Souhrada, J. & Spector, S.L. (1978). Bronchoconstrictive suggestion in asthma: a role for airways hyperreactivity and emotions. *American Review of Respiratory Disease*; Vol. 117, pp. 1029-1038.

Innes, N.J., Reid, A., Halstead, J., Watkin, S.W. & Harrison, B.D. (1998). Psychosocial risk factors in near-fatal asthma and in asthma deaths. *J R Coll Physicians Lond*, Vol. 32, pp. 430–434.

Irvine, L., Crombie, I.K., Clark, R.A., Slane, P.W., Feyerabend, C., Goodman, K.E. & Cater, J.I. (1999). Advising parents of asthmatic children on passive smoking: Randomised controlled trial. *BMJ*, Vol. 318, pp. 1456-1459.

Isenberg, S.A., Lehrer, P. & Hochron, S.M. (1992). The effects of suggestion and emotional arousal on pulmonary function in asthma: a review and a hypothesis regarding vagal mediation. *Psychosomatic Med*, Vol. 54, pp. 192-216.

Jasnoski, M.B.L., Bell, I.R. & Peterson, R. (1994). What connections exist between shyness, hay fever, anxiety, anxiety sensivity, and panic disorders? *Anxiety Stress Coping*, Vol. 7, pp. 19-34.

Juniper, E.F., Guiyatt, G.H., Cox, F.M., Ferrie, P.J. & King, D.R. (1999a). Mini Asthma Quality of Life. *Eur Respir J*, Vol. 14, pp. 32-38.

Juniper, E.F., O´Byrne, P.M., Guyatt, G.H., Ferrie, P.J. & King, D.R. (1999b). Development and validation of a questionnaire to measure asthma control. *Eur Respir J*, Vol. 14, pp. 902-907.

Kang, D.H., Coe, C.L., McCarthy, D.O., Jarjour, N.N., Kelly, E.A., Rodriguez, R.R., Busse, W.W. (1997). Cytokine profiles of stimulated blood lymphocytes in asthmatic and healthy adolescents across the school year. *Journal of Interferon and Cytokine Research*, Vol. 17, pp. 481-487.

Kelloway, J.S., Wyatt, R., DeMarco, J. & Adlis, S. (2000). Effect of salmentrol on patients adherence to their prescribed refills for inhaled corticosteroids. *Annals of Allergy, Asthma and Immunology*, Vol. 84, pp. 324-328.

Kinsman, R.A., Dirks, J.F. & Jones, N.F. (1982). Psychomaintenance of chronic physical illness. In: Millon, T. & Green, C.J. *Handbook of clinical Health Psychology*. New York: Plenum, pp. 435-465.

Kinsman, R.A., Luparello, T., O´Banion, K. & Spector, S. (1973). Multidimensional Analysis of the Subjective Symptomatology of Asthma. *Psychosomatic Medicine*, Vol. 35, No. 3, pp. 250-266.

Koch, C. & Laurent, G. (1999). Complexity and the nervous system. *Science*, Vol. 284, pp. 96-98.

Koivumaa-Honkanen, H.T., Honkanen, R., Vinamäki, H., Heikkilä, K., Kaprio, J. & Koskenvuo, M. (2000). Self-reported life satisfaction and 20-year mortality in healthy Finnish adults. *Am J Epidemiol*, Vol. 152, pp. 983-991.

Kotses, H., Bernstein, I.L., Bernstein, D.I., Reynolds, R.V.C., Korbee, L., Wigal, J.K., Ganson, E., Stout, C. & Creer, T.L. (1995). A self-management program for adult asthma. Part I: Development and evaluation. *Journal of Allergy and Clinical Immunology*, Vol. 95, pp. 529-540.

Landreville, P. & Veniza, J. (1994). Differences in appraisal and coping between elderly coronary artery disease patients high and low in depressive symptoms. *J Ment Health*, Vol. 3, pp. 79-90.

Lask, B. & Matthew, D. (1979). Childhood asthma. A controlled trial of family psychotherapy. *Archives of Disease in Childhood*, Vol. 54, pp. 116-119.

Lavoie KL, Bouthillier D, Bacon SL, Lemière, C., Martin, J., Hamid, Q., Ludwig, M., Olivenstein, R. & Ernst, P. (2010). Psychological distress and maladaptive coping styles in patients with severe versus moderate asthma. *Chest*, Vol. 137, No. 6, pp. 1324-31.

Lavoie, K.L., Bacon, S.L., Barone, S., Cartier, A., Ditto, B. & Labrecque, M. (2006). What is worse for asthma control and quality of life: depressive disorders, anxiety disorders, or both? *Chest*, Vol. 130, pp. 1039–1047.

Lehrer, P.M. (1998). Emotionally triggered asthma: A review of research literature and some hypotheses for self-regulation therapy. *Applied Psychophysiology and Biofeedback*, Vol. 23, pp. 13-41.

Lehrer, P.M., Feldman, J., Giardino, N., Song, H.S. & Schamaling, K. (2002). Psychological aspects of asthma. *Journal of Consulting and Clinical Psychology*, Vol. 70, No. 3, pp. 691-711.

Lehrer, P.M., Generelli, P. & Hochron, S. (1997). The effect of facial and trapezius muscle tension impedance in asthma. *Applied Psychophysiology and Biofeedbac*, Vol. 22, pp. 43-54.

Lehrer, P.M., Isenberg, S. & Hochron, S.M. (1993). Asthma and emotion: a review. *J Asthma*, Vol. 30, pp. 5-21.

Lehrer, P.M., Vaschillo, E., Vaschillo, B., Lu, S.E., Scardella, A., Siddique, M. & Habib, R.H. (2004). Biofeedback Treatment for Asthma. *Chest*, Vol. 126, pp. 352-361.

Lehrer, P.M., Vaschilo, E., Vaschilo, B., Lu, S.E., Eckeberg, D.L., Edelberg, R., Shih, W.J., Lin, Y., Kuusela, T.A., Tahvanainen, K.U. & Hamer, R.M. (2003). Heart rate variability biofeedback increases baroreflex gain and peak expiratory flow. *Psycosomatic Medicine*, Vol. 65, pp. 796-805.

Levenson, R.W. (1979). Effects of thematically relevant and general stressors on specificity of responding in asthmatic subjects. *Psychosom Med*, Vol. 41, pp. 28-39.

Levitan, H. (1985). Onset of asthma during intense mourning. *Psychosomatics*; Vol. 26, pp. 939-941.

Levy, S. (1984). Behavior and cancer. In: Light, R.J. & Pilemer, D.B. *Summing up: The science of reviewing research*. Cambridge, MA: Harvard University Press.

Luparello, T.J., Lyons, H.A., Bleecker, E.R. & McFadden, E.R. (1968). Influences of suggestion on airway reactivity in asthmatic subjects. *Psychosom Med*, Vol. 30, pp. 819-825.

MacKenzie, J.N. (1986). The production of "rose asthma" by artificial rose. *Am J Med Sci*, Vol. 91, pp. 45-47.

Manto, P.G. (1969). *An investigation of feedback mechanisms in stress-induced changes of autonomic balance*. Dissertação Académica: Rutgers University.

Martin, A.J., Campbell, D.A., Gluya, P.A., Coates, J.R., Ruffin, R.E., Roder, D.M., et al. (1995). Characteristics of near-fatal asthma in childhood. *Pediatric Pulmonology*, Vol. 20, pp. 1-8.

Martins, F. (1995). STAXI. In: Almeida, L., Simões, M. & Gonçalves, M. *Provas Psicológicas em Portugal*. Braga: APPORT.

Mathinson, D.A. (1993). Asthma in adults: diagnosis and treatment. In: Middleton, E., Rees, C.E., Ellis, E.F., Adkinson, N.F., Yunginger, J.W. & Busse, W.W. (Editors). *Allergy: principles and practice*. Vol 2. (4th ed.), pp. 1263-1300. St Louis (MO): Mosby.

Mayer-Gross, W., Slater, E. & Roth, M. (1969). *Clinical Psychiatry* (3rd ed.). London: Baillière, Tindall & Cassell.

McFadden, E.R., Luparello, T., Lyons, H.A. & Bleecker, E. (1969). The mechanism of action of sugestión in the induction of acute asthma attacks. *Psychosom Med*, Vol. 31, pp. 134-143.

McFarlane, W.R., Link, B., Dushay, R., et al. (1995). Psychoeducational multiple family groups: Four-year relapse outcome in schizophrenia. *Family Process*, Vol. 34, pp. 127-144.

McQuaid, E.L., Kopel, S.J. & Nassau, J.H. (2001). Behavioral adjustment in children with asthma: A meta-analysis. *J Dev Behav Pediatr*, pp. 430-490.

Miller, B.D. & Strunk, R.C. (1989). Circumstances surrounding the deaths of children due to asthma. *American Journal of Diseases of Children*, Vol. 143, pp. 1294-1299.

Miller, B.D. (1987). Depression and asthma: a potentially lethal mixture. *J Allergy Clin Immunol*, Vol. 80, pp. 481-486.

Miller, D.J. & Kotses, H. (1995). Classical conditioning of total respiratory resistance in humans. *Psychosomatic Medicine*, Vol. 57, pp. 148-153.

Mrazek, D.A., Schuman, W.B. & Klinnert, M. (1998). Early asthma onset: Risk of emotional and behavioral difficulties. *J Child Psychol Psychiatry*, Vol. 39, No. 2, pp. 247-254.

Neild, J.E. & Cameron, I.R. (1985). Bronchoconstriction in response to suggestion: its prevention by an inhaled anticholinergic agent. *BMJ*, Vol. 290, pp. 674.

Nouwen, A., Freeston, M.H., Labbé, R. & Boulet, R.P. (1999). Psychological factors associated with emergency room visits among asthmatic patients. *Behavior Modification*, Vo. 23, pp. 217-233.

Osowiecki, D.M. & Compas, B.E. (1999). A prospective study of coping, perceived control, and psychological adaptation to breast cancer. *Cogn Ther Res*, Vol. 23, pp. 169-80.

Picado, C., Montserrat, J.N., de Pablo, J., Plaza, V. & Agusti-Vidal, A. (1989). Predisposing factors to death after recovery from a life-threatning asthmatic attack. *J Asthma*, Vol. 26, No. 4, pp. 231-236.

Ponciano, E., Vaz Serra, A. & Relvas, J. (1982). Aferição da escala de auto-avaliação de ansiedade, de Zung, numa amostra de população portuguesa – I. – Resultados da aplicação numa amostra de população normal. *Psiquiatria Clínica*, Vol. 3, No. 4, pp. 191-202.

Ponciano, E., Vaz Serra, A. & Relvas, J. (1982). Aferição da escala de auto-avaliação de ansiedade, de Zung, numa amostra de população portuguesa – I. – Resultados da aplicação numa amostra de população normal. *Psiquiatria Clínica*, Vol. 3, No. 4, pp. 191-202.

Prueter, C. & Norra, C. (2005). Mood disorders and their treatment in patients with epilepsy. *J Neuropsychiatry Clin Neurosci*, Vol. 17, No. 1, pp. 20-8.

Put, C., Demedts, M., van den Bergh, O., Demyttenaere, K. & Verleden, G. (1999). Asthma symptoms: influence of personality versus clinical status. *Eur Respir J*, Vol. 13, pp. 751-756.

Rietveld, S.B.I. & Everaerd, W. (2000). Psychological confounds in medical research: the example of excessive cough in asthma. *Behav Res Ther*, Vol. 38, pp. 791-800.

Rimington, L.D., Davies, D.H., Lowe, D. & Pearson, M.G. (2001). Relationship between anxiety, depression, and morbidity in adult asthma patients. *Thorax*, Vol. 56, pp. 266-271.

Rumbak, M.J., Kelso, T.M., Arheart, K.L. & Self, T.H. (1993). Perception of anxiety as a contributing factor of asthma: indigent. *J Asthma*, Vol. 30, pp. 165-169.

Sandberg, S., Paton, J., Ahola, S., McCann, D.C., McGuinness, D., Hillary, C.R. & Oja, H. (2000). The role of acute and chronic stress in asthma attacks in children. *Lancet*, Vol. 356, No. 9234, pp. 982-7.

Santavirta, N. (1997). Coping, pain and disability in patients with chronic inflammatory and musculoskeletal diseases. Stockholm: Karolinska Institutet.

Santos, S.C. & Silva, D.R. (1997). Adaptação do State-Trait Anxiety Inventory (STAI) Form Y para a população portuguesa: Primeiros dados. *Revista Portuguesa de Psicologia*, Vol. 32, pp. 71-89.

Scharloo, M., Kaptein, A., Weinman, J., Hazes, J.M., Willems, L.N.A. (1998). Illness perceptions, coping and functioning in patients with rheumatoid arthritis, chronic obstructive pulmonary disease and psoriasis. *J Psychosom Res*, Vol. 44, pp. 537-85.

Scott, K.M., Von Korff, M., Ormel, J., Zhang, M.Y., Bruffaerts, R., Alonso, J., Kessler, R.C., Tachimori, H., Karam, E., Levinson, D., Bromet, E.J., Posada-Villa, J., Gasquet, I., Angermeyer, M.C., Borges, G., de Girolamo, G., Herman, A. & Haro, J.M. (2007) Mental disorders among adults with asthma: results from the World Mental Health Survey. *Gen Hosp Psychiatry*, Mar-Apr, Vol. 29, No. 2, pp. 123-33.

Silagy, C. (1999). Advising parents of asthmatic children on passive smoking: Ramdomized controlled trial. *Journal of Paediatrics*, Vol. 135, pp. 650-651.

Silva, D.R. & Campos, R. (1998). Alguns dados normativos do Inventário de Estado-Traço de Ansiedade Forma Y (STAI) de Spielberger para a população portuguesa. *Revista Portuguesa de Psicologia*, Vol. 33, pp. 71-89.

Silverglade, I., Tosi, D.J., Wise, P.S., D'Costa, A. (1994). Irrational beliefs and emotionality in adolescents with and without bronchial asthma. *Journal of General Psychology*, Vol. 121, pp.199-207.

Smith, J.R., Mildenhall, S., Noble, M.J., Shepstone, L., Koutantji, M., Mugford, M. & Harrison, B.D. (2005). The Coping with Asthma Study: a randomised controlled trial of a home based, nurse led psychoeducational intervention for adults at risk of adverse asthma outcomes. *Thorax*, Dec, Vol. 60, No. 12, pp. 1003-11.

Smith, J.R., Mugford, M., Holland, R., Noble, M.J. & Harrison, B.D. (2007). Psycho-educational interventions for adults with severe or difficult asthma: a systematic review. *J Asthma*, Apr, Vol. 44, No. 3, pp. 219-41.

Spielberger, C.D. & London, P. (1990). Blood pressure and injustice. *Psychology Today*, Vol. 1, pp. 48-51.

Spielberger, C.D. (1983). *Manual for the State-Trait Anxiety Inventory STAI (Form Y) ("Self Evaluation Questionnaire")*. Palo Alto: Consulting Psychologists Press, Inc.

Spielberger, C.D. (1988). *State-trait Anger Expression Inventory (STAXI)*. Odessa, FL: Psychological Assessment Resources.

Spinhoven, P., Peski-Oosterbaan, A.S., Van der Dooes, A.J., Willelms, N.J. & Sterk, P.J. (1997). Association of anxiety with perception of induced bronchoconstriction in patients with asthma. *Thorax*, Vol. 52, pp. 152.

Staudenmayer, H., Kinsman, R., Dirks, J.F., Spector, S.L. & Wangaard, C. (1979). Medical outcome in asthmatic patients: effects of airways hyperreactivity and symptom-focused anxiety. *Psychosomatic Medicine*, Vol. 41, pp. 109-118.

Steiner, H., Higgs, C.M.B., Fritz, G.K., Laszlo, G. & Harvey, J.E. (1987). Defense Style and the perception of asthma. *Psychosomatic Med*, Vol. 49, pp. 35-44.

Steinglass, P. (1998). Multiple family discussion groups for patients with chronic medical illness. *Families, Systems and Health*, Vol. 16, pp. 55-70.

Steinglass, P., Ostroff J., & Steinglass A.S. (2002). *Treatment Manual: The Ackerman/memorial Sloan-Kettering multiple family discussion group for cancer patients and their families.* Washington DC: George Washington University Rehabilitation Research and Training Centre.

Stout, C.K.H. & Creer, T.L. (1997). Improving perception of air flow obstruction in asthma patients. *Psychosomatic Med*, Vol. 59, pp. 201-206.

Strunk, R., Mrazek, D.A., Fuhrmann, G.S. & LaBrecque, J.F. (1985). Physiologic and psychological characteristics associated with deaths due to asthma in childhood. *J Am Med Assoc*, Vol. 254, No. 9, pp. 1193-1198.

Strunk, R.C., Nicklas, R.A., Milgrom, H., Ikle, D. (1999). Fatal and near-fatal asthma questionnaire: prelude to a national registry. *J Allergy Clin Immunol*, Vol. 104, pp. 763–768.

Suissa, S., Ernest, P., Benayoun, S., Baltzan, M. & Cai, B. (2000). Low-dose inhaled corticosteroids and the prevention of death from asthma. *N Engl J Med*, Vol. 343, pp. 332-336.

Sullivan, S.D., Elixhauser, A., Buist, S., Luce, B.R., Eisenberg, J. & Weiss, K.B. (1996). National asthma education and prevention program working group report on the cost effectiveness of asthma care. *Am J Respir Care Med*, Vol. 154, pp. 584-595.

Sun, H.W., Wang, J.P., Wang, S.Z., Wang, Y.Y., Song, Y.P., Yang, Z.H. & Wang, L.X. (2010). Effect of educational and psychological intervention on the quality of life of asthmatic patients. *Respir Care*, Vol. 55, No. 6, pp. 725-8.

Taitel, M.S., Kotses, H., Bernstein, I.L., Bernstein, D.I. & Creer, T.L. (1995). A self-management program for adult asthma. Part II: Cost-benefit analysis. *Journal of Allergy and Clinical Immunology*, Vol. 95, pp. 672-676.

ten Brinke, A., Ouwerkerk, M.E., Bel, E.H. & Spinhoven, P. (2001a). Similar psychological characteristics in mild and severe asthma. *Journal of Psychosomatic Research*, Vol. 50, pp. 7-10.

ten Brinke, A., Ouwerkerk, M.E., Zwinderman, A.H., Spinhoven, P. & Bel, E.H. (2001b). Psychopathology in patients with severe asthma is associated with increased health care utilization. *American Journal of Respiratory & Critical Care Medicine*, Vol. 163, pp. 1093-1096.

Thomas, M., Bruton, A., Moffat, M. & Cleland, J. (2011). Asthma and psychological dysfunction. *Prim Care Respir J*, Vol. 15.

Thomas, M., McKinley, R.K., Freeman, E. & Foy, C. (2001). Prevalence of dysfunctional breathing in patients treated for asthma in primary care: cross sectional survey. *BMJ*, Vol. 322, pp. 98-100.

van den Bergh, O., Stegen, K. & van de Woestijne, K.P. (1997). Learning to have psychosomatic complaints in psychosomatic patients. *Psychosomatic Medicine*, Vol. 59, pp. 13-23.

Vila, G., Nollet-Clemencon, C., Blic, J., Mouren-Simeoni, M.C. & Scheinmann, P. (2000). Prevalence of DSM IV anxiety and affective disorders in a pediatric population of asthmatic children and adolescents. *J Affect Disord*, Vol. 58, pp. 223-231.

Wainwright, N.W., Surtees, P.G., Wareham, N.J. & Harrison, B.D. (2007). Psychosocial factors and incident asthma hospital admissions in the EPIC-Norfolk cohort study. *Allergy*, Vol. 62, pp. 554-60.

Wamboldt, M.Z., & Levin, L.B.A. (1995). Utility of Multifamily Psychoeducational Groups for Medically - Ill Children and Adolescents. *Family Systems Medicine*, Vol. 13, pp. 151-161.

Weng, G., Bhalla, U.S. & Iyengar, R. (1999). Complexity in biological signaling systems. *Science*, Vol. 284, pp. 92-96.

Whitesides, G.M. & Ismagilov, G.M. (1999). Complexity in chemistry. *Science*, Vol. 284, pp. 89-92.

Wilson, S.R., Latini, D., Starr, N.J., Fish, L., Loes, L.M., Page, A. & Kubic, P. (1996). Education of parents of infants and very young children with asthma: a developmental evaluation of the wee wheezers program. *Journal of Asthma*, Vol. 33, No. 4, pp. 239-254.

Wöller, W., Kruse, J., Winter, P., Mans, E.J. & Alberti, L. (1993). Cortisone image and emotional support by key figures in patients with bronchial asthma. *Psychotherapy and Psychosomatics*, 59; 190-196.

Wright, R.J., Rodriguez, M. & Cohen, S. (1998). Review of psychosocial stress and asthma: an integrated biopsychosocial approach. *Thorax*, Vol. 53, pp. 1066-74.

Yellowlees, P.M. & Kalucy, R.S. (1990). Psychobiological aspects of asthma and the consequent research implications. *Chest*, Vol. 97, pp. 628-634.

Yellowlees, P.M. & Ruffin, R.E. (1989). Psychological defenses and coping styles in patients following a life-threatening attack of asthma. *Chest*, Vol. 95, pp. 1298-1303.

Yellowlees, P.M., Haynes, S., Potts, N. & Ruffin, R.E. (1988). Psychiatric morbidity in patients with life-threatening attack of asthma: initial report of a controlled study. *Med J Aust*, Vol. 149, pp. 246-249.

Yorke, J., Fleming, S.L. & Shuldham, C. (2007). Psychological interventions for adults with asthma: a systematic review. *A Respir Med,* Vol. 101, No. 1, pp. 1-14.

Zigmond, A.S.S.R. (1983). The hospital anxiety and depression scale. *Acta Psychiatr Scand,* Vol. 67, pp. 361-370.

Zung, W.W.K. (1971). A rating instrument for anxiety disorders. *Psychosomatics,* Vol. 6, pp. 371-379.

17

Obesity, Diet, Exercise and Asthma in Children

Luis Garcia-Marcos and Manuel Sanchez-Solis
University of Murcia,
Spain

1. Introduction

During the past decades, an increase in several pediatric morbid conditions has been well documented. Two of the most important of these conditions are obesity and asthma. While the increase of asthma prevalence has been explained in part by the so-called hygiene hypothesis, which claims for a shift from a Th1 to a Th2 environment (if the immunological system does not have to deal with infections -Th1- due to a much more aseptic environment, it will turn to an allergic predisposition -Th2) (von Mutius, 2007). However, this hypothesis does not explain the high prevalences among inner city populations (Platts-Mills et al., 2005) or developing countries as found in the International Study of Asthma and Allergies in Childhood (ISAAC) (Asher et al., 2006). On the other hand, the increased prevalence of obesity is most probably due to an imbalance between the energy intake (both in quantity as well as quality) and the expenditure, in which the lack of exercise is a key point. In this chapter we will explore the complex relationship between asthma, obesity diet and exercise in children.

2. Obesity and asthma are linked together

2.1 The epidemiological link

In this section some of the epidemiological evidence regarding the link between asthma and obesity is reviewed.

2.1.1 Obesity/overweight is associated and precedes asthma

Numerous studies support the epidemiological association between asthma and obesity. Though many of them are cross-sectional, thus making it difficult to establish a casual relationship, some have been specifically aimed at disentangling the first question of which is first in those two apparently connected diseases. The meta-analysis by Sutherland and Beuther (Beuther & Sutherland, 2007) included seven studies which fulfilled their criteria of including adult individuals followed for at least one year in which the main outcome variable was incident asthma and whose obesity was measured using body mass index (BMI). The aforementioned studies included more than 300,000 individuals and the result clearly demonstrated that BMI was associated to incident asthma in a dose-response manner: the association was higher with obesity than it was with overweight.

There are also a number of epidemiological clues which suggest that obesity in childhood precedes asthma later in life. For instance, in a Tasmanian cohort study (Burgess et al., 2007) of children recruited at the age of seven years, adiposity (defined as overweight at 7 years, or as highest quartile BMI) was associated with incident asthma between the ages of 21 and 32 years in girls, but not in boys. Although the number of subjects was low, the association was considerably high. Similarly, females who became overweight or obese between 6 and 11 years of age were seven times more likely to develop new asthma symptoms at ages 11 or 13, according to the Tucson Children Respiratory Study (Castro-Rodriguez et al., 2001). However, not all studies have found a higher association in girls. In fact, in the Children's Health Study (Southern California) the risk of new-onset asthma was higher in boys than in girls, although it was significant in both genders.

Not only do overweight or obesity seem to precede asthma but birth weight has also been shown to be related to later asthma. Although not all the reports coincide it does seem quite consistent that extreme high birth weights are strongly associated to asthma symptoms in school years (To et al., 2010). Furthermore, children with a predisposition for asthma may have a higher risk of developing asthma during childhood when their mothers are overweight before pregnancy, irrespective of the child's BMI (Scholtens et al., 2010). It is also of interest that infants breast fed for at least six moths have a better lung function, and this seems to be related to a lower weight gain. This was shown by Turner at al. (Turner et al., 2008) who followed 154 infants from birth. Maximal flow at functional residual capacity (V'maxFRC) was measured at 1 and 12 months of life: the change in V'maxFRC was inversely associated with change in weight. The group with lower V'maxFRC at 1 month and reduced change in V'maxFRC over infancy had the greatest weight gain and increased risk for asthma symptoms by the age of three years but not afterwards. Those authors concluded that postnatal weight gain may be indirectly associated with early transient asthma symptoms which might be the result of impaired lung growth during infancy, a situation which could be modifiable by breast feeding. A Danish cohort study in which lung function was measured at 6 weeks of age showed that infants in the upper quartile of BMI had lower $FEV_{0.5}$ (Bisgaard et al., 2009). To what extent this circumstance of the early years can be translated to older ages and established asthma is difficult to say, although a connection between obesity and architectural changes in the lung is suggestive, especially if the action of adipokines (which will be reviewed later in this chapter) is taken into account.

Taken together, epidemiological data indicate that body weight and asthma are related in some way, and that excess weight seems to precede asthma or asthma-related symptoms. This fact does not necessarily rule out that the two conditions develop in parallel with the former being apparent before. Furthermore, there are factors which modify the relationship between obesity and asthma. This has been shown in a cross-sectional study (Garcia-Marcos et al., 2008) including a very high number of children: although the association was highly significant for the whole group, it changed dramatically when the group was stratified between those asthmatics also suffering or not from rhinoconjunctivitis. Obesity was not a risk factor for those children with significant asthma who also suffered rhinoconjunctivitis. Although the study has limitations and rhinoconjunctivitis is not a perfect marker of atopy, it raises the question as to whether obesity may be related only to specific asthma phenotypes.

2.1.2 Obesity and asthma develop in parallel, especially in periods of fast growth and maturation

Rather than obesity being the cause of asthma, some findings support the hypothesis of parallel processes which may be related to a change of the environment in which children develop. It is probably when development is more intense (immediately after birth and during puberty) when those processes may be more obvious. Some facts support this view:

- Perinatal events (Jaakkola et al., 2006; Sukalich et al., 2006) or mother food consumption during pregnancy have an influence on later obesity and asthma (Chatzi et al., 2008; Castro-Rodriguez et al., 2010).
- Breast feeding and dietary habits during infancy and later on, are related to obesity and asthma (Matheson et al., 2007); (Moreno & Rodriguez, 2007).
- It is among pre-puberal girls where the association between obesity and asthma is most apparent (Castro-Rodriguez et al., 2001); (Garcia-Marcos et al., 2007), and obesity favours early menarche.
- Epidemiological studies show that females who became overweight or obese between 6 and 11 years of age were seven times more likely to develop new asthma symptoms at age 11 or 13 (Castro-Rodriguez et al., 2001). Moreover, the early onset of puberty has been associated with the persistence of asthma after puberty (Guerra et al., 2004).
- Obesity and asthma are linked conditions during puberty. Although both obesity and asthma can start early in the child life, it is probably around puberty when the connections between those conditions may be better revealed, as some epidemiological studies have shown (Castro-Rodriguez et al., 2001); (Herrera-Trujillo et al., 2005). Some mechanisms might explain this process. For instance, leptin is a key permissive factor (Navarro et al., 2007) -probably through the activation of kisspeptin neurons (Kauffman et al., 2007)- for the onset of puberty. Furthermore, the increase in body weight which occurs during the pubertal spurt induces a corresponding increase of circulating leptin, but also of interleukin (IL)-6 and tumour necrosis factor alpha (TNF-α).
- Several areas in the genome are common to mediators related both to asthma and obesity.

2.1.3 The association between obesity/overweight and bronchial hyperresponsiveness is conflicting

A recent review by Shore (Shore, 2010) lists eight studies dealing with the association of obesity and bronchial hyperresponsiveness (BHR) in adults and a further eight in children. Except for one, all the studies in adults were carried out using metacholine in the challenge test. In children, there were studies using metacholine (n=3), histamine (n=1) and exercise (n=3). The results do not point in the same direction even in the two longitudinal studies (one in adults and one in children). The study in adults reported that high initial BMI was un-linearly associated to later BHR; and weight gain was also associated linearly with the risk of later BHR. On the contrary, the study performed in children (Hancox et al., 2005) did not find any association. Interestingly, however, a high BMI was associated to asthma only in women. This might indicate that the link between obesity and asthma might not necessarily be mediated through airway inflammation revealed by metacholine challenge testing. The cross-sectional studies in children which used metacholine in the challenge test showed all types of results: no association; association only in males; or association only in females. On the contrary, all three cross-sectional studies using exercise as the challenge test found a positive association. The cross-sectional studies in adults (none of them using exercise) also found mixed results, including one study which observed that BMI increased BHR in non-asthmatics but not in asthmatics.

Although a number of factors such as gender, type of challenge test, non-linear association between BMI and BHR (which might counteract the effect of BMI if both low and high BMI are associated to BHR), age groups, asthma control, lack of control for diet, etc. may explain the discrepancy between studies, it seems quite clear that the evidence of an association (if any) between BMI and BHR is not as strong as it is for asthma diagnosis or asthma symptoms. It is interesting that the results are concordant only for the exercise challenge test which does not produce smooth muscle reactivity (as metacholine does) but provokes mast cell activation. It might be hypothesized that obese individuals either create a different osmolality of the airways (the mechanism thought to be responsible for BHR with exercise) while exercising, which in turn causes a higher mast cell activation; or have more mast cells in their airways; or they are more sensitive to osmolality. Although findings in animal models are difficult to translate to humans, it is of great interest that obese mice sensitized and challenged with ovoalbumin have increased numbers of mast cells in their lungs as compared to lean controls (Mito et al., 2002).

2.2 The clinical link

Further evidence that obesity and asthma are related to each other is the fact that BMI predicts asthma control as an independent factor. For instance, in a very recent study, Farah et al. (Farah et al., 2011) reported on asthma control in 49 asthmatic subjects before and after three months of treatment with high doses of inhaled corticosteroids. The effects of treatment were stratified according to BMI (normal, overweight and obese) and the degree of control was assessed by means of the asthma control questionnaire (ACQ-5) although other variables, such as forced expiratory volume during the first second (FEV1), airways resistance (Rrs) and reactance (Xrs) as measured by the forced oscillation technique, BHR to metacholine, and exhaled nitric oxide (FeNO), were also measured before and after treatment. After the treatment period neither FeNO (as a surrogate of bronchial eosinophilic inflammation) nor FEV1 predicted asthma control according to ACQ-5. The two independent predictors of ACQ-5 were Rrs and BMI. The authors conclude that BMI is a factor which determines asthma control and is independent of airway inflammation, lung function and BHR. Furthermore, after ICS treatment, BMI again predicts ACQ-5, and this seems independent of obesity-related changes in lung mechanics.

From a different angle, but adding some evidence to the argument, one study (Maniscalco et al., 2008) has shown that weight loss helps to control asthma in asthmatic individuals. In a series of 12 consecutive asthmatic females who had laparoscopic adjustable gastric banding and consecutively a significant weight loss, asthma control was significantly improved as compared to a control group. Interestingly, no changes in FeNO were found before and after the surgical procedure. Previously, another study showed that a small group of asthmatics (mainly women) significantly improved their asthma control after a very-low-calorie-diet period of 8 weeks (Hakala et al., 2000). In this case, spirometric variables significantly improved leading the authors to think that improvement may be due to better lung mechanics. To the best of our knowledge there are no controlled studies evaluating the effect of weight loss in obese children.

2.3 A genetic link?

There are some regions of the genome that are linked with both asthma and obesity, as occurs with chromosome 5q, 6, 11q13 and 12q (Tantisira & Weiss, 2001). Chromosome 5q contains genes coding the β_2-adrenergic receptor, which has been related to different asthma phenotypes, asthma severity and differential response to β_2-agonists (Hall et al., 1995). A change of Gln for Glu in this receptor has been also associated to obesity (Ishiyama-Shigemoto et al., 1999). Additionally, chromosome 5q contains the glucocorticoid receptor gene which has been involved in inflammatory responses associated to obesity and asthma. Chromosome 6 contains the gene for TNF-α, an interleukin which is important for both obesity and asthma. Another genome region which is linked with asthma and with obesity independently is that of chromosome 11q13 which contains genes for the uncoupling proteins UCP2-UCP3 (related to baseline metabolism) and for the low affinity receptor for IgE. To end, chromosome 12 contains the genes for inflammatory cytokines both related to asthma (such as IFN-γ, or nitric oxide synthase-1) and to obesity (such as signal transducer and activator of transcription protein 6 -STAT6-, or type 1 insulinoid growth factor) (Delgado et al., 2008). To what extent specific but very large areas of the genome are involved in the genesis of the parallel development of asthma and obesity is questionable. How epigenetic changes taking place under certain environments might influence genome areas related to both diseases is even more questionable.

2.4 The inflammation link

The hypothesis that the increase in the prevalence of asthma and obesity, being parallel, could be related to one another (Chinn & Rona, 2001) seems quite plausible. However, a definite link between the two conditions has yet to be definitely established, as it seems to be related to the age and gender of the studied population (Castro-Rodriguez et al., 2001; Chen et al., 2002; Garcia-Marcos et al., 2007), and also to the asthma phenotype (Garcia-Marcos et al., 2008; Gilliland et al., 2003). However, some of the epidemiological and experimental information reviewed in former sections seems to indicate that obesity may precede asthma. To explain this, several inflammatory mechanisms have been evoked:

2.4.1 Adipokines

Adipokines are cytokines produced by the adipose tissue. Some of them are associated both to obesity and to asthma.

2.4.1.1 Leptin

Leptin is mainly produced by white adipose tissue proportionally to the amount of such tissue. Leptin production is regulated by food intake: food consumption up regulates the *ob* gene, thus increasing leptin synthesis; conversely, fasting reduces leptin levels. Infection and sepsis and various pro-inflammatory cytokines including TNF-α and IL-1 increase leptin. Conversely to this acute response, chronic inflammation causes a reduction in leptin levels. Leptin is also moderated by sex hormones: while testosterone inhibits leptin production, ovarian sex steroids increase it, a fact which keeps up with gender-related dimorphism of this adipokine: leptin levels are higher in females than BMI and age-matched males. The main target organ for leptin is the hypothalamus in which it triggers efector pathways to suppress appetite and increase energy expenditure. Apart from the metabolic processes, leptin is also involved in other functions, including the immune response both innate and adaptative: it increases several pro-inflammatory cytokines, such as TNF-α, IL-6 and IL-12, and increases chemotaxis and the functioning of natural killer cells. Overall, leptin increases Th1 and suppresses Th2 response by acting on T regulatory cells (Treg). The leptin receptor gene (*db* gene) is expressed in the lung tissue of several animals and also in humans (Tsuchiya et al., 1999). Although the role of those receptors is not yet clear their presence indicates that the lung is a target organ for leptin. There is also some evidence that leptin can stimulate surfactant protein synthesis (Malli et al., 2010). However, the evidence that leptin influences lung growth and maturation comes from animal models, thus extrapolation to humans remains a major limitation. There also appears to be some role of leptin in respiratory function control, at least in mice (Groeben et al., 2004; Tankersley et al., 1996).

Asthmatic 12-year-old children who are overweight have higher levels of leptin than overweight children who are not asthmatics, despite there being no difference of BMI between the two groups (Mai et al., 2004). This has been also shown in preschool children with normal weight, although reduced to male gender (Guler et al., 2004). Very interestingly, however, is that leptin and BMI are both associated to asthma in adults in an independent way, so when adjusting for leptin levels there is still an association of BMI with asthma (Sood et al., 2006). Furthermore, in asthmatic children leptin and IgE serum levels are highly correlated to each other (Guler et al., 2004). Atopic asthmatic boys have higher leptin levels than non-atopic asthmatic boys. The extent to which leptin has the ability to recruit eosinophils into the lungs and to augment leukotriene synthesis by macrophages may actually be the explanation of its association with atopy still remains controversial (Mancuso et al., 2004; Wong et al., 2007). Further than allergic inflammation as a possible pathway to asthma mediated by leptin, this hormone seems to also have some up-regulatory effect on the sympathetic nervous system, although it does not seem to be important in regulating airway smooth muscle tone (Nair et al., 2008), a fact which might be in connection to the non-consistent findings related to the association between obesity and BHR. However, its is interesting that leptin and leptin receptor are significantly reduced in bronchial epithelial cells in patients with mild asthma which is uncontrolled and in severe treated asthmatics as compared to mild asthmatics under good control, and healthy controls. Additionally, leptin and leptin receptor expression correlated inversely with the thickness of the basement membrane, which is a salient feature of lung remodeling (Bruno et al., 2009).

2.4.1.2 Adiponectin

Adiponectin has an anti-inflammatory role, and decreases with increasing obesity. Contrary to this apparent anti-inflammatory role favoured by obesity, adiponectin is increased in other chronic inflammatory conditions such as rheumatoid arthritis, systemic lupus erythematosus or inflammatory bowel disease. Moreover, elevated levels of adiponectin in cord blood have been associated with an increased risk of asthma in children born from atopic mothers (Rothenbacher et al., 2007). More importantly, adiponectin decreases during puberty only in boys, and remains unchanged in girls (Andersen et al., 2007), a situation that would make gender a modifying factor in the association between obesity and asthma during puberty. Adiponectin and all its currently known receptors are expressed in multiple cell types in the lung (Hug et al., 2004; Miller et al., 2009; Takemura et al., 2007) which makes it a suitable candidate for an additional link between obesity and asthma. In ovoalbumin sensitized mice, administration of exogenous adiponectin protects against cell infiltration and cytokine levels. Serum adiponectin reduces allergic airway inflammation and BHR in mice (Shore et al., 2006). On the other hand and also in mice, adiponectin inhibits the proliferation of vessels associated to smooth muscles although it does not affect muscle itself (Medoff et al., 2009). These findings suggest that adiponectin is involved in allergic inflammation and pulmonary vascular remodeling in a mouse model of chronic asthma.

The number of studies in humans is scarce and the study by Rothenbacher et al. (Rothenbacher et al., 2007) seems to be contradictory to the animal model. Among children with a maternal history of atopy, lower level of adiponectin was associated to lower incidence of asthma or obstructive bronchitis during the first two years of life. Conversely, higher levels of cord serum adiponectin were associated to higher incidence of those respiratory conditions. Among those children without a maternal history of atopy, there was no association of the adipokine and the incidence of asthma or obstructive bronchitis. Other epidemiological studies in humans have rendered inconclusive results. In two cross-sectional studies with a relatively low number of school children, serum adiponectin was not associated to an ever diagnosis of asthma (Nagel et al., 2009) or to current asthma confirmed by metacholine challenge test (Kim et al., 2008). In two very large epidemiological studies in adults, although a clear association between higher BMI and asthma was found in both of them, adiponectin was only inversely associated with current asthma in premenopausal women in one. In a more recent study, 368 adolescent asthmatics were followed for one year: adiponectin was inversely associated to asthma symptoms and exacerbations and positively to FEV1/FVC but only in male subjects (Kattan et al., 2010). FeNO was not associated to serum adiponectin. Conversely, a study in adults did find that adiponectin was associated to lower values of FeNO in men but not in women. No further association of the adipokine and different asthma markers was found in any gender. (Sutherland et al., 2009).

2.4.1.3 Resistin

Resistin is also known as adipocyte-secreted factor or "found in inflammatory zone 3" (FIZZ3). It has recently been discovered and has been proposed as a link between obesity and diabetes. In contrast to mice, resistin is expressed in human adipocytes in low amounts; in fact it is in bone marrow where this adipokine is most expressed in humans (Filkova et al., 2009). Resistin has recently been shown to initiate a pro-inflammmatory state "in vitro" and "in vivo". Pro-inflammatory mediators such as TNF-α, IL-1β or IL-6 can strongly increase the expression of resistin in peripheral mononuclear cells. As stated above, resistin is minimally expressed in human adipose tissue, but adipocytes may be targets for it. Nagaev et al. have demonstrated that resistin, similarly to its action on peripheral blood mononuclear cells, can induce adipocytes to express IL-6 and TNF-α (Nagaev et al., 2006).

Resistin has been shown to be increased in the murine models of genetic as well as in diet-induced obesity. This has also been shown in humans. In an asthma cohort study on adult asthma, levels of resistin were higher in asthmatic patients as compared to controls, and resistin levels increased with increased severity of the disease (Larochelle et al., 2007). Conversely, atopic asthmatic children have lower resistin levels as compared to the non-atopic asthma and control groups (Kim et al., 2008). However, in a recent study (Arshi et al., 2010) in children of a similar age to those in the previous study (11 years) resistin levels were not different between a group of atopic asthmatics and a control group. In fact, its levels in the former study were about double than in the latter both in the control and in the atopic asthmatic groups. More recently, a study has shown that in a group of non-obese corticosteroid naïve adult female recently diagnosed asthmatics resistin predicted favourable anti-inflammatory effects of inhaled corticosteroids as assessed by levels of eosinophil cationic protein, eosinophil protein X and myeloperoxidase. Furthermore, an "in vitro" assay found that fluticasone significantly reduced resistin-induced IL-6 and TNF-α production in cultured monocytes/macrophages (Leivo-Korpela et al., 2011).

2.4.1.4 Adipsin

This adipokine is the rate-limiting enzyme in the alternate pathway of complement activation and is primarily expressed by adipocytes and monocytes/macrophages in humans. Adipsin has however been barely studied in asthma or allergic diseases. In a group of non-obese corticosteroid naïve adult female recently diagnosed asthmatics and with a positive bronchodilator tests, levels of adipsin were similar to the control group (Leivo-Korpela et al., 2011); however this adipokine has been reported to be significantly increased in individuals with seasonal allergic rhinitis, but only in males. Sublingual immunotherapy did not seem to affect adipsin levels (Ciprandi et al., 2009). Information regarding whether adipsin might have a role in asthma (if any) is still very scarce and we will have to wait until new studies publish their results.

2.4.1.5 Visfatin

Visfatin is identical to pre-B cell colony enhancing factor, a cytokine which is increased in the bronchoalveolar lavage fluid in animal models of acute lung injury and in neutrophils of septic patients. Exercise training with weight loss induced a significant reduction of plasma visfatin in non-diabetic women (Choi et al., 2007). Although this protein represents an additional link between obesity and inflammation, its role in asthma (if any) is still to be elucidated.

2.4.2 Immunologic properties of adipose tissue

The view of adipose tissue as a sole storage system has radically changed in the last decade. Further than being able to synthesize adipokines, adipocytes share some similarities with macrophages. In fact, preadipocytes can differentiate into macrophages, but the two cell types are distinct. On the other hand, about 10% of cells in the adipose tissue are macrophages. The number of macrophages in the adipose tissue is directly related to adiposity and to the size of adipocytes both in humans and in mice (Curat et al., 2004). Apart from secreting adipokines, adipocytes also secrete chemokines and cytokines, such as TNF-α, IL-6, Il-10, IL-1β and other factors such as monocyte chemoattractant protein-1 (MCP-1). It is thought that those mediators are secreted by the adipocyte itself since when adipose tissue is increased there is an up-regulation of genes related to inflammation. Indeed macrophages of the adipose tissue are an additional source of inflammatory mediators.

- TNF-α is the most important of cytokines produced by adipose tissue. It increases formation of Th2 cytokines such as IL-4 and Il-5, IL-6 and Il-1β by the bronchial epithelial cells. On the other hand, TNF-α increases the expression of leptin and adiponectin in cultured adipocytes (Kirchgessner et al., 1997). TNF-α is an important cytokine in the innate immune response and has been involved in the pathophysiology of several chronic inflammation diseases, including asthma (Thomas et al., 1995; Thomas & Heywood, 2002). This cytokine has an array of effects on the immunological system which have direct implications for the asthmatic response, such as recruitment of neutrophils, macrophages and mast cells; recruitment and activation of eosinophils; up-regulation of adhesion molecules both in the respiratory epithelium and on the vascular endothelium, which in turn can further increase inflammatory cell recruitment; proliferation and differentiation of fibroblasts (related to asthma remodeling and potentially to a more severe type of asthma); activation and increased release of cytokines by T cells of the Th2 arm; and induction of corticoisteroid resistance (Brightling et al., 2008).

- IL-6 is a proinflammatory cytokine which has a central role in host defence against infection and tissue injury. This interleukin derived from antigen presenting cells can induce production of IL-4 in naïve CD4+ cells, thus polarizing them into Th2 cells; i.e. to the allergic type of inflammation. This interleukin also modulates the intensity of the immune response by inhibiting Treg cell development. Additionally IL-6 promotes generation of Th17 cells (cells involved in autoimmune diseases) in mice, though its ability to do so in humans is subject to debate (Wilson et al., 2007). It has been recently shown that IL-6 levels are elevated in sputum of asthmatic patients as compared to healthy volunteers (Neveu et al., 2010).
- IL-10 is a cytokine with important regulatory function, having multiple biological effects in different cell-types. IL-10 modulates allergic disease in humans: the expression of IL-10 by antigen presenting cells in the airway of healthy subjects is important for inducing and maintaining tolerance to allergens (Commins et al., 2008).
- IL-1β is a potent mediator in response to infection and injury, and is increased in asthmatic airways as it is in other chronic inflammatory diseases. Apart from its pro-inflammatory effects, IL-1β has been shown to induce migration of vascular smooth muscle cells in culture and to provoke migration of endothelial cells. Its potential effects on the airway epithelial cell have been recently shown in cell cultures (White et al., 2008).

It should not be forgotten that apart from adipocytes, adipose tissue contains a considerable number of macrophages. Those cells are located in the white adipose tissue, which –as compared to brown adipose tissue which has as main role non-shivering thermogenesis- is the majority of adipose tissue and serves as energy storage. The number of macrophages in this tissue is proportional to adiposity and adipocyte size, both in mice and humans, and no difference exists between visceral and subcutaneous white fat (Weisberg et al., 2003).

2.4.3 Other endogenous molecules relating obesity with asthma

There are other hormones which may be related to obesity and asthma since they can be associated with processes related to food intake/body weight and inflammation.

2.4.3.1 Alpha-melanocyte stimulating hormone

Alpha-melanocyte stimulating hormone (α-MSH) belongs to a group of hormones called melanocortins, which include ACTH among others, with a common precursor (proopiomelanocortin). This hormone produces a significant down-regulation of pro-inflammatory cytokines such as IL-1β, IL-6 and TNF-α, as well as chemokines such as IL-8 and interferon gamma (IFN-γ). Furthermore, chemotaxis induced by IL-8 in human neutrophils and monocytes is blunted by α-MSH. Additionally, this hormone has been shown to induce IL-10 production (Brzoska et al., 2010). In a murine model, α-MSH was able to inhibit airway inflammation induced by aerosol sensitization and subsequent challenges with OVA. Additionally, the levels of two important interleukins related to the allergic response, IL-4 and IL-13, were highly decreased in the broncho-alveolar lavage fluid of mice treated with α-MSH. In agreement with the important role of IL-10 as an anti-inflammatory mediator, the action of α-MSH was dependent on the presence of IL-10, as IL-10 knock-out mice were resistant to treatment with α-MSH (Raap et al., 2003). In the context of an association between asthma and obesity, what is on interest of α-MSH is the fact that the hormone is included in one of the main mechanisms of energy balance. There are melanocortin receptors in the CNS and effects on food intake and on energy expenditure have been observed with treatments containing ligands of those receptors (Williams et al., 2000). Those receptors are hypothesized to be downstream mediators of the effects of leptin signaling: leptin increases the expression of the proopiomelanocortin gene in neurons of the nucleus tractus solitarius (Schwartz et al., 1997). Thus, α-MSH may play a role both in allergic inflammation and in food-intake control. In fact, the melanocortin system appears to be a common pathway for mediation of both leptin and ghrelin (Lebrethon et al., 2007).

2.4.3.2 Ghrelin

Ghrelin is not only a mere growth-hormone releasing factor but also an important appetite regulator, energy conservator and suppressor of the sympathetic nervous system. Ghrelin, secreted from the peripheral organ, has its regulatory region in the hypothalamic arcuate nucleus, where the regulatory region of appetite is located. Circulating ghrelin excites this region and stimulates food intake after passing through the blood-brain barrier. Additionally, this hormone can exert its action through receptors in the vagus nerve (Kojima & Kangawa, 2010). Apart from being an orexigenic hormone, ghrelin has an interesting association with IgE in humans. In a case-control study of obese school children, Matsuda et al. (Matsuda et al., 2006) found that ghrelin was inversely and significantly correlated with BMI but also with IgE both in allergic and non-allergic subjects as defined from a combination of asthma and skin symptoms. This correlation with IgE is higher among overweight patients as compared to normal weight ones, in which the correlation is still significant (Okamatsu et al., 2009). The strong inverse correlation between plasma ghrelin and serum IgE levels suggests that ghrelin may inhibit IgE production in some manner. In this context, it is of interest that in splenic murine T lymphocytes, mRNA levels of IL-4 and IL-10, which both increase IgE synthesis, are suppressed by ghrelin (Xia et al., 2004).

2.4.3.3 Eotaxin

Eotaxin is a key chemotactic agent responsible for the eosinophil-mediated bronchial inflammation. In their pivotal study, Vasudevan et al. (Vasudevan et al., 2006) showed that eotaxin circulating levels are increased in diet-induced obese mice. They also showed that after weight loss in humans eotaxin was significantly reduced. In a group of obese and non-obese Korean women it was shown that circulating eotaxin was similar in both groups, although women with central obesity had significantly higher levels of eotaxin than those without it. This study also showed that weight reduction after following an exercise program for 12 weeks was associated to a significant decrease in circulating eotaxin levels in the whole group (Choi et al., 2007).
Not only has eotaxin been studied in relation to obesity but also as to how this chemokine interacts with allergy inflammation in the context of obesity. In a murine allergy model (Calixto et al., 2010), diet-induced obesity enhanced eosinophil trafficking from bone marrow to lung tissues, and delayed their transit through the airway epithelium into the airway lumen. Consequently, eosinophils remain longer in lung peribronchiolar segments. Furthermore, Kim et al. (Kim et al., 2011) cultivated and differentiated pre-adypocites and investigated eotaxin expression during differentiation and found that levels of this chemokine increased as adipocytes differentiated. Eotaxin was further expressed when cultured cells were challenged with TNF-α and IL-4.

2.4.3.4 Plasminogen activator inhibitor 1

Remodeling of the airway is a key feature of asthma and is associated to a more severe type of disease. Plasminogen activator inhibitor 1 (PAI-1) is a potent inhibitor of both tissue-type plasminogen activator (t-PA) and urokinase-type plasminogen activator (u-PA). Both t-PA and u-PA are involved in the dissolution of fibrin and in the degradation of the extracellular matrix. Activated mast cells are a major source of PAI-1, and mast cell-derived PAI-1 is highly expressed in patients with fatal asthma (Cho et al., 2000). Furthermore, a gene polymorphism associated with PAI-1 levels is preferably transmitted to asthmatic patients; and deletion of PAI-1 prevents extracellular matrix deposition in a murine model of asthma (Cho et al., 2001); (Oh et al., 2002). In a very recent study (Cho et al., 2011), it was found that plasma levels of PAI-1 were significantly higher in obese subjects as compared to controls after adjusting for race and smoking status; furthermore, PAI-1 plasma levels were significantly and inversely correlated to forced vital capacity. Thus, it could be hypothesized that the reduction of FVC in obese patients may be in part mediated by PAI-1. Although research on the association of PAI-1 as a link between obesity and asthma is still very scarce, this is a field which warrants further investigation.

2.5 The mechanical link

The mechanical load of obesity might affect lung growth, leading to reduced pulmonary function. For instance, leptin-deficient mice which are obese very early in their development have substantially smaller lungs than normal ones (Shore et al., 2003). Maternal obesity in pregnancy increases the risk of pregnancy complications, caesarean sections and adverse birth outcomes, which have in turn been associated with respiratory illness in children. However, little is known of the effect of obesity in the mother during pregnancy with regard to respiratory diseases in the offspring. A recent Norwegian study (Haberg et al., 2009) (Norwegian and Child Study) which includes 100,000 pregnant mothers was able to analyse data from more than 33,000 mother-children pairs up to the age of 18 months of the infants and demonstrated that after adjustment for many factors including birth weight, preterm birth and pregnancy complications, infants born from obese mothers had a modest but significant increased risk (3.3%) of suffering from at least one episode of wheezing during the follow-up period. To what extent this finding is related to the low-grade inflammation status of mothers during pregnancy or to mechanical factors "in utero" and how they might affect lung development in the foetus is still to be determined. Furthermore, it is not known if this effect is maintained in later years.

Independently of its effects on lung development either in the fetal period or later on, obese subjects have a low functional residual capacity due to changes in the elastic properties of the chest wall (Shore & Johnston, 2006). At low volumes, the retractile forces of the lung parenchyma are reduced, thus airway smooth muscle has a lower load when functional residual capacity is reduced. Consequently it might shorten still further when activated (either by parasympathetic tone or broncho-constricting agents such as metacholine) (Naimark & Cherniack, 1960). However, some studies have noted that there is bronchial constriction in obese subjects after correcting for lung volume, which suggests that other mechanisms are involved. Apparently low tidal volume (which is common in obese individuals) may be one such mechanism: stretching of the airways smooth muscles causes cross-bridging of actin-myosin to detach, and the bigger the tidal volume (stretch) the easier it is for bronchodilation to occur. Low tidal volume facilitates more cross-bridging between actin and myosin, thus making airway smooth muscle stiffer and harder to stretch. Hence reduction of tidal volume in obese subjects could lead to a vicious circle in which small airway muscle strain leads to greater stiffness, and this leads to even less muscle strain in every breath (Shore, 2008). This paradigm is supported by the fact that both obese and asthmatic subjects have lower bronchodilation after deep breaths (Hakala et al., 1995; Skloot & Togias, 2003).

There could be additional mechanical explanations as to the reasons why airways in obese subjects are more easily constricted than in normal ones. Closure of small peripheral airways is common in obese individuals, especially in the supine posture (Hakala et al., 1995). Some authors have postulated that the frequent opening and closure of those airways may lead to the rupture of alveolar attachment to bronchioles, thus disconnecting airways from the attached parenchyma and exacerbating constriction (Milic-Emili et al., 2007). To what extent those less oxygenated areas could lead to higher artery pressures and pulmonary edema, further complicating the situation, is still very speculative although there is some evidence of edema in obese subjects and pulmonary hypertension in obese women (Bergeron et al., 2005); (Taraseviciute & Voelkel, 2006). Hypoxemia might exacerbate local hypoxia occurring in obese adipose tissue, a situation which contributes to the general inflammation of obesity (Hosogai et al., 2007; Ye et al., 2007). Situations related to obesity such as obesity hypoventilation syndrome or sleep disordered breathing could further aggravate this situation and although extreme and far from asthma, could add some clues to the mechanical associations between asthma and obesity.

2.6 The experimental link (animal models)

Three are several models in which the lung features of obese mice have been characterized. According to Shore (Shore, 2007), those are:

- *ob/ob* Mice: This is a type of mice which is not capable of synthesizing leptin, which is a satiety hormone formed in the adipose tissue. These mice eat in excess and are already obese at four weeks of age. These mice have smaller lungs than the wild type.
- *db/db* Mice: In this type of mice there is an altered leptin receptor in the hypothalamus ($Ob\text{-}R_b$) so the effect of leptin on satiety is lost. Thus, *db/db* mice are similar to *ob/ob* mice. As in the case of *ob/ob* mice, *db/db* mice have smaller lungs than the wild type.
- *Cpe^fat^* Mice: These mice have a missense mutation of the enzyme carboxipeptidase E (Cpe) which makes it inactive. Cpe cleaves neuropeptides such as corticotrophin-releasing factor and neuropeptide Y which control eating behaviours and energy consumption. In the absence of Cpe mice become obese but not as fast as *ob/ob* or *db/db* mice. These mice have lung size comparable to that of the wild type.
- Diet-induced obese mice: feeding recently weaned mice with a diet in which 45-60% of calories are derived from fat produces obesity. Obesity is milder than in the three prior models and lung size is again similar to that of the wild type.

Taken together, the results from the studies from animal models in obese mice suggest that obesity might be related to asthma in several ways. In the first place very early obese mice have smaller lungs and this might have implications both at the mechanical and at the ultra-structural level, in particular in the way lungs are alveolarized. Secondly, obesity either acquired very early or later on in the mice's lives increases BHR and this neither seems to be directly mediated by leptin nor is secondary to a prior inflammation. Lastly, obesity might have some effect on asthma through allergic sensitization as that hormone seems to increase sensitization, and thus BHR to allergen challenge (Shore et al., 2005), this being dependent on when obesity and sensitization develop.

2.7 A distinct asthma phenotype in the obese?

There seems to be enough epidemiological, clinical and mechanistic evidence that obesity and asthma "live" together in some individuals. Whether this comorbidity is a distinct phenotype as suggested by some authors; or obesity is a risk factor for asthma incidence and worse control, is difficult to say (Castro-Rodriguez & Garcia-Marcos, 2008; Lessard et al., 2008; Lugogo et al., 2010). However, both the mechanical, hormonal and immunological links between the two conditions suggest that obesity probably leads to asthma in many cases and could be in part responsible for the "asthma epidemic". Moreover, there are two other important factors -diet and exercise- which can favour both asthma and obesity in parallel. An official American Thoracic Society workshop report recently published concludes that obesity is a risk factor for asthma in all age groups and that asthma in the obese might represent a distinct phenotype with a more severe disease with a worse response to treatment (Dixon et al., 2010). The report states the urgent need to further investigate the mechanisms of asthma in this risk group and to develop new therapies directed to this specific population.

3. Diet as an independent factor in the development of asthma and obesity

Diet and exercise are probable common pathways for asthma and obesity irrespective of which of the two conditions starts first. This is quite well documented during the first months after birth. Infants who are breastfed have a different bacterial colonization of their intestine than those who are fed with artificial formulas (Harmsen et al., 2000). Similarly, children fed with the latter formulas gain weight more rapidly, although this does not seem to be translated into later obesity (Burdette et al., 2006). Although the information is still sparse, it is quite probable that the so-called microflora fingerprinting -which remains very stable throughout the years- is related to diet. Either by this mechanism which might be included into de hygiene hypothesis or by others, such as the antioxidant or pro-oxidant properties of some foods (Roberts et al., 2006), or the modulating properties of prebiotics -like fibers- to adjust intestinal microflora (Schley & Field, 2002), may have an effect on asthma and obesity.

There are currently enough studies to conclude that there is an association between consumption of some types of nutrients or foods and asthma. An ecological analysis of the European Community Respiratory Health Survey (ECRHS) showed a trend towards decreasing sensitization (specific IgE) prevalence with higher intakes of fruit and vitamins A and C (Farchi et al., 2003). Furthermore, other studies have found an association between consuming citrus/kiwi fruit and a lower last year prevalence of several asthma symptoms (Forastiere et al., 2000; Wickens et al., 2005); and also of rhinitis. The frequent intake of vegetables showed an inverse relationship with prevalence rates of asthma, allergic rhinoconjunctivitis and atopic eczema (Weiland et al., 1999). The intake of cereals has also been shown to be associated to a lower prevalence of asthma (Garcia-Marcos et al., 2007; To et al., 2004). A recent meta-analysis on food intake and asthma arrived at interesting conclusions (Nurmatov et al., 2011) in spite of the limitations of applying the meta-analysis technique to epidemiological studies which cannot be -by definition- perfectly controlled. With respect to individual nutrients, vitamins A, D, E and zinc seem to be protective, while vitamin C and selenium do seem to be neither a protective nor a risk factor. Higher consumption of fruit and vegetables are associated to a lower prevalence of asthma, with fruit having a higher impact. However the associations were not adjusted for obesity or exercise.

Two different groups, including ours, have very recently associated Mediterranean diet to a lower prevalence of asthma at different ages (Castro-Rodriguez et al., 2008; Chatzi et al., 2007; Garcia-Marcos et al., 2007) independently of exercise. Furthermore, Mediterranean diet also showed this protective effect in the offspring when the mother consumed it during pregnancy (Chatzi et al., 2008), although the effect might be restricted just to olive oil intake (Castro-Rodriguez et al., 2010). The reasons why this type of diet is associated with a lower prevalence of asthma could be explained in several ways. Considering that Mediterranean diet is rich in both antioxidants and *cis* monounsaturated fatty acids this is not an unexpected finding. Individually, a more frequent intake of seafood and also of cereals is associated with a lower prevalence of significant asthma. At 8-10 years of age atopy is a risk factor for a more severe asthma (Ponsonby et al., 2002), so it could be speculated that at least in part the protection offered by this diet is mediated through allergy modulation. The protection from asthma that Mediterranean diet seems to offer is probably due to a mixed effect of taking "protective" foods and avoiding "risky" foods. Protective foods may be those with antioxidant properties and rich in prebiotics, such as fibers (as in the Mediterranean diet); and risky foods may be those rich in *trans* fatty acids and unsaturated fat (as in fast foods) (Garcia-Marcos et al., 2007; Innis & King, 1999; von Kries et al., 2001). In fact, Mediterranean diet has been shown to increase the total antioxidant capacity in healthy adults (Pitsavos et al., 2005). Mediterranean diet has additionally been associated to a reduced prevalence of obesity. Due to its content in fibre and unsaturated fat (olive oil, fish) this diet is associated to better weight control (Schroder, 2007). On the contrary, fast food is related to an increase of calorie intake (Schmidt et al., 2005) and is greatly related to the school and family environment, especially during the transition to adulthood (Nelson et al., 2006)

3.1 Oxidant-antioxidant imbalance in asthma

Reactive oxygen species (ROS), formed in every cell during metabolic processes, are increased in asthma and can mediate pathophysiologic changes which are characteristic of this condition, such as initiating lipid peroxidation and favouring the release of arachidonic acid from cell membranes; contracting smooth muscle; increasing airway reactivity and vascular permeability; augmenting the synthesis and release of cytokines and chemokines; impairing the response to β_2 adrenergic drugs; and decreasing cholinesterase and neutral endopeptidase activities (Nadeem et al., 2008). Lungs have several antioxidant mechanisms including enzymatic (catalase, glutathione peroxidase ans superoxide dismutase) and non-enzymatic ones (vitamin C, E, albumin, uric acid, cerulopasmin and glutathione). Increased ROS generation is found when the activity of neutrophils, eosinophils, monocytes and macrophages is increased, as occurs in asthma (Kelly et al., 1988). Oxidative stress (a situation of imbalance between the production of ROS and the ability to detoxify the reactive intermediates or to repair the resulting damage) is an important consequence of asthma inflammation; is associated with an altered activity in anti-oxidation in lungs and blood; and also with airway reactivity (Katsumata et al., 1990; Nadeem et al., 2005; Sackesen et al., 2008).

There are numerous reports showing deficiencies of antioxidants in asthma: low levels of vitamin C in airway lining fluid, serum, plasma, whole blood and brochoalveolar lavage fluid; vitamin E in brochio-alveolar lavage fluid, red cells and plasma; or beta-carotene in serum (Kalayci et al., 2000; Kelly et al., 1999; Sackesen et al., 2008; Shanmugasundaram et al., 2001; Vural & Uzun, 2000; Wood et al., 2008). The cooperation of several antioxidants provides a better defense against ROS, so the total antioxidant capacity of serum is probably a better index than the measurement of a specific antioxidant. Again, antioxidant capacity in serum is reduced in asthmatics during exacerbations as compared with healthy individuals and is less reduced in subjects with stable asthma (Katsoulis et al., 2003). Very recently, oxidative stress has been shown to be increased in children with previous bronchilitis obliterans (Mallol et al., 2011) and although in this study the authors did not find correlation with lung function tests, several studies have indeed shown an inverse relationship between oxidative stress and lung function in asthmatics (Nadeem et al., 2005; Ochs-Balcom et al., 2006; Picado et al., 2001; Wood et al., 2000).

Taken together these results indicate that an oxidant-antioxidant imbalance could play a crucial role in the development of asthma symptoms and in the severity of the disease. Accordingly, certain diets may favor or protect from asthma depending upon their ability to maintain a better oxidant-antioxidant balance.

4. Exercise is an independent protective factor for asthma and obesity

Although it would be expected that asthmatics perform less exercise and severe asthmatic perform even less, it is not so straightforward that the lack of exercise favours obesity, which in turn favours asthma. Although this causal pathway may be present in some asthmatics, more exercise –independently of BMI- has been associated to a lower prevalence of mild asthma, although it does not influence severe asthma. If the association of asthma with exercise was a reverse causation effect it should be expected that at least in severe asthmatics, there was an inverse association, which does not seem the case when diet and BMI are controlled: in their study Garcia-Marcos et al. showed that after adjusting for BMI and Mediterranean diet exercise was not associated with severe asthma; and mild asthma was less prevalent among children who exercise more (Garcia-Marcos et al., 2007). Therefore, it might be hypothesized that at least in mild cases, the lack of exercise is associated to asthma. In this context, a very interesting and challenging hypothesis was proposed by Alexander in 2005 who maintains that the increase of asthma prevalence might be due in part to a "disuse contracture" which reminds of the mechanical link between obesity and asthma (Alexander, 2005). The following paragraphs are a brief explanation of that hypothesis.

Bronchial constriction and BHR are crucial features of asthma and are both driven by bronchial smooth muscle. When lumen is narrower than normal in a permanent way, there is also a reduction in the length of the annular components of the bronchii, namely smooth muscle fibres and collagen. Under-extension causes contracture: elastic components (smooth muscle and collagen) need a certain tension to operate correctly and when this is not provided by intermittent stretching they either fail to extend during growth (infants and schoolchildren) or reduce in length (adults) to a point in which habitual usage is enough to provoke a peak tension needed for effective functioning. This situation maybe reversible in its first stages but becomes permanent with time due to fixed cross-linking (Akeson et al., 1977). While this is typical of the joint tissues, it is most probably applicable to muscles and elastic tissues of the airways, which in continued growing (as in infancy and childhood) without stretching to their potential length the result would result in an increased thickness of the wall and narrowing of the lumen, which, in turn, will start a vicious cycle: thicker wall, less ability to stretch and more difficult distension to inspiration, less distension, less lumen and thicker wall again. If lumen is reduced to a critical point and according to Laplace's law, the product of atmospheric pressure times radius will not be able to counteract wall tension and bronchii would collapse. In this situation a very small increase of muscle tone will be enough to cause bronchial closure. Moreover, exercise increases respiratory rate and speed of airflow, thus reducing transmural pressure and further favouring collapse.

In summary, this hypothesis contemplates asthma as a lack of lung expansion by exercise during growth. While just a hypothesis, the idea of a lack of "sufficient" inspiration has been contemplated as a feasible explanation for the influence in asthma prevalence of TV watching. The ALSPAC study, after following a large sample of more than 5,000 children, found that new asthma cases, as diagnosed by a doctor, between the ages of 3.5 and 11.5 years were associated to the number of hours of TV watching after controlling for other risk factors including BMI: those watching more than 2h/day had double odds of having new onset asthma a compared to those watching 1-2h/day, while those watching less than 1h/day had just half the odds (Sherriff et al., 2009). While previous studies showed that new cases of asthma during adolescence are associated to lower fitness (Rasmussen et al., 2000; Vogelberg et al., 2007), sometimes confused by smoking, children in the ALSPAC study were too young to consider smoking-related TV watching as a plausible explanation. Sedentary lifestyle ("disuse contracture") is a more plausible explanation. Additionally, the ALSPAC group suggested as an additional explanation of their results that respiratory patterns associated to TV watching may also play a role: prolonged periods of watching a videotape are associated with lower sigh rates than while reading (Hark et al., 2005). Thus, "modern" as opposed to "classical" sedentary lifestyle maybe and additional factor favouring the "disuse contracture".

5. Conclusion

Obesity and asthma are linked together, a link which has been shown at different levels and has plausible pathways. However, it is still to be established if obesity causes asthma (or a specific asthma phenotype) or if the two conditions are part of a parallel development in the context of the western lifestyle in which sedentary habits and unhealthy diets (together with lower contact with germs and/or with "non-traditional" germs) may interact to favour an internal environment in which not only obesity and asthma, but other diseases such as type II diabetes or rheumatoid arthritis develop more easily.

The epidemiological and animal studies carried out to date have probably rendered all possible information and it is the time of more controlled trials. New pregnancy/birth cohort studies specifically designed to disentangle the interrelationship between asthma, obesity, exercise and diet are needed. Creative clinical trials will also have an important role here, although designing and performing them is a great challenge. The implications of the results of such studies on public health policies are crucial.

6. References

Akeson WH, Amiel D, Mechanic GL, Woo SL, Harwood FL, Hamer ML. (1977) Collagen cross-linking alterations in joint contractures: changes in the reducible cross-links in periarticular connective tissue collagen after nine weeks of immobilization, *Connect Tissue Res* 5(1): 15-19

Alexander CJ. (2005) Asthma: a disuse contracture?, *Med Hypotheses* 64(6): 1102-1104

Andersen KK, Frystyk J, Wolthers OD, Heuck C, Flyvbjerg A. (2007) Gender differences of oligomers and total adiponectin during puberty: a cross-sectional study of 859 Danish school children, *J Clin Endocrinol Metab* 92(5): 1857-1862

Arshi M, Cardinal J, Hill RJ, Davies PS, Wainwright C. (2010) Asthma and insulin resistance in children, *Respirology* 15(5): 779-784

Asher MI, Montefort S, Bjorksten B, Lai CK, Strachan DP, Weiland SK, Williams H. (2006) Worldwide time trends in the prevalence of symptoms of asthma, allergic rhinoconjunctivitis, and eczema in childhood: ISAAC Phases One and Three repeat multicountry cross-sectional surveys, *Lancet* 368(9537): 733-743

Bergeron C, Boulet LP, Hamid Q. (2005) Obesity, allergy and immunology, *J Allergy Clin Immunol* 115(5): 1102-1104

Beuther DA, Sutherland ER. (2007) Overweight, obesity, and incident asthma: a meta-analysis of prospective epidemiologic studies, *Am J Respir Crit Care Med* 175(7): 661-666

Bisgaard H, Loland L, Holst KK, Pipper CB. (2009) Prenatal determinants of neonatal lung function in high-risk newborns, *J Allergy Clin Immunol* 123(3): 651-657

Brightling C, Berry M, Amrani Y. (2008) Targeting TNF-alpha: a novel therapeutic approach for asthma, *J Allergy Clin Immunol* 121(1): 5-10

Bruno A, Pace E, Chanez P, Gras D, Vachier I, Chiappara G, La Guardia M, Gerbino S, Profita M, Gjomarkaj M. (2009) Leptin and leptin receptor expression in asthma, *J Allergy Clin Immunol* 124(2): 230-7, 237

Burdette HL, Whitaker RC, Hall WC, Daniels SR. (2006) Breastfeeding, introduction of complementary foods, and adiposity at 5 y of age, *Am J Clin Nutr* 83(3): 550-558

Burgess JA, Walters EH, Byrnes GB, Giles GG, Jenkins MA, Abramson MJ, Hopper JL, Dharmage SC. (2007) Childhood adiposity predicts adult-onset current asthma in females: a 25-yr prospective study, *Eur Respir J* 29(4): 668-675

Calixto MC, Lintomen L, Schenka A, Saad MJ, Zanesco A, Antunes E. (2010) Obesity enhances eosinophilic inflammation in a murine model of allergic asthma, *Br J Pharmacol* 159(3): 617-625

Castro-Rodriguez JA, Garcia-Marcos L. (2008) Wheezing and Asthma in childhood: an epidemiology approach, *Allergol Immunopathol (Madr)* 36(5): 280-290

Castro-Rodriguez JA, Garcia-Marcos L, Alfonseda Rojas JD, Valverde-Molina J, Sanchez-Solis M. (2008) Mediterranean diet as a protective factor for wheezing in preschool children, *J Pediatr* 152(6): 823-8, 828

Castro-Rodriguez JA, Garcia-Marcos L, Sanchez-Solis M, Perez-Fernandez V, Martinez-Torres A, Mallol J. (2010) Olive oil during pregnancy is associated with reduced wheezing during the first year of life of the offspring, *Pediatr Pulmonol* 45(4): 395-402

Castro-Rodriguez JA, Holberg CJ, Morgan WJ, Wright AL, Martinez FD. (2001) Increased incidence of asthmalike symptoms in girls who become overweight or obese during the school years, *Am J Respir Crit Care Med* 163(6): 1344-1349

Chatzi L, Apostolaki G, Bibakis I, Skypala I, Bibaki-Liakou V, Tzanakis N, Kogevinas M, Cullinan P. (2007) Protective effect of fruits, vegetables and the Mediterranean diet on asthma and allergies among children in Crete, *Thorax* 62(8): 677-683

Chatzi L, Torrent M, Romieu I, Garcia-Esteban R, Ferrer C, Vioque J, Kogevinas M, Sunyer J. (2008) Mediterranean diet in pregnancy is protective for wheeze and atopy in childhood, *Thorax* 63(6): 507-513

Chen Y, Dales R, Tang M, Krewski D. (2002) Obesity may increase the incidence of asthma in women but not in men: longitudinal observations from the Canadian National Population Health Surveys, *Am J Epidemiol* 155(3): 191-197

Chinn S, Rona RJ. (2001) Can the increase in body mass index explain the rising trend in asthma in children?, *Thorax* 56(11): 845-850

Cho S, Kang J, Lyttle C, Harris K, Daley B, Grammer L, Avila P, Kumar R, Schleimer R. (2011) Association of elevated plasminogen activator inhibitor 1 levels with diminished lung function in patients with asthma, *Ann Allergy Asthma Immunol* 106(5): 371-377

Cho SH, Hall IP, Wheatley A, Dewar J, Abraha D, Del Mundo J, Lee H, Oh CK. (2001) Possible role of the 4G/5G polymorphism of the plasminogen activator inhibitor 1 gene in the development of asthma, *J Allergy Clin Immunol* 108(2): 212-214

Cho SH, Tam SW, Demissie-Sanders S, Filler SA, Oh CK. (2000) Production of plasminogen activator inhibitor-1 by human mast cells and its possible role in asthma, *J Immunol* 165(6): 3154-3161

Choi KM, Kim JH, Cho GJ, Baik SH, Park HS, Kim SM. (2007) Effect of exercise training on plasma visfatin and eotaxin levels, *Eur J Endocrinol* 157(4): 437-442

Ciprandi G, De Amici M, Marseglia G. (2009) Serum adipsin levels in patients with seasonal allergic rhinitis: preliminary data, *Int Immunopharmacol* 9(12): 1460-1463

Commins S, Steinke JW, Borish L. (2008) The extended IL-10 superfamily: IL-10, IL-19, IL-20, IL-22, IL-24, IL-26, IL-28, and IL-29, *J Allergy Clin Immunol* 121(5): 1108-1111

Curat CA, Miranville A, Sengenes C, Diehl M, Tonus C, Busse R, Bouloumie A. (2004) From blood monocytes to adipose tissue-resident macrophages: induction of diapedesis by human mature adipocytes, *Diabetes* 53(5): 1285-1292

Delgado J, Barranco P, Quirce S. (2008) Obesity and asthma, *J Investig Allergol Clin Immunol* 18(6): 420-425

Dixon AE, Holguin F, Sood A, Salome CM, Pratley RE, Beuther DA, Celedon JC, Shore SA. (2010) An official American Thoracic Society Workshop report: obesity and asthma, *Proc Am Thorac Soc* 7(5): 325-335

Farah CS, Kermode JA, Downie SR, Brown NJ, Hardaker KM, Berend N, King GG, Salome CM. (2011) Obesity is a determinant of asthma control, independent of inflammation and lung mechanics, *Chest*

Farchi S, Forastiere F, Agabiti N, Corbo G, Pistelli R, Fortes C, Dell'Orco V, Perucci CA. (2003) Dietary factors associated with wheezing and allergic rhinitis in children, *Eur Respir J* 22(5): 772-780

Filkova M, Haluzik M, Gay S, Senolt L. (2009) The role of resistin as a regulator of inflammation: Implications for various human pathologies, *Clin Immunol* 133(2): 157-170

Forastiere F, Pistelli R, Sestini P, Fortes C, Renzoni E, Rusconi F, Dell'Orco V, Ciccone G, Bisanti L. (2000) Consumption of fresh fruit rich in vitamin C and wheezing symptoms in children. SIDRIA Collaborative Group, Italy (Italian Studies on Respiratory Disorders in Children and the Environment), *Thorax* 55(4): 283-288

Garcia-Marcos L, Arnedo PA, Busquets-Monge R, Morales Suarez-Varela M, Garcia dA, Batlles-Garrido J, Blanco-Quiros A, Lopez-Silvarrey VA, Garcia-Hernandez G, Aguinaga-Ontoso I et al . (2008) How the presence of rhinoconjunctivitis and the severity of asthma modify the relationship between obesity and asthma in children 6-7 years old, *Clin Exp Allergy* 38(7): 1174-1178

Garcia-Marcos L, Canflanca IM, Garrido JB, Varela AL, Garcia-Hernandez G, Guillen GF, Gonzalez-Diaz C, Carvajal-Uruena I, Arnedo-Pena A, Busquets-Monge RM et al . (2007) Relationship of asthma and rhinoconjunctivitis with obesity, exercise and Mediterranean diet in Spanish schoolchildren, *Thorax* 62(6): 503-508

Gilliland FD, Berhane K, Islam T, McConnell R, Gauderman WJ, Gilliland SS, Avol E, Peters JM. (2003) Obesity and the risk of newly diagnosed asthma in school-age children, *Am J Epidemiol* 158(5): 406-415

Groeben H, Meier S, Brown RH, O'Donnell CP, Mitzner W, Tankersley CG. (2004) The effect of leptin on the ventilatory responseto hyperoxia, *Exp Lung Res* 30(7): 559-570

Guerra S, Wright AL, Morgan WJ, Sherrill DL, Holberg CJ, Martinez FD. (2004) Persistence of asthma symptoms during adolescence: role of obesity and age at the onset of puberty, *Am J Respir Crit Care Med* 170(1): 78-85

Guler N, Kirerleri E, Ones U, Tamay Z, Salmayenli N, Darendeliler F. (2004) Leptin: does it have any role in childhood asthma?, *J Allergy Clin Immunol* 114(2): 254-259

Haberg SE, Stigum H, London SJ, Nystad W, Nafstad P. (2009) Maternal obesity in pregnancy and respiratory health in early childhood, *Paediatr Perinat Epidemiol* 23(4): 352-362

Hakala K, Mustajoki P, Aittomaki J, Sovijarvi AR. (1995) Effect of weight loss and body position on pulmonary function and gas exchange abnormalities in morbid obesity, *Int J Obes Relat Metab Disord* 19(5): 343-346

Hakala K, Stenius-Aarniala B, Sovijarvi A. (2000) Effects of weight loss on peak flow variability, airways obstruction, and lung volumes in obese patients with asthma, *Chest* 118(5): 1315-1321

Hall IP, Wheatley A, Wilding P, Liggett SB. (1995) Association of Glu 27 beta 2-adrenoceptor polymorphism with lower airway reactivity in asthmatic subjects, *Lancet* 345(8959): 1213-1214

Hancox RJ, Milne BJ, Poulton R, Taylor DR, Greene JM, McLachlan CR, Cowan JO, Flannery EM, Herbison GP, Sears MR. (2005) Sex differences in the relation between body mass index and asthma and atopy in a birth cohort, *Am J Respir Crit Care Med* 171(5): 440-445

Hark WT, Thompson WM, McLaughlin TE, Wheatley LM, Platts-Mills TA. (2005) Spontaneous sigh rates during sedentary activity: watching television vs reading, *Ann Allergy Asthma Immunol* 94(2): 247-250

Harmsen HJ, Wildeboer-Veloo AC, Raangs GC, Wagendorp AA, Klijn N, Bindels JG, Welling GW. (2000) Analysis of intestinal flora development in breast-fed and formula-fed infants by using molecular identification and detection methods, *J Pediatr Gastroenterol Nutr* 30(1): 61-67

Herrera-Trujillo M, Barraza-Villarreal A, Lazcano-Ponce E, Hernandez B, Sanin LH, Romieu I. (2005) Current wheezing, puberty, and obesity among mexican adolescent females and young women, *J Asthma* 42(8): 705-709

Hosogai N, Fukuhara A, Oshima K, Miyata Y, Tanaka S, Segawa K, Furukawa S, Tochino Y, Komuro R, Matsuda M et al . (2007) Adipose tissue hypoxia in obesity and its impact on adipocytokine dysregulation, *Diabetes* 56(4): 901-911

Hug C, Wang J, Ahmad NS, Bogan JS, Tsao TS, Lodish HF. (2004) T-cadherin is a receptor for hexameric and high-molecular-weight forms of Acrp30/adiponectin, *Proc Natl Acad Sci U S A* 101(28): 10308-10313

Innis SM, King DJ. (1999) trans Fatty acids in human milk are inversely associated with concentrations of essential all-cis n-6 and n-3 fatty acids and determine trans, but not n-6 and n-3, fatty acids in plasma lipids of breast-fed infants, *Am J Clin Nutr* 70(3): 383-390

Ishiyama-Shigemoto S, Yamada K, Yuan X, Ichikawa F, Nonaka K. (1999) Association of polymorphisms in the beta2-adrenergic receptor gene with obesity, hypertriglyceridaemia, and diabetes mellitus, *Diabetologia* 42(1): 98-101

Jaakkola JJ, Ahmed P, Ieromnimon A, Goepfert P, Laiou E, Quansah R, Jaakkola MS. (2006) Preterm delivery and asthma: a systematic review and meta-analysis, *J Allergy Clin Immunol* 118(4): 823-830

Kalayci O, Besler T, Kilinc K, Sekerel BE, Saraclar Y. (2000) Serum levels of antioxidant vitamins (alpha tocopherol, beta carotene, and ascorbic acid) in children with bronchial asthma, *Turk J Pediatr* 42(1): 17-21

Katsoulis K, Kontakiotis T, Leonardopoulos I, Kotsovili A, Legakis IN, Patakas D. (2003) Serum total antioxidant status in severe exacerbation of asthma: correlation with the severity of the disease, *J Asthma* 40(8): 847-854

Katsumata U, Miura M, Ichinose M, Kimura K, Takahashi T, Inoue H, Takishima T. (1990) Oxygen radicals produce airway constriction and hyperresponsiveness in anesthetized cats, *Am Rev Respir Dis* 141(5 Pt 1): 1158-1161

Kattan M, Kumar R, Bloomberg GR, Mitchell HE, Calatroni A, Gergen PJ, Kercsmar CM, Visness CM, Matsui EC, Steinbach SF et al . (2010) Asthma control, adiposity, and adipokines among inner-city adolescents, *J Allergy Clin Immunol* 125(3): 584-592

Kauffman AS, Clifton DK, Steiner RA. (2007) Emerging ideas about kisspeptin- GPR54 signaling in the neuroendocrine regulation of reproduction, *Trends Neurosci* 30(10): 504-511

Kelly C, Ward C, Stenton CS, Bird G, Hendrick DJ, Walters EH. (1988) Number and activity of inflammatory cells in bronchoalveolar lavage fluid in asthma and their relation to airway responsiveness, *Thorax* 43(9): 684-692

Kelly FJ, Mudway I, Blomberg A, Frew A, Sandstrom T. (1999) Altered lung antioxidant status in patients with mild asthma, *Lancet* 354(9177): 482-483

Kim HJ, Kim CH, Lee DH, Han MW, Kim MY, Ju JH, Do MS. (2011) Expression of eotaxin in 3T3-L1 adipocytes and the effects of weight loss in high-fat diet induced obese mice, *Nutr Res Pract* 5(1): 11-19

Kim KW, Shin YH, Lee KE, Kim ES, Sohn MH, Kim KE. (2008) Relationship between adipokines and manifestations of childhood asthma, *Pediatr Allergy Immunol* 19(6): 535-540

Kirchgessner TG, Uysal KT, Wiesbrock SM, Marino MW, Hotamisligil GS. (1997) Tumor necrosis factor-alpha contributes to obesity-related hyperleptinemia by regulating leptin release from adipocytes, *J Clin Invest* 100(11): 2777-2782

Kojima M, Kangawa K. (2010) Ghrelin: more than endogenous growth hormone secretagogue, *Ann N Y Acad Sci* 1200140-148

Larochelle J, Freiler J, Dice J, Hagan L. (2007) Plasma resistin levels in asthmatics as a marker of disease state, *J Asthma* 44(7): 509-513

Lebrethon MC, Aganina A, Fournier M, Gerard A, Parent AS, Bourguignon JP. (2007) Effects of in vivo and in vitro administration of ghrelin, leptin and neuropeptide mediators on pulsatile gonadotrophin-releasing hormone secretion from male rat hypothalamus before and after puberty, *J Neuroendocrinol* 19(3): 181-188

Leivo-Korpela S, Lehtimaki L, Vuolteenaho K, Nieminen R, Kankaanranta H, Saarelainen S, Moilanen E. (2011) Adipokine resistin predicts anti-inflammatory effect of glucocorticoids in asthma, *J Inflamm (Lond)* 8(1): 12-

Lessard A, Turcotte H, Cormier Y, Boulet LP. (2008) Obesity and asthma: a specific phenotype?, *Chest* 134(2): 317-323

Lugogo NL, Kraft M, Dixon AE. (2010) Does obesity produce a distinct asthma phenotype?, *J Appl Physiol* 108(3): 729-734

Mai XM, Bottcher MF, Leijon I. (2004) Leptin and asthma in overweight children at 12 years of age, *Pediatr Allergy Immunol* 15(6): 523-530

Malli F, Papaioannou AI, Gourgoulianis KI, Daniil Z. (2010) The role of leptin in the respiratory system: an overview, *Respir Res* 11152-

Mallol J, Aguirre V, Espinosa V. (2011) Increased oxidative stress in children with post infectious Bronchiolitis Obliterans, *Allergol Immunopathol (Madr)*

Mancuso P, Canetti C, Gottschalk A, Tithof PK, Peters-Golden M. (2004) Leptin augments alveolar macrophage leukotriene synthesis by increasing phospholipase activity and enhancing group IVC iPLA2 (cPLA2gamma) protein expression, *Am J Physiol Lung Cell Mol Physiol* 287(3): L497-L502

Maniscalco M, Zedda A, Faraone S, Cerbone MR, Cristiano S, Giardiello C, Sofia M. (2008) Weight loss and asthma control in severely obese asthmatic females, *Respir Med* 102(1): 102-108

Matheson MC, Erbas B, Balasuriya A, Jenkins MA, Wharton CL, Tang ML, Abramson MJ, Walters EH, Hopper JL, Dharmage SC. (2007) Breast-feeding and atopic disease: a cohort study from childhood to middle age, *J Allergy Clin Immunol* 120(5): 1051-1057

Matsuda K, Nishi Y, Okamatsu Y, Kojima M, Matsuishi T. (2006) Ghrelin and leptin: a link between obesity and allergy?, *J Allergy Clin Immunol* 117(3): 705-706

Medoff BD, Okamoto Y, Leyton P, Weng M, Sandall BP, Raher MJ, Kihara S, Bloch KD, Libby P, Luster AD. (2009) Adiponectin deficiency increases allergic airway inflammation and pulmonary vascular remodeling, *Am J Respir Cell Mol Biol* 41(4): 397-406

Milic-Emili J, Torchio R, D'Angelo E. (2007) Closing volume: a reappraisal (1967-2007), *Eur J Appl Physiol* 99(6): 567-583

Miller M, Cho JY, Pham A, Ramsdell J, Broide DH. (2009) Adiponectin and functional adiponectin receptor 1 are expressed by airway epithelial cells in chronic obstructive pulmonary disease, *J Immunol* 182(1): 684-691

Mito N, Kitada C, Hosoda T, Sato K. (2002) Effect of diet-induced obesity on ovalbumin-specific immune response in a murine asthma model, *Metabolism* 51(10): 1241-1246

Moreno LA, Rodriguez G. (2007) Dietary risk factors for development of childhood obesity, *Curr Opin Clin Nutr Metab Care* 10(3): 336-341

Nadeem A, Masood A, Siddiqui N. (2008) Oxidant--antioxidant imbalance in asthma: scientific evidence, epidemiological data and possible therapeutic options, *Ther Adv Respir Dis* 2(4): 215-235

Nadeem A, Raj HG, Chhabra SK. (2005) Increased oxidative stress in acute exacerbations of asthma, *J Asthma* 42(1): 45-50

Nagaev I, Bokarewa M, Tarkowski A, Smith U. (2006) Human resistin is a systemic immune-derived proinflammatory cytokine targeting both leukocytes and adipocytes, *PLoS One* 1e31-

Nagel G, Koenig W, Rapp K, Wabitsch M, Zoellner I, Weiland SK. (2009) Associations of adipokines with asthma, rhinoconjunctivitis, and eczema in German schoolchildren, *Pediatr Allergy Immunol* 20(1): 81-88

Naimark A, Cherniack RM. (1960) Compliance of the respiratory system and its components in health and obesity, *J Appl Physiol* 15377-382

Nair P, Radford K, Fanat A, Janssen LJ, Peters-Golden M, Cox PG. (2008) The effects of leptin on airway smooth muscle responses, *Am J Respir Cell Mol Biol* 39(4): 475-481

Navarro VM, Castellano JM, Garcia-Galiano D, Tena-Sempere M. (2007) Neuroendocrine factors in the initiation of puberty: the emergent role of kisspeptin, *Rev Endocr Metab Disord* 8(1): 11-20

Nelson MC, Gordon-Larsen P, North KE, Adair LS. (2006) Body mass index gain, fast food, and physical activity: effects of shared environments over time, *Obesity (Silver Spring)* 14(4): 701-709

Neveu WA, Allard JL, Raymond DM, Bourassa LM, Burns SM, Bunn JY, Irvin CG, Kaminsky DA, Rincon M. (2010) Elevation of IL-6 in the allergic asthmatic airway is independent of inflammation but associates with loss of central airway function, *Respir Res* 1128-

Nurmatov U, Devereux G, Sheikh A. (2011) Nutrients and foods for the primary prevention of asthma and allergy: systematic review and meta-analysis, *J Allergy Clin Immunol* 127(3): 724-733

Ochs-Balcom HM, Grant BJ, Muti P, Sempos CT, Freudenheim JL, Browne RW, McCann SE, Trevisan M, Cassano PA, Iacoviello L et al . (2006) Antioxidants, oxidative stress, and pulmonary function in individuals diagnosed with asthma or COPD, *Eur J Clin Nutr* 60(8): 991-999

Oh CK, Ariue B, Alban RF, Shaw B, Cho SH. (2002) PAI-1 promotes extracellular matrix deposition in the airways of a murine asthma model, *Biochem Biophys Res Commun* 294(5): 1155-1160

Okamatsu Y, Matsuda K, Hiramoto I, Tani H, Kimura K, Yada Y, Kakuma T, Higuchi S, Kojima M, Matsuishi T. (2009) Ghrelin and leptin modulate immunity and liver function in overweight children, *Pediatr Int* 51(1): 9-13

Picado C, Deulofeu R, Lleonart R, Agusti M, Mullol J, Quinto L, Torra M. (2001) Dietary micronutrients/antioxidants and their relationship with bronchial asthma severity, *Allergy* 56(1): 43-49

Pitsavos C, Panagiotakos DB, Tzima N, Chrysohoou C, Economou M, Zampelas A, Stefanadis C. (2005) Adherence to the Mediterranean diet is associated with total antioxidant capacity in healthy adults: the ATTICA study, *Am J Clin Nutr* 82(3): 694-699

Platts-Mills TA, Erwin E, Heymann P, Woodfolk J. (2005) Is the hygiene hypothesis still a viable explanation for the increased prevalence of asthma?, *Allergy* 60(Suppl 79): 25-31

Ponsonby AL, Gatenby P, Glasgow N, Mullins R, McDonald T, Hurwitz M. (2002) Which clinical subgroups within the spectrum of child asthma are attributable to atopy?, *Chest* 121(1): 135-142

Raap U, Brzoska T, Sohl S, Path G, Emmel J, Herz U, Braun A, Luger T, Renz H. (2003) Alpha-melanocyte-stimulating hormone inhibits allergic airway inflammation, *J Immunol* 171(1): 353-359

Rasmussen F, Lambrechtsen J, Siersted HC, Hansen HS, Hansen NC. (2000) Low physical fitness in childhood is associated with the development of asthma in young adulthood: the Odense schoolchild study, *Eur Respir J* 16(5): 866-870

Roberts CK, Barnard RJ, Sindhu RK, Jurczak M, Ehdaie A, Vaziri ND. (2006) Oxidative stress and dysregulation of NAD(P)H oxidase and antioxidant enzymes in diet-induced metabolic syndrome, *Metabolism* 55(7): 928-934

Rothenbacher D, Weyermann M, Fantuzzi G, Brenner H. (2007) Adipokines in cord blood and risk of wheezing disorders within the first two years of life, *Clin Exp Allergy* 37(8): 1143-1149

Sackesen C, Ercan H, Dizdar E, Soyer O, Gumus P, Tosun BN, Buyuktuncer Z, Karabulut E, Besler T, Kalayci O. (2008) A comprehensive evaluation of the enzymatic and nonenzymatic antioxidant systems in childhood asthma, *J Allergy Clin Immunol* 122(1): 78-85

Schley PD, Field CJ. (2002) The immune-enhancing effects of dietary fibres and prebiotics, *Br J Nutr* 87(Suppl 2): S221-S230

Schmidt M, Affenito SG, Striegel-Moore R, Khoury PR, Barton B, Crawford P, Kronsberg S, Schreiber G, Obarzanek E, Daniels S. (2005) Fast-food intake and diet quality in black and white girls: the National Heart, Lung, and Blood Institute Growth and Health Study, *Arch Pediatr Adolesc Med* 159(7): 626-631

Scholtens S, Wijga AH, Brunekreef B, Kerkhof M, Postma DS, Oldenwening M, de Jongste JC, Smit HA. (2010) Maternal overweight before pregnancy and asthma in offspring followed for 8 years, *Int J Obes (Lond)* 34(4): 606-613

Schroder H. (2007) Protective mechanisms of the Mediterranean diet in obesity and type 2 diabetes, *J Nutr Biochem* 18(3): 149-160

Schwartz MW, Seeley RJ, Woods SC, Weigle DS, Campfield LA, Burn P, Baskin DG. (1997) Leptin increases hypothalamic pro-opiomelanocortin mRNA expression in the rostral arcuate nucleus, *Diabetes* 46(12): 2119-2123

Shanmugasundaram KR, Kumar SS, Rajajee S. (2001) Excessive free radical generation in the blood of children suffering from asthma, *Clin Chim Acta* 305(1-2): 107-114

Sherriff A, Maitra A, Ness AR, Mattocks C, Riddoch C, Reilly JJ, Paton JY, Henderson AJ. (2009) Association of duration of television viewing in early childhood with the subsequent development of asthma, *Thorax* 64(4): 321-325

Shore SA. (2007) Obesity and asthma: lessons from animal models, *J Appl Physiol* 102(2): 516-528

Shore SA. (2008) Obesity and asthma: possible mechanisms, *J Allergy Clin Immunol* 121(5): 1087-1093

Shore SA. (2010) Obesity, airway hyperresponsiveness, and inflammation, *J Appl Physiol* 108(3): 735-743

Shore SA, Johnston RA. (2006) Obesity and asthma, *Pharmacol Ther* 110(1): 83-102

Shore SA, Rivera-Sanchez YM, Schwartzman IN, Johnston RA. (2003) Responses to ozone are increased in obese mice, *J Appl Physiol* 95(3): 938-945

Shore SA, Schwartzman IN, Mellema MS, Flynt L, Imrich A, Johnston RA. (2005) Effect of leptin on allergic airway responses in mice, *J Allergy Clin Immunol* 115(1): 103-109

Shore SA, Terry RD, Flynt L, Xu A, Hug C. (2006) Adiponectin attenuates allergen-induced airway inflammation and hyperresponsiveness in mice, *J Allergy Clin Immunol* 118(2): 389-395

Skloot G, Togias A. (2003) Bronchodilation and bronchoprotection by deep inspiration and their relationship to bronchial hyperresponsiveness, *Clin Rev Allergy Immunol* 24(1): 55-72

Sood A, Ford ES, Camargo CA, Jr. (2006) Association between leptin and asthma in adults, *Thorax* 61(4): 300-305

Sukalich S, Mingione MJ, Glantz JC. (2006) Obstetric outcomes in overweight and obese adolescents, *Am J Obstet Gynecol* 195(3): 851-855

Sutherland TJ, Sears MR, McLachlan CR, Poulton R, Hancox RJ. (2009) Leptin, adiponectin, and asthma: findings from a population-based cohort study, *Ann Allergy Asthma Immunol* 103(2): 101-107

Takemura Y, Ouchi N, Shibata R, Aprahamian T, Kirber MT, Summer RS, Kihara S, Walsh K. (2007) Adiponectin modulates inflammatory reactions via calreticulin receptor-dependent clearance of early apoptotic bodies, *J Clin Invest* 117(2): 375-386

Tankersley C, Kleeberger S, Russ B, Schwartz A, Smith P. (1996) Modified control of breathing in genetically obese (ob/ob) mice, *J Appl Physiol* 81(2): 716-723

Tantisira KG, Weiss ST. (2001) Complex interactions in complex traits: obesity and asthma, *Thorax* 56(Suppl 2): ii64-ii73

Taraseviciute A, Voelkel NF. (2006) Severe pulmonary hypertension in postmenopausal obese women, *Eur J Med Res* 11(5): 198-202

Thomas PS, Agrawal S, Gore M, Geddes DM. (1995) Recall lung pneumonitis due to carmustine after radiotherapy, *Thorax* 50(10): 1116-1118

Thomas PS, Heywood G. (2002) Effects of inhaled tumour necrosis factor alpha in subjects with mild asthma, *Thorax* 57(9): 774-778

To T, Guan J, Wang C, Radhakrishnan D, McLimont S, Latycheva O, Gershon AS. (2010) Is large birth weight associated with asthma risk in early childhood?, *Arch Dis Child*

To T, Vydykhan TN, Dell S, Tassoudji M, Harris JK. (2004) Is obesity associated with asthma in young children?, *J Pediatr* 144(2): 162-168

Tsuchiya T, Shimizu H, Horie T, Mori M. (1999) Expression of leptin receptor in lung: leptin as a growth factor, *Eur J Pharmacol* 365(2-3): 273-279

Turner S, Zhang G, Young S, Cox M, Goldblatt J, Landau L, Le Souef P. (2008) Associations between postnatal weight gain, change in postnatal pulmonary function, formula feeding and early asthma, *Thorax* 63(3): 234-239

Vasudevan AR, Wu H, Xydakis AM, Jones PH, Smith EO, Sweeney JF, Corry DB, Ballantyne CM. (2006) Eotaxin and obesity, *J Clin Endocrinol Metab* 91(1): 256-261

Vogelberg C, Hirsch T, Radon K, Dressel H, Windstetter D, Weinmayr G, Weiland SK, von Mutius E, Nowak D, Leupold W. (2007) Leisure time activity and new onset of wheezing during adolescence, *Eur Respir J* 30(4): 672-676

von Kries R, Hermann M, Grunert VP, von Mutius E. (2001) Is obesity a risk factor for childhood asthma?, *Allergy* 56(4): 318-322

von Mutius E. (2007) Allergies, infections and the hygiene hypothesis--the epidemiological evidence, *Immunobiology* 212(6): 433-439

Vural H, Uzun K. (2000) Serum and red blood cell antioxidant status in patients with bronchial asthma, *Can Respir J* 7(6): 476-480

Weiland SK, von Mutius E, Husing A, Asher MI. (1999) Intake of trans fatty acids and prevalence of childhood asthma and allergies in Europe. ISAAC Steering Committee, *Lancet* 353(9169): 2040-2041

Weisberg SP, McCann D, Desai M, Rosenbaum M, Leibel RL, Ferrante AW, Jr. (2003) Obesity is associated with macrophage accumulation in adipose tissue, *J Clin Invest* 112(12): 1796-1808

White SR, Fischer BM, Marroquin BA, Stern R. (2008) Interleukin-1beta mediates human airway epithelial cell migration via NF-kappaB, *Am J Physiol Lung Cell Mol Physiol* 295(6): L1018-L1027

Wickens K, Barry D, Friezema A, Rhodius R, Bone N, Purdie G, Crane J. (2005) Fast foods - are they a risk factor for asthma?, *Allergy* 60(12): 1537-1541

Williams DL, Kaplan JM, Grill HJ. (2000) The role of the dorsal vagal complex and the vagus nerve in feeding effects of melanocortin-3/4 receptor stimulation, *Endocrinology* 141(4): 1332-1337

Wilson NJ, Boniface K, Chan JR, McKenzie BS, Blumenschein WM, Mattson JD, Basham B, Smith K, Chen T, Morel F et al . (2007) Development, cytokine profile and function of human interleukin 17-producing helper T cells, *Nat Immunol* 8(9): 950-957

Wong CK, Cheung PF, Lam CW. (2007) Leptin-mediated cytokine release and migration of eosinophils: implications for immunopathophysiology of allergic inflammation, *Eur J Immunol* 37(8): 2337-2348

Wood LG, Fitzgerald DA, Gibson PG, Cooper DM, Garg ML. (2000) Lipid peroxidation as determined by plasma isoprostanes is related to disease severity in mild asthma, *Lipids* 35(9): 967-974

Wood LG, Garg ML, Blake RJ, Simpson JL, Gibson PG. (2008) Oxidized vitamin E and glutathione as markers of clinical status in asthma, *Clin Nutr* 27(4): 579-586

Xia Q, Pang W, Pan H, Zheng Y, Kang JS, Zhu SG. (2004) Effects of ghrelin on the proliferation and secretion of splenic T lymphocytes in mice, *Regul Pept* 122(3): 173-178

Ye J, Gao Z, Yin J, He Q. (2007) Hypoxia is a potential risk factor for chronic inflammation and adiponectin reduction in adipose tissue of ob/ob and dietary obese mice, *Am J Physiol Endocrinol Metab* 293(4): E1118-E1128

18

Asthma and Health Related Quality of Life in Childhood and Adolescence

Esther Hafkamp-de Groen and Hein Raat
Erasmus MC-University Medical Center Rotterdam
The Netherlands

1. Introduction

Asthma is the most frequent chronic disorder in childhood. Asthma puts a serious burden on children's health related quality of life, despite the availability of effective and safe treatment (Dalheim-Englund et al., 2004; Global Initiative for Asthma, 2010; Masoli et al., 2004; Mohangoo et al., 2005). The overall goal of asthma management is to achieve optimal disease control and health related quality of life improvements (Bateman et al., 2007; Pedersen et al., 2011). The World Health Organization has defined the term health related quality of life as the individual's perception of their position of life in the context of the culture and value systems in which they live and in relation to their goals, expectations and concerns (World Health Organization, 1993). The own perception is important because it emphasises that these are the impairments that patients themselves consider important. As in most medical conditions, the correlation between asthma control and health related quality of life is modest. Therefore, the impact that asthma has on a patient's health related quality of life cannot be inferred from the conventional clinical measures of asthma (e.g. spirometry); it must be measured directly (Juniper et al., 1999a, 1999b).

During the past decade, the use of health related quality of life as an essential outcome measure of childhood asthma treatment and management has increased (Merikallio et al., 2005). This review summarises recent literature on: 1) health related quality of life instruments for childhood asthma, 2) the impact of childhood asthma on children's health related quality of life, 3) the impact of children's asthma on caregiver's health related quality of life and 5) factors associated with health related quality of life in childhood asthma.

2. Health related quality of life instruments and childhood asthma

Several feasible, reliable and validated pediatric health related quality of life questionnaires are standardised and available to measure health related quality of life in asthmatic children (Fiese et al., 2005; Raat et al., 2006). Both generic and asthma-specific questionnaires are used to measure health related quality of life in school aged children. Generic health related quality of life questionnaires intend to measure all dimensions of health-related quality of life (Raat et al., 2006). Frequently applied generic health related quality of life questionnaires are: the Child Health Questionnaire (CHQ) (Gorelick et al., 2003), the Pediatric Quality of Life Inventory (PedsQL) (Varni et al., 2005), the TNO-AZL (Preschool) Children's Quality of Life questionnaire (TAPQoL/TACQoL) (Bunge et al., 2005), the Infant-Toddler Quality of

Life (ITQOL) questionnaire (Spuijbroek et al., 2011) and the KIDSCREEN/DISABKIDS questionnaires (Petersen et al., 2005). Asthma-specific health related quality of life questionnaires focus on those dimensions that are likely to be affected by asthma disease or treatment. The most prominent asthma-specific health related quality of life questionnaires are the Pediatric Asthma Quality of Life Questionnaire (PAQLQ) (Juniper et al., 1996; Raat et al. 2005), the How Are You (HAY) (Le Coq et al., 2000) instrument and the Childhood Asthma Questionnaire (CAQ) (Christie et al., 1993).

If children are unable to report about their own experience reliably, parents are appropriate sources of information about health related quality of life (Petsios et al., 2011). One study suggests that fathers may be better proxy reporters than mothers (Petsios et al., 2011). The correlation between child and parent reported quality of life improves with increasing age of the child (Annett et al., 2003). Although the agreement between child self-report and parent proxy report on health related quality of life has been showed as satisfactory, according to Petsios *et al.* (2011), parents may overestimate health related quality of life of their children with asthma. This has to be taken into account when interpreting results from parent reported health related quality of life questionnaires, in comparison with child self-reports.

The PAQLQ is the most frequently used disease-specific health related quality of life instrument with regard to childhood asthma. Therefore, using this instrument has the benefit for researchers that results can more easily be compared with previous findings. However, using the existing health related quality of life instruments may have some limitations. A recent study has investigated whether asthma-specific health related quality of life questionnaires actually include all relevant aspects of asthma-specific health related quality of life for children with asthma (Annett et al., 2003). They have found disagreement between distinct health related quality of life questionnaires on components of asthma-specific health related quality of life: only some components of the asthma symptoms domain and of the activity limitations domain are part of all questionnaires. Furthermore, according to Van den Bemt *et al.* (2010), not all essential components of asthma-specific health related quality of life, according to childhood asthma, are part of existing asthma-specific health related quality of life questionnaires.

When classifying health related quality of life questionnaires into standardised and individualised health related quality of life instruments, another limitation is revealed. In standardised health related quality of life instruments the questions and range of answers are predetermined and the same for all patients. As opposed to standardised health related quality of life instruments, individualised health related quality of life instruments allow patients to define their quality of life in relation to their goals and expectations. Carr & Higginson (2001) conclude that standardised health related quality of life questionnaires have limited ability to capture the health related quality of life of individual asthma patients.

The most appropriate approach to measure health related quality of life in asthmatic children would be to use a combination of parental and self-reports of both generic and asthma-specific health related quality of life by validated questionnaires (Raat et al., 2006). Whether such health related quality of life measures are truly patient centred and to what extent they actually represent the quality of life of individual or groups of asthmatic children should always be taken into account when one interprets study results (Carr & Higginson, 2001).

3. Impact of asthma on children's health related quality of life

Asthma might have physical, emotional and psychosocial impact on children's lives (Grootenhuis et al., 2007; Juniper, 1997; Merikallio et al., 2005; Sawyer et al., 2004). Important components of health related quality of life are the effects on, and consequences of asthma on peer relationships (e.g., being bullied), the dependence on medication, shortness of breath, cough, limitations in activities and limitations due to the response on cigarette smoke exposure (Van den Bemt et al., 2010). Compared to preschool children without asthma symptoms, preschool children with asthma symptoms have significantly lower health related quality of life scores for lung problems, sleeping, appetite, communication and positive mood health related quality of life scales (Mohangoo et al., 2005).

Most studies have focused on severity of symptoms to examine the impact of asthma symptoms on children's health related quality life; the results are conflicting (Everhart & Fiese, 2009). For example, disease severity is not consistently associated with children's health related quality of life in some studies (Erickson et al., 2002; Vila et al., 2003), whereas others report that children with moderate or severe asthma have a worse level of functioning in several domains of their health related quality of life compared to children with mild asthma (Annett et al., 2001; Merikallio et al., 2005; Mohangoo et al., 2007, 2011; Sawyer et al., 2000) suggesting there may be a 'dose-response' relationship between the frequency and intensity of children's asthma symptoms and their health related quality of life. Mohangoo *et al.* (2007, 2011) evaluated health related quality of life in infants and adolescents with asthma-like symptoms, such as attacks of wheezing and shortness of breath (Mohangoo et al., 2007, 2011). Asthma-like symptoms during the first year of life are associated with impaired health related quality of life at the age of 12 months. Also, the presence of at least four wheezing attacks during the past year was associated with impaired adolescents' health related quality of life. Frequent wheezing attacks mostly affect adolescents' general health, bodily pain, self esteem and mental health (Mohangoo et al., 2007). Previous studies have also found that wheezing attacks more often have a physical impact than a psychosocial impact (Merikallio et al., 2005).

As described earlier, one of the main goals of asthma management is to achieve good asthma control. Asthma control has been defined as the minimisation of night time and daytime symptoms, activity limitation, rescue bronchodilator use and airway narrowing (Global Initiative for Asthma, 2010). Poorly controlled asthma symptoms impair health related quality of life in children (Guilbert et al., 2011). An important issue is whether proper asthma management improves quality of life in asthma patients, and whether poor health related quality of life makes disease management harder. Studies have found that poor health related quality of life is predictive of subsequent asthma-related emergency department visits, which implicates poor asthma control (Magid et al, 2004). Pont *et al.* (2004) show that proper asthma management improves health related quality of life.

In short, children experience asthma as an interruption in daily life that influences them physically, emotionally and socially.

4. Impact of children's asthma on caregiver's health related quality of life

With childhood asthma, the family and particularly the primary caregiver may face a considerable burden. While there are several questionnaires for assessing parental/caregiver's health related quality of life not directly related to asthma (Osman &

Silverman, 1996), there is only one instrument to examine the specific impact of childhood asthma on parental/caregiver functioning: The Pediatric Asthma Caregiver's Quality of Life Questionnaire (PACQLQ) (Juniper et al., 1996).

Whereas some studies find no association between caregiver's health related quality of life and children's asthma symptoms (Annett et al., 2003), duration of asthma illness and asthma pre-treatment severity (Vila et al., 2003), other studies report that caregiver's and child's health related quality of life are significantly associated with each other (Dean et al., 2009, 2010; Garro, 2011; Halterman et al., 2004). Halterman *et al.* (2004) find that higher symptom levels with regard to childhood asthma are associated with lower parental health related quality of life. Further, when children's symptoms improve, parents show higher health related quality of life.

It should be considered how childhood asthma affects caregiver's health related quality of life. Caregivers of asthmatic children appear to be more compromised in their resistance to stress, mood, emotional stability, amount of spare time and leisure activities (Garro, 2011). Caregivers of children with uncontrolled asthma report significantly higher absenteeism than their controlled counterparts (Dean et al., 2009, 2010).

Both caregiver's health related quality of life, caregiver's perception of the child's asthma symptoms, and the child's health related quality of life may be important in diagnosis and control of established asthma in childhood (Skoner, 2002). While giving attention to the caregiver's health related quality of life, it should be taken into account that the profile of health related quality of life impairment is different in asthmatic children and in their parents (Farnik et al., 2010). Where activity limitation seems to be the most impaired domain in children, asthma symptom perception and emotional health appear to be the most affected health related quality of life domains in parents.

In addition to evaluation of the asthmatic child, the integral assessment of asthma requires the evaluation of caregiver's health related quality of life. Giving attention to caregiver's health related quality of life is needed in clinical practice in order to avoid possible interferences of the caregiver's distress in the optimization of child's asthma treatment outcomes (Majani et al., 2005).

5. Factors associated with health related quality of life in asthmatic children

As we described earlier, the frequency and severity of asthma attacks and effects of asthma management or treatment are associated with children's health related quality of life. Researchers have also investigated other variables in association to health related quality of life in childhood asthma (Annett et al., 2003; Erickson et al., 2002; Mrazek, 1992; Sawyer et al., 2000, 2001). Hospital admissions, absences from school, limitations of sport and other activities, sleeping problems (and fatigue) are associated with health related quality of life in asthmatic children (Mrazek, 1992). Erickson *et al.* (2002) show that both asthma morbidity and health related quality of life are related to socioeconomic status. Also, household income is most consistently associated with the health related quality of life of asthmatic children and their caregivers. Sawyer *et al.* (2001) report the impact of family functioning on health related quality of life in children with asthma. They have found that the degree to which children are upset by their asthma is related to general functioning of their families, and their symptom levels are associated with several dimensions of family functioning (Sawyer et al., 2000, 2001). Children living in families with more clearly defined roles, greater interest and concern for the well-being of each other and clearer rules have been

found to be less bothered by their asthma symptoms (Sawyer et al., 2000). A study by Annett *et al.* (2003) didn't find an association between health related quality of life of asthmatic children and family functioning, measured by the degree of cohesion among family members.
Results suggest that several factors may impact health related quality of life of asthmatic children. Important predictors of the health related quality of life of asthmatic children are socioeconomic status and family functioning. These findings implicate the need of specific attention to health related quality of life in asthmatic children from families with low socioeconomic status and poor family functioning.

6. Conclusion

Health care workers should be aware of the impact of asthma on children's life, their families and the factors associated with the health related quality of life of these children. Routine use of an health related quality of life questionnaire to evaluate health related quality of life in children with asthma symptoms and their caregivers should be recommended in health care. Specific application, for example, can be found in preventive child health care and in primary health care to prevent impairment of health related quality of life due to asthma symptoms and to realise adequate management of asthma symptoms. Attention should be given to health related quality of life in asthmatic children from families with low socioeconomic status and poor family functioning. Generally, a combination of parental and self-reports of both general and asthma-specific patient centred health related quality of life questionnaires should be applied. Further research should focus on which factors are responsible for the greatest burden on asthmatic children's health related quality of life and their caregivers' health related quality of life and how such risk factors should be prevented and managed.

7. References

Annett, RD.; Bender, BG.; Lapidus, J.; DuHamel, TR. & Lincoln, A. (2001). Predicting children's quality of life in an asthma clinical trial: What did children's reports tell us? *J Pediatr*, Vol.139, No.6, pp. 854-861, ISSN 0022-3476

Annett, RD.; Bender, BG.; DuHamel, TR. & Lapidus, J. (2003). Factors influencing parent reports on quality of life for children with asthma. *J Asthma*, Vol.40, No.5, pp. 577-587, ISSN 0277-0903

Bateman, E.D.; Bousquet, J.; Keech, ML.; Busse, WW.; Clark, TJ. & Pedersen, SE. (2007). The correlation between asthma control and health status: the GOAL study. *Eur Respir J*, Vol.29, No.1, pp. 56-63, ISSN 0903-1936

Bunge, EM.; Essink-Bot, ML.; Kobussen, MP.; Van Suijlekom-Smit, LW.; Moll, HA. & Raat, H. (2005). Reliability and validity of health status measurement by the TAPQOL. *Arch Dis Child*, Vol.90, No.4, pp. 351-358, ISSN 1468-2044

Carr, AJ. & Higginson, IJ. (2001). Are quality of life measures patient centred? *BMJ*, Vol.322, No.7298, pp. 1357-1360, ISSN 0959-8138

Christie, MJ.; French, D.; Sowden, A. & West, A. (1993). Development of child-centred disease-specific questionnaires for living with asthma. *Psychosom Med*, Vol.55, No.6, pp. 541-548, ISSN 0033-3174

Dalheim-Englund, AC.; Rydström, I.; Rasmussen, BH.; Moller, C. & Sandman, PO. (2004). Having a child with asthma-quality of life for Swedish parents. *J Clin Nurs*, Vol.13, No.3, pp. 386-395, ISSN 0962-1067

Dean, BB.; Calimlim, BC.; Kindermann, SL.; Khandker, RK. & Tinkelman, D. (2009). The impact of uncontrolled asthma on absenteeism and health-related quality of life. *J Asthma*, Vol.46, No.9, pp. 861-866, ISSN 1532-4303

Dean, BB.; Calimlim, BC.; Sacco, P.; Aguilar, D.; Maykut, R. & Tinkelman, D. (2010). Uncontrolled asthma: assessing quality of life and productivity of children and their caregivers using a cross-sectional Internet-based survey. *Health Qual Life Outcomes*, Vol.8, pp. 96, ISSN 1477-7525

Erickson, SR.; Munzenberger, PJ. & Plante, MJ.; Kirking, DM.; Hurwitz, ME. & Vanuya, RZ. (2002). Influence of sociodemographics on the health-related quality of life of pediatric patients with asthma and their caregivers. *J Asthma*, Vol.39, No.2, pp. 107-117, ISSN 0277-0903

Everhart, RS. & Fiese, BH. (2009). Asthma severity and child quality of life in pediatric asthma: A systematic review. *Patient Educ Couns*, Vol.75, No.2, pp. 162-168, ISSN 0738-3991

Farnik, M.; Pierzchała, W.; Brozek, G.; Zejda, JE. & Skrzypek, M. (2010). Quality of life protocol in the early asthma diagnosis in children. *Pediatr Pulmonol*, Vol.45, No.11, pp. 1095-1102, ISSN 1099-0496

Fiese, BH.; Wamboldt, FS. & Anbar, RD. (2005). Family asthma management routines: connections to medical adherence and quality of life. *J Pediatrics*, Vol.146, No.2, pp. 171-176, ISSN 0022-3476

Garro A. (2011). Health-related quality of life (HRQOL) in Latino families experiencing pediatric asthma. *J Child Health Care*, (Epub ahead of print), ISSN 1741-2889

Global Initiative for Asthma (GINA) Executive Committee. (2010). Global strategy for asthma management and prevention, In: Global Initiative for Asthma (GINA), Available from: www.ginasthma.org

Gorelick, MH.; Scribano, PV.; Stevens, MW. & Schultz, TR. (2003). Construct validity and responsiveness of the Child

Health Questionnaire in children with acute asthma. *Ann Allergy Asthma Immunol*, Vol.90, No.6, pp. 622-628, ISSN 1081-1206

Grootenhuis, MA.; Koopman, HM.; Verrips, EG.; Vogels, AG. & Last, BF. (2007). Health-related quality of life problems of children aged 8-11 years with a chronic disease. *Dev Neurorehabil*, Vol.10, No.1, pp. 27-33, ISSN 1751-8423

Guilbert, TW.; Garris, C.; Jhingran, P.; Bonafede, M.; Tomaszewski, KJ.; Bonus, T.; Hahn, RM. & Schatz, M. (2011). Asthma that is not well-controlled is associated with increased healthcare utilization and decreased quality of life. *J Asthma*, Vol.48, No.2, pp. 126-132, ISSN 1532-4303

Halterman, JS.; Yoos, HL.; Conn, KM.; Callahan, PM.; Montes, G.; Neely, TL. & Szilagyi, PG. (2004). The impact of childhood asthma on parental quality of life. *J Asthma*, Vol.41, No.6, pp. 645-653, ISSN 0277-0903

Juniper, EF.; Guyatt, GH.; Feeny, DH.; Ferrie, PJ.; Griffith, LE. & Townsend, M. (1996). Measuring quality of life in children with asthma. *Qual Life Research*, Vol.5, No.1, pp. 35-46, ISSN 0962-9343

Juniper, EF.; Guyatt, GH.; Feeny, DH.; Ferrie, PJ.; Griffith, LE. & Townsend, M. (1996). Measuring quality of life in the parents of children with asthma. *Qual Life Research*, Vol.5, No.1, pp. 27-34, ISSN 0962-9343

Juniper, EF. (1997). How important is quality of life in pediatric asthma? *Pediatr Pulmonology*, Suppl.15, pp. 17-21, ISSN 1054-187X

Juniper, EF.; Jenkins, C.; Price, MJ., Thwaites RMA. & James MH. (1999). Quality of life of asthma patients treated with salmeterol/fluticasone propionate combination product and budesonide (abstract). *Eur Respir J*, Vol.14, Suppl.30, pp. 370s

Juniper, EF.; Svensson, K.; O'Byrne, PM.; Barnes, PJ.; Bauer, CA.; Lofdahl, CG.; Postma, DS.; Pauwels, RA.; Tattersfield, AE. & Ullman, A. (1999). Asthma quality of life during 1 year of treatment with budesonide with or without formoterol. *Eur Respir J*, Vol.14, No.5, pp. 1038-104, ISSN 0903-1936

Le Coq, EM.; Colland, VT.; Boeke, AJ.; Boeke, P.; Bezemer, DP. & Van Eijk, JT. (2000). Reproducibility, construct validity, and responsiveness of the "How Are You?" (HAY), a self-report quality of life questionnaire for children with asthma. *J Asthma* , Vol.37, No.1, pp. 43-58, ISSN 0277-0903

Magid, DJ.; Houry, D.; Ellis, J.; Lyons, E. & Rumsfeld, JS. (2004). Health-related quality of life predicts emergency department utilization for patients with asthma. *Ann Emerg Med*, Vol.43, No.5, pp. 551-557, ISSN 1097-6760

Majani, G.; Baiardini, I.; Giardini, A.; Pasquali, M.; Tiozzo, M.; Tosca, M.; Cosentino, C.; La Grutta, S.; Marseglia, GL. &

Canonica, GW. (2005). Impact of children's respiratory allergies on caregivers. *Monaldi Arch Chest Dis*, Vol.63, No.4, pp. 199-203, ISSN 1122-0643

Masoli, M.; Fabian, D.; Holt, S. & Beasley, R. (2004). Global Initiative for Asthma (GINA) Program. The global burden of asthma: executive summary of the GINA Dissemination Committee report. *Allergy*, Vol.59, No.5, pp. 469-478, ISSN 0105-4538

Merikallio, VJ.; Mustalahti, K., Remes, ST., Valovirta, EJ. & Kaila, M. (2005). Comparison of quality of life between asthmatic and healthy school children. *Pediatr Allergy Immunol*, Vol.16, No.4, pp. 332-340, ISSN 0905-6157

Mohangoo, AD.; Essink-Bot, ML.; Juniper, EF.; Moll, HA.; De Koning, HJ. & Raat, H. (2005). Health-related quality of life in preschool children with wheezing and dyspnea: Preliminary results from a random general population sample. Qual Life Research, Vol. 14, No.8, pp. 1931-1936, ISSN 0962-9343

Mohangoo, AD.; De Koning, HJ.; Mangunkusumo, RT. & Raat, H. (2007). Health-Related Quality of Life in Adolescents with Wheezing Attacks. *J Adolesc Health*, Vol.41, No.5, pp. 464-471, ISSN 1879-1972

Mohangoo, AD.; De Koning, HJ.; De Jongste, JC.; Landgraf, JM.; Van der Wouden, JC.; Jaddoe, VW.; Hofman, A.; Moll, HA.; Mackenbach, JP. & Raat, H. (2011). Asthma-like symptoms in the first year of life and health-related quality of life at age 12 months: the Generation R study. *Qual Life Research*, In Press (Accepted: 2011-06-14), ISSN 1573-2649

Mrazek D. (1992). Psychiatric complications of pediatric asthma. *Ann Allergy*, Vol.69, No.4, pp. 285-293, ISSN 0003-4738

Osman, L. & Silverman, M. (1996). Measuring quality of life for young children with asthma and their families. *Eur Respir J*, Suppl.21, pp. 35s-41s, ISSN 0904-1850

Pedersen, SE.; Hurd, SS.; Lemanske, RF. (Jr); Becker, A.; Zar, HJ.; Sly, PD.; Soto-Quiroz, M.; Wong, G. & Bateman, ED. (2011). Global strategy for the diagnosis and management of asthma in children 5 years and younger. *Pediatr Pulmonol*, Vol.46, No.1, pp. 1-17, ISSN 1099-0496

Petersen, C.; Schmidt, S.; Power, M. & Bullinger, M. (2005). Development and pilot-testing of a health-related quality of life chronic generic module for children and adolescents with chronic health conditions: a European perspective. *Qual Life Research*, Vol.14, No.4, 1065-1077, ISSN 0962-9343

Petsios, K.; Priftis, KN.; Tsoumakas, C.; Hatziagorou, E.; Tsanakas, JN.; Galanis, P.; Antonogeorgos, G. & Matziou, V. (2011). Level of parent-asthmatic child agreement on health-related quality of life. *J Asthma*, Vol.48, No.3, pp. 286-297, ISSN 1532-4303

Pont, LG.; Van der Molen, T.; Denig, P.; Van der Werf, GT. & Haaijer-Ruskamp, FM. (2004). Relationship between guideline treatment and health-related quality of life in asthma. *Eur Respir J* , Vol.23, No.5, pp. 718-722, ISSN 0903-1936

Raat, H.; Bueving, H.J.; De Jongste, J.C.; Grol, MH.; Juniper, EF. & Van der Wouden, JC. (2005). Responsiveness, longitudinal- and cross-sectional construct validity of the Pediatric Asthma Quality of Life Questionnaire (PAQLQ) in Dutch children with asthma. *Qual Life Research*, Vol.14, No.1, pp. 265-272, ISSN 0962-9343

Raat, H.; Mohangoo, A.D. & Grootenhuis, M.A. (2006). Pediatric health-related quality of life questionnaires in clinical trials. *Curr Opin Allergy Clin Immunol*, Vol.6, No.3, pp. 180-185, ISSN 1528-4050

Sawyer, MG.; Spurrier, N.; Whaites, L.; Kennedy, D.; Martin, AJ. & Baghurst, P. (2000). The relationship between asthma severity, family functioning, and the health related quality of life of children with asthma. *Qual Life Research*, Vol.9, No.10, pp. 1105-1115, ISSN 0962-9343

Sawyer, MG.; Spurrier, N.; Kennedy, D. & Martin, J. (2001). The relationship between the quality of life of children with asthma and family functioning. *J Asthma*, Vol.38, No.3, pp. 279-284, ISSN

Sawyer, MG.; Reynolds, KE.; Couper, JJ.; French, DJ.; Kennedy, D.; Martin, J.; Staugas, R.; Ziaian, T. & Baghurst, PA. (2004). Health-related quality of life of children and adolescents with chronic illness – a two year prospective study. *Qual Life Research*, Vol.13, No.7, pp. 1309-1319, ISSN 0962-9343

Skoner D. (2002). Outcome measures in childhood asthma. *Pediatrics*, Vol.109, Suppl.2, pp. 393-398, ISSN 1098-4275

Spuijbroek, AT.; Oostenbrink, R.; Landgraf, JM.; Rietveld, E.; De Goede-Bolder, A.; Van Beeck, EF.; Van Baar, M.; Raat, H. & Moll, HA. (2011). Health-related quality of life in preschool children in five health conditions. *Qual Life Research*, Vol.20, No.5, pp. 779-786, ISSN 1573-2649

Van den Bemt, L.; Kooijman, S.; Linssen, V.; Lucassen, P.; Muris, J.; Slabbers, G. & Schermer, T. (2010). How does asthma influence the daily life of children? Results of focus group interviews. *Health Qual Life Outcomes*, Vol.8, pp. 5, ISSN 1477-7525

Varni, JW.; Burwinkle, TM.; Sherman, SA.; Hanna, K.; Berrin, SJ.; Malcarne, VL. & Chambers, HG. (2005). Health-related quality of life of children and adolescents with cerebral palsy: hearing the voices of the children. *Dev Med Child Neurol*, Vol.47, No.9, pp. 592-597, ISSN 0012-1622

Vila, G.; Hayder, R.; Bertrand, C.; Falissard, B.; De Blic, J.; Mouren-Simeoni, MC. & Scheinmann, P. (2003). Psychopathology and quality of life for adolescents with asthma and their parents. *Psychosomatics*, Vol.44, No.4, pp. 319-328, ISSN 0033-3182

World Health Organization (WHO), Division of Mental Health. (1993). Measurement of Quality of Life in Children. Available from: www.who.int/mental_health/media/en/663.pdf

Part 4

Treatment Strategies

19

Specific Immunotherapy and Central Immune System

Celso Pereira, Graça Loureiro, Beatriz Tavares and Filomena Botelho
Immunoallergology Department, Coimbra University Hospital, Portugal

1. Introduction

Despite the current knowledge, the mechanisms by which the specific immunotherapy (SIT) achieves clinical improvement remains unclear. However, it is now clear that the immune tolerance is one of the major targets of this kind of treatment. Immune tolerance depends on different mechanisms, including T-cell anergy, T-cell depletion by apoptosis, and active immune suppression (Akdis & Akdis, 2011). One of the goals of SIT is the induction of tolerance to allergens to which the patient is sensitized. IL-10 is probably a relevant cytokine induced by this treatment and is associated to regulatory T cells (T-regs) that actively control or suppress the function of other cells, generally in an inhibitory pattern (Frew, 2010).

The changes in microenvironment due to the decrease in histamine and PGE2 release by mast cell, and the IL-10 and TGF-β release by dendritic cells (DC) could switch the T-cell population into T-regs. These alterations will then lead to tolerance (Schmidt-Weber & Blaser 2005).

Much of the knowledge about SIT has been based on studies using subcutaneous route of administration (SCIT), but increasing data is now available based on studies using sublingual immunotherapy (SLIT).

The sublingual mucosa, where the deposition of the extract occurs, has very particular characteristics, quite different from the cellular subcutaneous tissue. The dendritic cells present in the buccal region are distinct from the Langerhans cells present in the skin. These cells present, constitutively, receptors with high affinity for IgE, $Fc\varepsilon RI^+$, MHC class I and II molecules, as well as co-stimulation molecules, namely CD40, CD80/B7.1 and CD86/B7.2 (Allam et al., 2006). There is also expression of CD14, a lipopolysaccharide (LPS) receptor, which is relevant for the modulation of Th2 and Th1.

In SLIT, the allergen is captured by the DC cell by *C-lectin* endocytosis receptors and/or by ligation to the IgE on the surface. After the internalization, the migration to the regional lymphoid nodules occurs, and it is then presented to the T cells (Geijtenbeek, 2006). A study that compares the DC population in the oral and nasal mucosa was able to demonstrate that only the DC myeloid type is profusely present in the oral region, in contrast with the nasal mucosa where both populations are present (Allam et al., 2006). Another very important difference is the high expression levels of FcεRI in the oral mucosa, which is almost absent in the skin's Langerhans cells (Allam et al., 2003). Furthermore, the expression levels of MHC class I and II molecules, CD40, CD80 and CD86 is significantly higher in oral DC than in the skin.

The integrity of the lamina propria in the oral mucosa, along with the highly reduced population of mast cells, eosinophils and basophils, are the factors that limit the contact of the allergen with submucosal areas or with circulating blood cells. All of these together constitute the excellent security profile characteristic of the SLIT (Moingeon et al., 2006). The DC seems to be crucial in the induction of the tolerance profile due to the production of IL-10 and TGF-β after activation, as well as an increase in indoleamine dioxygenase type 2 (IDO), necessary to the decrease in T cells proliferation.

The allergen absorption through the intact mucosa and the interaction with local dendritic cells could switch on the process leading to immune-tolerance. In addition to the local effect, the swallowed allergen could induce a supplementary outcome based on a GALT-related mechanism (Akdis et al., 2001). In fact, the first method of sublingual administration of SIT, in which the allergen was spat out, was significantly less effective. Most of the immunological changes and mechanisms that occur with sublingual administration of high allergen dosage have been recently demonstrated (Moingeon et al., 2006).

The aqueous extracts are highly effective, but induce more side-effects (local and systemic) than depot and modified vaccines (Larché et al., 2006). These have been developed in an attempt to reduce or remove allergenicity, while preserving or increasing the immunogenicity (Casanovas et al., 2005). Aqueous subcutaneous SIT is now the gold standard treatment for hymenoptera venom allergy and depot aeroallergen extracts for respiratory allergy (Wheeler & Woroniecki, 2004). The use of chemically modified allergens is not consensual. Although recent papers demonstrate a clinical benefit with allergoid therapy (Ibarrola et al., 2004), double blind placebo controlled studies comparing both extracts are still missing. On the other hand, the sublingual-swallowed administration of SIT in higher dosages had a clinical efficacy entirely demonstrated with similar immunological effects, namely the increase in allergen-blocking IgG, the induction of IgE-modulating $CD8^+$ T cells, the reduction of mast cells and eosinophils on the target mucosa, the decrease in inflammatory mediators, and a modulation on the inflammatory trafficking cells by reduced expression of adhesion molecules (Bousquet, 2006).

2. Kinetics of immunotherapy mechanism

The studies on the dynamics of SIT are of extreme relevance, because they represent the only approach available to define, on a biological point of view, the mechanism by which the therapeutics works. Despite the current advances contributing to the wide knowledge of the modulator effect, these studies are extremely rare, as a result of several ethical, technical and economical boundaries. Furthermore, there are also several difficulties in transposing the results from experimental studies using laboratory animals to Humans.

In a study using mice, the systemic activity of a modified aeroallergen, an allergoid administrated sublingually, was shown (Mistrello, 1994). However, before the study of an Italian group from Genoa in 1997, the kinetics and dynamics of the allergen in Humans was not known (Bagnasco, 1997). This study had the merit of assessing the response of the sublingual administration of a radioactively labeled allergen in a group of 9 healthy individuals (Bagnasco, 1997). *Par j* 1, the major *Parietaria judaica* allergen, was labeled with ^{123}I. In respect to the sublingual route, the application and deposition of the labeled allergen in 3 individuals was monitored for a period of 30 minutes before deglutition, by the acquisition of static images in the following 1, 2, 3, 5, 24 and 48 hours. In parallel, blood draws were collected for the determination of the radioactive counts at 5, 10, 20, 30 and 60 minutes, and then at 2, 3, 5 and 24 hours after the administration. A quantification of the same parameters in the urine was also performed. This study was able to demonstrate that the allergen was not degraded by the saliva and interestingly that there was no absorption by the sublingual mucosa.

The plasma radioactive activity only occurs after the deglutition of the allergen. Another surprising fact is that an enormous radioactive activity of the labeled allergen in the sublingual region is still detected, even after 48hours and despite the deglutition. Furthermore, the study also compared the same methodology either with nasal and oral (immediate deglutition) administration. The results from the application of the allergen in a nasal pulverization demonstrated activity in the superior region of the pharynx and proximal esophagus, and persistence of the labeled allergen until 36hours, with no bronchial deposition, but having activity in the plasma since the beginning. The oral route is simultaneous to the detection of immediate activity in the plasma, characterized by a pick at 2hours, followed by a decline, but with no identification of the labeled allergen. Probably there is protein degradation and only small peptides are absorbed at the level on the intestinal mucosa.

These results, done afterwards by the same group and obtained from healthy individuals, were crucial for the evaluation of the kinetics and dynamics of the allergen administration in 9 allergic patients with rhinitis (Bagnasco, 2001). The study compared the different alternatives of sublingual administration of the *Par j* 1 allergen labeled with ^{123}I. Namely non-modified allergen solution (drops), non-modified allergen in pills and modified allergen (allergoid) also in pills. The patients were monitored with dynamic acquisition in the first 20 minutes and static acquisitions of 5 minutes every hour until the 16th hour. Serial blood draws were also collected in order to quantify the radioactive plasmatic activity. The results confirmed persistent radioactive activity at the local of the administration of the allergen. For all the extracts, the plasmatic activity only occurs after deglutition. With the allergoid, the activity is higher, probably dependent of a lower enzymatic degradation and consequent lower possibility of intestinal absorption. The acquisitions in a gamma-rays camera only visualizes the activity after deglutition (1-5 minutes later), in the pharyngeal and esophagic region.

The same group of investigators studied the kinetics of the intranasal administration of *Par j* 1 labeled with ^{123}I in a group of 3 patients with allergic rhinitis, using a similar methodology although with distinct time points (Passalacqua, 2005). The radioactive activity in the nasal region disappears rapidly in allergic patients when compared to healthy individuals. The clinic inflammation controlled by the administration of the therapeutic allergen in these patients may condition an increase in the depuration or clearance of the mucosa. Plasmatic activity is also observed after an effective deglutition of the allergen. Despite the reduced number of patients used to conducted this study, the results are significantly distinct from the results observed when using the sublingual route, in which the radioactive activity persist at the local of administration, long after the deglutition of the therapeutic extract (Bagnasco, 2001).

The same Italian group responsible for the study with allergens administrated by non-injectable routes prompt the question of whether the results obtained up until that moment were restricted to specific characteristics of *Parietaria judaica*. Following this, the group published another study using a major allergen from *Dermatophagoides pteronyssinus*, the *Der p* 2 (Bagnasco, 2005). For the 7 patients with allergic rhinitis, the results were analogous to the ones mentioned above. This lead to the conclusion that the persistence of the radioactive activity at the local of administration of the allergen and the systemic absorption after the

deglutition is independent of the allergen used in the treatment and the chemical modification used.
The studies regarding the kinetics and dynamics of immune-therapy administrated by non-injectable routes were pioneer, even though its implementation was substantially more recent than conventional route, and interestingly they included the nasal route, which had no scientific validation for its efficacy (Bousquet, 1998; Alvarez-Cuesta, 2006). In respect to the subcutaneous route, our group has published in 2004 the first *in vivo* results regarding the dynamics of SIT in patients with allergic disease (Pereira, 2004).

3. Dynamics of the immunotherapy mechanism

The radioactive labeling of an allergen from the therapeutic extract is possible, but it would be restricted, exclusively, to one protein only. This could have been a strategy to evaluate the dynamics of the biological response to SIT. However, for patients under a maintenance treatment, the exclusion of some allergenic epitopes present in the therapeutic extracts would condition the interpretation of the results. Furthermore, it could, eventually, change the immunogenic structure of that epitope and as a consequence, the immune response that was induced. In these studies, the administration of the allergen extract, according to the maintenance scheme in place for each patient, would occur simultaneously with the reinjection of leucocytes labeled with ^{99m}Tc-HMPAO. The labeling of leucocytes with ^{99m}Tc-HMPAO is a technique that, on the theoretical level, has affinity for all the cellular elements of the white series (mononuclear and polymorphonuclear) and all of these have a specific contribution in the inflammatory process (Kumar, 2005; Peters, 1986).
The therapeutic allergenic extract injections always induce an inflammatory reaction at the local of the administration, detectable clinically by the presence of typical local signals. In the maintenance treatment, these symptoms have variable intensity and depend not only on the type of extract but also on the severity of the basal clinical features (Alvarez-Cuesta et al., 2006). The modified extracts and the extracts administrated sublingually are the ones that induce minor local secondary effects, as mentioned before. Therefore, although in a limited and controlled way, the SIT leads to an effective inflammatory allergic reaction in the area where the extract is applied, despite all the relevant immune-modulator mechanisms, which at the moment are well established for this therapeutic.
This local inflammatory allergic reaction will be, presumably, responsible by the dynamics of a response highly similar to the one observed in the allergic response in general (Pereira, 2009). Therefore, it can be admitted that the autologous reinjection of leucocytes will have a migration at that level by mechanisms dependent on the IgE-mediated mast cells activation (Bousquet, 1998; Alvarez-Cuesta et al., 2006).

3.1 Patients studied

Seventeen adult volunteer allergic patients were selected, 15 of them under maintenance therapeutic with specific immunotherapy. All were under a regular and programmed follow-up at the Immunoallergology department for the treatment of allergic pathology: respiratory allergy (bronchial asthma and rhinitis) and anaphylaxis (latex or hymenoptera venom). Until the date of selection of the patients, this treatment scheme has demonstrated clinical efficacy, translated by the complete remission of the symptoms, absent regular and preventive anti-allergic medication, no need of symptomatic medication in periods of worsening of the symptoms. Along with these criteria, it was also taken into account the favorable evolution of the laboratory parameters, namely reduction of the cutaneous reactivity to the responsible allergen by allergic diathesis in cutaneous prick tests using standardized extracts, and the reduction in the levels of the serum specific IgE, relatively to the beginning of the treatment. For the study of the dynamics of this therapeutic, samples from patients using different routes of administration of SIT and different allergenic extracts were also included. Patients were selected according to the type of allergen extract and route of administration of the SIT (Table 1).

Subcutaneous Administration Route		
	Aqueous subcutaneous extract (anaphylaxis)	
		4 patients: latex extract
		2 patients: Apis mellifera extract
	Subcutaneous depot extract (respiratory allergy)	
		2 patients: D pteronyssinus extract
		2 patients: pollen from Poaceae extract
	Subcutaneous modified allergen extract (respiratory allergy)	
		1 patient: pollen from Poaceae extract
		1 patient: pollen from Parietaria judaica extract
Sublingual Administration Route (respiratory allergy)		
	2 patients: D pteronyssinus extract	
	1 patient: pollen from Parietaria judaica extract	

Table 1. Patients under a specific immunotherapy treatment (extract, route of administration and allergic disease)

The control group included 2 patients allergic to *Dermatophagoides pteronyssinus*, with asthma and rhinitis, non-submitted to SIT and controlled with daily inhaled corticotherapy (fluticasone furoate). None of the selected patients presented any other concomitant pathology, namely inflammatory, which could interfere with the interpretation of the results. Furthermore, neither of the patients was under any other medication, besides the ones mentioned. All female patients were submitted to a quick urinary test to exclude pregnancy. All the studies were conducted under strict hospital vigilance, and the day of the immunotherapy administration was exactly the one previously defined in the maintenance therapeutic scheme. This study was, obviously, submitted for the approval of the Ethics Committee of the Institution, according to the "Declaration of Helsinki" of the World Medical Association (Helsinki 1964; Tokyo 1975; Venice 1983; Hong-Kong 1989).

3.2 Methodology for this study

A standard technique was used for the labeling of circulating leucocytes with ^{99m}Tc-HMPAO (Peters, 1986).

The allergen extracts used in the patients with subcutaneous immunotherapy (aqueous and depot) or submitted to sublingual *Dermatophagoides pteronyssinus* treatment were produced by the ALK-Abelló Laboratory (Madrid, Spain). For another patient in SLIT, the *Parietaria judaica* extract was provided by the Stallergenes Laboratory (Paris-France). In respect to the SCIT with modified extracts (allergoid), the glutaraldehyde-modified extract from pollens of

Poaceae was supplied by BIAL-Aristegui Laboratory (Bilbao, Spain) and the *Parietaria judaica* extract modified by depigmentation was provided by the Leti Laboratory (Madrid, Spain).
The maintenance dosage to which the patients were submitted on the day of the study corresponded to the one established on their treatment scheme, and was administrated on the pre-defined schedule. Two controls non-submitted to SIT with respiratory allergy to *Dermatophagoides pteronyssinus* were also studied. They were submitted, respectively to:
-0,5cc of bacterial aqueous extract by the subcutaneous route, immune stimulant inductor of a IgG response (Ribomunyl ®, Pierre Fabre Médicament, France), containing ribosomal fractions of *Klebsiella pneumoniae, Streptococcus pneumoniae, Streptococcus pyogenes, Haemophilus influenzae* and membrane fractions of *Klebsiella pneumoniae.*
-0,5cc of phenolated aqueous solution administrated by the subcutaneous route, diluting the solution from the ALK-Abelló Laboratory (Madrid, Spain).
Patients were positioned in dorsal decubitus, under a gamma camera. The puncture of the cubital vein with a caliber 14 catheter allowed the reinjection of the autologous leucocytes labeled with a radio-labeled pharmaceutical compound in fast bolus, followed by a venous wash with physiological serum. Simultaneously, the allergenic extract was administrated subcutaneously, according to the usual technique (Bousquet et al., 1998) in the external surface of the arm contralateral to the administration of the labeled cells. Both injections occurred at the same time, simultaneously to the beginning of the scintigraphic acquisition.
The 3 allergic patients submitted to SLIT were placed in dorsal decubitus under a gamma-rays camera, and drops containing the allergenic extract were administrated at the same time that the reinjection of radio labeled leucocytes in the cubital vein was performed. Three minutes later the allergen was swallowed, according to the usual protocol.
For the control group, the subcutaneous administration of the saline solution and the bacterial extract were performed the same way as for the patients in the active group.
In all the studies, the residual activity of the syringe containing the autologous cells that were reinjected was assessed, in order to quantify the radioactive dosage effectively administrated. The scintigraphic studies were performed under a gamma rays camera (GE XR, Milwaukee, USA) using a low energy and parallel cavities collimator coupled to a Camstar acquisition unity and to a eNTEGRA processing unity. The dynamic acquisition was obtained in an anterior side view of the head and neck to 64x64 resolution matrixes during 60 minutes (120 images x 30 seconds), followed by a static study at 60, 120, 180, 240, 300 and 360 minutes after the administration of the allergen and leucocytes labeled with ^{99m}Tc-HMPAO, during 5 minutes for each acquisition (256 x 256 resolution elements). The static images were obtained in anterior and posterior side views for the following projections: head and neck, thorax and abdomen. During the acquisitions, patients were asked to remain at rest, despite the induction of nasal symptoms, in order to maintain the geometry of the projections, and at the same time minimizing the distance to the detector.
A qualitative evaluation of the images obtained in the dynamic acquisition was then performed, either by sequential analysis or using a video of 120 images. The moment in which the activity in the nasal region started was determined, as well as the local of the administration and the subsequent focalizations of the inflammatory activity that was induced. In the same way, a qualitative evaluation of the focalized inflammatory activity on defined timings for the static acquisition was performed. For the quantitative results, a different approach was chosen, in respect to the type of image in study. For the dynamic images obtained from the head and neck, the regions of interest were drawn (ROIs, *region of interest*) at the local of the administration of the allergen extract and /or controls, the *background* area (muscle) and also the following areas: oropharynx, cranial calotte and

cervical lateral-external region of the neck. The dynamic acquisition was obtained in anterior view of the thorax and neck for matrixes with a resolution of 64 x 64 elements, during 60 minutes (120 images x 30 seconds), followed by a static study at 60, 120, 180, 240, 300 and 360 minutes for 5 minutes each acquisition (256 x 256 elements of resolution), after the administration of leucocytes labeled with ^{99m}Tc-HMPAO and the therapeutic allergen. The static images were obtained in anterior and posterior view for the thoracic projection and in anterior view for the abdominal projection.

A qualitative study of the images obtained in dynamic acquisition was then conducted by a sequential analysis or in a video of 120 images. The moment of the beginning of the activity at the local of the administration of the extract and in subsequent focalizations of the inflammatory activity that was induced was then determined. In the same way, a qualitative evaluation of the inflammatory activity focalized at defined timings for the static acquisition was performed. For the quantitative analysis a different approach was taken, regarding the type of image in study. For the dynamic thoracic images, ROIs were draw at the local of administration of the allergen and/or controls, as well as in the *background* area (muscle) and in possible focalizations (cervical, armpit and thoracic). For each ROI the total values, the average per pixel and the maximum values were determined. The uptake coefficient (UC, *uptake coefficient* ROI) was then calculated as the ratio between the maximum measurements of each ROI and the average value in the background area. For a best accuracy of the results it was also calculated the corrected uptake coefficient (UCC, *corrected uptake coefficient* ROI) by subtracting the uptake coefficient ROI in the background from the uptake coefficient ROI for each of the areas analyzed.

3.3 Results

The qualitative and quantitative results from patients submitted to specific treatment will be presented.

3.3.1 Qualitative results

All images from patients submitted to SIT were interpreted by analyzing the images with the same color scale, Figure 1. These crescent colors (from black to white) translate the inflammatory activity induced by the therapeutic action.

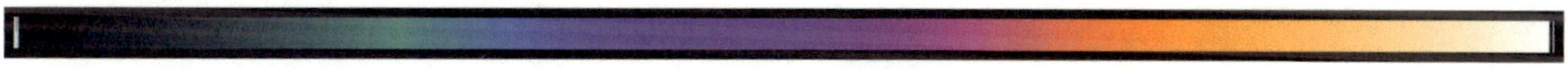

Fig. 1. Color scale from minimum activity (black) to maximum activity (white).

The studies regarding each type of SIT in analysis, namely regarding the type of extract and route of administration, are presented here (Figures 2 - 7). Besides the static images for the acquisitions of the thoracic and abdominal side view of each of the exemplified patients, an image from the dynamic sequence corresponding to the time point in which the beginning of the anti-inflammatory activity is observed at the site of administration of the extract will be presented. Furthermore, images obtained from two control patients will also be presented, namely with administration of a saline phenolated solution (SS) and a bacterial extract (BE). In all the studies the hepatosplenic region should be considered as an image of subtraction that should not be taken into account or interpreted. The spleen since it sequesters labeled erythrocytes, even though at residual levels, but always present in the pellet of isolated cells; the liver because it represents the preferential location for metabolization of the radio labeled pharmaceutical compound.

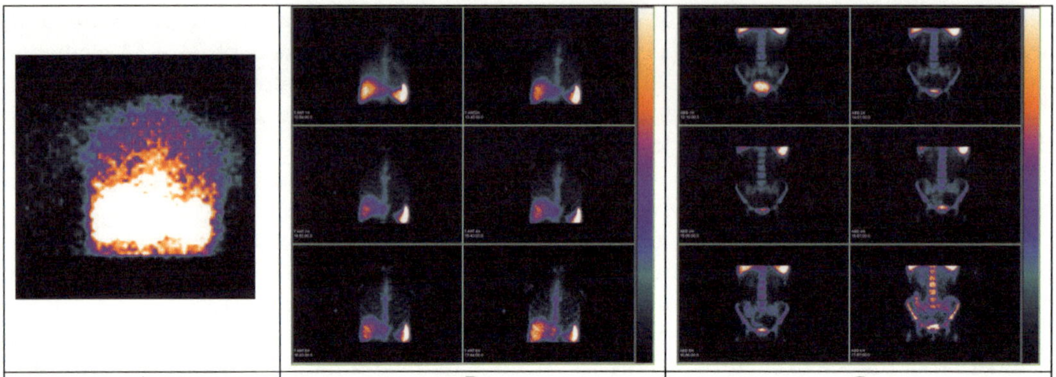

A B C

Fig. 2. Scintigraphic study of patient C1, control, with respiratory allergy to *Dermatophagoides pteronyssinus*, submitted to subcutaneous injection with bacterial extracts. Panel A shows the beginning of the activity at the external side of the arm after 45 minutes. Panels B and C show, respectively, thoracic and abdominal static acquisitions, in an anterior view.

For patient C1, submitted to subcutaneous injection with bacterial extract (BE), at 45 minutes we can observe inflammatory activity focalized at the site of administration. Furthermore, we observe focalizations, in the static studies, with inflammatory activity in bone structures (humeral head and iliac crest), as well as in the suprasternal region. The activity observed in the sternum and spinal cord (in anterior side view, not shown) should be interpreted with caution since there are superimposed structures with potential involvement. We do not observe intrapulmonary or intra-abdominal (intestinal) focalizations.
Regarding patient C2, submitted to subcutaneous injection of phenolate saline solution (SS) in the external face of the right arm, we notice minimum activity 50 minutes after the injection. For the static acquisitions we also observe activity localized to the structures described.

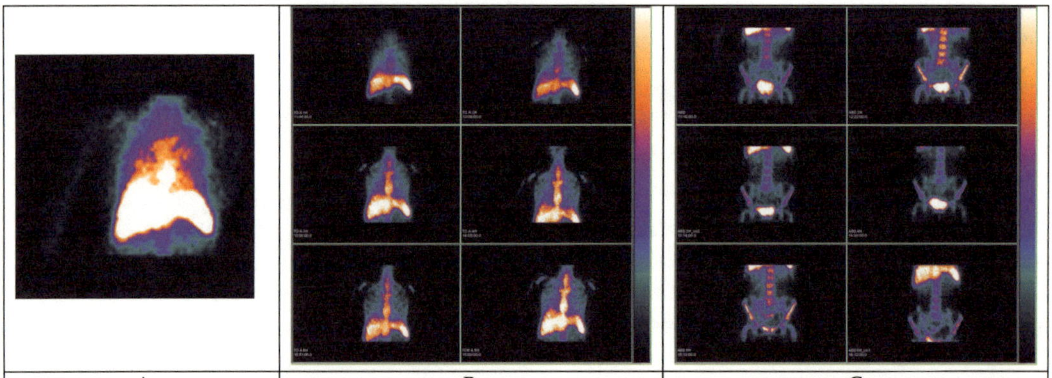

A B C

Fig. 3. Scintigraphic study of patient C2, control, with respiratory allergy to *Dermatophagoides pteronyssinus*, submitted to subcutaneous injection with phenolate saline solution. Panel A shows the beginning of the activity at the external side of the arm after 50 minutes. Panel Panels B and C show, respectively, thoracic and abdominal static acquisitions, in an anterior view.

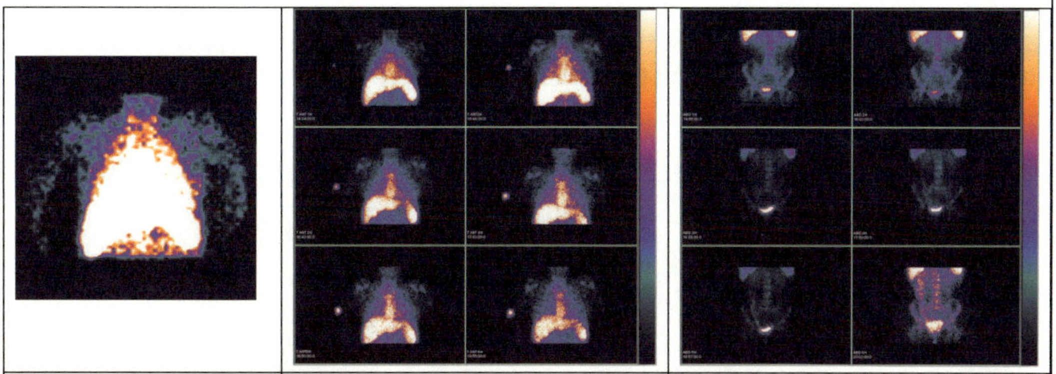

Fig. 4. Scintigraphic study of patient 6 (anaphylaxis to *Apis mellifera*), submitted to subcutaneous injection with aqueous extract. Panel A shows the beginning of the activity at the external side of the arm after 35 minutes. Panel Panels B and C show, respectively, thoracic and abdominal static acquisitions, in an anterior view.

For the patient (Figure 4), under treatment for anaphylaxis to hymenoptera venom, we observe inflammatory activity earlier at the local of administration of the therapeutic allergen extract, but the systemic involvement is also observed in all of the posterior scintigraphic images. Higher activity was detected in the bone structures, when compared to patient 3 with anaphylaxis to latex. We did not detect intra-abdominal (intestinal) focalizations in this patient. For these patients, as well as for all the other studies, the sternum bone structures and spinal cord will not be interpreted because of all the reasons already discussed.

For the patient allergic to pollens (Figure 5), the beginning of the inflammatory activity was detected at 35 minutes on the site of administration of the therapeutic extract. A systemic involvement in all the acquisitions was observed. In the armpit homolateral to the injection of the extract, we detect activity that persists throughout the study, similar to what happened in the cervical-lateral region of the neck. In the intestinal area we only observe focalizations at 60 and 120 minutes.

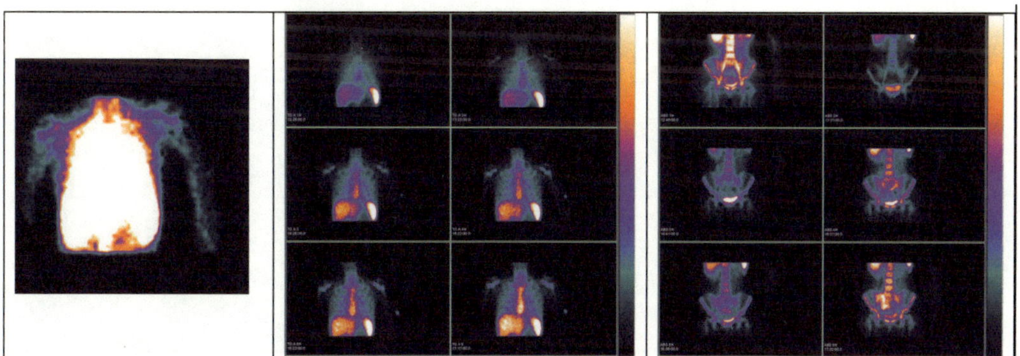

Fig. 5. Scintigraphic study of patient 8 with respiratory allergy (asthma and rhinitis) to grass pollen submitted to subcutaneous injection with depot extract. Panel A shows the beginning of the activity at the external side of the arm after 35 minutes. Panel Panels B and C show, respectively, thoracic and abdominal static acquisitions, in an anterior view.

For patient on figure 6, the inflammatory activity at the site of administration of the allergoid extract is highly reduced, when compared to the patients previously described. The systemic activity persists in all the structures considered, including the intra-abdominal area, from minute 60 to 120.

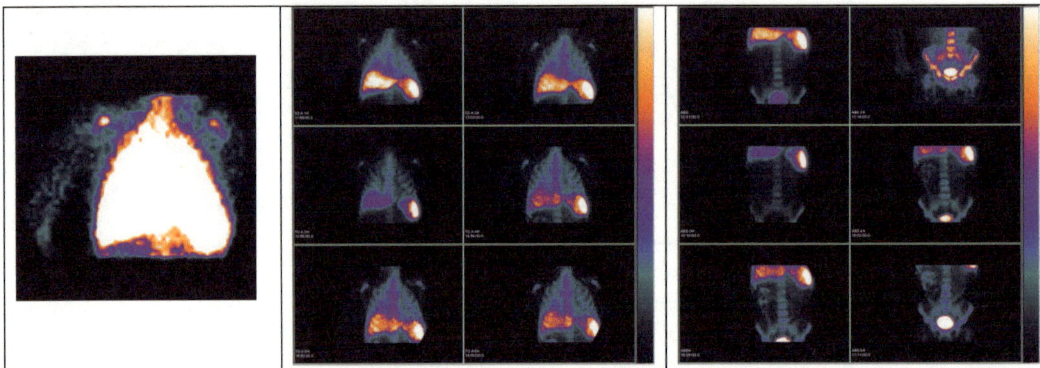

A	B	C

Fig. 6. Scintigraphic study of patient 11 with respiratory allergy (asthma and rhinitis) to grass pollens, submitted to subcutaneous injection of a glutaraldehyde modified extract. Panel A shows the beginning of the activity at the external side of the arm after 50 minutes. Panel Panels B and C show, respectively, thoracic and abdominal static acquisitions, in an anterior view.

The SLIT administration induced a very precocious beginning of activity when compared to the subcutaneous route. Patient from Figure 7, submitted to treatment with *D pt* extract, the inflammatory activity in the oropharynx occurred 3 minutes after the administration of the drop extract. We also observed a more relevant involvement of the cervical-lateral structures of the neck, which persisted throughout the trial. The systemic involvement was also present in this patient in different structures: intrapulmonary, bones and suprasternal region.

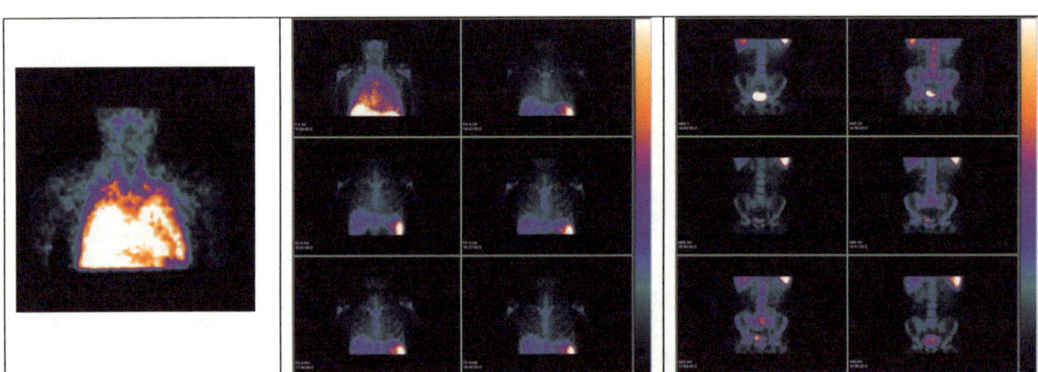

A	B	C

Fig. 7. Scintigraphic study of patient 13, with respiratory allergy (asthma and rhinitis) to *Dermatophagoides pteronyssinus*, submitted to sublingual administration. Panel A shows the beginning of the activity in the oral region after 3 minutes. Panel Panels B and C show, respectively, thoracic and abdominal static acquisitions, in an anterior view.

3.3.2 Quantitative analysis

All the scintigraphic studies were submitted to a quantitative evaluation in order to determine the corrected uptake coefficients. ROIs were draw in the areas with focalized activity, which included: local of administration of the allergenic extract, suprasternal region, humerus head and iliac crest. Besides this, every time intra-abdominal (intestinal) focalizations were present, the respective UCCs were calculated. Naturally, for each projection a ROI in the muscle area was draw, representing the background area.

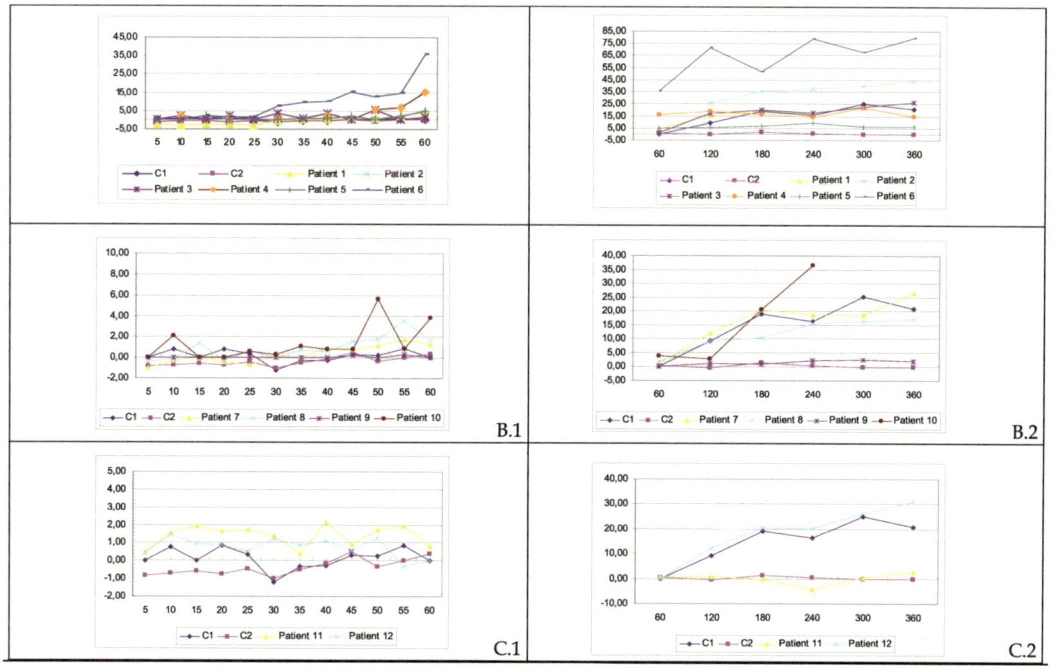

Fig. 8. Corrected uptake coefficients in the region of the administration of the allergenic therapeutic extract for the subcutaneous injectable treatments (1. Dynamic; 2. Static) throughout the study (expressed in minutes). A: aqueous extracts; B: depot extracts; C: chemically modified extracts (allergoid).

The beginning of the inflammatory activity for patients submitted to SCIT was different between the groups of patients in this study. The aqueous extracts for the treatment of anaphylaxis were the ones that induced higher UCCs, both in the dynamic and static evaluations. However, for the same type of extract, it seems that there are no relevant differences in respect to the type of allergen in the treatment, Figure 8.

Patients under treatment with the depot extracts showed intermediate levels between patients with aqueous extracts and allergoid. However, we should emphasize that a patient under depot extracts to dust mites showed a highly reduced UCC at the spot of the therapeutic injection, as well as a patient under treatment with pollinic extract modified with glutaraldehyde. The control patient submitted to BE, showed very significant UCCs at the local of administration in the evaluations made after the first 60 minutes. On the other side, for the patient submitted to SS, the quantification of the activity at the local of injection persisted always in much reduced levels.

For patients submitted to treatment with SLIT, the inflammatory activity is detected very early in the process, and persists throughout time at relatively constant levels, Figure 9. The patients allergic to dust mites showed higher levels when compared to the patient allergic to *Parietaria judaica*. However, for this patient, the study took place during the pollinic period, and therefore a reduced therapeutic dosage was administrated, which can justify, eventually, the results obtained.

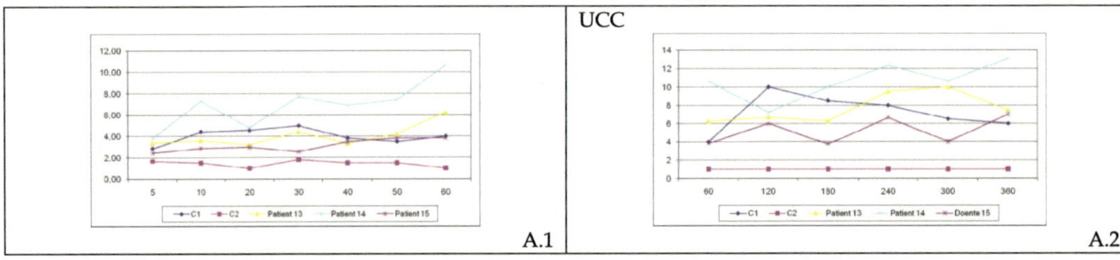

Fig. 9. Corrected uptake coefficients in the region of the administration of the sublingual allergenic therapeutic extract throughout the study (expressed in minutes). 1. Dynamic; 2. Static

The area located above the sternal furcula presented an early inflammatory activity, even during the dynamic studies. Since this region includes an extremely rich set of vascular structures, the effect of leukocyte recirculation maintained in the beginning of the study cannot be excluded. Therefore, it was decided to only evaluate the coefficients acquired with the static studies, Figure 10. Globally, the results are substantially higher than the control patient submitted to SS injection. Furthermore, it was also observed a slow increase during the experiment.

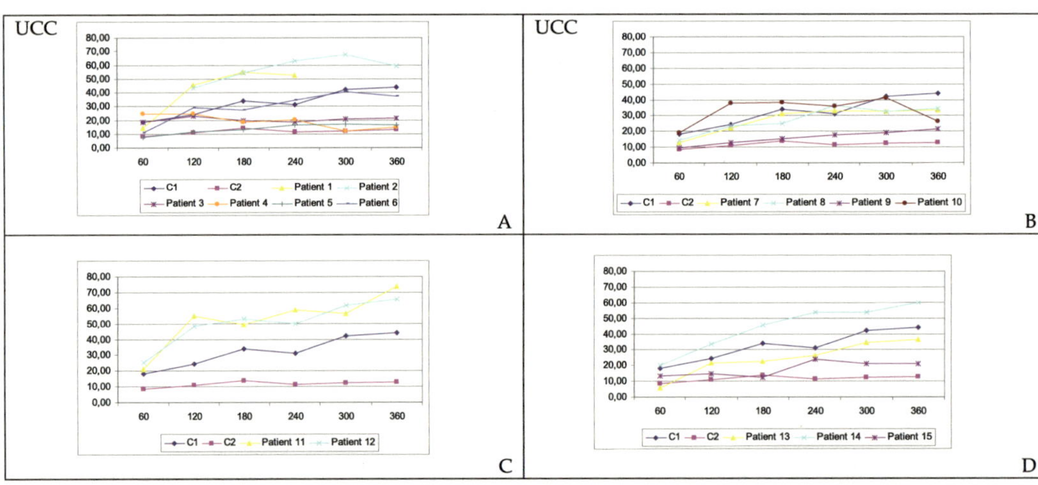

Fig. 10. Corrected uptake coefficients, taken at different time points during the experiment (minutes), obtained in the suprasternal region after the administration of the therapeutic extract. A: aqueous extracts; B: depot extracts; C: chemically modified extracts (allergoid); D: sublingual extracts

The evaluation of the UCCs in the bone structures localized in the humeral head and iliac crest was then performed, exclusively for static acquisitions, Figure 11.

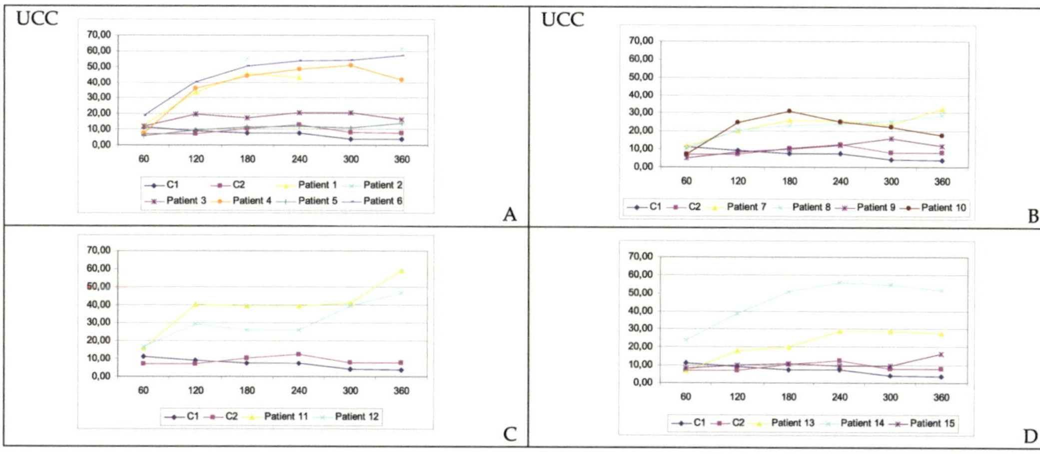

Fig. 11. Corrected uptake coefficients, taken at different time points during the experiment (minutes), obtained in the iliac crest after the administration of the therapeutic extract. A: aqueous extracts; B: depot extracts; C; chemically modified extracts (allergoid); D: sublingual extracts

The coefficients obtained in the two bone structures were similar and, globally, there was an apparent progressive increase throughout the experiment. However, regarding the type of extract and the method of administration, there wasn't a characteristic profile of the inflammatory activity in these structures. For the motives previously expressed, no other bone focalizations were considered.

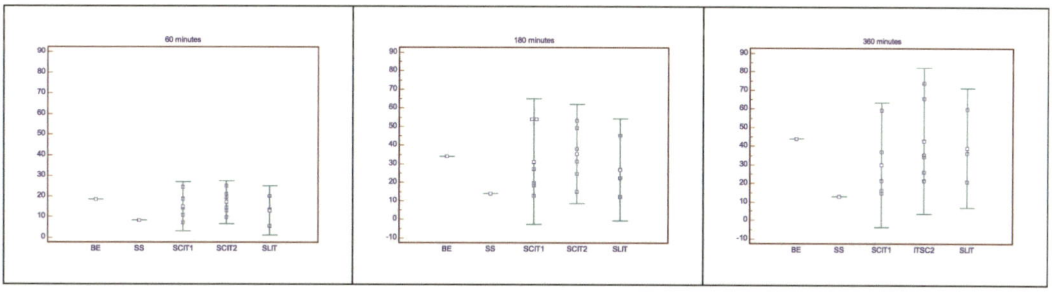

Fig. 12. Comparative results of the UCC obtained for the suprasternal of patients submitted to aqueous extracts (SCIT1) for the treatment of anaphylaxis; depot and allergoid extracts (SCIT2) for the treatment of respiratory allergy and sublingual aqueous extracts (SLIT), also for the treatment of respiratory allergy. The results obtained for control patients submitted to injection of bacterial extract (BE) or phenolated saline solution (SS). For all patients, samples were collected at 60, 180 and 360 minutes.

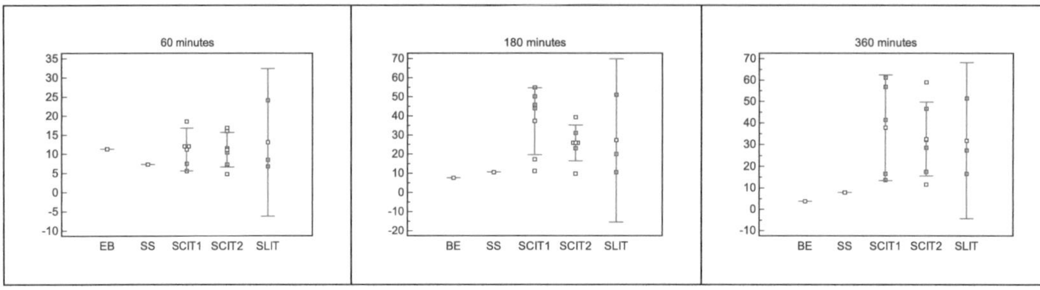

Fig. 13. Comparative results of the UCC obtained for the iliac crest of patients submitted to aqueous extracts (SCIT1) for the treatment of anaphylaxis; depot and alergoids extracts (SCIT2) for the treatment of respiratory allergy and sublingual aqueous extracts (SLIT), also for the treatment of respiratory allergy. The results obtained for control patients submitted to injection of bacterial extract (BE) or phenolated saline solution (SS). For all patients, samples were collected at 60, 180 and 360 minutes.

In the inflammatory focalization dependent of the ROI from the suprasternal region, no prevalence for a type of extract or method of administration of the treatment seems to exist, Figure 12. Similarly, it can be observed an increase in UCCs throughout the experiment. The same considerations can be applied to the inflammatory activity induced in the iliac crest, Figure 13.

3.4 Discussion

The administration of an allergenic therapeutical extract induces, always, an inflammatory reaction at the administration site that is characterized by the presence of clinically validated local symptoms. The modified extracts and the extracts delivered sublingually are the ones that induced lower secondary effects, as previously described. Although the main immunomodulator mechanism is already well established in SIT, it can dictate, in a limited and controlled approach, the effective inflammatory allergic reaction at the administration site. Therefore, we can admit that the autologous reinjection of leucocytes will have a migration dependent of the mast cell activation mediated by IgE (Togias, 2004; Kelly, 2007). This local inflammatory allergic reaction is, presumably, responsible for the dynamics of a response similar to allergy. Regarding the lymphocyte population, the circulatory migration to the tissue where the specific allergic reaction took place, is mediated by the expression of specific adhesion molecules that specify the type of cell implicated in the migration to the tissue (Togias, 2004). The migration of Th2 cells is associated to the expression of VCAM-1 and P-selectin, under effect of IL-4 and IL-13, that depends on the activation of lymphocyte transduction signals by transcription factors similar to STAT6 (Lukacs, 2000). On the other hand, the migration of Th1 cells seems to be dependent on the expression of STAT4, due to the effect of IL-12, and associated to the RANTES and ICAM-1 mechanism. In an interesting study with intradermic injection of allergenic peptides without the ability to induce an IgE response, it was possible to observe lymphocyte trafficking from the vascular department (Haselden, 1999). Also, the intervention of T-reg cell in the mechanisms of immunomodulation of SIT are well established either by inducing the population of Th1 cells or reducing the number of Th2 (Woodfolk, 2007; Francis, 2003).
Nevertheless, in these cells, it is not clear which is the specificity towards the allergen or what is the eligibility of the method of the induction (systemic or inhaled). Furthermore, it

was also not clear what is the dosage required for induction or what type of regulatory cells are induced (natural T-reg produced by the thymus and with an effect dependent of cellular contact or adaptive T-reg cells induced on the periphery and with the effect dependent of IL-10 or TGF-β) (Woodfolk, 2007). At the same time, other lymphocytes, such as $CD8^+$ e NKT cells, have the ability to respond to the allergen and represent other vectors involved in the SIT mechanisms (Woodfolk, 2007, Agea, 2005)).

As previously mentioned, DCs are considered central cells in inflammation and immune tolerance often reported in the SIT mechanisms. These cells represent the antigen presenting cells (APC) that, after migrating to the regional lymph node, induce an effective and differentiated immune response. Nevertheless, this is a very heterogeneous and diversified population, ubiquitously present, although in a reduced number when compared to other resident or circulation populations (von Bubnoff, 2002; Novak, 2004). Furthermore, it is known that myeloid DC cells can migrate from the blood to the tissues in order to capture antigens (Novak, 2004; Schmit-Weber, 2002, Allam, 2003). In specific situations, and under appropriated stimulus, the peripheral monocytes can differentiate into myeloid DC (von Bubnoff, 2002).

The skin and sublingual mucosa are, naturally, distinct. Therefore the mechanisms derived from the administration of the therapeutical allergenic extract should reflect this difference. The Langerhans cell (LC) is a DC myeloid cell (DC1) and are the most representative APCs in the skin. After a correct local stimulus, the monocyte chemotactic protein (MCP) determines the recruitment of LC progenitors from the bone marrow to the skin and the subsequent migration to the peripheral lymph nodes (Novak, 2004). The DC in the oral mucosa presents differences relatively to the skin, namely it expresses a higher number of MHCI and MCHII molecules, as well as the co-stimulation molecules CD40, CD80 and CD86 and also more FcγRIII (CD16), FcγRI (CD64) and FcεRI receptors (Allam, 2003). Several lymphoid structures are present in the oropharynx: tonsils, lymphatic ganglions and diffuse lymphoid tissue (Bienestock, 2005). It is well established that plasmacytoid DCs (DC2) are the APC most abundant in the Waldeyer's tonsillar ring and in the ganglion areas dependent on T cells, but that these cells are unable to effectively internalize the antigen (Novak, 2004). This is surely, a biologic characteristic of this region with consequences on the immune response on this area.

The subcutaneous tissue is, undoubtedly, composed by a population of resident cells that are biologically less active that the ones present in the oral mucosa. Nevertheless, the therapeutical administration of allergenic extracts by both ways has proven to be effective and able to induce an immunomodulator response in patients of IgE mediated allergy. This project did not intended to validate the efficacy of this therapy, broadly documented, but to study the dynamic of the resulting mechanism due to the administration of the therapeutical extract in patients maintained in the previously determined individual dosage. Theoretically, it would be extremely relevant to have monitored, under the same methodology, this treatment in different periods throughout the year, but the radioactive dosage accumulated would be ethically unacceptable.

In patients under subcutaneous injectable treatment, the anaphylaxis treatment with aqueous extracts induced the fastest signs of inflammatory activity in the administration site. The activity became visible 35 minutes after the administration, while with depot extracts, the activity was only visible between 40 and 45 minutes after the administration. In all patients, an increase in the intensity of the activities was observed throughout the observation period. The higher activity induced by the aqueous extracts did not translate into more exuberant clinical signs. The patients in SCIT to latex presented local clinical signs more pronounced than two patients allergic to *Apis*. In these two patients, the inflammatory activity was bigger and deeper, which can be explained by a higher amount of protein and the volume of extract administered.

In patients with respiratory allergy submitted to SCIT with depot extracts there were no evident differences connected to the extract composition, either mites or pollens.

Regarding the allergoid extracts, a reduced inflammatory activity was observed at the administration site, similarly to what was previously reported in the literature and demonstrated in daily clinical practice (Casanovas et al., 2005, 2007; Ariano et al., 1999). The modification of the allergenic with glutaraldehyde reduced the local inflammatory activity to levels similar to the ones observed in the control patients submitted to SS. In patient C1, asthmatic allergic to dust mites submitted to subcutaneous injection with BE, a local inflammatory activity was observed 45 minutes after the administration. This is an extract with immunomodulator activity, which induces the response of an IgG polyclonal antibody well documented in the literature (Clot, 1997). Although the local demonstration of activity was expected, the time necessary to observe activity was also extremely reduced.

The patient submitted to a phenolated solution presented a minimal local inflammatory activity only seen 60 minutes after the subcutaneous injection. Similarly to the patients studied in the previous chapter, it is considered that the irritation potential of this preservative can justify this result (Spiller et al., 1993).

In this study it was possible to assess and confirm the dynamics of the inflammation induced by the subcutaneous application of an allergenic extract. These results, although not surprising, were not unequivocally demonstrated, namely in terms of extension, depth of the adjacent region or evolution of the reaction along the course of the experiment. One advantage of the depot extracts when compared to the aqueous extracts, besides the safety profile, was the slower release of the allergenic protein (Wheeler & Woroniecki, 2004). In our patients we clearly observed a lower activity of these extracts, despite the fact that the patients with the aqueous extracts presented a worse level of basal allergic disease. The lymphocyte traffic seemed to be more intense and persistent with these extracts since the soluble allergenic is more readily available. In all patients submitted to SCIT, it is possible to observe systemic focalizations before the locally induced inflammatory activity. In the dynamic acquisition during the first 60 minutes, the anterior thoracic projection only permits to infer the potential activity in this view. In the intramedullary area of the humeral head is evident a significant intensity, surely dependent on the recirculation of cells representing all leukocyte cell populations.

In patients submitted to SCIT, the activity in bone structures and in thymic tissue presented a very intense activity that increased throughout the experiment. It should be noticed that these structures anatomically overlap to other organs from the central immune systems, but that in the peripheral immune lymphoid system, such as regional ganglion, and presumably in the region of the mediastinum, there is also evidence of activity. Furthermore, the mucosa immune system seems to be involved namely the pulmonary and less consistently the intestinal. The early involvement of the central lymphoid structures was an unexpected event, but was very consistent in all patients.

Obviously, with the methodology used it is not possible to determine the cell type and profile that is responsible by the activity induced by the migration from the circulation to a specific focalization. Nevertheless, given the actual knowledge regarding the mechanism that modulate this therapeutic, it is possible to admit that a diversified set of cells with different activation profiles and with divergent implications in the different structures.

The subcutaneous administration of the allergenic extract, particularly with aqueous extracts, defines an evident local inflammatory process. To this level, we admit that some conjunctive mast cells can be activated, although with limited intensity. As described in the literature, we also admit that the presence of conjunctive DCs, with IgE receptors, can favor this type of reaction. However, the most likely mechanism can depend on an effective presentation of the allergen to presenting cells and posterior migration to local-regional structures. This mechanism could explain the ganglion activity observed in the homolateral arm, with the involvement of other ganglion structures more distant, such as the ones present in the cervical lateral-external area.

On the other hand, we admit the influx from the circulation of DC or monocytes into the site of administration of the allergenic extract, since it is well known the ability of these cells to maturate into DCs or phagocytes. This dual mechanism, that simultaneously induce a biological defense from the aggression and favors an effective immune response, are probable local mechanisms. Therefore, the local administration of therapeutical allergens limits the local response that rapidly seems to have local-regional and systemic consequences. Probably, not only the biologic mediator produced *in situ*, as well as the following cell migration, presumably DCs, and the cellular limitations in venular structures in the proximity of the allergenic, allow the amplification of the systemic effect by mechanisms, possibly similar to the ones verified in the allergic reaction (Togias, 2004; Kelly, 2007).

The qualitative analysis of our SCIT patients corroborates, although indirectly, the complexity of the tolerance mechanisms, well described in the literature. The anatomic involvement of structures implicated with organs of the central immune system seems to sustain these effects. The activity observed in the bone marrow areas allow us to speculate that it could limit the modification of cellular profiles, namely lymphocyte, that has been documented in these patients (Denburg et al., 2000). Also, the demonstration of the contribution of regulatory cells can be sustained by our results given the involvement of the anatomic region reported to the thymic tissue, whose function persists throughout life (Arellano et al., 2006). Nevertheless, the pace of this process and the systemic involvement, evidenced by the focalization of the inflammatory activity, is clearly higher than expected, given the present knowledge. It should be noticed that this dynamic study evaluates, in a certain way, the biologic response in the whole organism. This contrasts with the usage of small biologic samples (such as tissues or humors), a procedure that is very common in most clinical and experimental studies.

We admit that the lungs are involved in the influx of leukocytes to the BALT, but it should be noticed that this is a preponderant location for the clinical symptoms that lead to treatment in patients with respiratory allergy.

In patients in SLIT, the beginning of the inflammatory activity in the site of administration was substantially earlier than the observed in patients in SCIT. In the two patients allergic to mites and in the patient allergic to *Parietaria judaica*, the activity was noticed 3 and 5 minutes after the respective induction. Despite this early onset of activity, no substantial differences were registered when the final results were compared, namely in the effects of regional or distant structures.

In fact, it seems evident that since the administration of the extract, a continuous increase of the local inflammatory activity as well as in cervical structures, particularly in the cervical lateral-external region. As described previously for SCIT patients, the venous recirculation at very early stages does not allow an effective validation of this effect, but the assessment in later periods, both in the dynamic or static acquisitions, there is an evident focalization in these cervical structures. For these patients, and with exception of the patient injected with extract modified with glutaraldehyde, and using the color scale, the intensity of the oropharynx is clearly inferior than the one verified in the injection site. Other clear difference, is the absence of a progressive increase of the inflammatory response focalized at the administration site verified in subsequent static evaluations. However, the systemic effect is very similar to the observed in patients under injectable treatment. We observe pulmonary focalizations as well as in regions reported to the organs from the immune central system. In these regions, the areas reported to the bones and in suprasternal, the images from the static studies support an increase of activity throughout the experiment.

In patients under SLIT, the extract was swallowed 3 minutes after the administration. It would be expected an intra-abdominal involvement, with intestinal focalizations. However, in none of these 3 patients that effect was observed. We admit that the extract can be completely degraded in the stomach, which would prevent an effect in the intestinal mucosa. Our results seem to corroborate the therapeutic inefficiency of the oral immunotherapy, which is not scientifically validated by the literature (Bousquet et al., 1998).

It is not possible to define and characterize the migrating population that focalizes in the distinct structures in patients under SLIT. Despite this, the available scientific knowledge allows us to assume that the allergenic persistence in the sublingual mucosa, as previously demonstrated (Bagnasco et al., 2005), allows the induction of the following immune response. As previously described, abundant lymphoid structures with specific biologic characteristics are present in this mucosa. The DC permits a fast transport to the tonsils and lymphatic ganglions in a magnitude that cannot be compared to the subcutaneous tissue. However, it is well established that the majority of DCs present in the tonsils are DC-2. These cells do not have the capacity to effectively internalize the allergenic protein and efficiently present it to the T-cell. Therefore, and although in smaller numbers, the DC-1 cells probably have a preponderant function. As a result, we admit that there might be an influx from the circulation of DC and monocytes, and that these, once in the mucosa, will differentiate and maturate. The early start of the activity will, presumably, result from the presence and availability of a biologically more active and diversified resident population. The reduced population of mast cells in the oral mucosa limits the local inflammatory response when compared to the subcutaneous administration. Therefore, and in theory, we can predict that the resulting mechanism derives from the activation of DCs and the presentation to lymphocytes in structures in the oral mucosa and that are dependent from the immune system. Thus, the therapeutical extract produces a powerful stimulus that initiates a local and systemic immune response, surely by regulating biologic mediators of cytokines and chemokines, as well as by limiting the entry of circulating cells from the vascular-lymphoid structures present in the oral mucosa.

The systemic effects in areas of the central immune system, similarly to what was observed for the injectable extracts, can corroborate the tolerance and immunomodulation, presently well documented in the therapeutical intervention.

In patients under injectable therapy, the UCCs results obtained in the homolateral armpit are higher that was expected by the exclusive visualization of the scintigraphic images. We admit that the results obtained in this focalization are, eventually, due to the migration of lymphatic cells from the administration site of the therapeutical extract to the ganglion structures present in the armpit region that allow a therapeutical amplification with natural systemic effect. In fact, functional studies in melanoma using a radio-labeled pharmaceutical compound administered intradermally evidenced the high rate of lymphatic migration to distant ganglion structures (Alazraki et al., 2002). Since the most important ganglion structures of the subcutaneous cellular tissue of the arm are located in the armpit, that the effective presentation of the allergenic protein to the T-cell in the lymph node is mediated by the DC and that the intralymphatic migration is very fast, the UCCs obtained in our patients are, probably, justified.

The eventual lymphatic migration proportions, are in fact, an amplification of the immune mechanism with characteristics that clearly favors tolerance. Therefore, it could lead not only to an effective diffusion of the response throughout the immune-lymphoid system, as well as a recirculation of cells from the allergenic administration site to distant central structures and organs that can allow the synergistic effects that concur with the immunomodulation of this therapy.

Therefore, the presumed ascending drainage justifies the precocious and persistent UCCs induced by the subcutaneous administration of the allergen in other vascular-lymphatic structures, anatomically located in the lateral-external region of the neck. Eventually, this process allows an amplification of the response to cervical structures with high biological activity. To this level, we do not observe significant differences of UCCs due to usage of different injectable extracts.

Although we verify focalization in the pulmonary region throughout the dynamic acquisition, we only calculated the coefficients in the static acquisition. The intense venous recirculation of leukocytes after the reinjection could falsify the results. However, all our patients presented intrapulmonary activity. Particularly in patients undergoing treatment for respiratory allergy, the influx of these cells to the targeted organ is compatible to the methods sensitivity. This way, the recirculation of leukocytes between the vascular compartment and the mucosa of the different organs of the immune system allow the convenient organic homeostasis that justifies the reduced numbers of pulmonary UCCs verified in control patients.

Given the results obtained in the patient submitted to BE, we presume that the unspecific bacterial immunomodulators have, besides favoring an IgG polyclonal response, a more central and selective regulator effect than the one presumed until now, but for which the clinically efficacy has been shown (Bousquet & Fiocchi, 2006). Regarding the patient allergic to dust mites submitted to SS injection, the reduced UCCs values were consistent throughout the experiment, and we presume that are derived from the organic recirculation of leukocytes, and correspond to the basal function of this tissue

The activity observed in the bone structures was confirmed by the UCCs calculated in the two considered ROIs. There were no differences in the results obtained in the medullary area of the humeral head or the iliac crest.

Our results suggest that either the bone marrow or the functional thymic tissue, organs from the central immune system, are preferential targets of the induction mechanism of SCIT, regardless of the type of allergenic extract. It should be noticed that in patients treated with modified extracts, allergoid, the dosage of allergenic used was substantially higher than the dosages in the depot extracts, and that the UCCs obtained in the regions associated with bone marrow were also higher. However, the size of the sample does not allow us to conclude if this treatment is more selective or effective. Nevertheless, we presume that given the previously described mechanisms, the bone marrow may participate in the SIT mechanism since earlier stages, right after the injection of the extracts.

In the suprasternal region, the UCCs were very similar in the different groups under active treatment and significantly distinct from the ones obtained in the patient submitted to SS injection. This data corroborates the eventual physiological dynamic of the leukocytes, possibly dependent of the persistent limitation of the medulla, even in cells apparently mature that were collected from the venous compartment.

In the intra-abdominal region, the UCCs obtained in the intestinal focalizations, observed occasionally in the scintigraphic images, confirmed the involvement of this mucosa. The calculations were only performed in focalizations areas during the first 4 hours, in order to minimize interferences due to faecal elimination.

For the three patients under sublingual treatment we do not have a control that we can compare to. Despite this, the values obtained in the asthma and rhinitis patients allergic to dust mites submitted to BE or SS in the nasal region (see previous chapter), are similar to the type of response verified in SLIT patients.

The capture and the inflammatory activity on the site of the administration of the therapeutic extract evidenced a very precocious activity that subdue in relatively high values throughout the experiment. These results are consistent with previously described dynamic studies (Bagnasco et al., 2005). The quantitative analysis does not evidence an increase of the local activity as seen in the majority of patients submitted to injectable extracts. In this mucosa, the presence of mast cells is extremely reduced which, despite the persistence of the extract (even after it was swallowed), does not induce a broader influx of circulating leukocytes due to this mechanism. Therefore, we presume that the much more limited activity observed can be due to circulating DCs and mast cells that have a recognized ability to mature and differentiate in the offended tissues. The readily availability of immune-lymphoid tissue in this localization will allow a fast amplification and dissemination of cells with the ability to induce an immunomodulator mechanism.

In patient 15, submitted to sublingual treatment with *Parietaria judaica* extracts, the UCCs obtained throughout the observation period were the lowest in these three patients. In fact, since the test was conducted during the pollinic period, we established a reduction of the allergenic dosage during the pollination period of this herb. It is a clinical procedure well established in the therapeutic with injectable extracts, although not consensual in sublingual treatment (Bousquet, 2006; Bousquet et al., 1998). Despite this, and since this patient lives in a geographic area with high levels of aeropalinologics, it was decided to reduce the maintenance dosage to 2/3 (10:15 drops). Eventually, this procedure had implications in the type of response that was evidenced, not only in the local activity as well as in the distant focalizations.

In patients under SLIT treatment, the UCCs obtained in the structures localized in the lateral-external region of the neck confirmed the analytic results from the scintigraphic images. The apparent descendent drainage in these vascular-lymphatic systems corroborates our proposal, particularly in the intrapulmonary capture. In the anatomic regions reported to the organs of the central immune system we observed UCCs with similar behavior than those verified in the patients under injectable treatment. Therefore, we presume that in SLIT there is also an early participation of the bone marrow and the functional thymic tissue.

4. Involvement of the organs from the immune system

In SCIT, we admit that the APC migration to ganglion structures is determinant to obtain a systemic effect and to acquire an immunomodulator and/or tolerance state. In patients submitted to SLIT, the inflammatory activity was observed in the first minutes, much earlier but with clearly lower gradients throughout the experiment. As previously described, the morphological characteristics of the conjunctive subcutaneous tissue and the oral, in particular from the sublingual region, are completely distinct. Therefore, the local availability of the whole array of the adjacent immuno-lymphatic-ganglion structures allows the effectiveness of the early stages of the mechanism. Paradoxically, the characteristics of the DCs present in the oral mucosa, mainly from the plasmacytoid type, are responsible for a less effective response (Novak et al., 2004). Previous work evidenced the presence of the allergenic extract in the sublingual mucosa long after it was swallowed, but it was extremely reduced 24 hours after that administration (Bagnasco et al., 2005). This difference, relatively to the subcutaneous administration, has natural implications in the periodicity of the therapeutical application. The amplification of the systemic effect seems to result from a descending involvement of structures presumably vascular-lymphatic in the lateral-external of the neck by a mechanism similar to SCIT.

Given the differences between the two administration methods and the type of therapeutic extract, the results obtained suggest a potentially selective influx of cells from the mononuclear-phagocyte system to the deposition site, similarly to the allergic reaction, which was documented in an interesting study done in ten patients submitted to an inhaled aggression (Upham et al., 2002). Naturally, the mediators produced locally will have a potential modulator effect in the adjacent vascular endothelium, which allows a possible immunomodulator effect in circulating leukocytes that allows a systemic involvement.

The recirculation and following focalization of intrapulmonary leukocytes was observed in all patients. The presence of the bronchus-associated lymphoid tissue (BALT) supports these results, in particular since this mucosa is a potential target in patients undergoing treatment of respiratory allergy. However, regarding the involvement of the intestinal mucosa, where the gut associated lymphoid tissue (GALT) is located, focalization of the inflammatory activity was occasionally observed. The SLIT with allergenic deglutition three minutes after the deposition did not produced any additional gain. In fact, we admit that the protein degradation can occur as result of the gastric enzymatic degradation as proposed in the literature (Bousquet et al., 1998).

The lymphocyte cellular modulation from a mainly Th2 profile into a lymphocyte profile mostly Th1, as well as the induction of T-lymphocytes with regulatory characteristics, are the most studied and documented mechanisms in the literature (Larché et al., 2006; Till et al., 2004; Canonica & Passalacqua, 2003). The complexity of the processes involved allows a constant effect throughout the treatment, but its dynamic mechanism is not well established. The need to extend in time the specific treatment translates the need to promote an immunologic memory *status*. The patients studied in this project were well documented, both clinically and laboratorial, and all were in maintenance treatment. Although we know several mechanisms involved, it is not known the dynamics and the regions implicated after the administration of the extract, nor in the induction stages or in maintenance periods.

It seems obvious the involvement of organs from the central immune system in the SIT action mechanisms. It also appears, given the results obtained in allergic patients submitted to specific provocation, that the participation of these organs could have a dynamic and pace with similar magnitude. These results look as redundant or expectable, but we had no previous knowledge about the location and timing of the immunomodulation process that has been so well characterized in the laboratory.

The induction of medullar cellular clones with phenotypes that favor the secretion type Th1 or clones precursors of DCs with tolerogenic characteristics are events that sustain the activity of the bone marrow, and is present at an early stage in patients undergoing treatment (van Helvoort et al., 2004; Moingeon et al., 2006). The essential function of several regulatory T-cells, well placed and with central function in the SIT mechanism, is an element that supports not only the intervention of bone marrow as well as the thymic activity (Schmidt-Weber & Blaser, 2005; Moingeon et al., 2006). Despite the anatomic involution, the organic function persists in adulthood (Hakim et al., 2005; Harris et al., 2005; Arellano et al., 2006). In this regard, we should notice that in one patient we had the opportunity to acquire a scintigraphic 21 hours after the simultaneous administration of leukocytes labeled with ^{99m}Tc-HMPAO and allergenic aqueous latex extract. In this patient we observe the persistence of the inflammatory activity in both the suprasternal and bone medullar areas, Figure 14.

It should be noticed that the half-life of the radio-labeled compound is 6 hours, and therefore the acquisition occurred at a time well past its half life. Nevertheless, the activity persisted at the administration site, allowing the therapeutic effect to continue, as well as activity in intra-bone areas and in the suprasternal region, which we judge representative the functional thymic tissue.

The study in this patient was done occasionally and was, in fact, a surprise, revealing activity that we supposed it was not possible due the anatomic physical conditionings. We proceeded with the quantitative evaluation that unequivocally contributed the qualitative assessment done in this patient. In Figure 15 we show the UCCs obtained for this patient after 6 hours (last programmed observation that coincides with ^{99m}Tc half-life) and 21 hours. Although the UCCs are lower after 21 hours when compared to the values obtained after 6 hours, it is evident that, despite after nearly four half-lives, the activity reported is very significant. We should highlight that the UCC in the ROI draw in the homolateral armpit maintains constant values of activity, which supports a continuous involvement.

The study in this patient, since it is not likely a continuous recirculation of leukocytes without focalization and influx to this organ, allows us to deduce that we were able to obtain an image of the functional thymic tissue.

Our results support the research developed since 1985 by a Canadian group that sustains the involvement of the central immune system's organs, mainly bone marrow, in the pathophysiology of the allergic inflammation (Denburg et al., 1998). The results obtained in experimental models and in humans with allergy are essential, regarding the participation of hematopoietic mechanisms during the response to an allergenic (Denburg et al., 1998; Denburg & van Eeden, 2006, Sehmi et al., 1996; Cyr & Denburg, 2001).

In a comparative study with 153 patients with pollinic rhinoconjunctivitis, the effect of the administration of SIT either subcutaneously or intralymphatic was compared (Senti et al., 2008). In the later group, the administration of the pollinic allergen directly in a inguinal lymphatic ganglion using ultrasound as a control, with only three injections separated by 4 weeks, in the response to a specific nasal induction 4 months after the last administration, required a dosage ten times higher than the one required in patients under SCIT treatment for three years and with a cumulative dosage drastically higher and with multiple allergenic injections. In addition to the clinical efficacy, the adverse effects were neglectable and the lymphatic intraganglionic injection was very well tolerated. This promising and innovative study can induce a complete reversion on the treatment of IgE mediated allergy. It should be noted that these results were obtained with conventional allergens. However we consider that the future use of highly selective peptides directly administered in immune structures can induce an even more elective therapeutical effect.

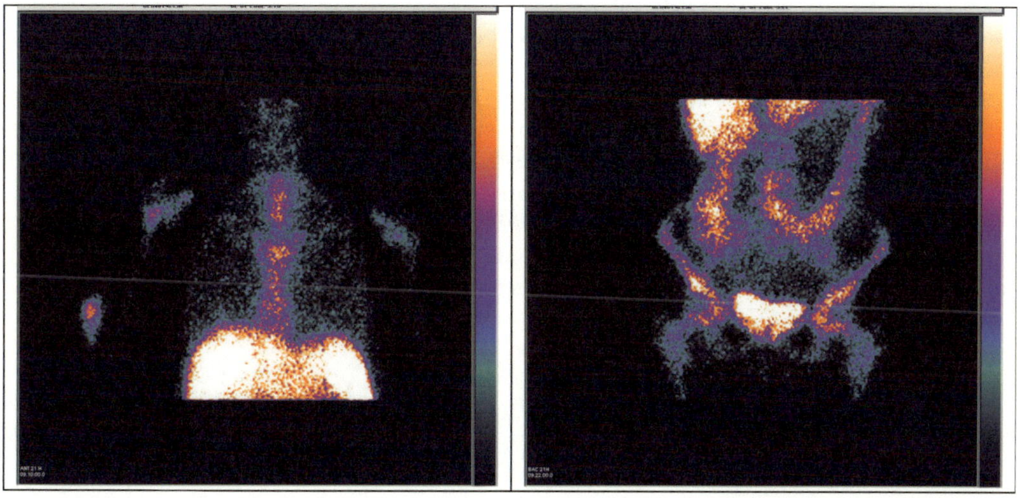

Fig. 14. Scintigraphic study in patient with anaphylaxis to latex, submitted to subcutaneous aqueous extract. Static acquisitions, anterior thoracic (A) and abdominal (B) views, 21 hours after the beginning of the study.

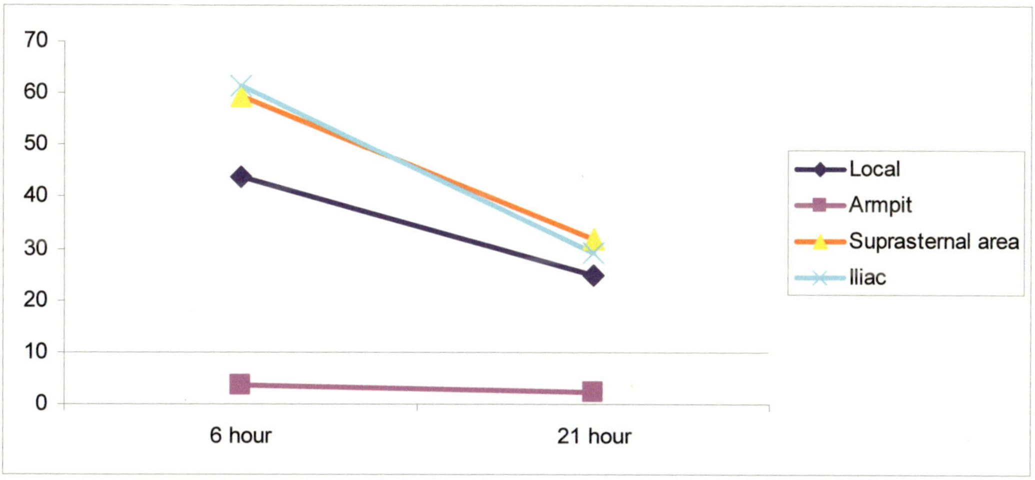

Fig. 15. Corrected uptake coefficient obtained in static acquisitions after 6 and 21 hours in different locations in patient with the diagnosis of latex anaphylaxis submitted to subcutaneous aqueous extract treatment.

5. Final remarks

SCIT limits the visualization of the inflammatory activity in systemic focalizations earlier than at the site of the extract administration. Generically, the local inflammatory activity evolves throughout time and is significantly broader than the one verified in the clinic, by the observation of the inflammatory signals. The pollinic extract modified with glutaraldehyde does not present nearly any inflammation at the injection site.

The involvement of the armpit's region homolateral to the administration of the extract occurs very early, which is compatible with the focalization of the inflammatory activity in immune ganglia structures. We admit an ascending drainage effect from the site of the extract's administration.

In patients submitted to SLIT, the visualization of the inflammatory activity is evident three minutes after the therapeutical extract's administration. In contrast to what was observed in SCIT patients, the inflammatory intensity, in the focalization, is relatively constant during the observation period, without an increase in later acquisitions. The SLIT also produced a very early systemic effect, namely with activity in the lateral-cervical region, where the presence of vascular-lymphatic structures have been reported. We admit that there is a descending drainage effect from the site of the extract's administration.

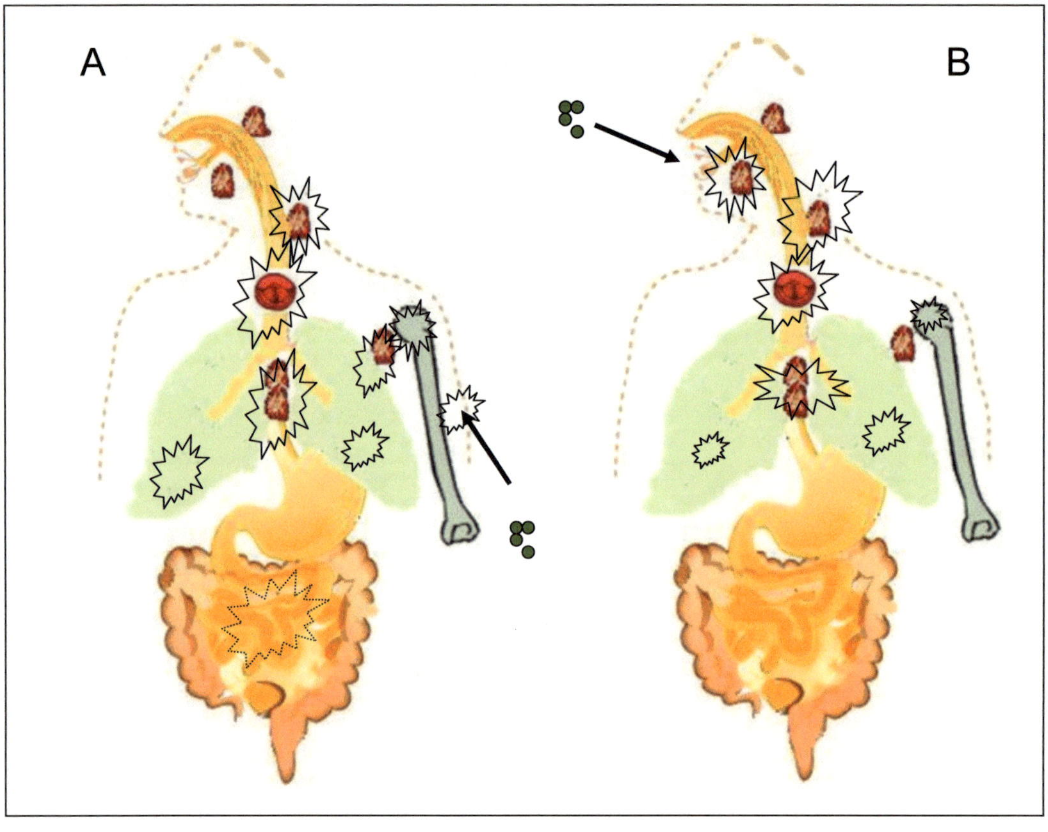

Fig. 16. Local and systemic events related to specific immunotherapy (A: subcutaneous; B: sublingual)

The visualization of the activity with intra-abdominal (intestinal) focalization was occasional, but exclusive to patients in SCIT. In patients undergoing SLIT, despite the swallowing of the extract, there was no focalization in this area three minutes after the extract's administration, Figure 16.

The anatomic regions reported to the central immune system (bone marrow and suprasternal area) evidenced a constant growth in UCCs during the experiment. The SIT triggers an early and continuous influx of leukocytes, from the circulation into the central immune organs, with potential implications in the immunomodulatory mechanism.

Regarding the response's magnitude in the bone marrow and functional thymic tissue, there were no apparent differences regarding the type of extract and the administration type during the first six hours after the administration of the therapeutical extract.

The persistence of the therapeutical extract administered subcutaneously indicates an inflammatory activity and a continuous influx of inflammatory cells. In the sublingual administration, the influx and local activity are lower, without any evidence of an increase in the inflammatory activity throughout the experiment. Therefore, patients under SLIT treatment will require administrations more frequent and with shorter breaks between administration in order to obtain a persistent therapeutic effect.

Our results reinforce the need for new and elective pharmacologic investigation strategies, focusing on the mainstay function of the central immune organs in the treatment of systemic inflammatory disease such as allergy. In fact, in face of the current knowledge of the immunological effects induced by SIT, namely the effect on T-regs with a long-lasting biological effect, this would only be possible if a central immune cellular modulation had occurred.

6. Acknowledgment

We would like to thank Dr Margarida Abrantes (IBILI, Medicine Faculty of Coimbra University. Portugal), Dr Daniel Machado (Immunoallergology Department, Coimbra University Hospital. Coimbra. Portugal), and Prof J Pedroso Lima (Nuclear Medicine Department, Coimbra University Hospital. Portugal) for all the performance and commitment to this project. The authors thank Dr Joana Branco and Dr André Faustino for the precious English writing assistance.

7. References

Agea, E.; et al. (2005). Human CD1-restricted T cell recognition of lipids from pollens. *The Journal Experimental Medicine,*.Vol.202, No.2, (July 2005), pp. 295-308, ISSN 0022-1007

Akdis, C.A. & Akdis, M. (2011) Mechanisms of allergen-specific immunotherapy. *The Journal of Allergy and Clinical Immunology,*.Vol.127, No.1, (January 2011), pp. 18-27, ISSN 0091-6749

Akdis, C.; et al. (2001). Mechanisms of IL10 induced T cell inactivation in allergic inflammation and normal response to allergens. *International Archives of Allergy and Immunology,* Vol.124, No.1-3, (January-March 2001), pp. 124: 180-182, ISSN 1018-2438

Allam, J.P.; et al. (2006). Comparative analysis of nasal and oral mucosa dendritic cells. *European journal of allergy and clinical immunology (Allergy),* Vol.61, No.2, (February 2006), pp. 166-172, ISSN 0105-4538

Allam, J.P.; et al. (2003). Characterization of dendritic cells from human oral mucosa: a new Langerhans_ cell type with high constitutive FcepsilonRI expression. *The Journal of Allergy and Clinical Immunology,* Vol. 112, No.1, (July 2003), pp. 141-148, ISSN 0091-6749

Alvarez-Cuesta E.; et al, (2006). Standards for pratical allergen- specific immunotherapy. *Allergy,* 2006; Vol. 61, Suppl.82, (October 2006), pp. 1-20, ISSN 0105-4538

Alazraki, N.; et al. (2002). Procedure guideline for lymphoscintigraphy and the use of intraoperative gamma probe for sentinel lymph node localization in melanoma of intermediate thickness. *Journal Nuclear Medicine*, Vol. 43, No.43, (October 2002), pp. 1414-1418, ISSN 0161-5505

Ariano, R., et al. (1999). Long-term treatment with allergoid immunotherapy with Parietaria. Clinical and immunologic effects in a randomized, controlled trial. *European journal of allergy and clinical immunology (Allergy)*, Vol.54, No.4, (April 1999), pp. 313-319, ISSN 0105-4538

Arellano, M.V.; et al. (2006). Thymic Function-Related Markers Within the Thymus and Peripheral Blood: Are They Comparable? *Journal of Clinical Immunolology*, Vol.26, No.1, (January 2006), pp. 96-100, ISSN 0271-9142

Bagnasco, M.; et al. (2005). Pharmacokinetics of Der p 2 allergen and derived monomeric allergoid in allergic volunteers. *International Archives of Allergy and Immunology*, Vol.138, No.3, (November 2005), pp. 197–202, ISSN 1018-2438

Bagnasco, M.; et al. (1997). Absortion and distribution kinetics of the major Parietaria judaica (Par j 1) administered by noninjectable routes in healthy human beings. *The Journal of Allergy and Clinical Immunology*, Vol.100, No.1, (July 1997), pp. 122-129, ISSN 0091-6749

Bagnasco, M.; et al. (2001). Pharmacokinetics of an allergen and a monomeric allergoid for oromucosal immunotherapy in allergic volunteers. *Clinical and Experimental Allergy*, Vol.31, No.1, (January 2001), pp. 54-60, ISSN 0954-7894

Bienestock, J. & McDermott, M.R.. (2005). Bronchus- and nasal-associated lymphoid tissues. Immunological Reviews. Vol.206, (August 2005), pp. 22-31, ISSN 0105-2896

Bousquet, J.. (2006). Sublingual immunotherapy: validated! *Allergy*, Vol.61, Suppl.81, (July 2006), pp. 5-31, ISSN 0105-4538

Bousquet, J. & Fiocchi, A. (2006). Prevention of recurrent respiratory tract infections in children using a ribosomal immunotherapeutic agent: a clinical review. *Paediatric Drugs*, Vol.8, No.4, pp. 235-243, ISSN 1174-5878

Bousquet, J.; et al. (1998). Allergen immunotherapy: therapeutic vaccines for allergic diseases. A WHO position paper. *The Journal of Allergy and Clinical Immunology*, Vol.102, No.4, (October 1998), pp. 558-562, ISSN 0091-6749

Canónica, G.W. & Passalacqua, G. (2003). Noninjection routes for immunotherapy. *Journal of Allergy and Clinical Immunology*, Vol.111, No.3, (March 2003), pp. 437-448, ISSN 0091-6749

Casanovas, M.; et al. (2005). Comparative Study of Tolerance between Unmodified and High Doses of Chemically Modified Allergen Vaccines of *Dermatophagoides pteronyssinus. International Archives of Allergy and Immunology*, Vol.137, No.3, (July 2005), pp. 211–218, ISSN 1018-2438

Casanovas, M.; et al. (2007). Safety of immunotherapy with therapeutic vaccines containing depigmented and polymerized allergen extracts. *Clinical and Experimental Allergy*, Vol. 37, No.3, (March 2007), pp. 434-440, ISSN 0954-7894

Clot, J. (1997). Pharmacology of ribosomal immunotherapy. *Drugs*, Vol. 54, Suppl.1, pp. 33-36, ISSN 0012-6667

Cyr, M.M. & Denburg, J.A.. (2001). Systemic aspects of allergic disease: the role of the bone marrow. *Current Opinion in Immunology*, Vol.13), No.6, (December 2001), pp. 727-732, ISSN 0952-7915

Denburg, J.A.; et al.. (1998). Hemopoietic mechanisms in allergic airway inflammation. *International Archives of Allergy and Immunology*, Vol.117, No.3, (November 1998), pp. 155-159, ISSN 1018-2438

Denburg, J.A.; et al.. (2000). Systemic aspects of allergic disease: Bone marrow responses. *The Journal of Allergy and Clinical Immunology*, Vol.106, Suppl.5.2, (November 2000), pp. S242-6, ISSN 0091-6749

Denburg, J.A. & van Eeden, S.F.. (2006). Bone marrow progenitors in inflammation and repair: new vistas in respiratory biology and pathophysiology. *The European Respiratory Journal*, Vol. 27, No.3, (March 2006), pp. 441-445, ISSN 0903-1936

Francis, J.N.; et al.. (2003). Induction of IL-101CD41CD251 T cells by grass pollen immunotherapy. *The Journal of Allergy and Clinical Immunology*, Vol.111, No.6, (June 2003), pp 1255-1261, ISSN 0091-6749

Frew, A.J.. (2010). Allergen immunotherapy. *The Journal of Allergy and Clinical Immunology*, Vol.125, No.2 (Suppl 2), (February 2010), pp. S306-133, ISSN 0091-6749

Geijtenbeek, T.B. et al.. (2002). Engering A, Van KY. DC-SIGN, a C-type lectin on dendritic cells that unveils many aspects of dendritic cell biology. *Journal of Leukocyte Biology*, Vol. 71, No.6, (June 2002), pp. 921–931, ISSN 0741-5400

Hakim, F.T.; et al.. (2005). Age-dependent incidence, time course, and consequences of thymic renewal in adults.*The Journal of Clinical Investigation*, Vol.115, No.4, (April 2005), pp. 930-939, ISSN 0021-9738

Harris, J.M.; et al.. (2005). Multiparameter evaluation of human thymic function: interpretations and caveats. *Clinical Immunology*, Vol. 115, No.2, (May 2005), pp. 138-146, ISSN 1521-6616

Haselden, B.M.; et al.. (1999). Immunoglobulin E-independent major histocompatibility complex-restricted T cell peptide epitope-induced late asthmatic reactions. *The Journal of Experimental Medicine*, Vol.189, No.12, (June 1999), pp. 1885-1894, ISSN 0022-1007

Ibarrola, I.; et al.. (2004). Biological characterization of glutaraldehyde-modified Parietaria judaica pollen extracts. *Clinical Experimental Allergy*, Vol. 34, No.2, (February 2004), pp. 303–309, ISSN 0954-7894

Kelly, M.; et al.. (2007). Modulating leukocyte recruitment in inflammation. *The Journal of Allergy and Clinical Immunology*, Vol.120, No.1, (July 2007), pp. 3-10, ISSN 0091-6749

Kumar V.. (2005) Radiolabeled white blood cells and direct targeting of micro-organisms for infection imaging. *The Quarterly Journal of Nuclear Medicine and Molecular Imaging*, Vol.49, No.4. (December 2005), pp. 325-338, ISSN 1824-4785

Lambrecht, B.N. & Hammad, H.. (2002) Myeloid dendritic cells make it to the top. *Clinical Experimental Allergy*, Vol.32, No.6, (June 2002), pp. 805-810, ISSN 0954-7894

Larché, M.; et al.. (2006). Immunological mechanisms of allergen-specific immunotherapy. Nature Reviews Immunology, Vol. 6, No.10, (October 2006), pp. 761-71, ISSN 1474-1733

Lukacs, N.. (2000). Migration of helper T-lymphocyte subsets into inflamed tissues. *The Journal of Allergy and Clinical Immunology*, Vol.106, No.5(Part 2), (November 2000), pp. S264-269, ISSN 0091-6749

Mistrello, G.; et al.. (1994). Modified Par j I allergen from P judaica pollen and its rate of absorption in rats. Immunology Letter,s Vol. 40, No.1, (April 1994), pp 31-36, ISSN 0165-2478

Moingeon, P.; et al.. (2006). Immune mechanisms of allergen-specific sublingual immunotherapy. *Allergy*, Vol. 61, No.2, (February 2006), pp. 151-165, ISSN 0105-4538

Novak, N.; et al.. (2004). The role of antigen presenting cells at distinct anatomic sites: they accelarate and they slow down allergies. *Allergy,* Vol. 59, No.1, (January 2004), pp. 5-14, ISSN 0105-4538

Passalacqua, G.; et al.. (2005). Pharmacokinetics of radiolabelled Par j 1 administered intranasally to allergic and healthy subjects. *Clinical and Experimental Allergy,* Vol. 35, No.7, (July 2005), pp. 880–883, ISSN 0954-7894

Pereira C. Dinâmica da inflamação alérgica e da imunoterapia específica. Contribuição para o seu estudo in vivo. PhD Thesis. Medicine Faculty from the University of Coimbra. 2009 (pp:1-516); University of Coimbra, Portugal.

Pereira, C.; et al.. (2004). Kinetics and dynamic evaluation of specific immunotherapy. *European annals of allergy and clinical immunology,* Vol.36, No.10, (December 2004), pp. 375-386. ISSN 1764-1489

Peters, A.M.; et al.. (1986). Clinical experience with 99m Tc-hexamethyl propylene-amine oxime for labelling leucocytes and imaging inflammation. *Lancet,* Vol. 25, No.2(8513), (October 1986), pp. 946-949, ISSN 0140-6736

Sehmi, R.; et al.. (1996). Increased levels of CD34+ hemopoietic progenitor cells in atopic subjects. *American Journal of Respiratory Cell Molecular Biology,* Vol.15, No.5, (November 1996), pp. 645-654, ISSN 1044-1549

Senti, G.; et al.. (2008). Intralymphatic allergen administration renders specific immunotherapy faster and safer: a randomized controlled trial. *Proceedings of the National Academy of Sciences of the United States of America,* Vol.105, No.46, (November 2008), pp. 17908-17912, ISSN 0027-8424

Schmit-Weber, C.B. & Blaser, K.. (2002). T-cell tolerance in allergic response. *Allergy,* Vol. 57, No.9, (September 2002), pp. 762-768, ISSN 0105-4538

Schmit-Weber, C.B. & Blaser, K.. (2005). New insights into the mechanisms of allergen-specific immunotherapy. *Current Opinion in Allergy Clinical Immunology,* Vol. 5, No.6, (December 2005), pp. 525-530, ISSN 1528-4050

Spiller, H.A.; et al.. (1993), A five year evaluation of acute exposures to phenol disinfectant (26%). *Journal of toxicology. Clinical toxicology,* Vol.31, No.2, pp. 307-313, ISSN 0731-3810

Till, S.J.; et al.. (2004). Mechanisms of immunotherapy. *The Journal of Allergy and Clinical Immunology,* Vol.113, No.6, (June 2004), pp. 1025-1034, ISSN 0091-6749

Togias, A.. (2004). Systemic effects of local allergic disease *The Journal of Allergy and Clinical Immunology,* Vol.113, No.1(Suppl 1), (January 2004), pp. S8-14, ISSN 0091-6749

Upham, J.W.; et al. (2002). Rapid response of circulating myeloid dendritic cells to inhaled allergen in asthmatic subjects. *Clinical Experimental Allergy,* Vol. 32, No.6, (June 2002), pp. 818-823, ISSN 0954-7894

von Bubnoff, D.; et al.. (2002). Antigen-presenting cells and tolerance induction. *Allergy,* Vol. 57, No.1, (January 2002), pp. 2-8, ISSN 0105-4538

van Helvoort, J.M.; et al.. (2004). Preferential expression of IgG2b in nose draining cervical lymph nodes and its putative role in mucosal tolerance induction. *Allergy,* Vol. 59, No.11, (November 2004), pp. 1211–1218, ISSN 0105-4538

Wheeler, A.W. & Woroniecki, S.R..(2004). Allergy vaccines- new approaches to an old concept. *Expert opinion on biological therapy,* Vol. 4, No.9, (September 2004), pp. 1473–11481, ISSN 1471-2598

Woodfolk, J.A.. (2007). T-cell responses to allergens. *The Journal of Allergy and Clinical Immunology,* Vol.119, No.2, (February 2007), pp. 280-294, ISSN 0091-6749

20

β_2-Adrenoceptor Agonists and Allergic Disease: The Enhancing Effect of β_2-Adrenoceptor Agonists on Cytokine-Induced TSLP Production by Human Lung Tissue Cells

Akio Matsuda and Kyoko Futamura
Department of Allergy and Immunology,
National Research Institute for Child Health and Development, Tokyo,
Japan

1. Introduction

1.1 β_2-adrenoceptor agonists and asthma

The adrenergic receptors (adrenoceptors) are a member of the G protein-coupled receptor superfamily of membrane proteins that are targets of the catecholamines, norepinephrine and epinephrine. To date, two main groups of adrenoceptors, α and β, with several subtypes have been identified. Many types of cells possess these receptors, and the binding of an agonist will generally cause a sympathetic response. Among them, β2-adrenoceptor agonists (β2-agonists) are widely used as bronchodilators in the treatment of bronchial asthma because of their potent bronchodilating effects on airway smooth muscle. In addition to being bronchodilators, they may also have anti-inflammatory properties, including inhibition of granulocyte functions (Yasui et.al., 2006). However, concerns have been raised regarding the use of β2-agonists on a regular daily basis rather than only as needed for rescue therapy. More specifically, continuous and repetitive β_2-agonist monotherapy has been considered to be associated with an increase in the degree of allergic inflammation (Cockcroft et.al., 1995), poor asthma outcomes (Paris et.al., 2008) and an increase in the risk of asthma death (Crane et.al., 1989; Nelson et.al., 2006). Although the precise molecular mechanisms underlying these undesirable effects of β_2-agonists are not fully understood, several studies have independently demonstrated that β_2-agonists have the potential to increase Th2 cytokine-mediated inflammation both *in vivo* and *in vitro*. For instance, Coqueret et.al. demonstrated that ovalbumin-sensitized mice treated with a daily injection of salbutamol showed increased anti-ovalbumin IgE levels in their serum, probably due to increased production of Th2 cytokines (Coqueret et.al., 1994). Panina-Bordignon et.al. demonstrated that β_2-agonists prevented Th1 development by selectively inhibiting IL-12 production (Panina-Bordignon et.al., 1997). More recently, Loza et.al. demonstrated that human Th2 cells express β_2-adrenergic receptor and that β_2-agonists augmented the accumulation of Th2 cells in human peripheral blood lymphocyte cultures subjected to bystander stimuli (Loza et.al., 2007). These findings suggest a mechanism by which β_2-agonist monotherapy may favor Th2 immune responses, which are believed to be involved in the pathogenesis of asthma.

1.2 TSLP and asthma

Thymic stromal lymphopoietin (TSLP) is an IL-7-like cytokine which was originally identified in the supernatant of a murine thymic stromal cell line (Friend et.al., 1994). Increasing evidence suggests that TSLP plays important roles in the pathogenesis of allergic diseases such as asthma and atopic dermatitis (Al-Shami te.al., 2005; Yoo et.al., 2005). The most clinically relevant role of TSLP is mediated by dendritic cells (DCs) through induction of OX40 ligand expression on DCs (Ito et.al., 2005; Liu, 2007a). Naïve T cells receiving antigen-presentation from TSLP-primed DCs develop into Th2 cells that produce IL-4, -5, -13 and TNF-α but not IL-10 (Ito et.al., 2005; Liu, 2007a; Soumelis et.al., 2002). These Th2 cells are now referred as to "inflammatory Th2 cells" in consideration of their potential for releasing the proinflammatory cytokine, TNF-α, in addition to Th2 cytokines (Orihara et.al.; 2008). Furthermore, mice with transgenic overexpression of TSLP in the lung develop severe airway inflammation, including massive infiltration by inflammatory cells, goblet cell hyperplasia and airway hyperresponsiveness (Zhou et.al., 2005). Mice with transgenic overexpression of TSLP in skin keratinocytes develop severe dermatitis with itching, which is similar to the clinical features of atopic dermatitis in humans (Yoo et.al., 2005). On the other hand, mice lacking the TSLP receptor exhibit strong Th1 responses and fail to develop an inflammatory lung response to antigens (Al-Shami te.al., 2005). Thus, TSLP is an important cytokine that is necessary and sufficient for initiation of allergic inflammation.

2. The enhancing effect of β_2-adrenoceptor agonists on cytokine-induced TSLP production by human lung tissue cells

2.1 Cytokine-induced production of TSLP by lung tissue cells

It is widely accepted that TSLP is expressed predominantly in epithelial cells of the lung, intestine and skin keratinocytes (Soumelis et.al., 2002; Liu et.al., 2007b). We confirmed an earlier report (kato et.al., 2007) that a combination of IL-4 and TNF-α synergistically induced TSLP production by normal human bronchial epithelial cells (NHBE) (Fig. 1A). Unlike NHBE, lung mesenchymal cells such as bronchial smooth muscle cells (BSMC) and normal human lung fibroblasts (NHLF) produced TSLP in response to TNF-α, but not IL-4 alone. However, like NHBE, those cells produced greater amounts of TSLP as a result of synergistic effects between IL-4 and TNF-α (Fig. 1B and 1C). Of note, these mesenchymal cells produce appreciable amounts of TSLP compared to NHBE, suggesting the possibility that lung mesenchymal cells are, like epithelial cells, important cellular sources of TSLP.

2.2 Effects of β_2-agonists on cytokine-induced TSLP production

We next examined the effects of β_2-agonists on the cytokine-induced TSLP production by the human lung tissue cells. Although β_2-agonists act mainly on airway smooth muscle as bronchodilators, they are also known to express anti-inflammatory effects on granulocytes (Yasui et.al., 2006), epithelial cells (Koyama et.al., 1999) and fibroblasts (Spoelstra et.al., 2002). As shown in Fig 2A, when NHBE were stimulated with a combination of IL-4 and TNF-α, simultaneous addition of various concentrations of two long-acting β_2-agonists, i.e., salmeterol and formoterol, and a short-acting β_2-agonist, salbutamol, showed significant enhancement of the cytokine-induced TSLP production. Optimal concentrations of these β_2-agonists were employed, and then the mRNA expression of TSLP in NHBE was measured by quantitative real-time PCR. TSLP mRNA expression was significantly enhanced by 10^{-10} M salmeterol, 10^{-10}

M formoterol and 10^{-8} M salbutamol (Fig. 2B), suggesting that the enhancing effects of β_2-agonists on TSLP production were transcriptionally-regulated. It should be noted that β_2-agonists enhanced TSLP production by airway smooth muscle cells and lung fibroblasts as well as bronchial epithelial cells (Fig. 2C and 2D). We suppose that the production of TSLP by these lung tissue cells is particularly important because dendritic cells have to migrate through these airway interstitial cells to lymphopoietic tissues in order to present antigen information to naïve T cells. Therefore, enhanced TSLP production by lung tissue cells in response to β_2-agonists may lead to exacerbation of allergic airway inflammation, and this may partly explain the undesirable clinical effects of continuous β_2-agonist monotherapy.

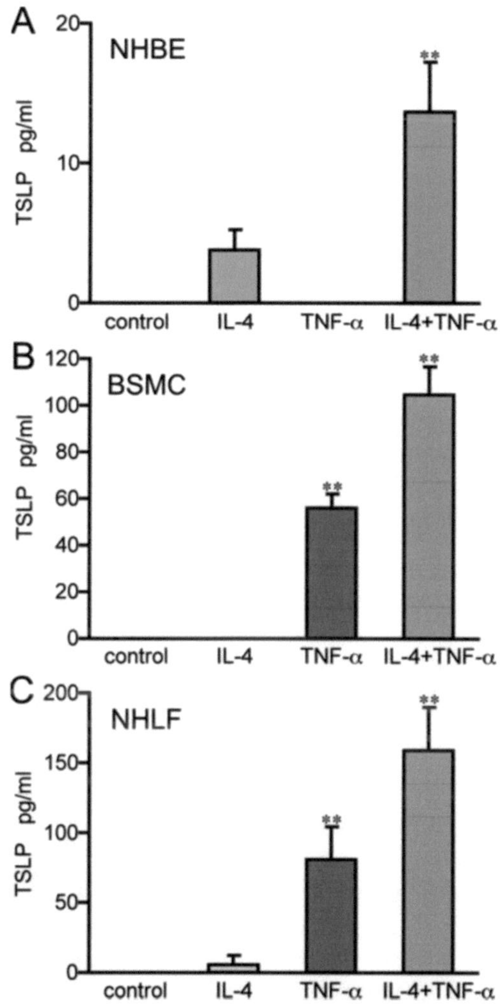

Fig. 1. Cytokines induce production of TSLP by lung tissue cells. NHBE (**A**), BSMC (**B**) and NHLF (**C**) were treated with 10 ng/ml IL-4 alone, 10 ng/ml TNF-α alone and a combination of both for 48 h. TSLP concentrations in the culture supernatants were quantified by ELISA. Data are shown as the mean ± SD of quadruplicate samples and are representative of at least three separate experiments. ** $p < .01$ compared with unstimulated control. Reprinted from Futamura et. Al., 2010.

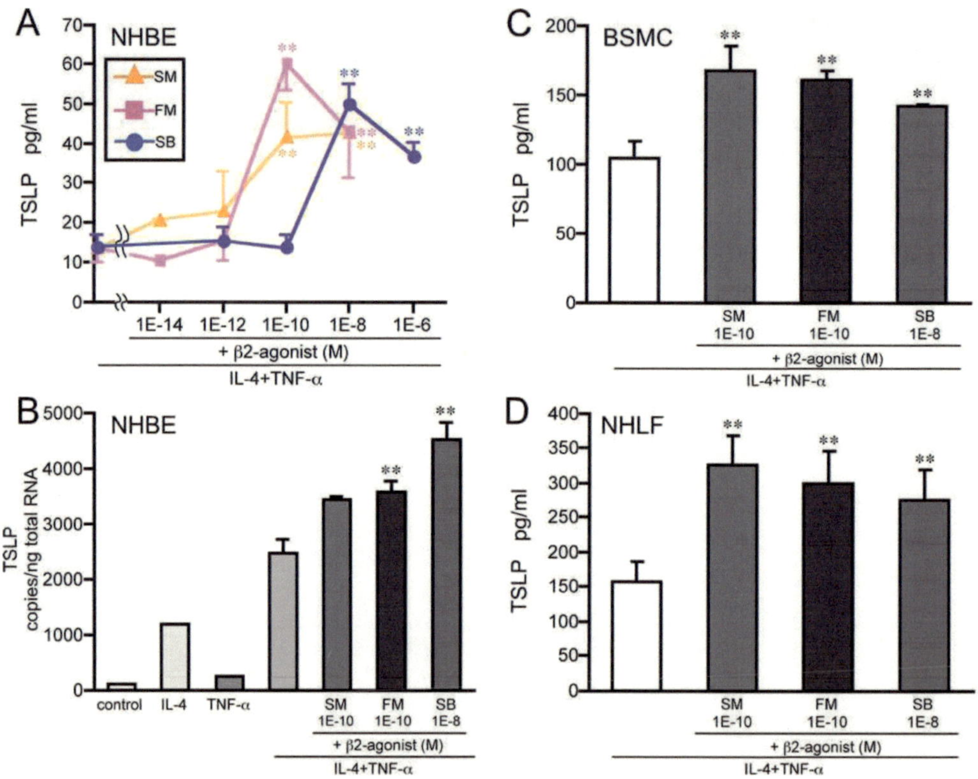

Fig. 2. β_2-agonists enhance cytokine-induced TSLP production by lung tissue cells. (**A**) NHBE were treated with different concentrations of two long-acting β_2-agonists, salmeterol (SM) and formoterol (FM), or a short-acting β_2-agonist, salbutamol (SB), in the presence of 10 ng/ml IL-4 and 10 ng/ml TNF-α for 48 h. TSLP concentrations in the culture supernatants were quantified by ELISA. (**B**) NHBE were treated with cytokines at 10 ng/ml in the presence and absence of the indicated concentrations of each β_2-agonist (SM, FM, SB) for 6 h. The copy numbers of TSLP mRNA are shown. BSMC (**C**) and NHLF (**D**) were treated with the indicated concentrations of each β_2-agonist (SM, FM, SB) in the presence of 10 ng/ml IL-4 and 10 ng/ml TNF-α for 48 h. TSLP concentrations in the culture supernatants were quantified by ELISA. All data are shown as the mean ± SD of quadruplicate samples and are representative of at least three separate experiments. ** $p < .01$ compared with IL-4 plus TNF-α. Reprinted from Futamura et. Al., 2010.

2.3 Effects of cAMP-elevating agents on cytokine-induced TSLP production

It is well known that binding of β_2-agonists to β_2-adrenoceptors activates adenylate cyclase, resulting in generation of intracellular cAMP. We therefore examined the role of intracellular cAMP in the enhancement of TSLP production. The cells were stimulated with three cAMP-elevating agents, i.e., 8-bromoadenosine cyclic monophosphate, dibutyryl adenosine cyclic monophosphate (hereinafter referred to as 8-Br cAMP and db cAMP, respectively) and forskolin (an adenylate cyclase activator). All three agents caused significant enhancement of cytokine-induced TSLP production by the lung tissue cells (Fig. 3). These results suggest that the enhancing effects of β_2-agonists on TSLP production were mediated via upregulation of intracellular cAMP in these cells.

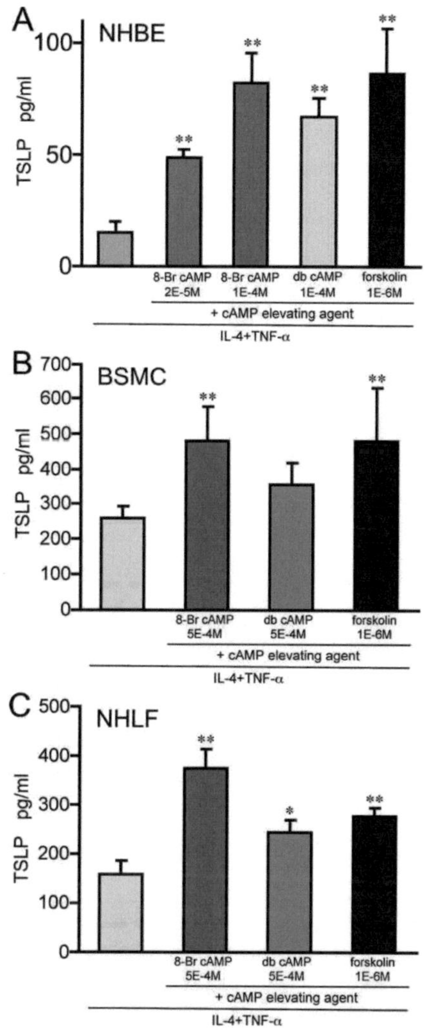

Fig. 3. Intracellular cAMP-elevating agents enhance cytokine-induced TSLP production by lung tissue cells. NHBE (**A**), BSMC (**B**) and NHLF (**C**) were treated with 10 ng/ml IL-4 and 10 ng/ml TNF-α in the presence and absence of the indicated concentrations of each cAMP-elevating agent (8-Br cAMP, db cAMP, forskolin) for 48 h. TSLP concentrations in the culture supernatants were quantified by ELISA. Data are shown as the mean ± SD of quadruplicate samples and are representative of at least three separate experiments. * $p < .05$ and ** $p < .01$ compared with IL-4 plus TNF-α. Reprinted from Futamura et. Al., 2010.

2.4 Effects of corticosteroid on cytokine-induced TSLP production

According to the recently updated guidelines for asthma management, the preferred treatment regimen for patients with intermittent asthma is an inhaled short-acting β_2-agonist, and the next step regimen is additional treatment with an inhaled corticosteroid. Therefore, we examined the effects of a corticosteroid, fluticasone, on the β_2-agonist-induced increase in TSLP production. Simultaneous addition of various concentrations of fluticasone caused dose-dependent, significant inhibition of both cytokine-induced (closed squares) and salmeterol-enhanced (closed triangles) TSLP production by NHBE (Fig. 4A, upper graph). Similar results were obtained in experiments using NHLF (Fig. 4A, lower graph) and BSMC (data not

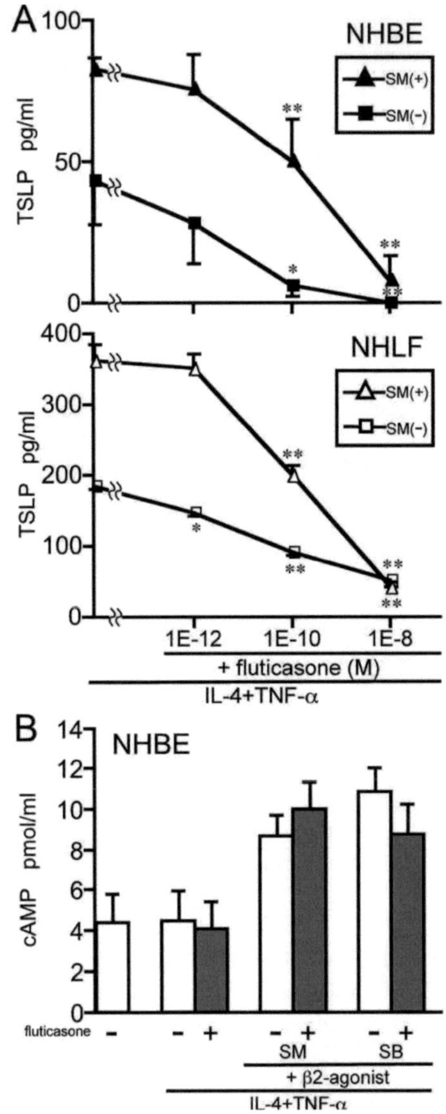

Fig. 4. Fluticasone inhibits TSLP production without affecting the intracellular cAMP level. (**A**) NHBE (upper graph) and NHLF (lower graph) were treated with 10 ng/ml IL-4 and 10 ng/ml TNF-α with and without 10^{-10} M salmeterol (SM) for 48 h. The effects of simultaneous addition of the indicated concentrations of fluticasone on the TSLP production are shown. Data are shown as the mean ± SD of quadruplicate samples and are representative of at least three separate experiments. * $p < .05$ and ** $p < .01$ compared to without fluticasone. (**B**) NHBE were treated with 10 ng/ml IL-4 and 10 ng/ml TNF-α with and without a β_2-agonist (10^{-10} M SM, 10^{-8} M SB) for 5 min. The effects of simultaneous addition of 10^{-8} M fluticasone on the intracellular cAMP levels are shown. Data are shown as the mean ± SD of triplicate samples and are representative of three separate experiments. Reprinted from Futamura et. al., 2010.

shown). Importantly, simultaneous treatment at the highest concentration of fluticasone (10^{-8} M), which can still considered to be clinically feasible, almost completely abrogated not only the cytokine-induced TSLP production but also the enhancement by the β_2-agonists.

2.5 Corticosteroid inhibition of TSLP production is not due to direct inhibition of cAMP signaling

In order to clarify how corticosteroids might inhibit TSLP production, we examined the effects of fluticasone and β_2-agonists on the intracellular cAMP level in NHBE. Addition of salmeterol or salbutamol significantly increased the cAMP level after 5 minutes of incubation. Addition of 10^{-8} M fluticasone showed no effect on the intracellular cAMP level whether in the presence or absence of a β_2-agonist (Fig. 4B), indicating that corticosteroid inhibition of TSLP production is not due to direct inhibition of cAMP signaling. These results also suggest that corticosteroids inhibit TSLP synthesis by acting on the downstream signaling pathway of cAMP.

To date, several mechanisms have been proposed to explain the synergistic action between corticosteroids and β_2-agonists: induction and protection of β_2-adrenoceptors by corticosteroids (Barnes, 2002), enhancement of translocation of glucocorticoid receptors into the nucleus by β_2-agonists (Usami et.al., 2005) and post-transcriptional regulation to suppress expression of inflammatory genes (Kaur et.al., 2008). Our results may shed new light on the mechanisms by which combination therapy using an inhaled β_2-agonist and an inhaled corticosteroid shows synergistic clinical efficacy in patients with asthma.

3. Future challenges

It remains to be clarified whether the enhancing effect of β_2-agonists on cytokine production is specific to TSLP or not. Koyama et. al. demonstrated that TNF-α-induced production of granulocyte-macrophage colony-stimulating factor (GM-CSF), CCL5 and IL-8 by a human bronchial epithelial cell line, BEAS-2B, was significantly inhibited by procaterol, a β_2-agonist (Koyama et. al., 1999). We confirmed that the cytokine-induced production of GM-CSF and CCL5, but not IL-8, by NHBE was significantly suppressed by β_2-agonist treatment (data not shown). On the other hand, it was reported that rhinovirus-induced IL-6 production by NHBE was increased by salmeterol (Edwards et. Al., 2007), and we also found that the cytokine-induced production of IL-6 as well as TSLP by NHBE was significantly enhanced by simultaneous treatment with β_2-agonists (data not shown). Thus, β_2-agonists are able to crucially modulate the production of various inflammatory mediators through mechanisms that need to be further elucidated.

4. Conclusion

In this study, we focused on the effects of β_2-agonists on the *in vitro* synthesis of TSLP, which is a key cytokine in the development of allergic diseases. We found that β_2-agonists significantly enhanced cytokine-induced TSLP production by cultured primary human lung tissue cells. This enhancement may be partly responsible for the undesirable clinical effects of continuous β_2-agonist monotherapy, and our other findings suggest that combination therapy with a corticosteroid might effectively inhibit TSLP-mediated allergic inflammation.

5. Acknowledgements

We would like to thank Dr. Kanami Orihara of the Department of Allergy and Immunology, National Research Institute for Child Health and Development, for her contribution in this work. This work was supported in part by grants from the National Institute of Biomedical Innovation (ID05-24 and ID05-41) and a grant from the Japan Health Science Foundation (KH51046).

6. References

Al-Shami, A.; Spolski, R.; Kelly, J.; Keane-Myers, A. & Leonard, W.J. (2005) A role for TSLP in the development of inflammation in an asthma model. J Exp Med 202:829-839.

Barnes, P.J. (2002) Scientific rationale for inhaled combination therapy with long-acting beta2-agonists and corticosteroids. Eur Respir J 19:182-191.

Cockcroft, D.W.; O'Byrne, P.M.; Swystun, V.A. & Bhagat, R. (1995) Regular use of inhaled albuterol and the allergen-induced late asthmatic response. J Allergy Clin Immunol 96:44-49.

Coqueret, O.; Petit-Frere, C.; Lagente, V.; Moumen, M.; Mencia-Huerta, J.M. & Braquet, P. (1994) Modulation of IgE production in the mouse by beta 2-adrenoceptor agonist. Int Arch Allergy Immunol 105:171-176.

Crane, J.; Pearce, N.; Flatt, A.; Burgess, C.; Jackson, R.; Kwong, T.; Ball, M. & Beasley, R. (1989) Prescribed fenoterol and death from asthma in New Zealand, 1981-83: case-control study. Lancet 1(8644):917-922.

Edwards, M.R.; Haas, J.; Panettieri, R.A.Jr.; Johnson, M. & Johnston, S.L. (2007) Corticosteroids and beta2 agonists differentially regulate rhinovirus-induced interleukin-6 via distinct Cis-acting elements. J Biol Chem 282:15366-15375.

Friend, S.L.; Hosier, S.; Nelson, A.; Foxworthe, D.; Williams, D.E. & Farr, A. (1994) A thymic stromal cell line supports in vitro development of surface IgM+ B cells and produces a novel growth factor affecting B and T lineage cells. Exp Hematol 22:321-328.

Futamura, K.; Orihara, K.; Hashimoto, N.; Morita, H.; Fukuda, S.; Sagara, H.; Matsumoto, K.; Tomita, Y.; Saito, H. & Matsuda, A. (2010) beta2-adrenoceptor agonists enhance cytokine-induced release of thymic stromal lymphopoietin by lung tissue cells. Int Arch Allergy Immunol 152:353-361

Ito, T.; Wang, Y.H.; Duramad, O.; Hori, T.; Delespesse, G.J.; Watanabe, N.; Qin, F.X.; Yao, Z.; Cao, W. & Liu, Y.J. (2005) TSLP-activated dendritic cells induce an inflammatory T helper type 2 cell response through OX40 ligand. J Exp Med 202:1213-1223.

Kato, A.; Favoreto, S. Jr.; Avila, P.C. & Schleimer, R.P. (2007) TLR3- and Th2 cytokine-dependent production of thymic stromal lymphopoietin in human airway epithelial cells. J Immunol 179:1080-1087.

Kaur, M.; Chivers, J.E.; Giembycz, M.A. & Newton, R. (2008) Long-acting beta2-adrenoceptor agonists synergistically enhance glucocorticoid-dependent transcription in human airway epithelial and smooth muscle cells. Mol Pharmacol 73:203-14.

Koyama, S.; Sato, E.; Masubuchi, T.; Takamizawa, A.; Kubo, K.; Nagai, S. & Isumi, T. (1999) Procaterol inhibits IL-1beta- and TNF-alpha-mediated epithelial cell eosinophil chemotactic activity. Eur Respir J 14:767-775.

Liu, YJ. (2007a) Thymic stromal lymphopoietin and OX40 ligand pathway in the initiation of dendritic cell-mediated allergic inflammation. J Allergy Clin Immunol 120:238-244.

Liu, Y.J.; Soumelis, V.; Watanabe, N.; Ito, T.; Wang, Y.H.; de Waal-Malefyt, Rd. R.; Omori, M.; Zhou, B. & Ziegler, S.F. (2007b) TSLP: an epithelial cell cytokine that regulates T cell differentiation by conditioning dendritic cell maturation. Annu Rev Immunol 25:193-219.

Loza, M.J.; Peters, S.P.; Foster, S.; Khan, I.U. & Penn, R.B. (2007) beta-Agonist enhances type 2 T-cell survival and accumulation. J Allergy Clin Immunol 119:235-244.

Nelson, H.S.; Weiss, S.T.; Bleecker, E.R.; Yancey, S.W. & Dorinsky, P.M. (2006) The Salmeterol Multicenter Asthma Research Trial: a comparison of usual pharmacotherapy for asthma or usual pharmacotherapy plus salmeterol. Chest 129:15-26.

Orihara, K.; Nakae, S.; Pawankar, R. & Saito, H. (2008) Role of regulatory and proinflammatory T-cell populations in allergic diseases. WAO (World Allergy Organization) Journal 1:9-14.

Panina-Bordignon, P.; Mazzeo, D.; Lucia, P.D.; D'Ambrosio, D.; Lang, R.; Fabbri, L.; Self, C. & Sinigaglia, F. (1997) Beta2-agonists prevent Th1 development by selective inhibition of interleukin 12. J Clin Invest 100:1513-1519.

Paris, J.; Peterson, E.L.; Wells, K.; Pladevall, M.; Burchard, E.G.; Choudhry, S.; Lanfear, D.E. & Williams, L.K. (2008) Relationship between recent short-acting beta-agonist use and subsequent asthma exacerbations. Ann Allergy Asthma Immunol 101:482-487.

Soumelis, V.; Reche, P.A.; Kanzler, H.; Yuan, W.; Edward, G.; Homey, B.; Gilliet, M.; Ho, S.; Antonenko, S.; Lauerma, A.; Smith, K.; Gorman, D.; Zurawski, S.; Abrams, J.; Menon, S.; McClanahan, T.; de Waal-Malefyt, Rd. R.; Bazan, F.; Kastelein, R.A. & Liu, Y.J. (2002) Human epithelial cells trigger dendritic cell mediated allergic inflammation by producing TSLP. Nat Immunol 2002;3: 673-680.

Spoelstra, F.M.; Postma, D.S.; Hovenga, H.; Noordhoek, J.A. & Kauffman, H.F. (2002) Additive anti-inflammatory effect of formoterol and budesonide on human lung fibroblasts. Thorax 57:237-241.

Usmani, O.S.; Ito, K.; Maneechotesuwan, K.; Ito, M.; Johnson, M.; Barnes, P.J. & Adcock, I.M. (2005) Glucocorticoid receptor nuclear translocation in airway cells after inhaled combination therapy. Am J Respir Crit Care Med 172:704-712.

Yasui, K.; Kobayashi, N.; Yamazaki, T.; Agematsu, K.; Matsuzaki, S.; Nakata, S. & Baba, A. (2006) Differential effects of short-acting beta2-agonists on human granulocyte functions. Int Arch Allergy Immunol 139:1-8.

Yoo, J.; Omori, M.; Gyarmati, D.; Zhou, B.; Aye, T.; Brewer, A.; Comeau, M.R.; Campbell, D.J. & Ziegler, S.F. (2005) Spontaneous atopic dermatitis in mice expressing an inducible thymic stromal lymphopoietin transgene specifically in the skin. J Exp Med 202:541-549.

Zhou, B.; Comeau, M.R.; De Smedt, T.; Liggitt, H.D.; Dahl, M.E.; Lewis, D.B.; Gyarmati, D.; Aye, T.; Campbell, D.J. & Ziegler, S.F. (2005) Thymic stromal lymphopoietin as a key initiator of allergic airway inflammation in mice. Nat Immunol 6:1047-1053.

21

Microbiota and Allergy: From Dysbiosis to Probiotics

Anne-Judith Waligora-Dupriet and Marie-José Butel
EA 4065 Département Périnatalité, Microbiologie, Médicament, Faculté des Sciences Pharmaceutiques et Biologiques, Université Paris Descartes, Sorbonne Paris Cité, France

1. Introduction

The update theory of hygiene implicates the gut microbiota in the increasing prevalence of allergy. Indeed, changes have been observed in the establishment of the gut microbiota over the last fifteen years, and dysbiosis has been demonstrated in allergic subjects by numerous clinical studies comparing the microbiota in subjects from countries with high and low prevalence of allergy, or subjects with or without allergic diseases. These results support the use of pro- and prebiotics to treat or prevent allergic diseases; however, randomized controlled trials, mainly concerning atopic dermatitis, rhinitis and asthma, provide conflicting data. The mechanism of action of probiotics has not been elucidated. Nevertheless, it appears that lactobacilli and bifidobacteria may mediate immune responses in a strain-specific way, and the interactions involved seem to include dendritic cells and detection of microbe-associated molecular patterns. Although these functional foods are promising, numerous issues, including the bacterial strains and doses to use, remain to be determined.

1.1 The update theory of hygiene implicates the gut microbiota

Over recent decades, the incidence of allergic diseases has been increasing in industrialized country whereas it is stable in developing countries (Mannino *et al.*, 1998). This dichotomy and the large differences in the prevalence of allergy between genetically similar populations suggest that environmental factors make a large contribution to the development of allergies (Asher *et al.*, 2010). Numerous studies agree on the importance of the T-helper CD4 lymphocyte population balance (Th1, Th2, Th17, T regulatory cells), and an imbalance towards Th2 is considered to be a major factor for the onset of allergic disease. Imbalances of this type have long been associated with the absence of triggers of the Th1 immune response during childhood. Indeed, the increase in incidence of allergic diseases in industrialized countries coincides with widespread vaccination, antibiotic usage, declining family size, improvements in household amenities, and higher standards of personal cleanliness, all of which have reduced the opportunity for cross infection between children over the past century (the hygiene hypothesis, proposed by Strachan in 1989). However, the reduction of Th1 responses as a consequence of modern lifestyle cannot alone explain the high prevalence of allergic diseases in industrialized countries. Moreover, epidemiologic studies show that the morbidity of autoimmune diseases, which are associated with a Th1 or Th17 profiles, are increasing and that helminthiasis, associated with a Th2 profile, are not associated with an increased risk of allergic disease (Bach, 2002). Recent work implicates therefore inadequate stimulation of either various regulatory T cell subsets, or Toll-like receptor (Okada *et al.*, 2010;Akdis *et al.*, 2004).

Commensal bacteria of the intestinal microbiota play a crucial role in development of the intestinal immune system and modulation of the T helper cell balance. Rautava *et al.* extended this "hygiene hypothesis" and suggested that the initial composition of the infant gut microbiota may be a key determinant in the development of atopic disease (Rautava *et al.*, 2004). Indeed, neonates are biased towards T helper type 2 responses with reference to adults (Adkins *et al.*, 2004;Protonotariou *et al.*, 2004), and the first bacteria to colonize the infant's gut are the first stimuli for post-natal maturation of the T-helper balance. The immature Th2-dominant neonatal response undergoes environment-driven maturation via microbial contact during the early postnatal period resulting in a gradual inhibition of the Th2 response and an increase of the Th1 response and prevention of allergic diseases. This hypothesis is consistent with various observations: the delayed colonization of the digestive tract associated with changes in lifestyle over the last 15 years (Campeotto *et al.*, 2007;Adlerberth and Wold, 2009); and evidence that caesarian section (Kero *et al.*, 2002;Laubereau *et al.*, 2004), prematurity (Agosti *et al.*, 2003), and exposure to antibiotics during pregnancy (McKeever *et al.*, 2002) —all factors which modify establishment of the gut microbiota— are associated with a higher risk of atopic disease.

2. The gut microbiota and its functions

The composition of microbial communities in the gut was first investigated through culture-based studies, leading to estimates of 400 to 500 different species in the adult human intestinal tract (Manson *et al.*, 2008). The dominant microbiota (10^9-10^{11} CFU.g^{-1}) is composed of obligate anaerobes, including Gram-negative bacilli such as *Bacteroides,* Gram-positive bacilli such as *Bifidobacterium, Eubacterium,* and Gram-positive cocci. The subdominant microbiota (10^6-10^8 CFU.g^{-1}) is composed of facultative anaerobes including various species of enterobacteria, notably *Escherichia coli*, and species of the *Enterococcus* and *Lactobacillus* genera. With population densities of below 10^6 CFU.g^{-1}, this microbiota is often extremely variable and transient.

The use of culture-independent approaches has provided novel insights into the gut microbiota community (Manson *et al.*, 2008). Many of the techniques used are based on analysis of 16S rRNA gene sequences, and studies have exploited combinations of 16S rRNA gene libraries, DNA microarrays, 16S rRNA gene fingerprinting, fluorescent *in* situ hybridization, and quantitative PCR. These culture-independent techniques have shown that the intestinal microbiota community is more complex than previously described. The proportion of bacteria in the adult intestine that can be cultured varies between 15 and 85% (Eckburg *et al.*, 2005); over 1200 bacterial species have been characterized (Rajilic-Stojanovic *et al.*, 2007), and current estimates are that there are up to 1000 bacterial species per individual and over 5000 different species in total in human intestines (Zoetendal *et al.*, 2008). Most of the gut microbiota are from only four major phyla (Tap *et al.*, 2009). *Firmicutes* and *Bacteroidetes* are the most abundant, and *Actinobacteria* - including bifidobacteria - and *Proteobacteria* are less abundant despite representing more than 1% of the total microbiota. Adult fecal microbiota has been demonstrated to be individual-specific and relatively stable over time (Rajilic-Stojanovic *et al.*, 2009). However, even though each individual harbors a unique microbiota, a number of microbial species are present in all individuals, consistent with the existence of a universal phylogenetic core to the human intestinal microbiota (Rajilic-Stojanovic *et al.*, 2009;Tap *et al.*, 2009).

The intestinal ecosystem develops rapidly during the neonatal stage of life. The intestine is sterile at birth and is colonized by bacteria following contact with the maternal microbiota and the surrounding environment. Little is known about the factors that lead to the establishment of particular bacterial strains. Colonizing bacteria originate mainly from the mother; the maternal gut microbiota is a major source and other sources include the microbiota of the vagina, perineum, and skin. Breast milk has also been demonstrated to be a source of lactic acid bacteria (Martin *et al.*, 2009;Gueimonde *et al.*, 2007). Infants encounter numerous bacteria in the environment including the microbiota of food and the microbiota of the skin of parents, siblings and nurses. Consequently, the number of bacterial species, mainly obligate anaerobes, increases with time in the infant gut. As a result of the diversity of exposure, there is substantial inter-individual variability in the composition and patterns of bacterial colonization during the first weeks of life (Penders *et al.*, 2006c;Palmer *et al.*, 2007;Vaishampayan *et al.*, 2010). However, by the end of the first year of life, the bacterial composition in the gut converges toward an adult-like microbiota profile (Palmer *et al.*, 2007). Various external factors can affect the pattern of bacterial colonization (for review see (Adlerberth and Wold, 2009;Vael and Desager, 2009;Campeotto *et al.*, 2007). Infants born by cesarean section are deprived of contact with their mother's gut and vaginal microbiota, which decreases bacterial diversity and colonization by obligate anaerobes, particularly bifidobacteria and *Bacteroides*. The mode of infant feeding also strongly affects bacterial establishment, with a dominant colonization by bifidobacteria being a characteristic distinguishing breastfed from formula-fed infants. However, improvements in infant formulas have led to there now being only minor differences in colonization according to feeding method (Adlerberth and Wold, 2009;Campeotto *et al.*, 2007). Finally, the establishment of gut microbiota in infants in industrialized countries appears to have been affected in modern times, most likely due to improved hygiene and general cleanliness in these countries, resulting in reduced bacterial exposure (Adlerberth and Wold, 2009;Campeotto *et al.*, 2007).

Although the gut microbiota community was for several decades mostly studied to elucidate pathogenic relationships, it is now clear that most microorganism-host interactions in the gut are, in fact, commensal or even mutualistic (Bik, 2009;Dethlefsen *et al.*, 2007). This complex ecosystem has various major functions (Fujimura *et al.*, 2010). Colonic fermentation of non-digestible dietary residues and endogenous mucus supplies energy and nutritive products to the bacteria. It also plays a role in the trophic functions of the intestinal epithelium (Wong *et al.*, 2006). The barrier effect, which involves secretion of antimicrobial molecules, competition for nutrients, and attachment to ecological niches, refers to a resistance to colonization by exogenous or opportunistic bacteria present at a low level in the gut (Stecher and Hardt, 2008). Finally, the gut microbial community has a major immune function. The contribution of the gut microbiota to immune system maturation has been demonstrated by the description of major abnormalities of the immune system in germ-free mice (Smith *et al.*, 2007). Intestinal IgA-secreting plasma cells are rare in germ-free animals, and the Peyer's patches are smaller and contain fewer lymphoid follicles than those in conventional mice. The T cell content of the mucosal immune system is also low in germ-free animals, and particularly the CD4+ cells of the lamina propria. Spleen and lymph nodes are relatively structureless with abnormal B- and T- cell zones. These morphologic features are associated with substantial functional abnormalities, such as hypogammaglobulinemia, a Th2 cell shift and defects in oral tolerance induction (Round *et al.*, 2010). Recent reviews have highlighted how the microbiota elicits innate and adaptative immune mechanisms that cooperate to protect the host and maintain intestinal homeostasis (Hooper and Macpherson, 2010;Garrett *et al.*, 2010). Colonization of germ-free mice by a single species of bacteria e.g. *Bacteroides fragilis* (Mazmanian *et al.*, 2005) or segmented filamentous bacteria (Gaboriau-Routhiau *et al.*, 2009), has been shown to be sufficient to restore the development of a multifaceted adaptative immune response. The capacity to stimulate steady-state gut T cell responses appears to be restricted to a small number of bacteria (Gaboriau-Routhiau *et al.*, 2009) and certain strains. Indeed, the immunostimulatory properties of *Bifidobacterium* are strain-specific (Medina *et al.*, 2007;Menard *et al.*, 2008) and only some strains of *Bifidobacterium* are able to induce Foxp3+ regulatory cells or be associated with protection from respiratory and oral allergy in mice (Lyons *et al.*, 2010). *B. infantis* restored the susceptibility to oral tolerance induction in germ-free mice only if the inoculation was at the neonatal stage (Sudo *et al.*, 1997). This suggests that there is a 'time window of opportunity' during the neonatal phase, consistent with observations with probiotics (Feleszko *et al.*, 2007).

3. Microbiota and allergy

The extended version of the hygiene hypothesis implicating the gut microbiota is supported by several clinical studies which have shown a relationship between allergic disease and gut microbiota. In particular, they have shown that the composition of the bacterial community in the feces differ between children who live in countries with high and low prevalence of allergy, as well between children with or without allergic diseases.

3.1 Is gut microbiota different between healthy individuals and allergic subjects? Case-control studies

Numerous studies have addressed the composition of the microbiota in healthy and allergic subjects. Some of the first studies (Bjorksten *et al.*, 1999;Sepp *et al.*, 1997) compared the microbiota between two-year old children in countries with high (Sweden) and low (Estonia) incidence of allergic diseases. Irrespective of country of residence, allergic children were colonized by fewer lactobacilli but had higher counts of aerobic bacteria, especially *Enterobacteriaceae* and staphylococci and lower counts of *Bacteroides*. A prospective study (Bjorksten *et al.*, 2001) found that children who developed atopic dermatitis and/or positive skin prick test results during the two first years of life were less often colonized with enterococci during the first month of life and with bifidobacteria during the first year of life. Furthermore, allergic infants had higher counts of clostridia at 3 months of age and lower counts of *Bacteroides* at 12 months. The prevalence of colonization with *Staphylococcus aureus* was also higher in allergic children than the reference group at 6 months old.

Case-control studies confirmed differences of the gut microbiota composition between allergic and healthy subjects but the differences identified concerned various particular genera and species, including *Bifidobacterium, Clostridium, Bacteroides, Lactobacillus* and *Enterobacteriaceae*. Indirect methods suggested an association between allergy and

Clostridium difficile. Allergic infants had higher fecal concentrations of the rarely detected i-caproic acid, which has been associated with the presence of *Clostridium difficile* (Bottcher *et al.*, 2000) and higher *C. difficile* IgG antibody levels at one year than non-allergic infants (Woodcock *et al.*, 2002). However, counting bacteria by FISH analysis indicated that colonization by *Clostridium* sp. was lower in allergic than reference subjects (Mah *et al.*, 2006) and no significant difference in *Clostridium* counts were found between preschool controls and children with allergy-associated atopic eczema/dermatitis syndrome (AAEDS) and non-allergic atopic eczema/dermatitis syndrome (NAAEDS) (Kendler *et al.*, 2006)

Numerous other studies reported quantitative differences in colonization with *Bifidobacterium*, a dominant genus in infant fecal microbiota which may have beneficial effects (Ventura *et al.*, 2004). The prevalence of *Bifidobacterium* has been found to be similar in healthy and allergic subjects, whatever the allergic disease (Stsepetova *et al.*, 2007;Waligora-Dupriet *et al.*, 2011), and for atopic dermatitis (Gore *et al.*, 2008), and wheezing (Murray *et al.*, 2005). However, the findings of one study are discordant (Sepp *et al.*, 2005) with none of the 5-year-old children with atopic dermatitis and only one child with bronchial asthma colonized with bifidobacteria. Besides, low levels of bifidobacterial colonization have been observed in infants suffering from atopic dermatitis (Kirjavainen *et al.*, 2001;Watanabe *et al.*, 2003;Mah *et al.*, 2006) and in infants suffering from atopic dermatitis and wheezing; note that these results have been contradicted by studies comparing healthy subjects with wheezing infants without other symptoms (Murray *et al.*, 2005) and with patients suffering from both atopic dermatitis and food allergy (Penders *et al.*, 2006a).

3.2 Does dysbiosis precede allergic symptoms? Prospective studies

Some prospective studies report that modifications of the composition of the intestinal microbiota can be detected before any atopic syndrome, suggesting that bacteria implicated in the maturation of the immune system may be important. The bacterial fatty acid profile in fecal samples differed significantly between 3-week-old infants in whom atopy was and was not developing. The stools of atopic subjects had more clostridia and tended to have fewer bifidobacteria than those of non atopic subjects, resulting in a reduced ratio of bifidobacteria to clostridia (Kalliomaki *et al.*, 2001a). The Koala Birth Cohort Study in the Netherlands confirmed these results by showing that gut dysbiosis precedes the manifestation of atopic symptoms and atopic sensitization (Penders *et al.*, 2007). In particular, *C. difficile* was associated with all atopic symptoms and sensitization. The presence of *Escherichia coli* was associated with a higher risk of developing (non-atopic) eczema, this risk increasing with increasing *E. coli* counts; infants colonized with *C. difficile* were at higher risk of developing atopic dermatitis, recurrent wheeze and allergic sensitisation. As *E. coli* was only associated with eczema and *C. difficile* was associated with all atopic outcomes, the underlying mechanisms may be different. Colonization with clostridia, including *C. difficile*, was associated with allergy development up to age 2 years in several studies (Kalliomaki *et al.*, 2001a;Bjorksten *et al.*, 2001;Penders *et al.*, 2007) but not in others (Adlerberth *et al.*, 2007;Sjogren *et al.*, 2009;Songjinda *et al.*, 2007). Fecal colonization at age 3 weeks with *Clostridium coccoides* subcluster XIVa species has been described as an early indicator of possible asthma later in life (Vael *et al.*, 2008;Vael *et al.*, 2011). However, Verhulst *et al.* (2008) found an association between antibiotics, anaerobic bacteria and wheezing during the first year of life, but increasing levels of *Clostridium* were protective against wheezing. These studies considered different *Clostridium* species and the genus *Clostridium* is a very heterogeneous group comprising several different clusters (Stackebrandt *et al.*, 1999). Indeed, it seems unlikely that all members of this genus exert the same effects on the human immune system (Penders *et al.*, 2007).

Children not developing allergy before age 2 years have been shown to be more frequently colonized with bifidobacteria than children developing allergy (Bjorksten *et al.*, 2001), but this decreased prevalence of *Bifidobacterium* in children suffering allergies was not confirmed in all studies (Songjinda *et al.*, 2007;Penders *et al.*, 2006a;Adlerberth *et al.*, 2007). Differences in patterns of colonization by bifidobacteria species have also been observed but no clear consensus exists. Young *et al* (2004) compared the populations of bifidobacteria in feces from children aged 25 to 35 days in Ghana (which has a low prevalence of atopy), New Zealand, and the United Kingdom (high-prevalence countries): almost all fecal samples from Ghana contained *Bifidobacterium longum* subsp *infantis* whereas those from the children living in the other countries did not. The authors suggested that place of birth influences the patterns of bifidobacterial species present. *B. adolescentis* has been found in the fecal microbiota of both allergic infants (Ouwehand *et al.*, 2001;He *et al.*, 2001) and non-allergic infants (Sjogren *et al.*, 2009). Similarly, *B. catenulatum/pseudocatenulatum* has been isolated from both allergic (Gore *et al.*, 2008) and non-allergic infants (Stsepetova *et al.*, 2007). Some authors report that restricted *Bifidobacterium* diversity is linked with allergy (Stsepetova *et al.*, 2007) but again, this was not confirmed in other studies at the species (Sjogren *et al.*, 2009;Waligora-Dupriet *et al.*, 2011) or strain level (Waligora-Dupriet *et al.*, 2011). It has been suggested that the intrinsic properties of bacterial strains may be pertinent. Indeed, *in vitro*, bifidobacterial species differentially affected expression of cell surface markers and cytokine production by dendritic cells harvested from cord blood. *B. bifidum*, *B. longum*, and *B. pseudocatenulatum*, species commonly detected in children in New Zealand and the United Kingdom increased the expression of the dendritic-cell activation marker CD83 and induce IL-10 production, whereas *B. infantis*, a species commonly isolated in Ghana, does not (Young *et al*, 2004). By contrast, heat-inactivated *B. longum* subsp *longum* and *B. adolescentis*, known as adult-type bifidobacteria, were significantly stronger inducers of pro-inflammatory cytokine (IL-12 and TNF-alpha) production by a murine macrophage cell line than *B. bifidum*, *B. breve*, and *B. longum* subsp *infantis* usually isolated from infants (He *et al.*, 2002). The Th1 stimulation profile induced by *B. adolescentis* (Karlsson *et al.*, 2004;He *et al.*, 2002) may intensify pathology in allergic infants (He *et al.*, 2002). However, the properties of intestinal bifidobacteria are highly strain-dependent (Matto *et al.*, 2004), and this is particularly true of immunostimulatory properties (Menard *et al.*, 2008;Medina *et al.*, 2007).

Bacteroidaceae are also associated with allergic development, although, as for clostridia and bifidobacteria, findings are contradictory. Indeed, *Bacteroides* colonization of the gut was not found to be linked to allergy in several studies (Adlerberth *et al.*, 2007;Kalliomaki *et al.*, 2001a; Bjorksten *et al.*, 2001; Sjogren *et al.*, 2009), but colonization with the *B. fragilis* group at age 3 weeks has been associated with a higher risk of developing asthma later in life (Vael *et al.*, 2008;Vael *et al.*, 2011). A high level of *Bacteroides* colonization positively correlated with IgE in children with atopic dermatitis (Kirjavainen *et al.*, 2002). Moreover, fecal *Bacteroides* strains induced high levels of Th2 cytokine production by peripheral blood monocyte cells from patients suffering from Japanese Cedar Pollinosis (Odamaki *et al.*, 2007).

Discrepancies between studies might be the consequence of the methods used to study the gut microbiota. Indeed, in the same study, some differences were observed with FISH but that were not detected by bacterial cultivation (Kalliomaki *et al.*, 2001a). These discrepancies are such that it is not possible to conclude about the association of particular species, genera or groups with the development of allergy, although it seems that the diversity of the gut microbiota is a major determinant in allergy risk. Interestingly, a large recent study did not find any relationships between the presence of various particular bacteria and allergy development up to 18 months of age (Adlerberth *et al.*, 2007), but showed that infants who developed allergy had a lower diversity in their gut microbiota at one week of age (Wang *et al.*, 2008).

Despite prospective studies showing that modifications of the gut microbiota composition can be detected before any atopic syndrome, these epidemiological studies cannot demonstrate which of these factors appears first. Atopy could be linked to a mucosal state favoring some bacterial populations to the detriment of others. In a mouse model of food allergy, mice with high and low anaphylaxis scores showed differences in intestinal microbiota composition: high responders exhibited less staphylococcus colonization (Rodriguez *et al.*, 2011). The composition of the intestinal bacteria fluctuated significantly during the pollen season in adults with IgE-dependent pollinosis, with colonization by the *Bacteroides fragilis* group increasing with pollen dispersal, especially at the end of the pollen season (Odamaki *et al.*, 2007). It is clear that the cause-and-effect relationship between the composition of the microbiota and allergic diseases remains to be determined.

4. Probiotics and allergic diseases

Despite discrepancies between studies, there is mounting evidence of a relationship between the intestinal microbiota and allergy. It therefore follows that a modulation of the gut microbiota may help prevent allergic diseases and this notion supports the use of probiotics, prebiotics and synbiotics. Probiotics are currently defined as "live microorganisms which when administered in adequate amounts confer a health benefit on the host" (FAO/WHO, 2001; FAO/WHO 2001, 2002). The most widely used probiotics are lactic acid bacteria, specifically *Lactobacillus* and *Bifidobacterium* species (Williams, 2010). The yeast *Saccharomyces boulardii* is also used. Although the efficacy of probiotics is sometimes debatable, they offer substantial potential benefits to health and are safe for human use.

The mechanisms of action of "probiotic" strains in allergic diseases may include modulation of the gut microbiota, maturation of the gut barrier, stimulation of the immune system and immunomodulation. However, the effects of probiotics described in experimental models need to be confirmed for human use through randomized controlled trials. We conducted bibliographic searches in the PubMed/Medline database for the following terms (all field): allergy AND probiotic*", and results limited to randomized controlled trials identified 99 publications.

4.1 Clinical impact of probiotics in atopic/allergic diseases

4.1.1 Probiotics in the treatment of atopic dermatitis

Fifty studies have evaluated clinical consequences of probiotics in the treatment of atopic dermatitis (AD) in infants and children, and between them have studied about 1100 subjects. AD is a chronic highly pruritic inflammatory skin disease including IgE- and non-IgE-mediated mechanisms. It commonly occurs during early infancy but can persist or even start in adulthood. It includes a wide clinical spectrum from minor forms to major symptoms including erythrodermic rash and can be associated with other atopic diseases such as food allergy, asthma, and allergic rhinitis. To evaluate the effects of probiotics on AD, a rigorous definition of study participants is necessary. The diagnosis of AD is currently based on diagnostic criteria scales developed by Hanifin and Rafka in 1980 and by the "United Kingdom Working party" in 1994 (*in* Roguedas-Contios and Misery, 2011). It is equally important that diseases outcome measures used in treatment studies are both valid and reliable. Three of the various eczema outcome measures have been shown to be reliable: SCORing Atopic Dermatitis (SCORAD), the Eczema Area and Severity Index (EASI) and the Patient Oriented Eczema Measure (POEM). SCORAD is commonly used in studies of probiotics. It combines an estimation of the intensity and extent of the eczema with a subjective itch. However, it assesses a clinical state of the disease at a particular time point without taking into account overall severity or evolution of the disease (Société Française de Dermatologie, 2005). Some quality of life scales are also used, for example the Infant Dermatitis Quality Of Life (IDQOL), Dermatitis Family Impact (DFI), and Dermatitis Family Impact Questionnaire (DFIQ) scores (Gerasimov *et al.*, 2010; Weston *et al.*, 2005) scores.

The age range of subjects included varies between studies: around weaning (median 5 months old) (Brouwer *et al.*, 2006;Isolauri *et al.*, 2000;Kirjavainen *et al.*, 2003;Viljanen *et al.*, 2005b;Gruber *et al.*, 2007), around 1 year old (Weston *et al.*, 2005;Folster-Holst *et al.*, 2006), and around 5 years old (Rosenfeldt *et al.*, 2003, 2004; Sistek *et al.*, 2006; Woo *et al.*, 2010). Seven of these publications describe effects of *Lactobacillus rhamnosus* GG LGG in infants but report contradictory results (Brouwer *et al.*, 2006;Isolauri *et al.*, 2000;Kirjavainen *et al.*, 2003;Viljanen *et al.*, 2005b;Gruber *et al.*, 2007;Folster-Holst *et al.*, 2006;Nermes *et al.*, 2011). Two of them (Isolauri *et al.*, 2000;Kirjavainen *et al.*, 2003) showed a significant decrease of the SCORAD score, but both these studies included only small groups of infants (27 and 35). Moreover, the heat-inactivated LGG used in Kirjavainen's study induced adverse gastrointestinal symptoms and diarrhea leading to the recruitment of patients being stopped after the pilot phase (Kirjavainen *et al.*, 2003). Six other studies, similar in terms of subjects included and protocol, did not find any improvement in SCORAD scores following LGG supplementation (Folster-Holst *et al.*, 2006;Brouwer *et al.*, 2006;Gruber *et al.*, 2007;Viljanen *et al.*, 2005b;Nermes *et al.*, 2011;Rose *et al.*, 2010). Other probiotic strains have been studied, and *Bifidobacterium lactis* Bb12 (Isolauri *et al.*, 2000), *L. sakei* KCTC 10755B0 and *L. fermentum* VRI-003 (Weston *et al.*, 2005) induced significant decreases in SCORAD scores. In the last of these studies, the effects of *L. fermentum* VRI-003 were found to persist two months after the end of supplementation. Four studies used a *L. rhamnosus* strain (not LGG) alone (Brouwer *et al.*, 2006) or mixed with *L. reuteri* (Rosenfeldt *et al.*, 2003) or with other *Lactobacillus sp.* and *Bifidobacterium sp.* (Viljanen *et al.*, 2005b;Sistek *et al.*, 2006). These studies did not detect significant SCORAD score improvement although in the crossover study of Rosenfeldt *et al* (2003), which included children older than those in the other studies, patients felt better according to their subjective evaluations. Nevertheless, a pronounced decrease in SCORAD score was observed in patients with a positive skin prick-test response and increased IgE levels (Viljanen *et al.*, 2005b;Rosenfeldt *et al.*, 2003;Sistek *et al.*, 2006). The administration of a probiotic mixture containing *L. acidophilus* DDS-1, *B. lactis* UABLA-12, and fructo-oligosaccharide was associated with a significant clinical improvement in children with AD and in particular a large decrease in SCORAD score and increase in quality of life score relative to the placebo group (Gerasimov *et al.*, 2010). This was not the case with a mixture of *B. breve* M-16V and galacto-/fructooligosaccharide (Immunofortis) (van der Aa *et al.*, 2010), even though this synbiotic mixture seemed to prevent asthma-like symptoms in infants with

AD (van der Aa *et al.*, 2011). To conclude, investigations of probiotics for the treatment of AD provide promising results, but are not conclusive, as confirmed by meta-analyzes (Lee *et al.*, 2008;Osborn and Sinn, 2007) such that they do not provide sufficient basis to recommend the use of such products.

4.1.2 Probiotics in the treatment of rhinitis and respiratory allergic diseases

Eleven studies have evaluated clinical effects of probiotics in the treatment of allergic diseases of the respiratory tract, *i.e.* rhinitis and asthma, and altogether included about 890 subjects.

Lactobacillus paracasei-33, whether or not heat-inactivated, improved quality of life of patients with allergic rhinitis: both frequency and intensity of symptoms were significantly lower in the LP-33 group than the placebo group, after the 30-day treatment (Wang *et al.*, 2004;Peng & Hsu, 2005). Likewise, *Lactobacillus casei* DN114 001 decreased the occurrence of rhinitis episodes and improved the health status of children with allergic rhinitis (Giovannini *et al.*, 2007). For patients with Japanese cedar pollen allergy, LGG and *Lactobacillus gasseri* TMC0356 reduced nasal symptoms (Kawase *et al.*, 2009), and *B. longum* BB536 was able to relieve eye symptoms (Ishida *et al.*, 2005;Xiao *et al.*, 2007). The degree of eosinophil infiltration into the respiratory mucosa correlates directly with the intensity of allergic rhinitis and can be used as an objective marker of the disease. A mixture of *L. acidophilus* NCFMTM and *B. lactis* Bl-04 reduced nasal eosinophil infiltration (Ouwehand *et al.*, 2009) as did *Bacillus clausii* which also reduced the number of days on which antihistamine was used in children with allergic rhinitis due to pollen sensitization (Ciprandi *et al.*, 2005a). However, *L. rhamnosus* ATCC53103 was not beneficial to teenagers and young adults allergic to birch pollen or ingested apple and who had intermittent symptoms of atopic allergy and/or mild asthma (Helin *et al.*, 2002). Similarly, *L. casei* Shirota was not found to reduce symptoms of Japanese cedar pollen allergy (Tamura *et al.*, 2007), although the strain did reduce serum concentrations of IL-5, IL-6, IFN-γ and specific IgE in subjects with allergic rhinitis (Ivory *et al.*, 2008). In children with recurrent wheeze and an atopic family history, LGG had no clinical effect on asthma-related events, and only a small effect on allergic sensitization (Rose *et al.*, 2010); likewise, long-term consumption of fermented milk containing *L. casei* had no detectable effect in asthmatic children (Giovannini *et al.*, 2007)

4.1.3 Probiotics in the primary prevention of allergic diseases

The prevention of allergy through an early administration of probiotics is appealing.

Four studies investigating probiotic supplementation begun during pregnancy. The first study to be published was by the team of Isolauri and reported promising results on preventive effects of LGG (Kalliomaki *et al.*, 2001b). LGG was given prenatally to 132 mothers who had at least one first-degree relative (or partner) with atopic eczema, allergic rhinitis, or asthma, and postnatally for 6 months to their infants. Two years later, the frequency of atopic eczema in infants given probiotics was half that of those on placebo (Kalliomaki *et al.*, 2001b). The reduction was greatest for infants who were exclusively breastfed, and therefore who did not receive the probiotic directly until 3 months of age (LGG being given to the mother) (Rautava *et al.*, 2002a). Administration of probiotics to the mother during pregnancy and breast-feeding appeared to be a safe and effective method for enhancing the immunoprotective potential of breast milk and preventing atopic eczema in the infant. The protective effect of LGG extended beyond infancy until 7 years old

(Kalliomaki *et al.*, 2003; 2007). Infants most likely to benefit from probiotics might be those with an elevated cord blood IgE concentration (Rautava *et al.*, 2002a), despite such high IgE levels not appearing as a risk factor for atopic diseases (Bergmann *et al.*, 1998). However, LGG had no impact on sensitization: there was no difference between LGG and placebo groups at 2, 4 and 7 year old as concerns the numbers of infants with high levels of specific IgE and/or positive prick test results (Kalliomaki *et al.*, 2001b; 2003; 2007).

The preventive effect of LGG was not confirmed in a similar study by Kopp *et al.* (2008) with 94 mother-infant couples. The discrepancies between the data of Kalliomaki *et al* and the data of Kopp *et al* cannot be explained by the minor differences between the study designs, but could be linked to the study populations. The German cohort (Kopp *et al*) was at higher risk of allergy than the Finnish cohort (Kalliomaki *et al*), the infants had older siblings, and the genetic contexts were different. Two other preventive studies considered prenatal and postnatal supplementation with probiotics. An investigation of *L reuteri* ATCC55730 supplementation for infants with a family history of allergic disease did not confirm a preventive effect against infant eczema but found a decreased prevalence of IgE-associated eczema during the second year. The effect was larger in the subgroup of children of allergic mothers (Abrahamsson *et al.*, 2007). Infants receiving *L rhamnosus* HN001 had a significantly lower risk of eczema than infants receiving placebo, but this was not the case for *B animalis* subsp *lactis* and there was no significant effect of these two strains on atopy (Wickens *et al.*, 2008). Taylor *et al* (2006a; 2006b; 2007a; 2007b) and of Soh *et al* (2009) studied newborns given, from birth to 6 months of life, *L. acidophilus* LAVRI-A1 (178 infants) and a mixture of *L. rhamnosus* LPR and *B. longum* BL999 (253 infants), respectively, and did not find any reduction of the risk of AD in high-risk infants as assessed from the numbers of patients affected, SCORAD score or IgE sensitization. Moreover, *L. acidophilus* was associated with increased allergen sensitization (Taylor *et al.*, 2007a). Likewise, supplementation with LGG during pregnancy and early infancy did not alter the severity of atopic dermatitis in affected children and was associated with an increased rate of recurrent episodes of wheezing and bronchitis (Kalliomaki *et al.*, 2003; 2007; Kopp *et al.*, 2008).

4.2 Mechanisms of probiotic action in atopic/allergic diseases in human

Although no unambiguous clinical benefits were observed in several studies, probiotics may nevertheless have useful effects on microbiota composition, the immune system and the gut barrier in infants and in children.

4.2.1 Effects of probiotics on microbiota composition

Any effects of probiotic microorganisms on health and well-being may potentially be due, at least in part, to modulation of the intestinal microbiota. However, few of the studies on probiotics and allergic diseases assessed the consequences of probiotic use on gut microbiota composition. From the available evidence, it seems that probiotics have no impact on microbiota. In the treatment of rhinitis with *L. acidophilus* NCFMTM, fecal probiotic cell counts correlated positively with fecal acetic, propionic and butyric acid concentrations (Ouwehand *et al.*, 2009), suggesting that the presence of *L. acidophilus* NCFMTM increases microbial fermentation in the colon. However, the colonization pattern did not differ between groups that consumed the probiotic strains and placebo. Similarly, no modification of the gut microbiota was observed following LGG supplementation in infants with AD (Kirjavainen *et al*, 2003). The fecal microbiota fluctuated in subjects with Japanese cedar pollinosis during the pollen season and supplementation with BB536 yogurt modulated the microbiota in a manner that may possibly contribute to the alleviation of allergic symptoms (Odamaki *et al*, 2007).

4.2.2 Gut immunity and barrier effect

Probiotics may modulate local immune systems. Treatment with LGG resulted in a trend towards elevated fecal IgA levels, and this effect was significant in IgE-associated cow-milk allergy infants, suggesting maturation of intestinal immunity and triggering of a mechanism to protect the gut from the offending food (Viljanen *et al.*, 2005a). In older subjects with a mature immune system and suffering from allergic rhinitis, fecal IgA concentrations increased in the placebo group during the pollen season; this increase was prevented by *L. acidophilus* NCFMTM (Ouwehand *et al.*, 2009).
Probiotics have also been reported to decrease the levels of fecal inflammatory markers, but this is controversial: findings differ between studies and strains used. Treatment of AD with LGG was associated with a decrease of TNF-α and α-antitrypsin levels suggesting that LGG may alleviate inflammation in the gut. Indeed, TNF-α is a proinflammatory cytokine for both Th1- and Th2-type cells, and a marker of local inflammation. The presence of α-antitrypsin indicates protein loss in the intestine and is a marker of mucosal integrity. These results were not confirmed in the studies by Folster-Holt *et al* (2006) and Brouwer *et al* (2006) who did not observe any differences in α-antitrypsin, or calprotectin, or eosinophilic cationic protein levels between infants receiving or not receiving LGG. Accumulation of eosinophilic cationic protein at sites of allergic inflammation demonstrates local eosinophil degranulation in the gut. Specific lactobacilli (*L. rhamnosus* 19070-2 and *L reuteri* DSM 12246) might reverse increased small intestinal permeability (such permeability is involved in the pathogenesis of atopic dermatitis) thereby stabilizing the intestinal barrier function and decreasing gastrointestinal symptoms in children with AD (Rosenfeldt *et al.*, 2004).

4.2.3 Th1/Th2 balance

Certain strains of *Lactobacillus* and *Bifidobacterium* can modulate cytokine production.
Bacillus clausii modulated the cytokine pattern in the nasal mucosa in allergic children with recurrent respiratory infections. In particular, *B. clausii* restored physiological Th1 polarization and induced T-regulatory cell responses, as documented by increased levels of IL-10 and tumor growth factor (TGF)-β after treatment (Ciprandi *et al.*, 2005b). TGF-β is a regulatory cytokine which may be responsible for a decrease in local inflammation (Shull *et al.*, 1992). Interestingly, Rautava *et al* (2002b) observed high TGF-β2 concentrations in breast-milk from mothers who had received LGG for prevention of allergic disease. The authors concluded that, first, direct supplementation of infant after birth is not necessary, and second that probiotics could increase the protective effects of breast milk.
The effects on the Th1-Th2 balance of probiotic strains used for the treatment of AD in early infancy have been evaluated in several studies. Pohjavuori *et al.* (2004) were able to demonstrate greater IFN-γ production in anti-CD3/anti-CD28-stimulated *in vitro* peripheral blood mononuclear cells (PBMC) from infants treated with LGG than placebo. A different modulatory effect was observed with a mix of four bacterial strains including LGG: a significant increase in secretion of IL-4 in infants with cow milk allergy. By contrast, production of the predominant Th1 cytokine INF-γ, and the Th2 cytokines IL-4 or IL-5 after polyclonal or specific anti-CD3/anti-CD28 stimulation, was unaffected by supplementation

with *L rhamnosus, LGG* (Brouwer *et al.*, 2006) or a lactobacillus mix (Rosenfeldt *et al.*, 2003). A decrease in circulating IgA-, IgG- and IgM-secreting cells and an increase in memory B cells during LGG supplementation has been described (Nermes *et al.*, 2011).
The oral administration of particular probiotic strains to patients with atopic dermatitis can modulate the cytokine pattern *in vivo* at site other than the intestine. *L. casei* Shirota reduced serum concentrations of IL-5, IL-6, IFN-γ and specific IgE in subjects with allergic rhinitis (Ivory *et al.*, 2008) but was not found to be effective in reducing the symptoms of Japanese cedar pollen allergy (Tamura *et al.*, 2007). Probiotics can be involved in both antagonistic and synergistic relationships with each other, and with members of the gut ecosystem. Indeed, mixtures of bacteria induced a response in human dendritic cells different to those of the component bacteria in isolation: antagonistic immunosuppressive effects were observed with certain strains of *Lactobacillus* and *Bifidobacterium* but synergistic effects were observed when these *Lactobacillus* and *Bifidobacterium* strains were combined with *E. coli* and *K. pneumoniae* strains (Zeuthen *et al.*, 2006).

5. Conclusion

Despite some promising results, the role of probiotics in the treatment and the prevention of allergy and related diseases has not been clearly demonstrated. Indeed, clinical trials provide various contradictory findings that do not allow probiotic supplementation to be included in the guidelines for the management of allergic diseases. These conflicting data may be however attributable to the differences between studies. The populations studied have been very diverse in terms of size, age, sensitization and allergic disease, environment, and genetic background. Study designs included different probiotics in term of strains, preparations (alive/ killed; one strain/mixture/synbiotics), doses, duration of supplementation, and period of administration (prental/postnatal). In addition to these issues, progress in our basic knowledge of probiotic strains, in strain selection, and in understanding their mechanisms of action is needed to give credibility to the health claims made for probiotics and especially for the design of efficacious therapeutic agents.

6. References

Abrahamsson, T.R., Jakobsson, T., Bottcher, M.F., Fredrikson, M., Jenmalm, M.C., Bjorksten, B., and Oldaeus, G. (2007) Probiotics in prevention of IgE-associated eczema: a double-blind, randomized, placebo-controlled trial. *J Allergy Clin Immunol* 119: 1174-1180. ISSN: 0091-6749

Adkins, B., Leclerc, C., and Marshall-Clarke, S. (2004) Neonatal adaptive immunity comes of age. *Nat Rev Immunol* 4: 553-564. ISSN: 1474-1733

Adlerberth, I., Strachan, D.P., Matricardi, P.M., Ahrne, S., Orfei, L., Aberg, N. *et al.* (2007) Gut microbiota and development of atopic eczema in 3 European birth cohorts. *J Allergy Clin Immunol* 120: 343-350. ISSN: 0091-6749

Adlerberth, I., and Wold, A.E. (2009) Establishment of the gut microbiota in Western infants. *Acta Paediatr* 98: 229-238. ISSN: 0803-5253

Agosti, M., Vegni, C., Gangi, S., Benedetti, V., and Marini, A. (2003) Allergic manifestations in very low-birthweight infants: a 6-year follow-up. *Acta Paediatr Suppl* 91: 44-47. ISSN: 0803-5253

Akdis, M., Verhagen, J., Taylor, A., Karamloo, F., Karagiannidis, C., Crameri, R. *et al.* (2004) Immune responses in healthy and allergic individuals are characterized by a fine balance between allergen-specific T regulatory 1 and T helper 2 cells. *J Exp Med* 199: 1567-1575. : 0022-1007

Asher, M.I., Stewart, A.W., Mallol, J., Montefort, S., Lai, C.K., Ait-Khaled, N., and Odhiambo, J. (2010) Which population level environmental factors are associated with asthma, rhinoconjunctivitis and eczema? Review of the ecological analyses of ISAAC Phase One. *Respir Res* 11: 8. ISSN: 1465-9921

Bach, J.F. (2002) The effect of infections on susceptibility to autoimmune and allergic diseases. *N Engl J Med* 347: 911-920. ISSN: 0028-4793

Bergmann, R.L., Bergmann, K.E., and Wahn, U. (1998) Can we predict atopic disease using perinatal risk factors? *Clin Exp Allergy* 28: 905-907. ISSN: 0954-7894

Bik, E.M. (2009) Composition and function of the human-associated microbiota. *Nutr Rev* 67 Suppl 2: S164-S171. ISSN: 0029-6643

Bjorksten, B., Naaber, P., Sepp, E., and Mikelsaar, M. (1999) The intestinal microflora in allergic Estonian and Swedish 2-year-old children. *Clin Exp Allergy* 29: 342-346. ISSN: 0954-7894

Bjorksten, B., Sepp, E., Julge, K., Voor, T., and Mikelsaar, M. (2001) Allergy development and the intestinal microflora during the first year of life. *J Allergy Clin Immunol* 108: 516-520. ISSN: 0091-6749

Bottcher, M.F., Nordin, E.K., Sandin, A., Midtvedt, T., and Bjorksten, B. (2000) Microflora-associated characteristics in faeces from allergic and nonallergic infants. *Clin Exp Allergy* 30: 1590-1596. ISSN: 0954-7894

Brouwer, M.L., Wolt-Plompen, S.A., Dubois, A.E., van der, H.S., Jansen, D.F., Hoijer, M.A. *et al.* (2006) No effects of probiotics on atopic dermatitis in infancy: a randomized placebo-controlled trial. *Clin Exp Allergy* 36: 899-906. ISSN: 0954-7894

Campeotto, F., Waligora-Dupriet, A.J., Doucet-Populaire, F., Kalach, N., Dupont, C., and Butel, M.J. (2007) [Establishment of the intestinal microflora in neonates]. *Gastroenterol Clin Biol* 31: 533-542. ISSN: 0399-8320

Ciprandi, G., Vizzaccaro, A., Cirillo, I., and Tosca, M.A. (2005a) *Bacillus clausii* effects in children with allergic rhinitis. *Allergy* 60: 702-703. ISSN: 0105-4338

Ciprandi, G., Vizzaccaro, A., Cirillo, I., and Tosca, M.A. (2005b) *Bacillus clausii* exerts immuno-modulatory activity in allergic subjects: a pilot study. *Eur Ann Allergy Clin Immunol* 37: 129-134. ISSN: 1764-1384

Dethlefsen, L., McFall-Ngai, M., and Relman, D.A. (2007) An ecological and evolutionary perspective on human-microbe mutualism and disease. *Nature* 449: 811-818. ISSN: 0028-0836

Eckburg, P.B., Bik, E.M., Bernstein, C.N., Purdom, E., Dethlefsen, L., Sargent, M. *et al.* (2005) Diversity of the human intestinal microbial flora. *Science* 308: 1635-1638. ISSN: 0036-8075

FAO/WHO. Health and nutritional properties of probiotics in food includion powder milk with live lactic acid bacteria. 30 (suppl 2), S23-S33. 2001. Argentina. http://www.who.int/foodsafety/publications/fs_management/probiotics/en/index.html

FAO/WHO Working group. Guidelines for the evaluation of probiotics in food. 2002. London, 30 avril-1er mai. http://www.who.int/entity/foodsafety/publications/fs_management/probiotics2/en/index.html

Feleszko, W., Jaworska, J., Rha, R.D., Steinhausen, S., Avagyan, A., Jaudszus, A. *et al.* (2007) Probiotic-induced suppression of allergic sensitization and airway inflammation is associated with an increase of T regulatory-dependent mechanisms in a murine model of asthma. *Clin Exp Allergy* 37: 498-505. ISSN: 0954-7894

Folster-Holst, R., Muller, F., Schnopp, N., Abeck, D., Kreiselmaier, I., Lenz, T. *et al.* (2006) Prospective, randomized controlled trial on *Lactobacillus rhamnosus* in infants with moderate to severe atopic dermatitis. *Br J Dermatol* 155: 1256-1261. ISSN: 0007-0963

Fujimura, K.E., Slusher, N.A., Cabana, M.D., and Lynch, S.V. (2010) Role of the gut microbiota in defining human health. *Expert Rev Anti Infect Ther* 8: 435-454. ISSN: 1478-7210

Gaboriau-Routhiau, V., Rakotobe, S., Lecuyer, E., Mulder, I., Lan, A., Bridonneau, C. *et al.* (2009) The key role of segmented filamentous bacteria in the coordinated maturation of gut helper T cell responses. *Immunity* 31: 677-689. ISSN:1074-7613

Garrett, W.S., Gordon, J.I., and Glimcher, L.H. (2010) Homeostasis and inflammation in the intestine. *Cell* 140: 859-870. ISSN: 0092-8674

Gerasimov, S.V., Vasjuta, V.V., Myhovych, O.O., and Bondarchuk, L.I. (2010) Probiotic supplement reduces atopic dermatitis in preschool children: a randomized, double-blind, placebo-controlled, clinical trial. *Am J Clin Dermatol* 11: 351-361. ISSN: 1175-0561

Giovannini, M., Agostoni, C., Riva, E., Salvini, F., Ruscitto, A., Zuccotti, G.V., and Radaelli, G. (2007) A randomized prospective double blind controlled trial on effects of long-term consumption of fermented milk containing Lactobacillus casei in pre-school children with allergic asthma and/or rhinitis. *Pediatr Res* 62: 215-220. ISSN: 0031-3998

Gore, C., Munro, K., Lay, C., Bibiloni, R., Morris, J., Woodcock, A. *et al.* (2008) *Bifidobacterium pseudocatenulatum* is associated with atopic eczema: A nested case-control study investigating the fecal microbiota of infants. *J Allerg Clin Immunol* 121: 135-140. ISSN 0091-6749

Gruber, C., Wendt, M., Sulser, C., Lau, S., Kulig, M., Wahn, U. *et al.* (2007) Randomized, placebo-controlled trial of *Lactobacillus rhamnosus GG* as treatment of atopic dermatitis in infancy. *Allergy* 62: 1270-1276. ISSN 0105-4338

Gueimonde, M., Laitinen, K., Salminen, S., and Isolauri, E. (2007) Breast milk: a source of bifidobacteria for infant gut development and maturation? *Neonatology* 92: 64-66. ISSN: 1661-7800

He, F., Morita, H., Ouwehand, A.C., Hosoda, M., Hiramatsu, M., Kurisaki, J. *et al.* (2002) Stimulation of the secretion of pro-inflammatory cytokines by *Bifidobacterium* strains. *Microbiol Immunol* 46: 781-785. ISSN: 0385-5600

He, F., Ouwehand, A.C., Isolauri, E., Hashimoto, H., Benno, Y., and Salminen, S. (2001) Comparison of mucosal adhesion and species identification of bifidobacteria isolated from healthy and allergic infants. *FEMS Immunol Med Microbiol* 30: 43-47. ISSN: 0928-8244

Helin, T., Haahtela, S., and Haahtela, T. (2002) No effect of oral treatment with an intestinal bacterial strain, *Lactobacillus rhamnosus* (ATCC 53103), on birch-pollen allergy: a placebo-controlled double-blind study. *Allergy* 57: 243-246. ISSN 0105-4338

Hooper, L.V., and Macpherson, A.J. (2010) Immune adaptations that maintain homeostasis with the intestinal microbiota. *Nat Rev Immunol* 10: 159-169. ISSN: 1474-1733

Ishida, Y., Nakamura, F., Kanzato, H., Sawada, D., Yamamoto, N., Kagata, H. *et al.* (2005) Effect of milk fermented with *Lactobacillus acidophilus* strain L-92 on symptoms of Japanese cedar pollen allergy: a randomized placebo-controlled trial. *Biosci Biotechnol Biochem* 69: 1652-1660. ISSN: 0916-8451

Isolauri, E., Arvola, T., Sutas, Y., Moilanen, E., and Salminen, S. (2000) Probiotics in the management of atopic eczema. *Clin Exp Allergy* 30: 1604-1610. ISSN 0954-7894

Ivory, K., Chambers, S.J., Pin, C., Prieto, E., Arques, J.L., and Nicoletti, C. (2008) Oral delivery of *Lactobacillus casei* Shirota modifies allergen-induced immune responses in allergic rhinitis. *Clin Exp Allergy* 38: 1282-1289. ISSN 0954-7894

Kalliomaki, M., Kirjavainen, P., Eerola, E., Kero, P., Salminen, S., and Isolauri, E. (2001a) Distinct patterns of neonatal gut microflora in infants in whom atopy was and was not developing. *J Allergy Clin Immunol* 107: 129-134. ISSN 0091-6749

Kalliomaki, M., Salminen, S., Arvilommi, H., Kero, P., Koskinen, P., and Isolauri, E. (2001b) Probiotics in primary prevention of atopic disease: a randomised placebo-controlled trial. *Lancet* 357: 1076-1079. ISSN: 0140-6736

Kalliomaki, M., Salminen, S., Poussa, T., Arvilommi, H., and Isolauri, E. (2003) Probiotics and prevention of atopic disease: 4-year follow-up of a randomised placebo-controlled trial. *Lancet* 361: 1869-1871. ISSN: 0140-6736

Kalliomaki, M., Salminen, S., Poussa, T., and Isolauri, E. (2007) Probiotics during the first 7 years of life: a cumulative risk reduction of eczema in a randomized, placebo-controlled trial. *J Allergy Clin Immunol* 119: 1019-1021. ISSN 0091-6749

Karlsson, H., Larsson, P., Wold, A.E., and Rudin, A. (2004) Pattern of cytokine responses to gram-positive and gram-negative commensal bacteria is profoundly changed when monocytes differentiate into dendritic cells. *Infect Immun* 72: 2671-2678. ISSN: 0019-9567

Kawase, M., He, F., Kubota, A., Hiramatsu, M., Saito, H., Ishii, T. *et al.* (2009) Effect of fermented milk prepared with two probiotic strains on Japanese cedar pollinosis in a double-blind placebo-controlled clinical study. *Int J Food Microbiol* 128: 429-434. ISSN: 0168-1605

Kendler, M., Uter, W., Rueffer, A., Shimshoni, R., and Jecht, E. (2006) Comparison of fecal microflora in children with atopic eczema/dermatitis syndrome according to IgE sensitization to food. *Pediatr Allergy Immunol* 17: 141-147. ISSN: 0905-6157

Kero, J., Gissler, M., Gronlund, M.M., Kero, P., Koskinen, P., Hemminki, E., and Isolauri, E. (2002) Mode of delivery and asthma -- is there a connection? *Pediatr Res* 52: 6-11. ISSN: 0031-3998

Kirjavainen, P.V., Apostolou, E., Arvola, T., Salminen, S.J., Gibson, G.R., and Isolauri, E. (2001) Characterizing the composition of intestinal microflora as a prospective treatment target in infant allergic disease. *FEMS Immunol Med Microbiol* 32: 1-7. ISSN: 0928-8244

Kirjavainen, P.V., Arvola, T., Salminen, S.J., and Isolauri, E. (2002) Aberrant composition of gut microbiota of allergic infants: a target of bifidobacterial therapy at weaning? *Gut* 51: 51-55. ISSN: 0017-5749

Kirjavainen, P.V., Salminen, S.J., and Isolauri, E. (2003) Probiotic bacteria in the management of atopic disease: underscoring the importance of viability. *J Pediatr Gastroenterol Nutr* 36: 223-227. ISSN: 0277-2126

Kopp, M.V., Hennemuth, I., Heinzmann, A., and Urbanek, R. (2008) Randomized, double-blind, placebo-controlled trial of probiotics for primary prevention: no clinical effects of *Lactobacillus* GG supplementation. *Pediatrics* 121: e850-e856. ISSN: 0031-4005

Laubereau, B., Filipiak-Pittroff, B., von, B.A., Grubl, A., Reinhardt, D., Wichmann, H.E., and Koletzko, S. (2004) Caesarean section and gastrointestinal symptoms, atopic dermatitis, and sensitisation during the first year of life. *Arch Dis Child* 89: 993-997. ISSN: 0003-9888

Lee, J., Seto, D., and Bielory, L. (2008) Meta-analysis of clinical trials of probiotics for prevention and treatment of pediatric atopic dermatitis. *J Allergy Clin Immunol* 121: 116-121. ISSN 0091-6749

Lyons, A., O'Mahony, D., O'Brien, F., MacSharry, J., Sheil, B., Ceddia, M. *et al.* (2010) Bacterial strain-specific induction of Foxp3+ T regulatory cells is protective in murine allergy models. *Clin Exp Allergy* 40: 811-819. ISSN 0954-7894

Mah, K.W., Bjorksten, B., Lee, B.W., Van Bever, H.P., Shek, L.P., Tan, T.N. *et al.* (2006) Distinct pattern of commensal gut microbiota in toddlers with eczema. *Int Arch Allergy Immunol* 140: 157-163. ISSN: 1018-2438

Mannino, D.M., Homa, D.M., Pertowski, C.A., Ashizawa, A., Nixon, L.L., Johnson, C.A. *et al.* (1998) Surveillance for asthma--United States, 1960-1995. *MMWR CDC Surveill Summ* 47: 1-27. ISSN: 0892-3787

Manson, J.M., Rauch, M., and Gilmore, M.S. (2008) The commensal microbiology of the gastrointestinal tract. *Adv Exp Med Biol* 635: 15-28. ISSN: 0065-2598

Martin, R., Jimenez, E., Heilig, H., Fernandez, L., Marin, M.L., Zoetendal, E.G., and Rodriguez, J.M. (2009) Isolation of bifidobacteria from breast milk and assessment of the bifidobacterial population by PCR-denaturing gradient gel electrophoresis and quantitative real-time PCR. *Appl Environ Microbiol* 75: 965-969.ISSN: 0099-2240

Matto, J., Malinen, E., Suihko, M.L., Alander, M., Palva, A., and Saarela, M. (2004) Genetic heterogeneity and functional properties of intestinal bifidobacteria. *J Appl Microbiol* 97: 459-470. ISSN: 1364-5072

Mazmanian, S.K., Liu, C.H., Tzianabos, A.O., and Kasper, D.L. (2005) An immunomodulatory molecule of symbiotic bacteria directs maturation of the host immune system. *Cell* 122: 107-118. ISSN: 0092-8674

McKeever, T.M., Lewis, S.A., Smith, C., and Hubbard, R. (2002) The importance of prenatal exposures on the development of allergic disease: a birth cohort study using the West Midlands General Practice Database. *Am J Respir Crit Care Med* 166: 827-832. ISSN: 1073-449X

Medina, M., Izquierdo, E., Ennahar, S., and Sanz, Y. (2007) Differential immunomodulatory properties of *Bifidobacterium longum* strains: relevance to probiotic selection and clinical applications. *Clin Exp Immunol* 150: 531-538. ISSN: 0009-9104

Menard, O., Butel, M.J., Gaboriau-Routhiau, V., and Waligora-Dupriet, A.J. (2008) Gnotobiotic mouse immune response induced by *Bifidobacterium* sp. strains isolated from infants. *Appl Environ Microbiol* 74: 660-666. ISSN: 0099-2240

Murray, C.S., Tannock, G.W., Simon, M.A., Harmsen, H.J., Welling, G.W., Custovic, A., and Woodcock, A. (2005) Fecal microbiota in sensitized wheezy and non-sensitized non-wheezy children: a nested case-control study. *Clin Exp Allergy* 35: 741-745. ISSN 0954-7894

Nermes, M., Kantele, J.M., Atosuo, T.J., Salminen, S., and Isolauri, E. (2011) Interaction of orally administered *Lactobacillus rhamnosus* GG with skin and gut microbiota and humoral immunity in infants with atopic dermatitis. *Clin Exp Allergy* 41: 370-377. ISSN 0954-7894

Odamaki, T., Xiao, J.Z., Iwabuchi, N., Sakamoto, M., Takahashi, N., Kondo, S. *et al.* (2007) Fluctuation of fecal microbiota in individuals with Japanese cedar pollinosis during the pollen season and influence of probiotic intake. *J Investig Allergol Clin Immunol* 17: 92-100. ISSN: 1018-9068

Okada, H., Kuhn, C., Feillet, H., and Bach, J.F. (2010) The 'hygiene hypothesis' for autoimmune and allergic diseases: an update. *Clin Exp Immunol* 160: 1-9. ISSN: 0009-9104

Osborn, D.A., and Sinn, J.K. (2007) Probiotics in infants for prevention of allergic disease and food hypersensitivity. *Cochrane Database Syst Rev*: CD006475. ISSN: 1469-493X

Ouwehand, A.C., Isolauri, E., He, F., Hashimoto, H., Benno, Y., and Salminen, S. (2001) Differences in *Bifidobacterium* flora composition in allergic and healthy infants. *J Allergy Clin Immunol* 108: 144-145. ISSN 0091-6749

Ouwehand, A.C., Nermes, M., Collado, M.C., Rautonen, N., Salminen, S., and Isolauri, E. (2009) Specific probiotics alleviate allergic rhinitis during the birch pollen season. *World J Gastroenterol* 15: 3261-3268. ISSN: 1007-9327

Palmer, C., Bik, E.M., DiGiulio, D.B., Relman, D.A., and Brown, P.O. (2007) Development of the human infant intestinal microbiota. *PLoS Biol* 5: e177. ISSN: 1544-9173

Penders, J., Stobberingh, E.E., Thijs, C., Adams, H., Vink, C., van, R.R., and van den Brandt, P.A. (2006a) Molecular fingerprinting of the intestinal microbiota of infants in whom atopic eczema was or was not developing. *Clin Exp Allergy* 36: 1602-1608. ISSN 0954-7894

Penders, J., Thijs, C., Vink, C., Stelma, F.F., Snijders, B., Kummeling, I. *et al.* (2006b) Factors influencing the composition of the intestinal microbiota in early infancy. *Pediatrics* 118: 511-521. ISSN: 0031-4005

Penders, J., Thijs, C., van den Brandt, P.A., Kummeling, I., Snijders, B., Stelma, F. *et al.* (2007) Gut microbiota composition and development of atopic manifestations in infancy: the KOALA Birth Cohort Study. *Gut* 56: 661-667. ISSN: 0017-5749

Peng, G.C., and Hsu, C.H. (2005) The efficacy and safety of heat-killed *Lactobacillus paracasei* for treatment of perennial allergic rhinitis induced by house-dust mite. *Pediatr Allergy Immunol* 16: 433-438. ISSN: 0905-6157

Pohjavuori, E., Viljanen, M., Korpela, R., Kuitunen, M., Tiittanen, M., Vaarala, O., and Savilahti, E. (2004) *Lactobacillus* GG effect in increasing IFN-gamma production in infants with cow's milk allergy. *J Allergy Clin Immunol* 114: 131-136. ISSN 0091-6749

Protonotariou, E., Malamitsi-Puchner, A., Rizos, D., Papagianni, B., Moira, E., Sarandakou, A., and Botsis, D. (2004) Age-related differentiations of Th1/Th2 cytokines in newborn infants. *Mediators Inflamm* 13: 89-92. ISSN: 0962-9351

Rajilic-Stojanovic, M., Heilig, H.G., Molenaar, D., Kajander, K., Surakka, A., Smidt, H., and De Vos, W.M. (2009) Development and application of the human intestinal tract chip, a phylogenetic microarray: analysis of universally conserved phylotypes in the abundant microbiota of young and elderly adults. *Environ Microbiol* 11: 1736-1751. ISSN:1462-2912

Rajilic-Stojanovic, M., Smidt, H., and De Vos, W.M. (2007) Diversity of the human gastrointestinal tract microbiota revisited. *Environ Microbiol* 9: 2125-2136. ISSN:1462-2912

Rautava, S., Kalliomaki, M., and Isolauri, E. (2002a) Probiotics during pregnancy and breast-feeding might confer immunomodulatory protection against atopic disease in the infant. *J Allergy Clin Immunol* 109: 119-121. ISSN 0091-6749

Rautava, S., Kalliomaki, M., and Isolauri, E. (2002b) Probiotics during pregnancy and breast-feeding might confer immunomodulatory protection against atopic disease in the infant. *J Allergy Clin Immunol* 109: 119-121. ISSN 0091-6749

Rautava, S., Ruuskanen, O., Ouwehand, A., Salminen, S., and Isolauri, E. (2004) The hygiene hypothesis of atopic disease--an extended version. *J Pediatr Gastroenterol Nutr* 38: 378-388. ISSN: 0277-2126

Rodriguez, B., Prioult, G., Bibiloni, R., Nicolis, I., Mercenier, A., Butel, M.J., and Waligora-Dupriet, A.J. (2011) Germ-free status and altered caecal subdominant microbiota are associated with a high susceptibility to cow's milk allergy in mice. *FEMS Microbiol Ecol* 76: 133-144. ISSN: 0168-6496

Roguedas-Contios, A.M., and Misery, L. (2011) What is Intrinsic Atopic Dermatitis? *Clin Rev Allergy Immunol*. ISSN: 1080-0549

Rose, M.A., Stieglitz, F., Koksal, A., Schubert, R., Schulze, J., and Zielen, S. (2010) Efficacy of probiotic *Lactobacillus* GG on allergic sensitization and asthma in infants at risk. *Clin Exp Allergy* 40: 1398-1405. ISSN 0954-7894

Rosenfeldt, V., Benfeldt, E., Nielsen, S.D., Michaelsen, K.F., Jeppesen, D.L., Valerius, N.H., and Paerregaard, A. (2003) Effect of probiotic *Lactobacillus* strains in children with atopic dermatitis. *J Allergy Clin Immunol* 111: 389-395. ISSN 0091-6749

Rosenfeldt, V., Benfeldt, E., Valerius, N.H., Paerregaard, A., and Michaelsen, K.F. (2004) Effect of probiotics on gastrointestinal symptoms and small intestinal permeability in children with atopic dermatitis. *J Pediatr* 145: 612-616. ISSN: 0022-3476

Round, J.L., O'Connell, R.M., and Mazmanian, S.K. (2010) Coordination of tolerogenic immune responses by the commensal microbiota. *J Autoimmun* 34: J220-J225. ISSN: 0896-8411

Sepp, E., Julge, K., Mikelsaar, M., and Bjorksten, B. (2005) Intestinal microbiota and immunoglobulin E responses in 5-year-old Estonian children. *Clin Exp Allergy* 35: 1141-1146. ISSN 0954-7894

Sepp, E., Julge, K., Vasar, M., Naaber, P., Bjorksten, B., and Mikelsaar, M. (1997) Intestinal microflora of estonian and swedish infants. *Acta Paediat* 86: 956-961. ISSN: 0803-5253

Shull, M.M., Ormsby, I., Kier, A.B., Pawlowski, S., Diebold, R.J., Yin, M. *et al.* (1992) Targeted disruption of the mouse transforming growth factor-beta 1 gene results in multifocal inflammatory disease. *Nature* 359: 693-699. ISSN: 0028-0836

Sistek, D., Kelly, R., Wickens, K., Stanley, T., Fitzharris, P., and Crane, J. (2006) Is the effect of probiotics on atopic dermatitis confined to food sensitized children? *Clin Exp Allergy* 36: 629-633. ISSN 0954-7894

Sjogren, Y.M., Jenmalm, M.C., Bottcher, M.F., Bjorksten, B., and Sverremark-Ekstrom, E. (2009) Altered early infant gut microbiota in children developing allergy up to 5 years of age. *Clin Exp Allergy* 39: 518-526. ISSN 0954-7894

Smith, K., McCoy, K.D., and Macpherson, A.J. (2007) Use of axenic animals in studying the adaptation of mammals to their commensal intestinal microbiota. *Semin Immunol* 19: 59-69. ISSN: 1044-5323

Société Française de Dermatologie (2005) Conférence de consensus "Prise en charge de la dermatite atopique de l'enfant". *Ann Dermatol Venereol* 132: 1S19-1S33. ISSN: 0151-9638

Soh, S.E., Aw, M., Gerez, I., Chong, Y.S., Rauff, M., Ng, Y.P. *et al.* (2009) Probiotic supplementation in the first 6 months of life in at risk Asian infants--effects on eczema and atopic sensitization at the age of 1 year. *Clin Exp Allergy* 39: 571-578. ISSN 0954-7894

Songjinda, P., Nakayama, J., Tateyama, A., Tanaka, S., Tsubouchi, M., Kiyohara, C. *et al.* (2007) Differences in developing intestinal microbiota between allergic and non-allergic infants: a pilot study in Japan. *Biosci Biotechnol Biochem* 71: 2338-2342. ISSN: 0916-8451

Stackebrandt, E., Kramer, I., Swiderski, J., and Hippe, H. (1999) Phylogenetic basis for a taxonomic dissection of the genus *Clostridium*. *FEMS Immunol Med Microbiol* 24: 253-258. ISSN: 0928-8244

Stecher, B., and Hardt, W.D. (2008) The role of microbiota in infectious disease. *Trends Microbiol* 16: 107-114. ISSN: 0966-842X

Strachan, D.P. (1989) Hay fever, hygiene, and household size. *BMJ* 299: 1259-1260. ISSN: 0959-8138

Stsepetova, J., Sepp, E., Julge, K., Vaughan, E., Mikelsaar, M., and De Vos, W.M. (2007) Molecularly assessed shifts of *Bifidobacterium* ssp. and less diverse microbial communities are characteristic of 5-year-old allergic children. *FEMS Immunol Med Microbiol* 51: 260-269. ISSN: 0928-8244

Sudo, N., Sawamura, S., Tanaka, K., Aiba, Y., Kubo, C., and Koga, Y. (1997) The requirement of intestinal bacterial flora for the development of an IgE production system fully susceptible to oral tolerance induction. *J Immunol* 159: 1739-1745. ISSN: 0022-1767

Tamura, M., Shikina, T., Morihana, T., Hayama, M., Kajimoto, O., Sakamoto, A. *et al.* (2007) Effects of probiotics on allergic rhinitis induced by Japanese cedar pollen: randomized double-blind, placebo-controlled clinical trial. *Int Arch Allergy Immunol* 143: 75-82. ISSN: 1018-2438

Tap, J., Mondot, S., Levenez, F., Pelletier, E., Caron, C., Furet, J.P. *et al.* (2009) Towards the human intestinal microbiota phylogenetic core. *Environ Microbiol* 11: 2574-2584. ISSN: 1462-2912

Taylor, A., Hale, J., Wiltschut, J., Lehmann, H., Dunstan, J.A., and Prescott, S.L. (2006a) Evaluation of the effects of probiotic supplementation from the neonatal period on innate immune development in infancy. *Clin Exp Allergy* 36: 1218-1226. ISSN 0954-7894

Taylor, A.L., Dunstan, J.A., and Prescott, S.L. (2007a) Probiotic supplementation for the first 6 months of life fails to reduce the risk of atopic dermatitis and increases the risk of allergen sensitization in high-risk children: a randomized controlled trial. *J Allergy Clin Immunol* 119: 184-191. ISSN 0091-6749

Taylor, A.L., Hale, J., Hales, B.J., Dunstan, J.A., Thomas, W.R., and Prescott, S.L. (2007b) FOXP3 mRNA expression at 6 months of age is higher in infants who develop atopic dermatitis, but is not affected by giving probiotics from birth. *Pediatr Allergy Immunol* 18: 10-19. ISSN: 0905-6157

Taylor, A.L., Hale, J., Wiltschut, J., Lehmann, H., Dunstan, J.A., and Prescott, S.L. (2006b) Effects of probiotic supplementation for the first 6 months of life on allergen- and vaccine-specific immune responses. *Clin Exp Allergy* 36: 1227-1235. ISSN 0954-7894

Vael, C., and Desager, K. (2009) The importance of the development of the intestinal microbiota in infancy. *Curr Opin Pediatr* 21: 794-800. ISSN: 1040-8703

Vael, C., Nelen, V., Verhulst, S.L., Goossens, H., and Desager, K.N. (2008) Early intestinal Bacteroides fragilis colonisation and development of asthma. *BMC Pulm Med* 8: 19. ISSN: 1471-2466

Vael, C., Vanheirstraeten, L., Desager, K.N., and Goossens, H. (2011) Denaturing gradient gel electrophoresis of neonatal intestinal microbiota in relation to the development of asthma. *BMC Microbiol* 11: 68. ISSN: 1471-2180

Vaishampayan, P.A., Kuehl, J.V., Froula, J.L., Morgan, J.L., Ochman, H., and Francino, M.P. (2010) Comparative metagenomics and population dynamics of the gut microbiota in mother and infant. *Genome Biol Evol* 2: 53-66. ISSN: 1759-6653

van der Aa, L.B., Heymans, H.S., van Aalderen, W.M., Sillevis Smitt, J.H., Knol, J., Ben, A.K. *et al.* (2010) Effect of a new synbiotic mixture on atopic dermatitis in infants: a randomized-controlled trial. *Clin Exp Allergy* 40: 795-804. ISSN 0954-7894

van der Aa, L.B., van Aalderen, W.M., Heymans, H.S., Henk Sillevis, S.J., Nauta, A.J., Knippels, L.M. *et al.* (2011) Synbiotics prevent asthma-like symptoms in infants with atopic dermatitis. *Allergy* 66: 170-177. ISSN 0105-4338

Ventura, M., van, S.D., Fitzgerald, G.F., and Zink, R. (2004) Insights into the taxonomy, genetics and physiology of bifidobacteria. *Antonie van Leeuwenhoek* 86: 205-223. ISSN: 0003-6072

Verhulst, S.L., Vael, C., Beunckens, C., Nelen, V., Goossens, H., and Desager, K. (2008) A longitudinal analysis on the association between antibiotic use, intestinal microflora, and wheezing during the first year of life. *J Asthma* 45: 828-832. ISSN: 0277-0903

Viljanen, M., Kuitunen, M., Haahtela, T., Juntunen-Backman, K., Korpela, R., and Savilahti, E. (2005a) Probiotic effects on faecal inflammatory markers and on faecal IgA in food allergic atopic eczema/dermatitis syndrome infants. *Pediatr Allergy Immunol* 16: 65-71. ISSN: 0905-6157

Viljanen, M., Savilahti, E., Haahtela, T., Juntunen-Backman, K., Korpela, R., Poussa, T. *et al.* (2005b) Probiotics in the treatment of atopic eczema/dermatitis syndrome in infants: a double-blind placebo-controlled trial. *Allergy* 60: 494-500. ISSN 0105-4338

Waligora-Dupriet, A.J., Campeotto, F., Romero, K., Mangin, I., Rouzaud, G., Menard, O. *et al.* (2011) Diversity of gut *Bifidobacterium* species is not altered between allergic and non-allergic French infants. *Anaerobe*. ISSN: 1075-9964

Wang, M., Karlsson, C., Olsson, C., Adlerberth, I., Wold, A.E., Strachan, D.P. *et al.* (2008) Reduced diversity in the early fecal microbiota of infants with atopic eczema. *J Allergy Clin Immunol* 121: 129-134. ISSN 0091-6749

Wang, M.F., Lin, H.C., Wang, Y.Y., and Hsu, C.H. (2004) Treatment of perennial allergic rhinitis with lactic acid bacteria. *Pediatr Allergy Immunol* 15: 152-158. ISSN: 0905-6157

Watanabe, S., Narisawa, Y., Arase, S., Okamatsu, H., Ikenaga, T., Tajiri, Y., and Kumemura, M. (2003) Differences in fecal microflora between patients with atopic dermatitis and healthy control subjects. *J Allergy Clin Immunol* 111: 587-591. ISSN 0091-6749

Weston, S., Halbert, A., Richmond, P., and Prescott, S.L. (2005) Effects of probiotics on atopic dermatitis: a randomised controlled trial. *Arch Dis Child* 90: 892-897. ISSN: 0003-9888

Wickens, K., Black, P.N., Stanley, T.V., Mitchell, E., Fitzharris, P., Tannock, G.W. *et al.* (2008) A differential effect of 2 probiotics in the prevention of eczema and atopy: a double-blind, randomized, placebo-controlled trial. *J Allergy Clin Immunol* 122: 788-794. ISSN 0091-6749

Williams, N.T. (2010) Probiotics. *Am J Health Syst Pharm* 67: 449-458. ISSN: 1079-2082

Wong, J.M., de, S.R., Kendall, C.W., Emam, A., and Jenkins, D.J. (2006) Colonic health: fermentation and short chain fatty acids. *J Clin Gastroenterol* 40: 235-243. ISSN: 0192-0790

Woo, S.I., Kim, J.Y., Lee, Y.J., Kim, N.S., and Hahn, Y.S. (2010) Effect of *Lactobacillus sakei* supplementation in children with atopic eczema-dermatitis syndrome. *Ann Allergy Asthma Immunol* 104: 343-348. ISSN: 1081-1206

Woodcock, A., Moradi, M., Smillie, F.I., Murray, C.S., Burnie, J.P., and Custovic, A. (2002) *Clostridium difficile*, atopy and wheeze during the first year of life. *Pediatr Allergy Immunol* 13: 357-360. ISSN: 0905-6157

Xiao, J.Z., Kondo, S., Yanagisawa, N., Miyaji, K., Enomoto, K., Sakoda, T. *et al.* (2007) Clinical efficacy of probiotic *Bifidobacterium longum* for the treatment of symptoms of Japanese cedar pollen allergy in subjects evaluated in an environmental exposure unit. *Allergol Int* 56: 67-75. ISSN: 1323-8930

Young, S.L., Simon, M.A., Baird, M.A., Tannock, G.W., Bibiloni, R., Spencely, K. *et al.* (2004) Bifidobacterial species differentially affect expression of cell surface markers and cytokines of dendritic cells harvested from cord blood. *Clin Diagn Lab Immunol* 11: 686-690. ISSN: 1071-412X

Zeuthen, L.H., Christensen, H.R., and Frokiaer, H. (2006) Lactic acid bacteria inducing a weak interleukin-12 and tumor necrosis factor alpha response in human dendritic cells inhibit strongly stimulating lactic acid bacteria but act synergistically with gram-negative bacteria. *Clin Vaccine Immunol* 13: 365-375. ISSN: 1556-6811

Zoetendal, E.G., Rajilic-Stojanovic, M., and De Vos, W.M. (2008) High-throughput diversity and functionality analysis of the gastrointestinal tract microbiota. *Gut* 57: 1605-1615. ISSN: 0017-5749

22

Natural Products and Dermatological Hypersensitivity Diseases

Clayton MacDonald and Marianna Kulka
Institute for Nutriscience and Health, National Research Council, Canada

1. Introduction

The management of dermatological hypersensitivity diseases is a lifelong struggle for most patients. Often, patients are advised to avoid triggers and aggregating factors that lead to flare ups which eventually becomes second nature to them. However, when the symptoms of these conditions become unbearable and conventional medicine no longer provides relief, an increasing proportion of allergy patients are looking to alternative treatments for comfort. Natural products are compounds isolated from natural sources (usually plants or animals) that have potentially beneficial bioactivity. However, many types of compounds can be defined as natural bioactives including synthesized molecules that are based upon naturally occurring compounds. As such, we will define the term "natural bioactive" as any compound whose parent compound structure occurs in nature. Medical research is exploring these compounds as potential treatment sources for a myriad of conditions, including the dermatological hypersensitivity diseases. With the growing interest in natural health products it could be possible that disease sufferers, by self exploring alternative treatments, are potentially leading the search towards the next new approved and medically accepted treatment.

2. Current treatments and management in dermatological hypersensitivity diseases

The management of atopic and hypersensitivity diseases are initially addressed by life style modifications. With all hypersensitivity diseases, be it food allergies, contact hypersensitivity, or allergic asthma, suffers quickly become aware of their disease triggers and begin a lifelong course of avoidance (Custovic *et al.*, 1998). Unknown triggers can be identified medically using a skin prick/patch test. This involves a controlled dermal exposure to the known and the most frequent allergens, and triggers are identified from the resultant skin reactions (Li, 2002). Pharmacological treatments are added into the treatment schedule as the severity of disease progresses, following well-developed treatment ladders (algorithms) (Schmitt *et al.*, 2008). As the patient moves into the stronger classes of treatments in these schedules, the associated side effects become more severe, influencing treatment decisions, ultimately compliance rate and exploration of alternative treatments.

2.1 Life style modifications and diet

The effect of diet on allergies and atopic diseases mitigation has been well studied, but has produced conflicting results (Allan & Devereux, 2011; Devereaux & Yusuf, 2003; Finch *et al.*,

2010; Wichers, 2009). In children with a family history of atopic diseases, research has been focused towards the effects of maternal diet during pregnancy, lactation, and then subsequently in the infant when and which foods are introduced. Of particular interest is the effect of probiotics on the development of allergies which will be discussed below (section 4.2.4). In patients with food allergies triggers are eliminated from the diet, however other foods have been suggested which might be beneficial to allergy suffers. Some of these compounds include poly-unsaturated fatty acids (PUFA); Vitamins C (Chang *et al.*, 2009), D, E, Zinc, Selenium. However, these findings have been meet with mixed results (Finch *et al.*, 2010).

2.2 Medical treatment

Medical treatments are initiated as the severity of symptoms become worse and the disease becomes intolerable (Schmitt *et al.*, 2008). For each condition, drug classes have been recommended to be added in a specific order/time in the treatment schedule. However, due to the nature of these conditions treatment is individually tailored depending on patient response and their tolerance of the side effects. These patients follow a defined treatment plan consisting of pharmacological classes, based on their indications and complications. When treatment is initiated for a patient, the success of treatment always needs to balance with the side effect the treatment has on patient quality of life. (R. Finkel *et al.*, 2009). The following is a brief overview of some conventional treatments for hypersensitivity disease such as sterioids and anti-histamines. Some of these compounds originated from natural sources but have been modified extensively to improve both their efficacy and potency. As such, these medications are not strictly considered "naturally sourced." In section 3 below, we will address "naturally sourced" treatments for comparison.

2.2.1 Corticosteroids

Corticosterioids are a class of steroid hormones that are frequently used as a first line treatment in many immunological and dermatological diseases (Richard Finkel, 2009). They can be classified as short to long acting (1-55+ hours) and are applied topically or systematically. They are very effective at mitigating inflammation; however, their side effects limit their long term use. Many of the new treatments are being sought as corticosteroids sparing alternatives (Del Rosso & Friedlander, 2005).

Mechanism of Action: Corticosteroids bind intracellular receptors forming dimers that bind to the glucocorticoid response element of the promoter region of steroid responsive genes, which up regulates 10-100 genes (Bolognia *et al.*, 2008). They also act by inhibiting nuclear factor kB (NF-κB) which dramatically decreases the inflammatory response through the down regulation of certain cytokines, cell adhesion molecules and other inflammatory mediators. (Ex: TNFα, GM-CSF, several interleukins (ex. Il-1, IL-2, IL-6, Il-8); Intercellular adhesion molecule-1 and E-selectin; cyclooxygenase, etc). (D'Acquisto *et al.*, 2002; Richard Finkel, 2009)

Topical Benefits: Reduced itching, improvements in sleep, appearance of skin, self-esteem and quality of life (Miller & Eichenfield, 2006):. *Side effects*(Miller & Eichenfield, 2006) Short Term – stinging on application (for potent preparations); Medium to Long Term – local complications (i.e. skin thinning, striate, glaucoma from periocular use, contact sensitization and tolerance), etc. ; Systemic effects – suppression of the hypothalamic-pituitary-adrenal axis, Cushing's syndrome, decreased immunity.

Systemic Benefits (Miller & Eichenfield, 2006): Relief from itching, skin redness and infiltration and reduced oozing; *Side Effects*(Miller & Eichenfield, 2006): Short term - increased appetite, psychosis and dyspepsia; Long term - hypertension, osteoporosis, adrenal suppression, striate and muscle atrophy, Cushing's Syndrome, decreased immunity.

2.2.2 Emollients

Emollients are creams designed to alleviate the symptoms of pruritus in dermatitis (Bolognia *et al.*, 2008). They are normally applied daily and act by coating the skin and creating an artificial barrier. They are composed of either water free or water-in-oil ointments with urea (10-20%) or lactic acid (5-12%). The underlying principle of this treatment is to 'correct' the barrier defect of the skin in AD. *Benefits:* Reduce skin dryness, itching and penetration of skin by irritants and allergens; prevention of skin cracking; possible reduced need for topical corticosteroids, possible enhanced response when used with topical corticosteroids. *Side Effects:* Possible stinging on application (R. Finkel *et al.*, 2009).

2.2.3 Topical calcineurin inhibitors

These compounds are among the newest class of immunomodulatory compounds that have been approved for use in inflammatory skin diseases (2000) (Grassberger *et al.*, 2004). Members of this class include Pimecrolimus, Tacrolimus and Ascomycin. All originated as natural products isolated from the fermentation products of the bacteria *Streptomyces sp. (Richard Finkel, 2009).* This class has the advantage of treating AD refractory to corticosteroids and reducing the amount of corticosteroids required in severe cases (Spergel & Leung, 2006).

Mechanism of Action: Inhibits calcineurin phosphatase by binding to FK506 binding protein which then complexes to calcineurin preventing its activation (Assmann *et al.*, 2000). Activated calcineurin dephosphorylates the cytoplasmic subunit of the nuclear factor of activated T cells (NFAT), which then translocates to the nucleus where it forms a complex that assists in transcription of numerous cytokines (ex. Th1: IL2, INFϒ; Th2: IL4, IL5) (Grassberger *et al.*, 1999; Sakuma *et al.*, 2001).

Indications: (Bolognia et al., 2008)

Pimecrolmus - Mild to moderate atopic dermatitis, other inflammatory dermatoses

Tacrolimus - Moderate to severe atopic dermatitis, other inflammatory dermatoses

Benefits: Reduced itching and improvements in sleep, appearance of skin, self-esteem and quality of life (Grassberger *et al.*, 2004; Miller & Eichenfield, 2006)

Adverse Effects

Short term - mild stinging or burning upon application; normally improves after a week

Long term - (>5 years) - Tacrolimus: safety unknown, use with caution with excess exposure to UV light; Pimecrolimus: safety profile based on 5 years of use appears good.

2.2.4 Immunomodulators

This class of drugs/compounds function by attenuating the immune response underlying the hypersensitivity reaction. Some of these compounds have been used as immunosuppressants in transplant medicine while others are either components of the immune system or a new class of treatments known as 'biological agents' which are artificially created monoclonal antibody designed to target errant members of the immune system (R. Finkel *et al.*, 2009). Interestingly some of the immunosuppressants have their origin as natural products including: cyclosporine (isolotaed from fungus *Tolypocladium inflatum*), mycophenolate mofetil (isolated from fungus *Penicillium stoloniferum*) tacrolimus (isolated from *Streptomyces tsukubaensis*) as well as others (R. Finkel *et al.*, 2009).

Interferon γ

Was investigated for use in atopic dermatitis due to its pathological dysregulation, and was found to be effective in short term (Hanifin *et al.*, 1993) and long term studies (Stevens *et al.*, 1998). However, its low response rate and high costs deter its regular use and implementation.

Biological Agents – Monoclonal Antibodies

These agents are biologically engineered antibodies directed against specific targets in the immune system. Some of these agents have made it to market for specific conditions (see table1). Omalizumab is a humanized mouse monocolonal antibody targeting the IgE Fc Region. It binds free IgE but not IgE bound to FcεRI on masts cells, so in this way it sequesters free IgE without activating bound IgE and causing mast cell degranulation (Presta *et al.*, 1993). Omalizumab has been approved by the FDA for use in severe recalcitrant asthma (Strunk & Bloomberg, 2006) and has been investigated for severe cases of atopic dermatitis with positive results (Lane *et al.*, 2006).

AGENT	**TARGET / MOA**	**CONDITION**
Alefacept, Efalizumab	T-cell activation, T-cell trafficking	Psoriasis
Etanercept, Infliximab, Adalimumab	TNFα	Psoriasis
Anakinra	IL-1	Rheumatoid arthritis
Rituximab	CD20 (B-cells)	B-cell mediated skin diseases

Table 1. Examples of Biological Agents employed in Dermatological Conditions

Immunosuppresants: Cyclosporine, methotrexate, Mycophenolate mofetil

These drugs act by modulating different functions of the immune system and decreasing their activity. These drugs while very potent in activity require caution in use, because of associated side effects including nephro- , neuro-, and hepatictoxicity (R. Finkel *et al.*, 2009).

2.2.5 Other medical treatments

Anti-Microbial:

This class of pharmaceuticals are commonly used against infections caused by pathological secondary barrier defects in the epidermis. Infections can be caused by intense scratching leading to excoriations or due to immune suppression from other treatments. Common infections associated with atopic dermatitis include bacterial (*S. aurues),* viral (*Molluscum contagiosum, HSV*) and fungal (*Candida sp., Malassezia sp.*) (Bolognia *et al.*, 2008).

Retinoids

Retinoids are related to Vitamin A and act by binding nuclear receptors (RAR, RXR) which directly and indirectly up regulate gene expression responsible for immune and inflammatory responses and proliferation and differentiation of epithelial cells (Bolognia *et al.*, 2008). Retinoids require careful consideration before use due to side effects including local effects, systemic, psychological but more importantly teratogenic effects (David *et al.*, 1988).

Anti-Histamines

This class of drugs has multiple therapeutic targets including allergic and inflammatory conditions, motion sickness and nausea, gastric acid secretion and others (Richard Finkel, 2009). They play a role in urticaria prevention (Jauregui *et al.*, 2007) and symptomatic treatment in other mast cell conditions (Herman & Vender, 2003; Montoro *et al.*, 2007) especially for edema control and pruritus.

Mast Cell Stabilizers

Members of this class of drugs include cromolyn and nedocromil, and are used in mast cell mediated allergic conditions. They function by inhibiting the IgE mediated release of histamine by stabilization of the membrane (Corin, 2000).

2.2.6 Other treatments

In addition to medicinal treatments prescribed by practitioners are a series of physical and alternative treatments. Very popular with dermatological treatment is the use of UV light and tanning beds, especially for psoriasis. Although the mechanism of action is unknown, it is thought that UV activates Psoralen which inhibits cellular proliferation. In certain conditions practitioners may prescribe Ichthyotherapy in which small fish (doctor fish) are employed to remove dead skin from lesions. Coal tar (mixture of hydrocarbons) is used as an emollient and remains a popular treatment in many dermatological centers (Bolognia *et al.*, 2008).

3. The use of Complementary and Alternative Medicine (CAM)

Complementary and Alternative Medicine (CAM): Group of diverse medical and health care interventions, practices, products or disciplines that are not generally considered as part of conventional medicine (NCCAM, 2011)

Complementary Medicine: Any of a range of medical therapies that fall beyond the scope of scientific medicine but may be used alongside it in the treatment of disease and ill health (NCCAM, 2011)

Alternative Medicine: Medical therapies that are used in lieu of conventional therapy (NCCAM, 2011),

(Note: There are many definitions that have been put forward for CAM, these are the ones designated by the National Center for Complementary and Alternative Medicine (USA)).

Recognition of the rising interest and potential importance of Traditional Medicine (TM) and CAM lead the WHO to survey its membership on their respective national attitudes and regulatory status of this branch of health care. They found in 2005 that 71% of respondents have laws, legislative mandates and National regulatory bodies in place for TM/CAM (WHO, 2005). In 1991, the United States created the Office of Alternative Medicine to scientifically scrutinize alternative health practices for the benefit of public and health professionals knowledge. By 1998, due to increasing interest of the subject, this department was expanded into the National Center for Complementary and Alternative Medicine as a member institute of the United States Institutes of Health. It was from this department that a systematic classification of Complementary and Alternative Medicines was formed and grouped into 5 categories (Molassiotis *et al.*, 2005), see Table 1. It is from the biological based therapies and the Alternative Medical systems that sources of natural products are being explored for as potential disease treatments and being entered into clinical trials. It should be noted that treatments from the other groups have entered clinical trials for certain conditions with mixed results including massage (Schachner *et al.*, 1998), acupuncture (Salameh *et al.*, 2008), meditation (Chida *et al.*, 2007), prayer and others.

CLASSIFICATION		EXAMPLES
I	Alternative Medical Systems	Traditional Chinese Medicine, Ayruveda
II	Mind-Body Interventions	Meditation, Prayer, Healing or Support Groups
III	Biological Based Therapies	Herbs, Dietary Supplements, Vitamins
IV	Manipulation and Body Based	Massage, Chiropractive, Osteopathy
V	Energy Therapies	Qi Gong, Reiki

Table 2. Classification of CAM devised by Center for Complementary and Alternative Medicine

3.1 Demographics of CAM use in industrialized nations

There has been a well-recognized trend in the increasing use of CAM among the general public (Harris & Rees, 2000; Su & Li, 2011). In the 2002 US National Health Interview Survey (NHIS) of 31,044 adults, 36% of adults reported using CAM in the previous 12 months, and if a life time prevalence was included, this figure rose to 50% (Barnes *et al.*, 2004). The results from the 2007 survey saw the 12 month prevalence figure rise to 38.6% and among those positive respondents, the most common CAM was listed as 'natural products' (Barnes *et al.*, 2008). Earlier smaller scale national surveys conducted by Eisenberg *et al.* found prevalence rates of 33.8% in 1990 and 42.1% in 1997, although these values are higher (possibly due to the small samples size) it is generally agreed that CAM use is continually increasing (Eisenberg *et al.*, 1998). The NHIS surveys identified some demographic characteristics common among users which have been confirmed from other studies. CAM use is more prevalent among women, adults with higher education, those who engaged in leisure time and physical activity, those who had one or more existing health conditions and have made frequent medical visits in the past year (Barnes *et al.*, 2008; Eisenberg *et al.*, 1998; Metcalfe *et al.*, 2010; Sirois & Gick, 2002). Other identified factors are higher socioeconomic status, being married, those who wished to take a more active role in health care decision making and most interestingly those with a chronic health condition (Metcalfe *et al.*, 2010; Wiles & Rosenberg, 2001). The popularity of CAM use is also recognized in other industrialized countries ; the rates for Canada are estimated at 12-20% (Gavin & Boon, 2005) and 46% in Germany and 49% in France where alternative treatments are well engrained in the national consciousness (Fisher & Ward, 1994). The trend of increasing CAM can be identified from Germany (West) with its 12 months prevalence almost doubling since the 1970's (See Figure

1) (Dixon *et al.*, 2003). It should be kept in perspective when looking at the trends of TM/CAM use that (as defined by the WHO) up to 80% of the world's population uses TM/CAM as their sole source of health care in the places where Western health care is inaccessible ((World Health Organization., 2009).

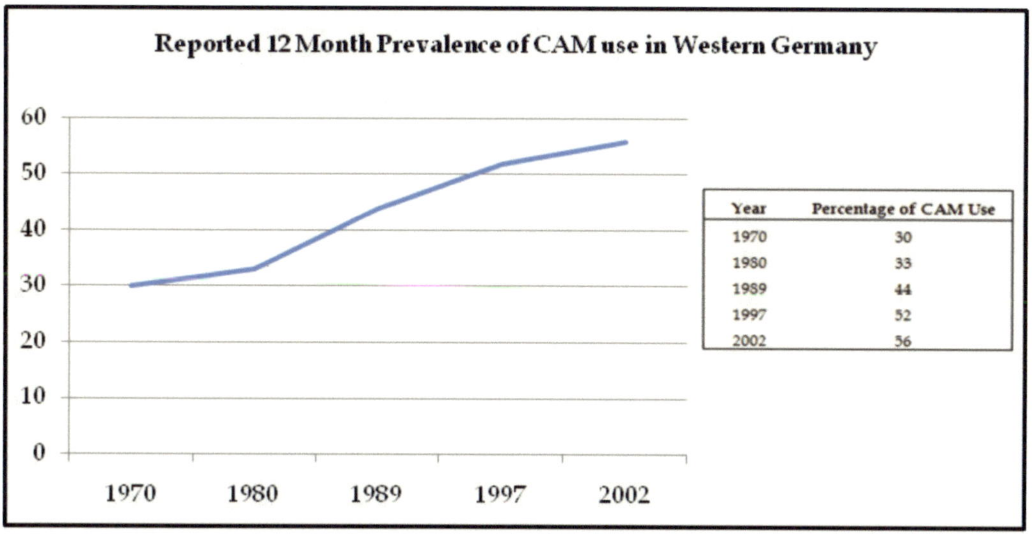

Fig. 1. Reported Use of CAM in Western Germany from 1970s to 2002

3.2 Patient and user attitude toward CAM

There have been many attempts to identify the reasons and motivations as to why members of the public are exploring alternative options for their well-being and health care. A large European study of 956 Cancer patients in 12 countries, found a prevalence rate of CAM use of 38.2% (Range of 14.8% to 73.1%). From those who reported using CAM therapy they were investigated first, for their motivation and second, how found out about them. The most common motivation for CAM use was to increase their body's ability to fight disease (50.7%), followed by improved physical well-being (40.6%), and improvement of emotional well-being (35.2%). Sources of information about CAM were identified as friends (56.5%), family (29.1%), media (28.4%) and only 18.6% said their physician was the source (Molassiotis *et al.*, 2005). Use of CAM is associated with greater number of physical symptoms and with symptoms of greater intensity, longer disease duration (Sirois & Gick, 2002). The reasons for people to explore alternative treatment are varied, but what should be recognized is that are they exploring them. By having members of the public vetting these treatments in terms of personal satisfaction gives health care workers a unique opportunity by looking at the usage trends in members of the public as potential treatments sources.

3.3 Health care practitioners attitude towards CAM

The number of visits to practitioners of alternative therapies is now higher than the number of visits to all US primary care physicians (Pagan & Pauly, 2005). Physician and health care professionals response to CAM has been varied with differences depending on country, region, age, experience and even sex. In a literature review by Sewitch *et al* found that characteristics of physicians whom are more likely to recommend CAM are younger, female, less experienced; while those less likely to recommend CAMs were older, male, more experienced physicians (Sewitch & Rajput, 2010). Older physicians are less likely to use CAMs themselves or recommend it to their family (Kurtz *et al.*, 2003). It should be noted that physicians are the most skeptical and least likely to recommend CAMs to patients, of all members of the health care profession. Rural health care providers offered CAM more frequently than their urban colleagues (Brems *et al.*, 2006). Between 60-80% of surveyed physicians express interest in CAM therapy (Corbin Winslow & Shapiro, 2002; Milden & Stokols, 2004) but few as 14% have recommended it their patients. Among physicians there is prejudice about the different types if CAMs, established practices such as acupuncture, chiropractor tend to be surveyed as the most likely to be beneficial to the patient; While reiki, bioelectromagnetics, aromatherapy have been ranked by doctors as having the least potential to be beneficial or event harmful to the patient (Levine *et al.*, 2003).

3.4 CAM and allergies

In a German study of 351 subjects with hypersensitivity (hay fever, asthma, atopic eczema, food allergies), 93 (26%) were found to be users of CAM. Of the 93 users, 94% previously were treated conventionally before starting CAM while 3 users used CAM before starting conventional treatment. Of those treated conventionally the majority (85%) were treated more than 10 years before trying CAM, they also score the efficacy of conventional medicine lower in their experience. Their reported motivations for using CAM were: conviction that CAM has less side effects (78%), wish to try everything (72%), unsatisfying results from conventional medicine (66%), and belief CAM is more natural (61%) (Schafer *et al.*, 2002) . In a review of 7 surveys of dermatological patients who used CAM they found life time prevalence of 35-65% (Ernst, 2000); among all the surveys they found severity of illness and length of disease had the greatest influence on CAM use. In Europe approximately 30% of patients with allergies report using CAM and this rises to approximately 50% of patients whom required in-patient treatment (Schafer, 2004). The use CAM is related to the severity of the symptoms of their conditions, patients who identify with having poor control are more likely to explore alternative treatments.

4. Search for natural products

Natural products are compounds that have been isolated from a living organism that have been found to be biologically active. A large proportion of the medicines in our current pharmacopeia have either originate as natural products or are inspired by a natural product using it chemical structure as framework on which to build on (Newman & Cragg, 2007). These compounds are being explore for, from all facets of nature including CAMs, our foodstocks, and on an increasing scale the marine sources. The remainder of the chapter will explore some of the natural products undergoing clinical trials for the treatment of Atopic dermatitis. Atopic dermatitis was selected due to its complex pathology, its association with the atopic march and the availability of an animal model which will be discussed below. The test compounds will be discussed below in the context of atopic dermatitis; however some of them are being tested in other related dermatological conditions.

4.1 Clinical trials

Any medicinal compound before entering into an approved treatment system (i.e. National Pharmacopeia) requires rigorous study and clinical trials, which have a defined set of trial steps, before they can be approved for use by National Regulatory bodies. In the United States this task is mandated by the Food and Drug Administration (FDA), in Canada by Health Canada and in the European Union by the European Medicines Agency (Rawson, 2000). All drug approvals required an evidence based approach to qualify their efficacy, evaluate the potential toxicity, and to prevent any unforeseen harm to patients. It is interesting to note that estimates now have the cost of marketed drugs from the R&D stage to consumer use at 500 million to 1 billion dollars and at a time frame of up to 10-15 years (DiMasi *et al.*, 2003). Only about 1 out of 1000 drugs from the animal testing stage (or preclinical phase) make it into clinical trials and from there only 1 in 5-10 eventually become approved. In this manner only 21 new drugs were approved by the FDA in 2010, 25 in 2009 and 21 in 2008 (Kaitin & DiMasi, 2011). However if natural compounds are identified from CAM treatment sources already employed by members of the public they may provide new treatment options which can enter rigorous evidence based trials which have already been vetted by members of the public.

Pre-Clinical Studies / Phase 0: Pre-clinical studies are conducted as *In vitro* (cell culture) and *In Vivo* (animal studies) as initial investigations into suspected potential biological activity. Phase 0 studies are human trials using microdoses to determine if its biological effects are what is expected (Υσηα Ρανι, 2009)

Phase I: Small scale study of 20-100 healthy subjects, testing the safety, pharmacodynamics and pharmacokinetics of the study compound (Streiner & Normam, 2009), consists usually of either single or multiple ascending doses trials.

Phase II: Following the safety approval of drugs in Phase I, these are a small studies of 50-300 diseased subjects , designed to assess dosing requirements, efficacy, (Streiner & Normam, 2009) and safety profiles in people with the condition.

Phase III: Randomized controlled multicenter trials on large group of diseased patients with the target condition, this study are used to determine if the study compound has targeted therapeutic effects (R. Finkel *et al.*, 2009).

Phase IV: These studies occur after the drug has enter the market and is known as Post-Marketing Surveillance. They determine if any adverse events happen in large group of patients which were not previously identified. This phase is important is identifying any rare adverse events which occur in large treatment populations. This monitoring is responsible from removing from market approved drug which later have been found to be potentially harmful, examples are Troglitazone (Cohen, 2006; Gale, 2006) and Vioxx (Karha & Topol, 2004).

4.2 Atopic Dermatitis

Atopic dermatitis (AD) has been recognized since at least the 1500s (Wallach *et al.*, 2005) with its first formal medical description in 1933(Wise & Sulzberger, 1933). This condition is currently a popular target of medical research due to its increasing incidence (Peroni *et al.*, 2008; H. Williams, 1992), distressing rash and intense pruritic symptoms(Hanifin & Rajka, 1980), leading to general negative effects on the patients quality of life (Kiebert *et al.*, 2002) and its being refractory to treatment, along with a host of other reasons . With is long recognition in recent medical history, has led to many treatment options being made available. If any new product is found to possess immunomodulatory effects they tend to be investigated as possible treatments for AD. The remainder of this chapter will look at Natural Products and Natural Preparations undergoing clinical trials for the treatment of AD.

PHASE	PARAMETERS
Pre-Clinical	In-Vitro (Cell Culture) and In Vivo (Animal Studies), determines biological activity, toxicity, etc
I	Small group health subjects; Pharmacokinetic and Pharmacodynamic properties, Single Ascending Dose, Multiple Ascending Doses
II	Small group diseased subjects, determine dosing requirements, drug efficacy
III	Larger group diseased subjects; Randomized Controlled Multicenter trials
IV	Post Marketing Surveillance Trial

Table 3. Phases of Clinical Trials

4.2.1 Animal Models: NC/Nga mice

One of the advantages of research into treatment for atopic dermatitis has been the development of an animal model that has been accepted to be representative of the disease (Suto *et al.*, 1999). Using this model, researchers are able to easily test products prior to proceeding to human clinical trials. NC/Nga mice are a strain that originated from the Japanese fancy mice (Nishiki-Nezumi), established as an inbred strain in 1955 (Matsuda *et al.*, 1997). Researchers noticed the development of spontaneous dermatitis like lesions that appeared just before or after weaning but the cause and pathogenesis had been unclear. A study was conducted to compare these lesions to those of human Atopic Dermatitis (Suto *et al.*, 1999). Mice raised in specific pathogen free (SPF) air controlled bioclean rooms did not develop lesion, but when moved to air uncontrolled rooms, spontaneously several different type of lesions developed after 8 weeks. These mice developed clinical signs similar to AD: itching, erythema and hemorrhage, edema, superficial erosion, deep excoriation, scaling and dryness of the skin, and retarded growth. Infectious causes were ruled out by co-rearing with BALB/c mice which did not develop lesions. The histopathological changes which were consistent with Atopic Dermatitis as well as clinical labs values such as IgE hyperproduction (Matsuda *et al.*, 1997), overproduction of Th2 specific cytokines (Suto *et al.*, 1999; Vestergaard *et al.*, 1999). A literature search conducted in May 2011 resulted in 245 and 185 articles when the following keywords were used together: NC/Nga Mice, Atopic Dermatitis.

4.2.2 Animal trials

The following is a list of compounds (albeit not exhaustive) investigated using the NC/Nga mice model as potential treatments for Atopic Dermatitis. All were oral feeding studies in which the test compound was compared to a control. The efficacies of test compounds were determined by the improvement in symptoms of skin erythema, edema, excoriations, dryness, and scratching behavior. Other parameters measured depended on the trial and included plasma Ig levels, cytokines and chemokine profiles, and evaluation of skin biopsies. All of these studies had positive outcomes based on the design parameters and were recommended by their research teams for use in human clinical trials.

Rumex Japonicus Houtt

Rumex is an herb used in the traditional medical systems originating from Eastern Asian countries (Japan, Korea, China) for the treatment of various skin diseases including AD (H. S. Lee *et al.*, 2006). Previous studies have shown that it contains components with anti-oxidant and antibacterial properties (Elzaawely *et al.*, 2005). Identified Bioactive compounds include anthraquinone derivatives: emodin, chrysophanol, physcion. These compounds studied from other natural sources are reported to have antibacterial, antifungal, anti-inflammatory, immunosuppressive and antiviral properties (H. S. Lee *et al.*, 2006) After 42 days, mice treated with the test compound were found to have significant decreases in the severity of all symptoms when compared to the control, particularly the scratching behavior, which is the most distressing symptom of AD. There was a decrease in plasma IgE and IL4 (which mediate type I hypersensitivity) and noticeable decrease of inflammatory changes in the skin biopsies. The results were more pronounced in the higher concentration groups indicating this compound causes a dose response (H. S. Lee *et al.*, 2006).

PG 102 – Actinidia Arguta

Actinidia Argurta, commonly known as Hardy Kiwi, is a fruit native to Korea, Northern China and Siberia. Compound PG102 and isolated from this fruit by Park *et al.* in 2005 and found to have oral immune modulating effects in mice (Park *et al.*, 2005). A follow up study conducted to determine the effect on the NC/Nga mice model (Park *et al.*, 2007), found that after 9 weeks, PG102 showed statistically significant beneficial effect on AD symptoms and scratching behavior, while noted immunomolecular effects showed a decrease in IgE, IgG, IL4 while IL12 was increased. Other reported effects including the prevention of eosinophilia, decreased levels of eotaxin and TARC, inhibiting the infiltration of inflammatory cells into the dermis, preventing the thickening of the epidermis and dermis and reduced expression of Th2 mediated cytokines and chemokines (Park et al., 2007). All of these effects are beneficial in attenuating the pathophysiological changes seen in Atopic dermatitis. Kim *et al.* tested the extract for efficacy compared to dexamethasone (corticosteriod) and tacrolimus and found PG102 attenuated the physical symptoms of AD similar to dexamethasone and more efficiently than tacrolimus. It also had positive effects on the molecular inflammatory markers as well (ex. IgE, IL4, INFϒ and others). However, all three compounds affected the physical changes in the dermis in a similar manner (Kim *et al.*, 2009). The initial results indicated this compound shows a promising potential for future use as an oral dietary supplement for the long term treatment of AD.

Saururus Chinensis Baill

Saururus is a perennial herbaceous plant used in Korean folk medicine for the treatment of various conditions such as edema, jaundice, gonorrhea and used has been employed as an antipyretic, diuretic, and anti-inflammatory agent (Choi *et al.*, 2008). It has been shown to have anti-oxidant activity (Y. S. Lee *et al.*, 2004) and has been used in the management of various skin diseases including AD in Eastern countries. It contains flavonoids (quercetin, quercitrin, isoquercitrin, rutin) as active components which are reported as possessing number of biological effects: antiallergic, anti-inflammatory, antiviral, antiproliferative, anticarcinogenic (Scalbert & Williamson, 2000). After 63 days this compound was found to significantly improve skin severity scores and improved itching behavior, with the higher concentration preforming better. Molecular evaluation found a decrease in IgE but no changes in IL4.

Lyophyllum Decastes

Lyophyllum is an edible mushroom cultivated in Japan that is commonly known as 'Fried Chicken Mushroom'. In a previous study, 11 polysaccharide extracts were found to have anti-tumour activity (Ukawa *et al.*, 2000) particularly (1-3)B-D-Glucan and (1-6)B-D-Glucan. In 2006, it was examined for its potential effect on the AD mice model (Ukawa *et al.*, 2007) using a 6 week feeding study. At the end of the study the treatment group had significant decreases in skin severity scores, as well as decreases in serum IgE, Histamine, and IL-4.

Persimmon Leaf Extract

Persimmon is the edible fruit of the Diospyros kaki Thunberg (Ebenanceae) tree which grows in China, Korea and Japan (Matsumoto *et al.*, 2002). Kaempferol, a flavonoid contained in the leaf, was found to inhibit antigen and calcium ionophore A23187 induced histamine release. Kaempferol-3-glucoside (astraglandin) has been shown to have anti-pruritic effects(Ishiguro & Oku, 1997). Kotani *et al.* found the leaf extract inhibited the release of histamine from human basophilic cell line KU812 (M Kotani, 1999) promoting them to study the effect on NC/Nga model (Kotani *et al.*, 2000). A 14 week oral feeding study using both Persimmon Leaf extract and Astraglandin alone found both were effective in decreasing the severity of skin scores, inhibiting IgE, IL4, IL13 and Histamine release (Kotani *et al.*, 2000). A similar follow up study was conducted confirming these earlier results and included measurement of Transepidermal water loss (TEWL) (Major pathology in AD due to dermal barrier dysfunction) and was found to be improved by the extract (Matsumoto *et al.*, 2002).

Konjac Glucomannan

Konjac is a plant found in eastern Asia and is very popular in Japan as cooking supplement. Two compounds of interest have been isolated from this product and tested as possible treatments: Konjac glucomannan which has been tested in mice and Konjac ceramide which entered human trials (see section 4.2.4). Glucomannan, a dietary fiber isolated from the tubers of *Amorphophallus konjac,* is a highly viscous polysaccharide composed of glucose and mannose residues (Onishi *et al.*, 2005). During the 1970's dietary fibers were investigated as part of the epidemiology of colon cancer (Burkitt, 1971a, 1971b). During mice feeding studies it was observed that serum IgE levels decreased and IgA and IgG increased(Lim *et al.*, 1997) indicating dietary fibers indirectly influenced immunoglobulin production. This theory was investigated in NC/Nga mouse model during an 8 week controlled feeding trial. Skin severity symptoms were significantly improved and scratching events were decreased to 1/3 to 1/6 of controls. Serologically it almost totally suppressed IgE levels and decreased the total Immunoglobulin, with a noted decreased in IL-4 and INFϒ. Since the compound suppressed both Th1 and Th2 related cytokines it's mechanism of action cannot be attributed to Th1/Th2 polarization (Onishi *et al.*, 2004, 2005). Follow up studies found that it decreased scratching behvaiour in a dose dependent manner (OnishiKawamotoSuzuki *et al.*, 2007), and prevented IgE class switching in Balb/c mice following injection of keratinocyte extract (Oomizu *et al.*, 2006). It was also found to suppress allergic rhinitis like inflammation following nasal challenge with ovalabumin (OnishiKawamotoUeda *et al.*, 2007).

Gyokuheifusan

This is a traditional Chinese Medicine formulation that has been used for the treatment of allergic and respiratory disease (ex. infections, allergic rhinitis, asthma, and others) (Fang *et al.*, 2005).This preparation contains three herbal medications: *Astragalus membranaceus, Atractylodes ovata, Saposhinkovia divaricate*. In a study on the immunomodulatory effects of the formulation on allergic asthma, it was found to reduce the severity of asthma through normalization of INFϒ/IL4 ratio (Th1/Th2 balance) (Fang *et al.*, 2005). These results were hypothesized to extent to AD, after a 4 week oral feeding treatment placebo control study it was found that dermatitis severity scores were improved significantly, as well as IgE and the IFNϒ/IL4 balance (Nakatsukasa *et al.*, 2009).

COMPOUND	PARAMETER IMPROVEMENT	MOLECULAR IMPROVEMENTS
Rumex Japonicus Houtt	Skin Severity Scores, Scratching Behaviour, Skin inflammatory Changes	Decrease IgE, IL4
PG102 - *Actinidia Arguta*	Skin Severity Scores, Scratching Behaviour; Prevented eosinophilia, inflammatory cells entering dermis	Decrease IgE, IgG, IL4, TARC, Eotaxin; Increase IL12; Reduce expression of Th2 mediated cytokines
Saururis Chinensis Baill	Skin Severity Scores, Scratching Behaviour	Decrease IgE
Lyophyllum Decastes	Skin Severity Scores, Scratching Behaviour	Decrease IgE, IL4, Histamine
Persimmon Leaf Extract	Skin Severity Scores, Transepidermal Water Loss	Decrease IgE, IL4, IL13, Histamine,
Konjac Glucomannan	Skin Severity Scores, Scratching Behaviour	Decrease IgE, Ig, IL4, INFϒ
Gyokuheifusan	Skin Severity Scores	Decrease IgE, IFNϒ/IL4 balance

Table 4. Summary of Treatments Tested in Animal Models

4.2.3 Human clinical trials

When clinical trials are conducted for Atopic Dermatitis subjective symptoms such as erythema and pruritus, must be converted to objective and uniform results so that they may be compared with other studies. The following are some of the most commonly used systems and those employed in the following studies:

Transepidermal Water Loss (TEWL) (Pinnagoda et al., 1990): This is a measure of integrity of stratum corneum's water barrier function; it provides information about the integrity of the skin, which becomes compromised in AD and may be influenced and improved with treatment. It is measured using tewameter, with units expressed as $g/m^2/h$; with improvement indicated by a lower value.

Blood flow volume (BFV) :Measured as a parameter of inflammation using Laser Blood Flow Monitor; Arbitrary unit with improvement indicated by lower values.

Skin Color (a^* Value): Erythema quantified by skin color reflectance it is measured using colorimeter

Visual Scoring - Visual judgment made by clinical investigator, scored 0-5

SCORAD (SCORing Atopic Dermatitis) (SCORAD, 1993): Standardized method for reporting dermatitis severity first published in 1993 by the European Task Force on Atopic Dermatitis, allows dermatitis severity to be reported numerically ranging from 0-103.

$$\text{SCORAD Calculation} = A/5 + 7\,(B/2) + C$$

	PARAMETER	TOTAL SCORE
A	*SPREAD/BODY SURFACE AREA*	100
	Judge based on rule of 9 for body surface area	
B	*INTENSITY*	18
	Erythema (1-3) Edema (1-3) Oozing/Crusting (1-3) Excoriation (1-3) Lichenification (1-3)	
C	*SUBJECTIVE SYMPTOMS*	20
	Pruritus (1-10) Insomnia (1-10)	

Table 5. Parameters for SCORAD Calculation

4.2.4 Human clinical of trials of natural products

WBI-1001 (IPBD: 2-isopropyl-5-[(E)-2-phenylethenyl] benzene-1,3-diol)

This compound is derived from a metabolite of a unique group of bacterial symbiots of entomopathogenic nematodes. It was found to inhibit inflammatory cytokine secretion by activated T cells including: TNFα, INF ϒ as well as inhibit allergic contact dermatitis in a mouse edema model (Bissonnette *et al.*, 2010). A phase 2A, double blind, vehicle controlled study resulted in statistically significant improvement in SCORAD, pruritus, and the amount of affected body surface area. These improvements were reached after 3-5 weeks of treatment. A 12 week Phase IIb trial was conducted (NCT01098734) as of June 9th 2011, the results are still pending publication.

Konjac Ceramide

Konjac ceramide is the second compound of interest isolated from konjac. Ceramides are a normal component of the lipid membrane, and their deficiency has been suggested as one of the pathological factors resulting in skin barrier disruption (Imokawa *et al.*, 1991), having being previously studied in the treatment of dermatitis (Berardesca *et al.*, 2001). Glucosylceramides are isolated, purified and produced as a nutritional supplement (Kimata, 2006) and oral intake has been found to decrease transepidermal water loss in normal adults (Miyanishi *et al.*, 2005). Konjac due to its high concentration of ceramide was studied for its effect on AD as an oral supplement. Following a 4 week oral feeding trial in 50 children, the SCORAD index was significantly improved when compared to the control group. INFϒ and IL-12 were significantly increased while IL-4 and IL-13 were decreased indicating a skewing of the cytokine pattern towards a Th1 type. Interestingly in this study, ceramide was found to attenuate allergen specific response to HDM (house dust mite) and JCP (Japanese cedar pollen) by improving skin symptoms and wheal response but had no effect following dermal challenge of Egg white, histamine or buckwheat (Kimata, 2006).

Borage Oil: Gamma-Linolenic Acid

In patients with AD, an abnormality in metabolism of polysaturated fatty acids (PUFA) is commonly observed (Wright, 1991). PUFA are structural components of cell membrane phospholipids which are important in maintaining membrane fluidity (Wright, 1991), as well as being important as precursors for pharmacologically active immunological agents (ie Eicosanoids) (R. Finkel *et al.*, 2009). Borage oil contains a high content (24%) of ϒ-linolenic acid (GLA) which is a metabolite of linoleic acid, one of the essential fatty acids. It is postulated an abnormality in essential fatty acid metabolism affects production of GLA and its incorporation into membranes, occurs in AD (Horrobin, 2000; Wright, 1991). Previous studies have shown GLA supplementation lead to improvements in multiple diseases including seborrheic dermatitis in children (Tollesson & Frithz, 1993). In a small Japanese study in a pediatric population, undershirts coated with Borage oil were given to 32 children in a double-blind, placebo controlled study (Kanehara *et al.*, 2007) . After 2 weeks it was found that there was a statistically significant improvement in symptoms of itch and erythema, but no improvement papules, erosions, and trans-epidermal water loss (Kanehara *et al.*, 2007). In a literature review of 12 trials (oral and topical) on the efficacy of Borage Oil in the treatment of AD by Foster *et al.* in 2010 found that 5 studies show statistically significant improvement, while 5 showed borage oil to be ineffective and 2 studies were shown only to have partial response (Foster *et al.*, 2010). The efficacy of borage oil in the treatment of AD remains questionable, a previous product EpoGam used for treatment of AD was removed from market in 2002 in the UK when it was found to be ineffective. This product contained primrose oil which contains lower concentration of GLA then borage oil but was based on the same pathophysiologic principle(H. Williams, 2003). Borage oil while providing some benefit in some studies requires future study to determine its efficacy and it remains to be determine if it will be steroid sparing.

Emollient Therapy

Emollient therapy is a mainstay in the management of the symptoms of AD (Szczepanowska *et al.*, 2008). While studies into the prevention of AD are less common, Simpson *et al.* proposed that 'skin barrier protection from birth using bland emollients is a safe and feasible strategy for AD prevention' (Simpson *et al.*, 2010). This was based on the results from previous studies that found use of petrolatum early in life may be protective against AD development, there was trend towards increased TEWL and skin hydration before development of AD, use of emollients in premature infants protects against skin inflammation and emollients are effective at preventing flares in established AD (Simpson *et al.*, 2010). In 20 high risk infants (based on the ISSAC criteria (Asher *et al.*, 2006)) emollient therapy was initiated in the first week of life in order to maintain intact skin barrier. After 2 years it was found that only 15% of subject developed AD when conservative estimates of high risk infants would be positive for AD in the range of 30-50% suggesting this treatment could have both a protective and preventative effect (Simpson *et al.*, 2010).

Probiotics

Living or inactivated organisms that are claimed to exert beneficial effects on health when ingested are referred to as Probiotics (Schrezenmeir & de Vrese, 2001). The use of probiotic and prebiotics in the field of allergology is a controversial subject, with the results of prenatal and postnatal supplementation for the prevention of atopic dermatitis having mixed results (J. Lee *et al.*, 2008). Probiotic intestinal colonization is theorized to affect the Th1/Th2 immunological maturation prior to the establishment of atopic dermatitis (Gruber *et al.*, 2010). Physiologically the normal gut milieu has an immune system that is balance between protective mucosal immunity and systemic tolerance. In food allergies the balance is impaired and oral tolerance of dietary antigens is not achieved. Risk Factors for the development of food allergy include immature gut barrier and type II Th2 cell skewed cytokine profile are present in early infancy. This may lead to atopic sensitization as antigen uptake is aberrant and Th2 cells further produce IL4 a cytokine essential for B cell differentiation into IgE producing cells and IL5 which is important for eosinophils . Normal bacterial flora at birth is shown to counterbalance the Th2 activity and promote oral tolerance. The predilection of bacteria to promote the differentiation of Th1 cell lineage may be due to specific CpG motif characteristics of bacterial DNA which has been show to induce polycolonal B-cell activation and secretion of Th1 Cytokines IL6, IL12 and interferon Y (Passeron *et al.*, 2006).The guts of infants born in poor areas of developing countries where allergy prevalence is lower, are colonized earlier by enterobacteria, enterococcim lactobacilli, and eubacteria and displays a higher turnover of different E. coli strains in the intestinal microflora ((Matricardi *et al.*, 2003). In a meta-analysis of 21 studies (1997-2007) by Lee *et al.* (2007) containing 1898 subjects looking at Probiotics in the prevention of atopic dermatitis found a risk reduction of 61% in the development of atopic dermatitis in high risk infants (J. Lee *et al.*, 2008). Newer studies have found conflicting results (Boyle *et al.*, 2011) so its use remains controversial. Strains of bacteria that have been investigated include *Lactobacillus rhamnosus GG* (Gruber *et al.*, 2007), *Bifidobacterium lactis (Kukkonen et al., 2007), Mycobacterium vaccae* and others (Matricardi *et al.*, 2003). In studies of the use of the Probiotics following the establishment of AD has been met with mixed results. In one study it was found that while probiotics did improve SCORAD results they were not statistically significant when compared to placebo (Viljanen *et al.*, 2005) . Other studies have shown the probiotics following established AD in children did improve SCORAD (Passeron *et al.*, 2006) .

St. John's Wort Cream

St. John Wort is a family of plants with worldwide distribution accounting for about 370 species. It has been use as a herbal treatment for depression (Rapaport *et al.*, 2011), ADHD (Chan, 2008) and other psychological condition, however without proven clinical effects. It has been traditionally used for the topical treatment of wounds, burns, nerve lesions and has used as a remedy for eczematous skin conditions (Schempp *et al.*, 2000). Hypericin is a major component of St. John wort and has been found to have bioactive properties exhibiting dose dependent photosensitizing activity (Schempp *et al.*, 2000). Hyperforin, a second compound, was found to have anti-bacterial activity (Gurevich *et al.*, 1971). After a 7 day topical trial, the treatment compound was found to significantly improved SCORAD scores. Colony forming units of *S. aureus* were measured, and found to be decreased by the treatment compound when compared to control, however not significantly. No molecular markers of inflammation were measure in this study.

Herbal Preparations – Traditional Chinese Medicine

Multiple trials have been conducted using formulas of traditional Chinese medicine. These formulas have a long history of use and documentation within their medical systems. The difficulty in investigating these compounds are due to the manner of preparation and individuality of the treatment. In a 2007 study by Hon *et al.* of a five herb formulation (*Flos lonicerae, Herba menthae, Cortex moutan, Rhizoma atractylodis, Cortex phellodendri)* in a placebo controlled 12 week oral feeding trial found that while the treatment group and placebo group both improved symptoms there was no statistically significance between the two. However in the treatment group, the number of days of corticosteroids use during the month was significantly decreased, improving the quality of life of the subject (Hon *et al.*, 2007). In a follow up study it was found the formulation suppressed brain-derived neurotrophic factor (BDNF), Thymus and activation regulated chemokine (TARC), INF-ϒ, and TNFα (Leung *et al.*, 2008).

COMPOUND	PARAMETER IMPROVEMENT	MOLECULAR IMPROVEMENTS
WBI-1001	SCORAD, Pruritus, Body Surface Area	Inhibited TNFα, Increased INF ϒ
Konjac Ceramide	SCORAD, Transepidermal Water loss, Allergen specific response	Increased INFϒ, IL12; Decreased IL4, IL13
Borage Oil	SCORAD?, Itch, Erythema	Metabolism of PUFA
Emollient Therapy	Prevention of AD	
Probiotics		
St. John's Wort Cream	SCORAD, Decreased *Staph. Aureus* CFUs	
TCM		

Table 6. Summary of Treatments Tested in Human Clinical Trials

4.2.5 Approved compounds

The calcineurin inhibitors are among the most recent example of natural products that had been identified having potential biological activity, then successfully proceeded through the clinical trial phase and have been approved for use in the treatment of AD and other dermatological hypersensitivity conditions. The following natural product concoction is the most recent treatment approved for use in AD by the FDA. Using an understanding of the pathophysiology of AD, compounds were selected that targeted different facets of the pathology to work in concert in the treatment of AD.

Atopiclair MAS063D (Atopiclair)

Hydrolipidic cream developed for the management of Atopic dermatitis, containing moisturizing elements and natural products (Belloni *et al.*, 2005): The agent contains a combination of the bioactive compounds from *Vitis vinifera,* glycyrrhetinic acid and Hyaluronic acid. Hyaluronic acid is barrier forming and hydrating agent, traditionally used as lubricant in surgery (Manuskiatti & Maibach, 1996). It is a naturally occurring glycosaminoglycan in the body found in healthy connective tissue and induces tissue hydration (traditionally used as lubricant in other areas of medicine - ocular surgery, orthopedic surgery). Telmesterine and extracts from *vitis viniferia* have been found to have anti protease activities, (inhibiting harmful enzymes that exuded by damaged skin; and antioxidant effects protecting against free radicals (Belloni *et al.*, 2005). Procyanidins found in *vitis viniferia* have been examined at the vascular endothelium, where they help to prevent oxidative damage, they also form a barrier to protect against elastase, collagenase, hyaluronidase, and B-glucuronidase. Glycyrrhetinic acid is a compound found to have anti-inflammatory activity (Teelucksingh *et al.*, 1990) In 2003, the first vehicle controlled, double blind study of Atopiclair was conducted in a study group of 20 subjects with contact dermatitis. Subjects applied vehicle to one arm and treatment compound to the other and were measured at 24, 48 and 72 hours. Results from this compound were promising, with significant improvements in Transepidermal water loss (by 50%), Blood flow volume, Skin color, Visual Scoring. Only itch magnitude results fell below significance but showed improvement (Hongbo Zhai, 2003). In a follow up study in 2004, Atopiclair was tested in patients with Atopic Dermatitis and found significant improvement in all patients after 22 days. Statistically significant improvements were measure in total body surface area affected, Itch score, SCORAD value, and Quality of sleep. In an informal survery following the study 93% of subjects responded positively to the product (Belloni *et al.*, 2005). Following this study Atopiclair was approved by the FDA for the use in the treatment of atopic dermatitis (Abramovitis & Perlmutter, 2007).

5. Conclusions

Natural Products have been identified as potential sources of bioactive compounds used in the treatment of immune disorders. Historically some of the major and most important pharmaceutical compounds have their origin as natural products (Newman & Cragg, 2007). Penicillin, discovered as a metabolite of mold in a petri dish, revolutionized the manner in which medicine has been practiced since wide spread implementation following World War II (R. Finkel *et al.*, 2009). Many of the classes of treatment compounds currently being used in immunology and dermatology have originated from natural products. It might hold true that the next revolutionary treatment might likewise have its origin from the natural world, potentially being already explored by patients looking into CAMs.

It is inevitable that nature will continue to provide pharmaceutical active compounds that will be used in all practices and disciplines of medicine. It is those conducting the exploration for these compounds to keep an open mind to the possibility that an already employed alternative medicine might provide the next clue or even a source unknown.

6. References

Abramovitis, W, & Perlmutter, A. (2007). Atopiclair: its position within a topical paradigm for the treatment of atopic dermatitis. *Expert Rev. Dermatol, 2*(2), 115-119.

Allan, K., & Devereux, G. (2011). Diet and asthma: nutrition implications from prevention to treatment. *J Am Diet Assoc, 111*(2), 258-268.

Asher, M. I., Montefort, S., Bjorksten, B., Lai, C. K., Strachan, D. P., Weiland, S. K., et al. (2006). Worldwide time trends in the prevalence of symptoms of asthma, allergic rhinoconjunctivitis, and eczema in childhood: ISAAC Phases One and Three repeat multicountry cross-sectional surveys. *Lancet, 368*(9537), 733-743.

Assmann, T., Homey, B., & Ruzicka, T. (2000). Applications of tacrolimus for the treatment of skin disorders. *Immunopharmacology, 47*(2-3), 203-213.

Barnes, P.M., Bloom, B., & Nahin, R.L. (2008). Complementary and alternative medicine use among adults and children: United States, 2007. *Natl Health Stat Report*(12), 1-23.

Barnes, P.M., Powell-Griner, E., McFann, K., & Nahin, R.L. (2004). Complementary and alternative medicine use among adults: United States, 2002. *Adv Data*(343), 1-19.

Belloni, G., Pinelli, S., & Veraldi, S. (2005). A randomised, double-blind, vehicle-controlled study to evaluate the efficacy and safety of MAS063D (Atopiclair) in the treatment of mild to moderate atopic dermatitis. *Eur J Dermatol, 15*(1), 31-36.

Berardesca, E., Barbareschi, M., Veraldi, S., & Pimpinelli, N. (2001). Evaluation of efficacy of a skin lipid mixture in patients with irritant contact dermatitis, allergic contact dermatitis or atopic dermatitis: a multicenter study. *Contact Dermatitis, 45*(5), 280-285.

Bissonnette, R., Chen, G., Bolduc, C., Maari, C., Lyle, M., Tang, L., et al. (2010). Efficacy and safety of topical WBI-1001 in the treatment of atopic dermatitis: results from a phase 2A, randomized, placebo-controlled clinical trial. *Arch Dermatol, 146*(4), 446-449.

Bolognia, Jean, Jorizzo, Joseph L., & Rapini, Ronald P. (2008). *Dermatology* (2nd ed. / edited by Jean L. Bolognia, Joseph L. Jorizzo, Ronald P. Rapini ; associate and artwork editor, Julie V. Schaffer. ed.). St. Louis, Mo. ; London: Mosby Elsevier.

Boyle, R. J., Ismail, I. H., Kivivuori, S., Licciardi, P. V., Robins-Browne, R. M., Mah, L. J., et al. (2011). Lactobacillus GG treatment during pregnancy for the prevention of eczema: a randomized controlled trial. *Allergy, 66*(4), 509-516.

Brems, C., Johnson, M. E., Warner, T. D., & Roberts, L. W. (2006). Patient requests and provider suggestions for alternative treatments as reported by rural and urban care providers. *Complement Ther Med, 14*(1), 10-19.

Burkitt, D. P. (1971a). Epidemiology of cancer of the colon and rectum. *Cancer, 28*(1), 3-13.

Burkitt, D. P. (1971b). Possible relationships between bowel cancer and dietary habits. *Proc R Soc Med, 64*(9), 964-965.

Chan, E. (2008). St. John's Wort does not show benefit for ADHD in short trial. *J Pediatr, 153*(5), 724.

Chang, H. H., Chen, C. S., & Lin, J. Y. (2009). High dose vitamin C supplementation increases the Th1/Th2 cytokine secretion ratio, but decreases eosinophilic infiltration in bronchoalveolar lavage fluid of ovalbumin-sensitized and challenged mice. *J Agric Food Chem, 57*(21), 10471-10476.

Chida, Y., Steptoe, A., Hirakawa, N., Sudo, N., & Kubo, C. (2007). The effects of psychological intervention on atopic dermatitis. A systematic review and meta-analysis. *Int Arch Allergy Immunol, 144*(1), 1-9.

Choi, M. S., Kim, E. C., Lee, H. S., Kim, S. K., Choi, H. M., Park, J. H., et al. (2008). Inhibitory effects of Saururus chinensis (LOUR.) BAILL on the development of atopic dermatitis-like skin lesions in NC/Nga mice. *Biol Pharm Bull, 31*(1), 51-56.

Cohen, J. S. (2006). Risks of troglitazone apparent before approval in USA. *Diabetologia, 49*(6), 1454-1455.

Corbin Winslow, L., & Shapiro, H. (2002). Physicians want education about complementary and alternative medicine to enhance communication with their patients. *Arch Intern Med, 162*(10), 1176-1181.

Corin, R. E. (2000). Nedocromil sodium: a review of the evidence for a dual mechanism of action. *Clin Exp Allergy, 30*(4), 461-468.

Custovic, A., Simpson, A., Chapman, M. D., & Woodcock, A. (1998). Allergen avoidance in the treatment of asthma and atopic disorders. *Thorax, 53*(1), 63-72.

D'Acquisto, F., May, M. J., & Ghosh, S. (2002). Inhibition of nuclear factor kappa B (NF-B): an emerging theme in anti-inflammatory therapies. *Mol Interv, 2*(1), 22-35.

David, M., Hodak, E., & Lowe, N. J. (1988). Adverse effects of retinoids. *Med Toxicol Adverse Drug Exp, 3*(4), 273-288.

Del Rosso, J., & Friedlander, S. F. (2005). Corticosteroids: options in the era of steroid-sparing therapy. *J Am Acad Dermatol, 53*(1 Suppl 1), S50-58.

Devereaux, P. J., & Yusuf, S. (2003). The evolution of the randomized controlled trial and its role in evidence-based decision making. *J Intern Med, 254*(2), 105-113.

DiMasi, J. A., Hansen, R. W., & Grabowski, H. G. (2003). The price of innovation: new estimates of drug development costs. *J Health Econ, 22*(2), 151-185.

Dixon, Anna, Riesberg, Annette, Weinbrenner, Susanne, Saka, Omer, Grand, Julian Le, & Busse, Reinhard. (2003). Complementary and Alternative Medicine in the UK and Germany: *Research and Evidence on Supply and Demand* (pp. 128). London: Anglo-German Foundation for the Study of Industrial Society

Eisenberg, D. M., Davis, R. B., Ettner, S. L., Appel, S., Wilkey, S., Van Rompay, M., et al. (1998). Trends in alternative medicine use in the United States, 1990-1997: results of a follow-up national survey. *JAMA, 280*(18), 1569-1575.

Elzaawely, A. A., Xuan, T. D., & Tawata, S. (2005). Antioxidant and antibacterial activities of Rumex japonicus HOUTT. Aerial parts. *Biol Pharm Bull, 28*(12), 2225-2230.

Ernst, E. (2000). The usage of complementary therapies by dermatological patients: a systematic review. *Br J Dermatol, 142*(5), 857-861.

Fang, S. P., Tanaka, T., Tago, F., Okamoto, T., & Kojima, S. (2005). Immunomodulatory effects of gyokuheifusan on INF-gamma/IL-4 (Th1/Th2) balance in ovalbumin (OVA)-induced asthma model mice. *Biol Pharm Bull, 28*(5), 829-833.

Finch, J., Munhutu, M. N., & Whitaker-Worth, D. L. (2010). Atopic dermatitis and nutrition. *Clin Dermatol, 28*(6), 605-614.

Finkel, R., Clark, M., & Cubeddu, L. (2009). *Pharmacology* (4th ed.). Philadelphia: Lippincott Williams & Wilkins.

Finkel, Richard. (2009). *Pharmacology* (4th ed.). Baltimore: Lippincott Williams & Wilkins.

Fisher, P., & Ward, A. (1994). Complementary medicine in Europe. *BMJ, 309*(6947), 107-111.

Foster, R. H., Hardy, G., & Alany, R. G. (2010). Borage oil in the treatment of atopic dermatitis. *Nutrition, 26*(7-8), 708-718.

Gale, E. A. (2006). Troglitazone: the lesson that nobody learned? *Diabetologia, 49*(1), 1-6.

Gavin, J. A., & Boon, H. (2005). CAM in Canada: places, practices, research. *Complement Ther Clin Pract, 11*(1), 21-27.

Grassberger, M., Baumruker, T., Enz, A., Hiestand, P., Hultsch, T., Kalthoff, F., et al. (1999). A novel anti-inflammatory drug, SDZ ASM 981, for the treatment of skin diseases: in vitro pharmacology. *Br J Dermatol, 141*(2), 264-273.

Grassberger, M., Steinhoff, M., Schneider, D., & Luger, T. A. (2004). Pimecrolimus -- an anti-inflammatory drug targeting the skin. *Exp Dermatol, 13*(12), 721-730.

Gruber, C., van Stuijvenberg, M., Mosca, F., Moro, G., Chirico, G., Braegger, C. P., et al. (2010). Reduced occurrence of early atopic dermatitis because of immunoactive prebiotics among low-atopy-risk infants. *J Allergy Clin Immunol, 126*(4), 791-797.

Gruber, C., Wendt, M., Sulser, C., Lau, S., Kulig, M., Wahn, U., et al. (2007). Randomized, placebo-controlled trial of Lactobacillus rhamnosus GG as treatment of atopic dermatitis in infancy. *Allergy, 62*(11), 1270-1276.

Gurevich, A. I., Dobrynin, V. N., Kolosov, M. N., Popravko, S. A., & Riabova, I. D. (1971). [Antibiotic hyperforin from Hypericum perforatum L]. *Antibiotiki, 16*(6), 510-513.

Hanifin, J. M., & Rajka, G. (1980). Diagnositic features of atopic dermatitis. *Acta Derm Venereol (Stockh), Suppl 92*, 44-47.

Hanifin, J. M., Schneider, L. C., Leung, D. Y., Ellis, C. N., Jaffe, H. S., Izu, A. E., et al. (1993). Recombinant interferon gamma therapy for atopic dermatitis. *J Am Acad Dermatol, 28*(2 Pt 1), 189-197.

Harris, P., & Rees, R. (2000). The prevalence of complementary and alternative medicine use among the general population: a systematic review of the literature. *Complement Ther Med, 8*(2), 88-96.

Herman, S. M., & Vender, R. B. (2003). Antihistamines in the treatment of dermatitis. *J Cutan Med Surg, 7*(6), 467-473.

Hon, K. L., Leung, T. F., Ng, P. C., Lam, M. C., Kam, W. Y., Wong, K. Y., et al. (2007). Efficacy and tolerability of a Chinese herbal medicine concoction for treatment of atopic dermatitis: a randomized, double-blind, placebo-controlled study. *Br J Dermatol, 157*(2), 357-363.

Hongbo Zhai, Clarissa D Villarama, Zeba Hasan Hafeez, Howard I Maiback. (2003). Efficacy of a Topical Agent, MAS063D ('Atopiclair'), in the Treatment of Sodium Lauryl Sulphate-Induced Irritant Contact Dermatitis. *Exog Dermatol, 2*, 301-305.

Horrobin, D. F. (2000). Essential fatty acid metabolism and its modification in atopic eczema. *Am J Clin Nutr, 71*(1 Suppl), 367S-372S.

Imokawa, G., Abe, A., Jin, K., Higaki, Y., Kawashima, M., & Hidano, A. (1991). Decreased level of ceramides in stratum corneum of atopic dermatitis: an etiologic factor in atopic dry skin? *J Invest Dermatol, 96*(4), 523-526.

Ishiguro, K., & Oku, H. (1997). Antipruritic Effect of Flavonol and 1,4-Naphthoquinone Derivatives form *Impatiens balsamina* L. *Phytotherapy Research, 11*, 343-347.

Jauregui, I., Ferrer, M., Montoro, J., Davila, I., Bartra, J., del Cuvillo, A., et al. (2007). Antihistamines in the treatment of chronic urticaria. *J Investig Allergol Clin Immunol, 17 Suppl 2*, 41-52.

Kaitin, K. I., & DiMasi, J. A. (2011). Pharmaceutical innovation in the 21st century: new drug approvals in the first decade, 2000-2009. *Clin Pharmacol Ther, 89*(2), 183-188.

Kanehara, S., Ohtani, T., Uede, K., & Furukawa, F. (2007). Clinical effects of undershirts coated with borage oil on children with atopic dermatitis: a double-blind, placebo-controlled clinical trial. *J Dermatol, 34*(12), 811-815.

Karha, J., & Topol, E. J. (2004). The sad story of Vioxx, and what we should learn from it. *Cleve Clin J Med, 71*(12), 933-934, 936, 938-939.

Kiebert, G., Sorensen, S. V., Revicki, D., Fagan, S. C., Doyle, J. J., Cohen, J., et al. (2002). Atopic dermatitis is associated with a decrement in health-related quality of life. *Int J Dermatol, 41*(3), 151-158.

Kim, J. Y., Lee, I. K., Son, M. W., & Kim, K. H. (2009). Effects of orally administered Actinidia arguta (Hardy Kiwi) fruit extract on 2-chloro-1,3,5-trinitrobenzene-induced atopic dermatitis-like skin lesions in NC/Nga mice. *J Med Food, 12*(5), 1004-1015.

Kimata, H. (2006). Improvement of atopic dermatitis and reduction of skin allergic responses by oral intake of konjac ceramide. *Pediatr Dermatol, 23*(4), 386-389.

Kotani, M., Matsumoto, M., Fujita, A., Higa, S., Wang, W., Suemura, M., et al. (2000). Persimmon leaf extract and astragalin inhibit development of dermatitis and IgE elevation in NC/Nga mice. *J Allergy Clin Immunol, 106*(1 Pt 1), 159-166.

Kukkonen, K., Savilahti, E., Haahtela, T., Juntunen-Backman, K., Korpela, R., Poussa, T., et al. (2007). Probiotics and prebiotic galacto-oligosaccharides in the prevention of allergic diseases: a randomized, double-blind, placebo-controlled trial. *J Allergy Clin Immunol, 119*(1), 192-198.

Kurtz, M. E., Nolan, R. B., & Rittinger, W. J. (2003). Primary care physicians' attitudes and practices regarding complementary and alternative medicine. *J Am Osteopath Assoc, 103*(12), 597-602.

Lane, J. E., Cheyney, J. M., Lane, T. N., Kent, D. E., & Cohen, D. J. (2006). Treatment of recalcitrant atopic dermatitis with omalizumab. *J Am Acad Dermatol, 54*(1), 68-72.

Lee, H. S., Kim, S. K., Han, J. B., Choi, H. M., Park, J. H., Kim, E. C., et al. (2006). Inhibitory effects of Rumex japonicus Houtt. on the development of atopic dermatitis-like skin lesions in NC/Nga mice. *Br J Dermatol, 155*(1), 33-38.

Lee, J., Seto, D., & Bielory, L. (2008). Meta-analysis of clinical trials of probiotics for prevention and treatment of pediatric atopic dermatitis. *J Allergy Clin Immunol, 121*(1), 116-121 e111.

Lee, Y.S., Baek, Y.I., Kim, J.R., Cho, H.K., Sok, D.E., & Jeong, H.S. (2004). Antioxidant activities of a new lignan and a neolignan from *Saururus chinensisis*. *Bioorganic & Medicinal Chemistry Letters, 14*, 5623-5628.

Leung, T. F., Wong, K. Y., Wong, C. K., Fung, K. P., Lam, C. W., Fok, T. F., et al. (2008). In vitro and clinical immunomodulatory effects of a novel Pentaherbs concoction for atopic dermatitis. *Br J Dermatol, 158*(6), 1216-1223.

Levine, S. M., Weber-Levine, M. L., & Mayberry, R. M. (2003). Complementary and alternative medical practices: training, experience, and attitudes of a primary care medical school faculty. *J Am Board Fam Pract, 16*(4), 318-326.

Li, J. T. (2002). Allergy testing. *Am Fam Physician, 66*(4), 621-624.

Lim, B., Yamada, K., Nonaka, M., Kuramoto, Y., Hung, P., & Sugano, M. (1997). Dietary fibers modulate indices of intestinal immune function in rats. *J Nutr, 127*(5), 663-667.

M Kotani, A Fujita, T Tanaka. (1999). Inhibitory effects of persimmon leaf extract on allergic reaction in human basophilic leukemic cells and mice. *J Jpn Soc Nutr Food Sci, 52*, 147-151.

Manuskiatti, W., & Maibach, H. I. (1996). Hyaluronic acid and skin: wound healing and aging. *Int J Dermatol, 35*(8), 539-544.

Matricardi, P., Bjorksten, B., Bonini, S., Bousquet, J., Djukanovic, R., Dreborg, S., et al. (2003). Microbial products in allergy prevention and therapy. *Allergy, 58*(6), 461-471.

Matsuda, H., Watanabe, N., Geba, G. P., Sperl, J., Tsudzuki, M., Hiroi, J., et al. (1997). Development of atopic dermatitis-like skin lesion with IgE hyperproduction in NC/Nga mice. *Int Immunol, 9*(3), 461-466.

Matsumoto, M., Kotani, M., Fujita, A., Higa, S., Kishimoto, T., Suemura, M., et al. (2002). Oral administration of persimmon leaf extract ameliorates skin symptoms and transepidermal water loss in atopic dermatitis model mice, NC/Nga. *Br J Dermatol, 146*(2), 221-227.

Metcalfe, A., Williams, J., McChesney, J., Patten, S. B., & Jette, N. (2010). Use of complementary and alternative medicine by those with a chronic disease and the general population--results of a national population based survey. *BMC Complement Altern Med, 10*, 58.

Milden, S. P., & Stokols, D. (2004). Physicians' attitudes and practices regarding complementary and alternative medicine. *Behav Med, 30*(2), 73-82.

Miller, Alicia D, & Eichenfield, Lawrence F. (2006). Evolving management of atopic dermatitis. *Expert Review of Dermatology, 1*(1), 31-41.

Miyanishi, K., Shiono, N., Shirai, H., Dombo, M., & Kimata, H. (2005). Reduction of transepidermal water loss by oral intake of glucosylceramides in patients with atopic eczema. *Allergy, 60*(11), 1454-1455.

Molassiotis, A., Fernadez-Ortega, P., Pud, D., Ozden, G., Scott, J. A., Panteli, V., et al. (2005). Use of complementary and alternative medicine in cancer patients: a European survey. *Ann Oncol, 16*(4), 655-663.

Montoro, J., Sastre, J., Jauregui, I., Bartra, J., Davila, I., del Cuvillo, A., et al. (2007). Allergic rhinitis: continuous or on demand antihistamine therapy? *J Investig Allergol Clin Immunol, 17 Suppl 2*, 21-27.

Nakatsukasa, Hiroko, Tago, Fumitoshi, Okamoto, Takuya, Tsukimoto, Mitsutoshi, & Kojima, Shuji. (2009). Therapeutic Effects of Gyokuheifusan on NC/Nga Mouse Model of Allergic Dermatitis. *Journal of Health Science, 55*(4), 516-524.

NCCAM. (2011). *Exploring the science of complementary and alternative medicine : third strategic plan, 2011-2015*. Bethesda, Md.: U.S. Dept. of Health and Human Services, National Institutes of Health.

Newman, D. J., & Cragg, G. M. (2007). Natural products as sources of new drugs over the last 25 years. *J Nat Prod, 70*(3), 461-477.

Onishi, N., Kawamoto, S., Nishimura, M., Nakano, T., Aki, T., Shigeta, S., et al. (2004). The ability of konjac-glucomannan to suppress spontaneously occurring dermatitis in NC/Nga mice depends upon the particle size. *Biofactors, 21*(1-4), 163-166.

Onishi, N., Kawamoto, S., Nishimura, M., Nakano, T., Aki, T., Shigeta, S., et al. (2005). A new immunomodulatory function of low-viscous konjac glucomannan with a small particle size: its oral intake suppresses spontaneously occurring dermatitis in NC/Nga mice. *Int Arch Allergy Immunol, 136*(3), 258-265.

Onishi, N., Kawamoto, S., Suzuki, H., Santo, H., Aki, T., Shigeta, S., et al. (2007). Dietary pulverized konjac glucomannan suppresses scratching behavior and skin inflammatory immune responses in NC/Nga mice. *Int Arch Allergy Immunol, 144*(2), 95-104.

Onishi, N., Kawamoto, S., Ueda, K., Yamanaka, Y., Katayama, A., Suzuki, H., et al. (2007). Dietary pulverized konjac glucomannan prevents the development of allergic rhinitis-like symptoms and IgE response in mice. *Biosci Biotechnol Biochem, 71*(10), 2551-2556.

Oomizu, S., Onishi, N., Suzuki, H., Ueda, K., Mochizuki, M., Morimoto, K., et al. (2006). Oral administration of pulverized Konjac glucomannan prevents the increase of plasma immunoglobulin E and immunoglobulin G levels induced by the injection of syngeneic keratinocyte extracts in BALB/c mice. *Clin Exp Allergy, 36*(1), 102-110.

Pagan, J. A., & Pauly, M. V. (2005). Access to conventional medical care and the use of complementary and alternative medicine. *Health Aff (Millwood), 24*(1), 255-262.

Park, E. J., Kim, B., Eo, H., Park, K., Kim, Y., Lee, H. J., et al. (2005). Control of IgE and selective T(H)1 and T(H)2 cytokines by PG102 isolated from Actinidia arguta. *J Allergy Clin Immunol, 116*(5), 1151-1157.

Park, E. J., Park, K. C., Eo, H., Seo, J., Son, M., Kim, K. H., et al. (2007). Suppression of spontaneous dermatitis in NC/Nga murine model by PG102 isolated from Actinidia arguta. *J Invest Dermatol, 127*(5), 1154-1160.

Passeron, T., Lacour, J. P., Fontas, E., & Ortonne, J. P. (2006). Prebiotics and synbiotics: two promising approaches for the treatment of atopic dermatitis in children above 2 years. *Allergy, 61*(4), 431-437.

Peroni, D. G., Piacentini, G. L., Bodini, A., Rigotti, E., Pigozzi, R., & Boner, A. L. (2008). Prevalence and risk factors for atopic dermatitis in preschool children. *Br J Dermatol, 158*(3), 539-543.

Pinnagoda, J., Tupker, R. A., Agner, T., & Serup, J. (1990). Guidelines for transepidermal water loss (TEWL) measurement. A report from the Standardization Group of the European Society of Contact Dermatitis. *Contact Dermatitis, 22*(3), 164-178.

Presta, L. G., Lahr, S. J., Shields, R. L., Porter, J. P., Gorman, C. M., Fendly, B. M., et al. (1993). Humanization of an antibody directed against IgE. *J Immunol, 151*(5), 2623-2632.

Rapaport, M. H., Nierenberg, A. A., Howland, R., Dording, C., Schettler, P. J., & Mischoulon, D. (2011). The treatment of minor depression with St. John's Wort or citalopram: Failure to show benefit over placebo. *J Psychiatr Res, 45*(7), 931-941.

Rawson, N. S. (2000). Time required for approval of new drugs in Canada, Australia, Sweden, the United Kingdom and the United States in 1996-1998. *CMAJ, 162*(4), 501-504.

Sakuma, S., Higashi, Y., Sato, N., Sasakawa, T., Sengoku, T., Ohkubo, Y., et al. (2001). Tacrolimus suppressed the production of cytokines involved in atopic dermatitis by direct stimulation of human PBMC system. (Comparison with steroids). *Int Immunopharmacol, 1*(6), 1219-1226.

Salameh, F., Perla, D., Solomon, M., Gamus, D., Barzilai, A., Greenberger, S., et al. (2008). The effectiveness of combined Chinese herbal medicine and acupuncture in the treatment of atopic dermatitis. *J Altern Complement Med, 14*(8), 1043-1048.

Scalbert, A., & Williamson, G. (2000). Dietary intake and bioavailability of polyphenols. *J Nutr, 130*(8S Suppl), 2073S-2085S.

Schachner, L., Field, T., Hernandez-Reif, M., Duarte, A. M., & Krasnegor, J. (1998). Atopic dermatitis symptoms decreased in children following massage therapy. *Pediatr Dermatol, 15*(5), 390-395.

Schafer, T. (2004). Epidemiology of complementary alternative medicine for asthma and allergy in Europe and Germany. *Ann Allergy Asthma Immunol, 93*(2 Suppl 1), S5-10.

Schafer, T., Riehle, A., Wichmann, H. E., & Ring, J. (2002). Alternative medicine in allergies - prevalence, patterns of use, and costs. *Allergy, 57*(8), 694-700.

Schempp, C. M., Ludtke, R., Winghofer, B., & Simon, J. C. (2000). Effect of topical application of Hypericum perforatum extract (St. John's wort) on skin sensitivity to solar simulated radiation. *Photodermatol Photoimmunol Photomed, 16*(3), 125-128.

Schmitt, J., Meurer, M., Schwanebeck, U., Grahlert, X., & Schakel, K. (2008). Treatment following an evidence-based algorithm versus individualised symptom-oriented treatment for atopic eczema. A randomised controlled trial. *Dermatology, 217*(4), 299-308.

Schrezenmeir, J., & de Vrese, M. (2001). Probiotics, prebiotics, and synbiotics--approaching a definition. *Am J Clin Nutr, 73*(2 Suppl), 361S-364S.

SCORAD. (1993). Severity scoring of atopic dermatitis: the SCORAD index. Consensus Report of the European Task Force on Atopic Dermatitis. *Dermatology, 186*(1), 23-31.

Sewitch, M. J., & Rajput, Y. (2010). A literature review of complementary and alternative medicine use by colorectal cancer patients. *Complement Ther Clin Pract, 16*(1), 52-56.

Simpson, E. L., Berry, T. M., Brown, P. A., & Hanifin, J. M. (2010). A pilot study of emollient therapy for the primary prevention of atopic dermatitis. *J Am Acad Dermatol, 63*(4), 587-593.

Sirois, F. M., & Gick, M. L. (2002). An investigation of the health beliefs and motivations of complementary medicine clients. *Soc Sci Med, 55*(6), 1025-1037.

Spergel, J. M., & Leung, D. Y. (2006). Safety of topical calcineurin inhibitors in atopic dermatitis: evaluation of the evidence. *Curr Allergy Asthma Rep, 6*(4), 270-274.

Stevens, S. R., Hanifin, J. M., Hamilton, T., Tofte, S. J., & Cooper, K. D. (1998). Long-term effectiveness and safety of recombinant human interferon gamma therapy for atopic dermatitis despite unchanged serum IgE levels. *Arch Dermatol, 134*(7), 799-804.

Streiner, DL , & Normam, GL. (2009). Drug Trial Phases. *Community Oncology, 6*(1), 36-40.

Strunk, R. C., & Bloomberg, G. R. (2006). Omalizumab for asthma. *N Engl J Med, 354*(25), 2689-2695.

Su, D., & Li, L. (2011). Trends in the use of complementary and alternative medicine in the United States: 2002-2007. *J Health Care Poor Underserved, 22*(1), 296-310.

Suto, H., Matsuda, H., Mitsuishi, K., Hira, K., Uchida, T., Unno, T., et al. (1999). NC/Nga mice: a mouse model for atopic dermatitis. *Int Arch Allergy Immunol, 120 Suppl 1*, 70-75.

Szczepanowska, J., Reich, A., & Szepietowski, J. C. (2008). Emollients improve treatment results with topical corticosteroids in childhood atopic dermatitis: a randomized comparative study. *Pediatr Allergy Immunol, 19*(7), 614-618.

Teelucksingh, S., Mackie, A. D., Burt, D., McIntyre, M. A., Brett, L., & Edwards, C. R. (1990). Potentiation of hydrocortisone activity in skin by glycyrrhetinic acid. *Lancet, 335*(8697), 1060-1063.

Tollesson, A., & Frithz, A. (1993). Borage oil, an effective new treatment for infantile seborrhoeic dermatitis. *Br J Dermatol, 129*(1), 95.

Ukawa, Y., Ito, H., & Hisamatsu, M. (2000). Antitumor effects of (1-->3)-beta-D-glucan and (1-->6)-beta-D-glucan purified from newly cultivated mushroom, Hatakeshimeji (Lyophyllum decastes Sing.). *J Biosci Bioeng, 90*(1), 98-104.

Ukawa, Y., Izumi, Y., Ohbuchi, T., Takahashi, T., Ikemizu, S., & Kojima, Y. (2007). Oral administration of the extract from Hatakeshimeji (Lyophyllum decastes sing.) mushroom inhibits the development of atopic dermatitis-like skin lesions in NC/Nga mice. *J Nutr Sci Vitaminol (Tokyo), 53*(3), 293-296.

Υσηα Ρανι, MYP Ναιδι. (2009). Phase 0 - Microdosing strategy in clinical trials. *Indian Journal of Pharmacology, 40*(6), 240-242.

Vestergaard, C., Yoneyama, H., Murai, M., Nakamura, K., Tamaki, K., Terashima, Y., et al. (1999). Overproduction of Th2-specific chemokines in NC/Nga mice exhibiting atopic dermatitis-like lesions. *J Clin Invest, 104*(8), 1097-1105.

Viljanen, M., Savilahti, E., Haahtela, T., Juntunen-Backman, K., Korpela, R., Poussa, T., et al. (2005). Probiotics in the treatment of atopic eczema/dermatitis syndrome in infants: a double-blind placebo-controlled trial. *Allergy, 60*(4), 494-500.

Wallach, D., Coste, J., Tilles, G., & Taieb, A. (2005). The first images of atopic dermatitis: an attempt at retrospective diagnosis in dermatology. *J Am Acad Dermatol, 53*(4), 684-689.

WHO. (2005). *National policy on traditional medicine and regulation of herbal medicines : report of a WHO global survey*. Geneva: World Health Organization.

Wichers, H. (2009). Immunomodulation by food: promising concept for mitigating allergic disease? *Anal Bioanal Chem, 395*(1), 37-45.

Wiles, J., & Rosenberg, M. W. (2001). 'Gentle caring experience'. Seeking alternative health care in Canada. *Health Place, 7*(3), 209-224.

Williams, H. (1992). Is the prevalence of atopic dermatitis increasing? *Clin Exp Dermatol, 17*(6), 385-391.

Williams, H. . (2003). Evening primrose oil for atopic dermatitis. *BMJ, 327*(7428), 1358-1359.

Wise, F., & Sulzberger, MG. (1933). *In Year Book of Dermatology and Syphiolology*.

World Health Organization. (2009). *Report of the WHO Interregional Workshop on the Use of Traditional Medicine in Primary Health Care : Ulaanbaatar, Mongolia, 23-26 August 2007*. Geneva: World Health Organization.

Wright, S. (1991). Essential fatty acids and the skin. *Br J Dermatol, 125*(6), 503-515.

23

Preventive Phytotherapy of Anaphylaxis and Allergic Reactions

Elaine A. Cruz[1], Michelle F. Muzitano[1],
Sonia S. Costa[2] and Bartira Rossi-Bergmann[3]
[1]*Faculdade de Farmacia, Macae Campus,*
[2]*Nucleo de Pesquisa de Produtos Naturais,*
[3]*Instituto de Biofísica Carlos Chagas Filho,*
Universidade Federal do Rio de Janeiro,
Brazil

1. Introduction

Anaphylactic shock is an extreme and life-threatening allergic reaction that requires immediate action to prevent death from airway and blood pressure collapse. The acute management comprises the use of epinephrine (adrenaline), the first-line medication of choice, and H1-antihistaminic drugs in doses that will depend on the severity of symptoms, in order to preserve the airway function and maintain the blood pressure and oxygenation at acceptable levels (Kemp & Lockey, 2002). On the other hand, long-term management comprises identification of precipitants (e.g.: Medications, foods, latex, insect venom) and their avoidance, and also immunotherapy.

One of the main mediators that are released and associated the many anaphylactic symptoms is histamine. H1-antihistamines are commonly used to relieve anaphylactic cutaneous symptoms such as itching, flushing, and urticaria, but play little role in the relief of bronchospasm or gastrointestinal symptoms, and fail to relieve upper airway edema or hypotension. Moreover, in usual doses, antihistamines alone do not prevent the explosive release of histamine and other mediators of inflammation from mast cells and basophils that culminate in the anaphylactic shock.

Since bronchospasm, hypotension and edema are not reversed immediately with antihistamines, a rapid administration of epinephrine is required to revert these symptoms. It has potent life-saving β-1 adrenergic vasoconstrictor effects on the small arterioles and precapillary sphincters leading to decreased mucosal edema, thereby preventing and relieving upper airway obstruction, and also to increased blood pressure, thereby preventing and relieving shock. (Kemp et al, 2008). Its strong effect on β-1 adrenergic receptors activation lead to increased rate and force of cardiac contractions, while activation of β-2 adrenergic receptors leads to increased bronchodilation and decreased release of histamine, tryptase, and other mediators of inflammation from mast cells and basophils (T.C. Westfall & D.P. Westfall, 2006). The adverse effects of epinephrine therapy involve pallor, headache (β -1 adrenergic receptors), palpitations (β-1 adrenergic receptors), tremor, vasodilation, increased release of mediators (β-2 adrenergic receptors) and anxiety (central CNS stimulation) that altogether

may impose severe risk to patients with cardiac, central nervous system or thyroid diseases. On the other hand, glucocorticoids, that down-regulate β-2 while up-regulating β-1 adrenergic receptors and are mainstays in the treatment of asthma, have been shown not to reverse anaphylaxis symptoms (Simons, 2006). Therefore, in view of the hyper-acute nature of anaphylactic shock that limits adequate therapy, prevention is still the most adequate measure. Current prevention of anaphylaxis is based on allergen desensitization through specific immunotherapy of patients with high-risk of type I hypersensitivity reactions that involve immunoglobulin E (IgE)–mediated release of histamine and other mediators. The immunotherapy comprises the administration of increased doses of low-concentrated specific allergen solution that induce peripheral tolerance associated with differentiation of IL-10 and TGF-β - producing $CD4^{+}CD25^{+}$ regulatory T cells (Francis et al , 2003; Jutel et al, 2003). The efficacy of immunotherapy is also associated with an increase of antigen-specific IgG antibodies that block IgE effects on mast cells and basophils (Akdis & Blaser, 2000).
Table 1 summarizes the current measures available to treat and prevent anaphylactic shock:

DRUG	PHASE OF MANAGEMENT	EFFECTS
EPINEFRINE	Acute	Vasoconstriction, increased peripheral vascular resistance, increased blood pressure and relief of hypotension and shock; decreased mucosal edema and relief of upper airway obstruction and angioedema (effects through β-1 adrenergic receptors). Bronchodilation, decreased release of mediators (effects through β-2 adrenergic receptors).
H1-ANTIHISTAMINES	Acute	Relief of itching, flushing, urticaria, bronchospasm and gastrointestinal symptoms.
β2-ADRENERGIC AGONIST	Acute	Reversion of bronchospasm by relaxing of airway smooth muscle and reduction of asphyxia.
GLUCOCORTICOIDS	Acute	Inhibition of cytokine and arachidonic acid derivates production.
IMMUNOTHERAPY	Long-term	Induction of antigen-specific tolerance and increase of blockers antigen-specific IgG antibodies production.

Table 1. Summary of management of anaphylactic shock

2. Plants as sources of anti-allergic substances

Over the years, ethnobotanical studies allowed the association of plants with a diversity of biological activities and the discovery of new pharmaceutical drugs (Farnsworth et al., 1994). In the period 1981 to 2006, 52% of the small molecules discovered and in the development process were natural products or had their origins in natural products (Newman et al., 2007).

There have been many reports on the anti-allergic effects of some plants and natural compounds (Table 2).

SPECIES	EXTRACT	EXPERIMENTAL MODEL	EFFECT	REFERENCE
Ailanthus altissima	Swingle	Rat	Inhibits production of histamine, TNF, IL-6, and IL-8, and nuclear NF-κB/Rel A	Kang et al., 2010
Albizzia lebbeck	Bark aqueous extract	Guinea pig	Inhibits ileum contraction and bronchospasm	Barua et al.,1997
Baliospermum montanum	Leaf chloroform and ethanol extracts	Rat	Inhibits mast cell degranulation	Venkatesh et al., 2010
Calotropis gigantea	Methanol extract	Rat	Inhibits paw edema	Ghaisas et al., 2011
Camellia japonica	Leaf extract. (quercetin and eugenol)	Rat	Inhibits Src-family kinase and degranulation in mast cells, and passive cutaneous anaphylaxis.	Lee et al., 2008
Crinum glaucum	Aqueous extract	Guinea pig	Inhibits ileum contractions	Okpo and Adeyemi, 2002
Euphorbia hirta	Ethanol extract	Rat and mouse	Inhibits paw edema, passive cutaneous and systemic anaphylaxis, TNF-α and IL-6.	Youssouf et al.,2007
Garcinia brasiliensis	7-epiclusianone	Guinea pig	Inhibits allergen-evoked intestinal spasm	Neves et al., 2007
Impatiens balsamina	Petal ethanol extract (flavonols and naphthoquinones)	Mouse	Prevents blood pressure fall and fatal anaphylactic shock	Ishiguro et al.,1997; Fukumoto et al.,1996
Impatiens textori	Flower ethanol extract (apigenin, and luteolin)	Mouse	Inhibits scratching behavior and blood pressure decrease.	Ueda et al., 2005
Kalanchoe pinnata	Aqueous extract (quercitrin)	Mouse	Inhibits bronchospasm, fatal anaphylactic shock, IgE, eosinophilia, IL-5, IL-10, IL-13 and TNF-α, and histamine release.	Cruz et al, 2011, Cruz et al., 2008
Macrocystis pyrifera seaweed	Alginic acid	Rat	Inhibits histamine release, IL-1β and TNF-α, but not IL-6 or IL-8 production.	Jeong et al., 2006

SPECIES	EXTRACT	EXPERIMENTAL MODEL	EFFECT	REFERENCE
Matricaria recutita	Methanol extract	Rat	Reduces compound 48/80 induced anaphylaxis and histamine release	Chandrashekhar et al., 2011
Oryza sativa	Methanol extract	Rat	Reduces histamine release	Kim et al., 1999
Picrorhiza kurroa	Root and rhizome glycoside fraction	Guinea pig, mouse and rat.	Inhibits passive cutaneous anaphylaxis, ileum contraction but not bronchospasm induced by histamine.	Baruah et al., 1998
Porcirus trifoliata	Aqueous extract	Rat	Inhibits histamine release	Lee et al., 1996
Prunus mahaleb	Ethanol extract (oleic and linoleic acids)	Guinea pigs	Ovalbumin-induced bronchospasm	Shams et al., 2007
Rhus javanica	Gall aqueous extract	Rat and mouse	Decrease histamine release, TNF-α and IL-6 secretion.	Kim et al., 2005

Table 2. Anti-anaphylactic natural products

Chamomile (*Matricaria recutita,* Asteraceae) is one of the medicinal plants whose methanol extract containing flavonoids, tannins, terpenoids and coumarines has reported properties against compound 48/80 induced anaphylaxis in rats (Chandrashekhar et al., 2011). Not only plants but also seaweeds containing alginic acid (Jeong et al., 2006) and honeybees-produced propolis have been marketed for their anticipated anti-allergic effects (revised by Sforcin, 2007). Propolis consists of approximately 300 plant-derived compounds including flavonoids, phenolic acids, cinnamic acid derivatives, terpenoids, cellulose and amino acids. It has demonstrated protection against OVA-sensitized airway inflammatory reaction associated with inihibition of mast cell degranulation, and chrysin and kaempferol present in the ethanol extract appears to be the main anti-allergic compounds (Nakamura et al., 2010). Since 2005, there have been a number of double-blind, placebo-controlled clinical studies in China investigating the efficacy and safety of Chinese herbal products. The major findings of four promising herbal remedies, comprising at least three plant species, were revised by Li and Brown (2009).

Most of the plant products that fight inflammation belong to the chemical groups of alkaloids, coumarins, polyphenols, terpenoids and flavonoids. In particular, flavonoids such as quercetin, luteolin, fisetin and apigenin have been described with potent immunomodulatory properties. Studies on structure-activity relationship of 45 flavonoids showed that oberall they were more potent in inhibiting the production of IL-4 which is largely associated with allergic reactions (Revised by Kawai et al. 2007). Comalada et al. (2006) studied the structure–activity relationship for several flavonoids using primary bone marrow-derived mouse macrophages. They observed that some flavonoids inhibit TNF-α production as well as *i*NOS expression and nitric oxide (NO) production in LPS-activated macrophages, an effect that has been associated with the inhibition of the NF-κB pathway.

Suppression of of NF-κB nuclear factor activation by *Ailanthus altissima* swingle has also been associated with the reduced production of TNF-α, IL-6, and IL-8 pro-inflammatory cytokines and reduced histamine release during induced anaphylaxis (Kang et al., 2010). Flavonoids are known to have potent antiallergic activity (Kawai et al, 2007). For instance, luteolin and quercetin flavonoids (Figure 1) are potent inducers of the anti-inflammatory cytokine IL-10. Structure–activity relationship showed that four hydroxylations at positions 5, 7, 30 and 40, together with the double bond at C2–C3 and the position of the B ring at 2, seem to be necessary for the highest anti-inflammatory effect.

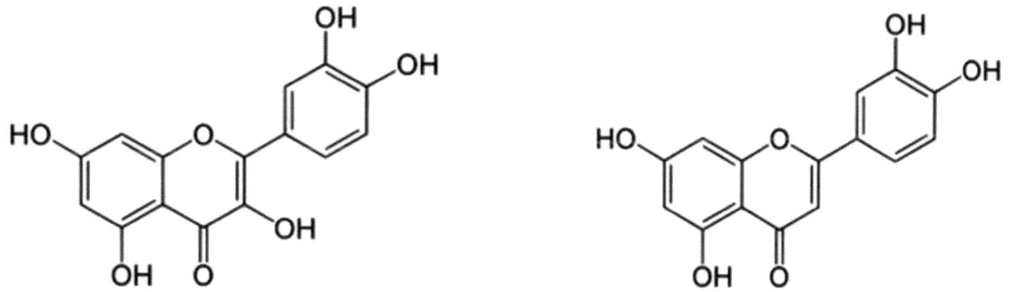

Quercetin Luteolin

Fig. 1. Chemical structures of quercetin and luteolin flavonoids.

Due to the problematic curative therapeutics, preventive therapy may be an alternative life-saving therapy in highly allergic individuals prone to anaphylactic shock. It depends primarily on optimal management of risk factors, avoidance of allergen and other anaphylactic sensitizers (food, insect stings, plants and drugs), and immunomodulation. Since induced immunotolerance therapy involving the administration of increasing doses of a specific allergen has had limited success, and currently available immunosuppressive drugs are not safe enough to be continuously administered as a prophylactic measure, new anti-anaphylactic substances are highly needed in the market. In view of the enormous diversity of chemicals produced, medicinal plants are particularly interesting for the discovery of new anti-allergic agents as the safety of continuous consumption (e.g. herbal infusions) is popularly testified. This is the case of the plant *Kalanchoe pinnata*, whose potential use as source of anti-anaphylactic substances is described below in more detail.

3. The *Kalanchoe pinnata* example

Kalanchoe pinnata (Kp, syn *Bryophyllum pinnatum* Kentz., *Bryophyllum calycinum* Salisb., Crassulaceae) (Figure 2), is widely used in folk medicine in the form of infusions, juices and compresses to treat rheumatoid arthritis, gastric ulcer and in skin disorders (Lucas and Machado, 1946; Lorenzi and Abreu-Matos, 2008). It is native of Madagascar, Kp is now found in several countries such as India, China, and Brazil (Allorge-Boiteau, 1996).

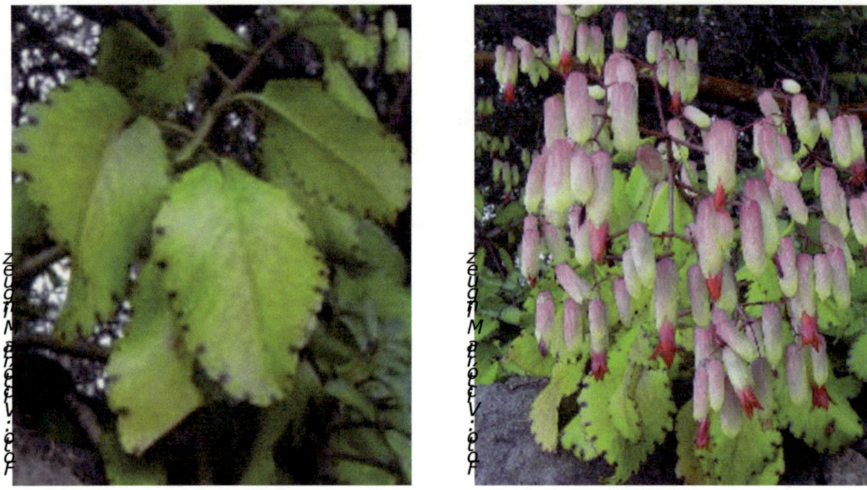

Fig. 2. *Kalanchoe pinnata* (Crassulaceae) : Leaves and Inflorescences

Antiparasitic (anti-leishmania), antibacterial, hepatoprotective and immunomodulatory activities have been described for Kp leaf extracts (Da Silva et al. 1995; Akinpelu, 2000; Muñoz et al. 2000; Yadav and Dixit, 2003; Rossi-Bergmann et al. 1994; Almeida et al., 2000). Exploratory toxicological studies in mice and humans have indicated absence of chronic and acute oral toxicity (Torres-Santos et al., 2003, Sousa et al., 2005). The clinical safety of Kp was also suggested during a study in 67 pregnant women (25 to 35 weeks of gestation) and their neonates (Plangger et al., 2006), corroborating its popular acceptance and pharmaceutical potential.

Kp contains substances belonging to different chemical classes, including: terpenes (Siddiqui et al. 1989; Gaind et al., 1972), bufadienolidos (Yamagishi et al., 1989; Supratman et al., 2001) and flavonoids (Gaind and Gupta, 1971; Ichikawa, 1986; Muzitano et al., 2006a, 2006b and 2009). Kp flavonoids are significantly more abundant when the leaves are collected during the summer (Muzitano et al., 2011). Quercitrin (quercetin 3-*O*-α-L-rhamnopyranoside), kaempferol 3-*O*-α-L-arabinopyranosyl (1→2)-α-L-rhamnopyranoside (kapinnatoside), quercetin 3-*O*-α-L-arabinopyranosyl (1→2)-α-L-rhamnopyranoside and 4′,5-dihydroxy-3′,8-dimethoxyflavone 7-*O*-β-D-glucopyranoside were isolated from a bioactive flavonoid fraction obtained from a Kp aqueous extract (Muzitano et al., 2006a, 2006b and 2009).

3.1 The anti-anaphylactic effect of the aqueous extract of *Kalanchoe pinnata*

The anti-anaphylactic activity of the aqueous extract of Kp leaves given orally to ovalbumin (OVA)-sensitized mice indicated the potent immunomodulatory action, preferentially inhibiting Th2-type immune responses known to be committed with enhanced susceptibility to cutaneous leishmaniasis and to allergies (Rossi-Bergmann et al, 1994; Da Silva et al 1999, Cruz et al 2008, Gomes et al 2009). Despite the early reports on the antihistaminic activity of Kp using the experimental models of isolated guinea pig ileum contraction and vasodilatation in rats (Nassis et al, 1992); its fatty acid associated suppressive activity on T cells (Rossi-Bergmann et al, 1994, Almeida *et al*, 2000).), and its Th2-suppressive and iNOS-suppressive association with oral protection against cutaneous and visceral leishmaniasis

(Da-Silva *et al*, 1995, Da-Silva *et al*, 1999, Gomes et al. 2009), only recently the therapeutic effect of Kp in allergy was more deeply explored.

The antianaphylactic activity o Kp was studied using a murine model of OVA-induced anaphylactic shock. The intraplantar injection of OVA (2.5 mg/kg) into pre-sensitised mice elicited a severe systemic anaphylactic response with death occurring within 15 min-30 min of allergen challenge. This extreme allergic reaction was effectively prevented with 400 mg/Kg of oral Kp during the 14-day sensitization process that maintained alive 100% for over 48 h of follow-up. Intraperitoneal injections with 200 mg/kg of Kp every other day during the same period of time was also effective, but to a lesser extent (80% of survival), similar to observed with 12.5 mg/Kg of i.p. cyclosporin A, an immunosuppressive drug also having anti-allergic effect. Interestingly, a single i.p. dose of 200 mg/Kg of Kp 3 h prior to OVA challenge was sufficient to protect 60% of the animals, suggesting that not only immunosuppression but also modulation of acute events related to shock was critical for protection.

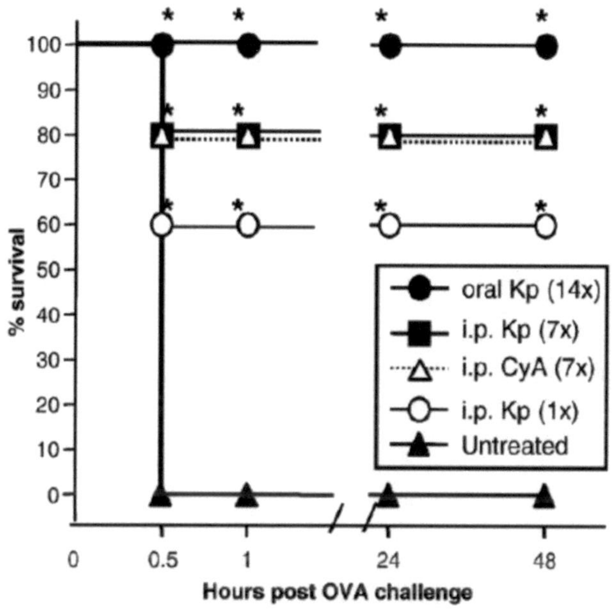

Fig. 3. Pre-treatment with Kp prevents fatal anaphylactic shock. BALB/c mice (n=5) were sensitized with OVA in adjuvant on days 1 and 7, and were challenged with 50 µg of OVA on day 14. During the sensitization period, they were treated as follows: i) by the oral route (daily doses of 400 mg/Kg of Kp for 14 days), ii) by the intraperitoneal route (7 doses of 200 mg/Kg of Kp or 12.5 mg/Kg of Cyclosporin in alternate days; or a single dose of 200 mg/Kg of Kp 3 h before OVA challenge). Controls were left untreated. Upon challenge on day 14, death events were monitored for up to 48 h and recorded as shown. The results are expressed as the percentage of surviving animals. *p<0.01 compared to untreated group.

As allergic parameters, the effect of Kp treatment on the number of circulating eosinophils and in allergen-specific IgE response was investigated. The OVA-induced enhanced eosinophilia was prevented by Kp, especially in animals receiving multiple oral or i.p. doses, although a single i.p. dose of Kp could be effective (Figure 4A). The raised production of OVA-specific IgE in sensitized mice was prevented by Kp therapy, particularly in animals on the oral regimen (Figure 4B).

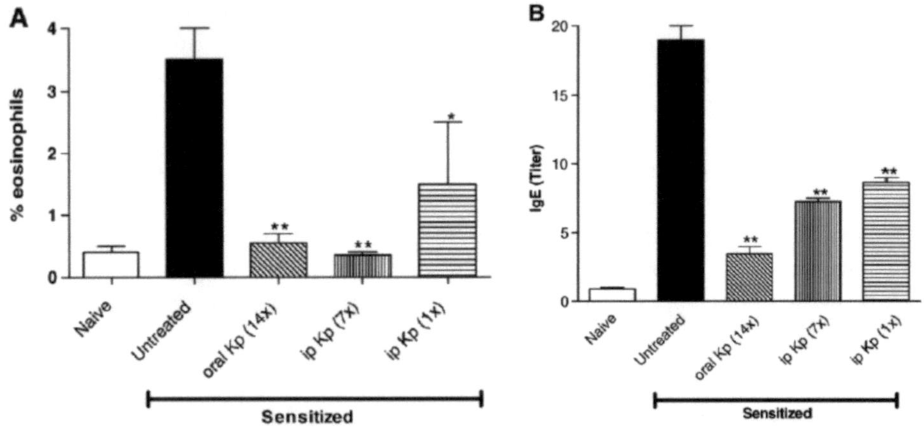

Fig. 4. Decreased eosinophilia and OVA-specific IgE levels in Kp-treated mice. Mice were sensitized and treated with Kp as for Fig. 1. A group of animals was bled 1 h before allergen challenge for the percentage of eosinophils in total leukocytes (top) and for individual assessment of the serum levels of anti-OVA IgE (bottom). Means±S.D (n=4). *p≤0.05 and **p≤0.01 in relation to untreated controls.

3.2 Quercitrin as an important anti-anaphylactic component of *Kalanchoe pinnata*

Like the aqueous extract, the isolated quercitrin flavonoid (Figure 5) was found to to be active in mice against cutaneous leishmaniasis caused by *Leishmania amazonensis* infection (Muzitano et al, 2006). Since cutaneous leishmaniasis, like allergy, is a disease driven by Th2-type immune responses, quercitrin was tested in the mouse model of OVA-induced anaphylactic shock. The animals were treated daily with oral quercitrin during the 14-day OVA-sensitization, with a dose 5% of that used with Kp (400 mg/Kg), compatible with its content in the aqueous extract. We observed that oral treatment with quercitrin conferred resistance to fatal anaphylactic shock in 75% of the animals, as compared with 0% of resistance in untreated sensitized animals (Figure 6), suggesting that quercitrin is an important anti-anaphylactic component of Kp.

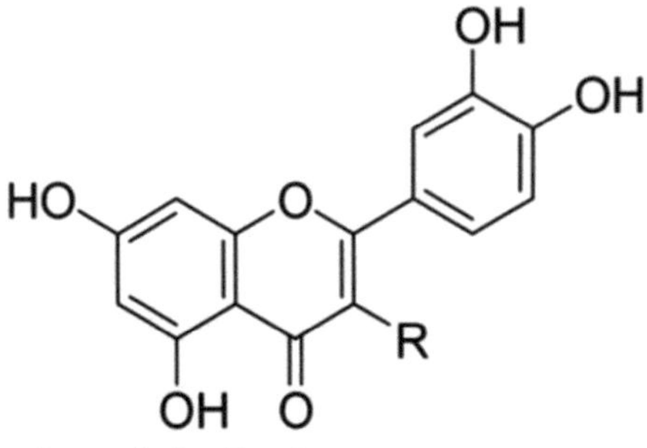

Quercitrin: R= O-α-ramnopyranose

Fig. 5. Chemical structure of quercitrin.

To better analyze the modulatory effect on Th2-type T cells, IL-5 and IL-10 cytokines were measured in the cell culture supernatants. Treatment of sensitized mice with oral or i.p. Kp reduced the capacity of their cells to respond to OVA with IL-5 and IL-10 production (Fig. 7). The production of TNF-α was also inhibited by Kp treatment, and like IL-10, this effect was more pronounced when the i.p. route was used, indicating that cytokines that contribute to allergy are down regulated during i.p, and to a lesser extent oral Kp treatments. The importance of the TNF-α was confirmed in mice deficient in TNFR1, and corroborated with other studies on *Ailanthus altissimain* and *Euphorbia hirta* (Table 2).

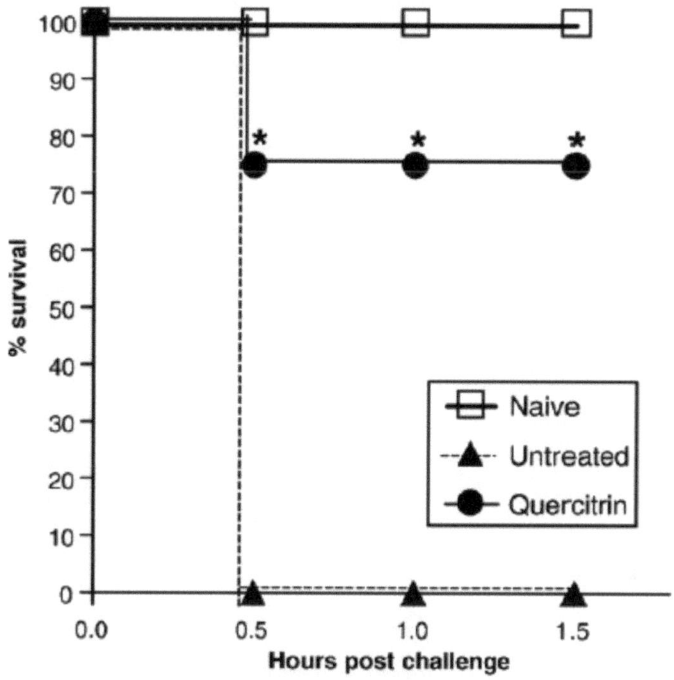

Fig. 6. Pre-treatment with quercitrin partially prevents death due to anaphylactic shock. BALB/c mice (n=8) were sensitized as for Fig. 1. During the sensitization period, they were daily treated with 20 mg/Kg of quercitrin by the oral route, during 14 days. Controls were left untreated. Naive were untreated non-immunized mice. Upon challenge on day 14, death events were monitored for up to 90 min and recorded as shown. The results are expressed as the percentage of surviving animals. *pb0.01 compared to untreated group.

The effect of Kp on histamine release by anti-DNP IgE-sensitized mast cells challenged with DNP was also investigated, and a significant inhibition of secreted histamine was found in cells that were pre-treated with Kp prior to DNP challenge (Fig. 8).

As mentioned above, cutaneous leishmaniasis and allergy are pathologies associated with expanded Th2-type immune responses, and they are benefited from the oral treatment with Kp. Although blockade of histamine release may ultimately contribute to the anti-anaphylactic effect of Kp, it is conceivable that downregulation of Th2-type immune responses is more critical for the resistance phenotype. The immunological effects of Kp are summarized in Figure 9.

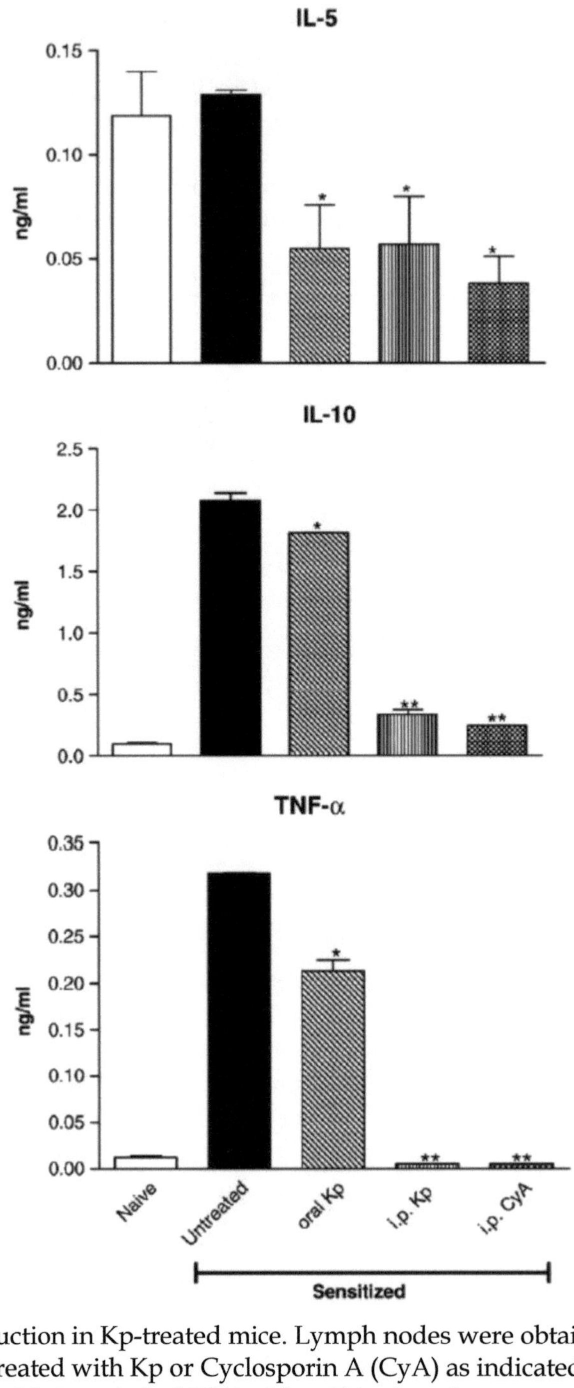

Fig. 7. Cytokine production in Kp-treated mice. Lymph nodes were obtained from mice that were sensitized and treated with Kp or Cyclosporin A (CyA) as indicated, and the cells restimulated in vitro with 1 mg/ml of OVA. After 48 h, the culture supernatants were collected for the determination of IL-5, IL-10 and TNF-α levels by ELISA.Means±S.D. (n=5). *p≤0.05 and **p≤0.01 in relation to untreated controls.

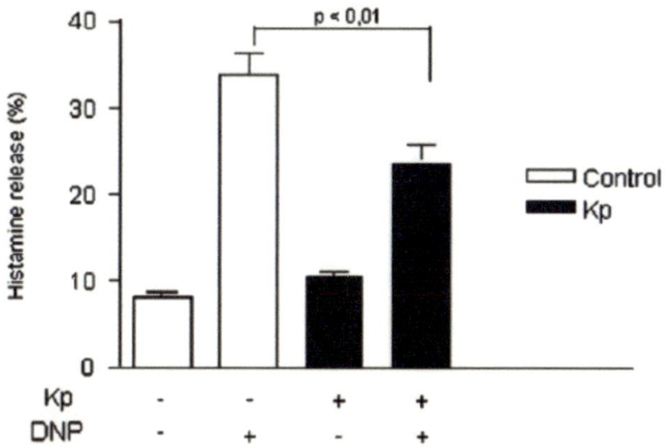

Fig. 8. Prevention of mast cell histamine release by Kp in vitro. Rat peritoneal mast cells were sensitized in vitro with anti-DNP IgE and then incubated with 500 μg/ml of Kp for 30 min prior to the 1-hour challenge with 50 μg/ml of DNP/BSA. Histamine was measured in the supernatants by a fluorimetric assay and expressed as the percentage of total histamine in cell lysates. Means±S.D (n=4).

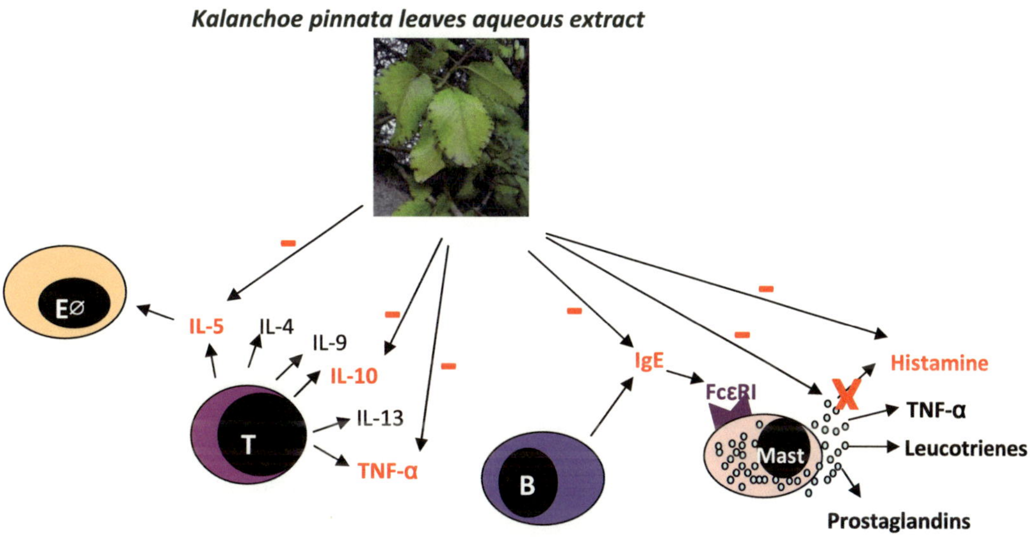

Eϕ: eosinophil, **B:** B lymphocyte, **TH2:** TH2 lymphocyte, **Mast:** mast cell.

Fig. 9. Anti-anaphylactic mechanisms of Kp. Anaphylactic shock is mediated by immunological mechanisms involving the production of Th2 cytokines (IL-4, IL-5, IL-9 and IL-13), the production of antigen-specific IgE antibodies, the recruitment and activation of eosinophils (through IL-5) and mast cells. The subsequent contact with antigen causes crosslinking of IgE molecules that are linked to the surface of mast cells via Fcε RI receptor and subsequent degranulation. After crosslinking, there is a systemic release of inflammatory mediators that responsible for the symptoms and the severity of anaphylaxis. Treatment with aqueous extract of Kp inhibits the production of IgE, the production of IL-10, IL-5 and TNF-α, degranulation of mast cells and histamine release.

The safety of Kp to humans is substantiated by the fact that it is widely consumed in the popular medicine, and that a human case of cutaneous leishmaniasis displayed unaltered serum toxicological parameters following oral treatment (Torres-Santos et al, 2003). For its effectiveness in mice and expected clinical safeness, quercitrin-containing Kp or quercitrin alone are potential candidates for clinical tests aiming at a prophylactic therapy for hypersensitive people under the risk of anaphylactic shock.

Anaphylaxis is a life-threatening allergic condition. Promising preventive measures include allergen nonspecific and allergen-specific immunotherapy. A range of plant species, including *Kalanchoe pinnata*, contain promising anti-allergic substances. Flavonoids extracted from *K. pinnata*, particularly quercitrin that down regulate Th2-type immune responses and also inflammatory reactions primarily induced by TNF-α, that together lead to overt release of histamine and other mediators by mast cells and basophils, culminating with anaphylactic shock.

4. References

Akdis, C.A. & Blaser, K. (2000). Mechanisms of allergen-specific immunotherapy. *Allergy*, 55, pp. (522-530).

Akinpelu, D.A. (2000). Antimicrobial activity of *Bryophyllum pinnatum* leaves. *Fitoterapia*, 71, pp. (193-194).

Allorge-Boiteau, L. (1996). Madagascar centre de spéciation et d'origine du genre *Kalanchoe* (Crassulaceae). In: *Biogéographie de Madagascar*. LOURENÇO, W.R. Editions de l'ORSTOM, Paris.

Almeida, A.P., Da Silva, A.G., Souza, M.L.M., Lima, L.M.T.R. Rossi-Bergmann, B., Gonçalves De Moraes, V.L. & Costa, S.S. (2000). Isolation and chemical analysis of a fatty acid fraction of *Kalanchoe pinnata* with a potent lymphocyte suppressive activity. *Planta Medica*, 66, pp. (134-137).

Barua, C.C., Gupta, P.P., Patnaik, G.K., Kulshrestha, D.K. & Dhawan, B.N. (1997). Studies on antianaphylactic activity of fractions of Albizzia lebbeck. *Current Science*, 72, 6, *pp.* (397-399).

Baruah, C.C., Gupta, P.P., Nath, A, Patnaik, L.G.K. &; Dhawan, B.N. (1998). Anti-allergic and anti-anaphylactic activity of picroliv - A standardised iridoid glycoside fraction of Picrorhiza kurroa. *Pharmacological Research*, 38, 6, pp. (487-492).

Chandrashekhara, V.M., Halagalia, K.S., Nidavania, R.B., Shalavadia, M.H., Ganapatyb, S., Biswasa, D. & Muchchandia, V.M. (2011). Anti-allergic activity of German chamomile (Matricaria recutita L.) in mast cell mediated allergy model. *Journal of Ethnopharmacology*, 137, 1, pp. (336-340).

Comalada, M., Ballester, I., Bailón, E., Sierra, S., Xaus, J., Gálvez, J., De Medina, F.S. & Zarzuelo, A. (2006). Inhibition of pro-inflammatory markers in primary bone marrow-derived mouse macrophages by naturally occurring flavonoids: Analysis of the structure-activity relationship. *Biochemical Pharmacology*, 72, pp. (1010-1021).

Costa, S.S., Muzitano, M.F., Camargo, L.M.M. & Coutinho, M.A.S. (2008). Therapeutic Potential of *Kalanchoe* Species: Flavonoids and other Secondary Metabolites. *Natural Product Communications*, 3, pp. (2151-2164).

Cruz, E.A., Da-Silva, S.A.G, Muzitano, M.F., E Silva, P.M.R., Costa, S.S. & Rossi-Bergmann, B. (2008). Immunomodulatory Immunomodulatory pretreatment with *Kalanchoe pinnata* extract and its quercitrin flavonoid effectively protects mice against fatal anaphylactic shock. *International Immunopharmacology*, 8, 12, pp. (1616-1621).

Cruz, E.A., Reuter, S., Martin, H., Dehzad, N., Muzitano, M.F., Costa, S.S., Rossi-Bergmann, B., Buhl, R., Stassen, M. & Taube, C. (2011). *Kalanchoe pinnata* inhibits mast cell activation and prevents allergic airway disease. *Phytomedicine.* (Jul 2011).

Da-Silva, S.A.G., Costa, S.S., Mendonça, S.C.F., Silva, E.M., Moraes, V.L.G. & Rossi-Bergmann B. (1995). Therapeutic effect of oral Kalanchoe pinnata leaf extract in murine leishmaniasis. *Acta Tropica*, 60, pp. (201–210).

Da-Silva, S.A.G., Costa, S.S. & Rossi-Bergmann, B. (1999). The anti-leishmanial effect of *Kalanchoe* is mediated by nitric oxide intermediates. *Parasitology*, 118, pp. (575-582).

Farnsworth, N.R. (1994). Ethnopharmacology and drug development. *Ciba Foundation Symptoms*, 185, pp. (42–51).

Francis, J.N., Till, S.J. & Durham, S.R. (2003). Induction of IL-10+CD4+CD25+ T cells by grass pollen immunotherapy. *J. Allergy Clin. Immunology*, 111, pp. (1255-1261).

Fukumoto, H., Yamaki, M., Isoi, K. & Ishiguro, K. (1996). Antianaphylactic effects of the principal compounds from the white petals of Impatiens balsamina L. *Phytotherapy Research*, 10, 3, pp. (202-206).

Gaind, K.N. & Gupta, R.L. (1972). Alkanes, alkanols, triterpenes and sterols of *Kalanchoe pinnata*. *Phytochemistry*, 11, pp. (1500-1502).

Gaind, K.N. & Gupta, R.L. Flavonoid glycosides from *Kalanchoe pinnata*. (1971). *Planta Medica*, 20, pp. (368-373).

Ghaisas, M.M., Kumar, D., Sarda, A.P. & Bhamre, S.S. (2011). Anti-anaphylactic and Mast Cell Stabilizing Effect of Calotropis gigantea Extract. *Latin American Journal of Pharmacy*, 30, 2, pp. (363-367).

Gomes, D.C.O., Muzitano, M.F., Costa, S.S. & Rossi-Bergmann, B. (2009). Effectiveness of the immunomodulatory extract of *Kalanchoe pinnata* against murine visceral leishmaniasis. *Parasitology*, 137, pp. (613-618).

Ichikawa, M., Ogura, M. & Iijima, T. Antiallergic flavone glycoside from *Kalanchoe pinnatum*. Patent 61, 118, 396 [86, 118, 319] (Cl. CO7H17/07), Apl 84/240, 282, 14 nov 1984; 4p-Chemical Abstracts, 105, 178423q, 1986.

Ishiguro, K. & Fukumoto, H. (1997). A practical and speedy screening method for murine anaphylaxis: On the antianaphylactic effect of Impatiens balsamina L. *Phytotherapy Research*, 11, 1, pp. (48-50).

Jeong, H.J., Lee, S.A., Moon, P.D., Na, H.J., Park, R.K., Um, J.Y., Kim, H.M. & Hong, S.H. (2006). Alginic acid has anti-anaphylactic effects and inhibits inflammatory cytokine expression via suppression of nuclear factor-kappa B activation. *Clinical and Experimental Allergy*, 36, 6, pp. (785-794).

Jutel, M., Akdis, M., Budak, F., Aebischer-Casaulta, C., Wrzyszcz, M., Blaser, K. & Akdis, C.A. (2003). IL-10 and TGF-beta cooperate in the regulatory T cell response to mucosal allergens in normal immunity and specific immunotherapy. *European Journal of Immunology*, 33, pp. (1205-1214).

Kang, T.H., Choi, I.Y., Kim, S.J., Moon, P.D., Seo, J.U., Kim, J.J., An, N.H., Kim, S.H., Kim, M.H., Um, J.Y., Hong, S.H., Kim, H.M. & Jeong, H.J. (2010). Ailanthus altissima swingle has anti-anaphylactic effect and inhibits inflammatory cytokine expression via suppression of nuclear factor-kappaB activation. *In Vitro Cellular & Developmental Biology-Animal*, 46, 1, pp. (72-81).

Kawai, M., Hirano, T., Higa, S., Arimitsu, J., Maruta, M., Kuwahara, Y., Ohkawara, T., Hagihara, K., Yamadori, T., Shima, Y., Ogata, A., Kawase, I. & Tanaka, T. (2007). Flavonoids and Related Compoundsas Anti-Allergic Substances. *Allergology International*, 56, pp. (113-123).

Kemp, S.F., Lockey, R.F. & Simons, F.E.R. (2008). Epinephrine: the drug of choice for anaphylaxis: a statement of the World Allergy Organization. *Allergy*, 63, pp. (1061–1070).

Kemp, S.F. & Lockey, R.F. (2002). Anaphylaxis: A review of causes and mechanisms. *Journal of Allergy and Clinical Immunology*, 110, pp. (341-348).

Kim, H.M., Yi, D.K. & Shin, H.Y. (1999). The evaluation of antianaphylactic effect of Oryza sativa L-in rats. *American Journal of Chinese Medicine*, 27, 1, pp. (63-72).

Kim, S.H., Park, H.H., Lee, S., Jun, C.D., Choi, B.J., Kim, S.Y., Kim, S.H., Kim, D.K., Park, J.S., Chae, B.S. & Shin, T.Y. (2005). The anti-anaphylactic effect of the gall of Rhus javanica is mediated through inhibition of histamine release and inflammatory cytokine secretion. *International Immunopharmacology*, 5, 13-14, pp. (1820-1829).

Lee, J.H., Kim, J.W., Ko, N.Y., Mun, S.H., Kim, D,K., Kim, J.D., Kim, H.S. Lee, K.R., Kim, Y.K., Radinger, M., Her, E. & Choi, W.S. (2008). Camellia japonica suppresses immunoglobulin E-mediated allergic response by the inhibition of Syk kinase activation in mast cells. *Clinical and Experimental Allergy*, 38, 5, pp. (794-804).

Lee, Y.M., Kim, D.K., Kim, S.H., Shin, T.Y. & Kim, H.M. (1996). Antianaphylactic activity of Poncirus trifoliata fruit extract. *Journal of Ethnopharmacology*, 54, 2-3, pp. (77-84).

Li, X.M. & Brown, L. (2009). Efficacy and mechanisms of action of traditional Chinese medicines for treating asthma and allergy. *Journal of Allergy and Clinical Immunology*, 123, pp. (297-306).

Li, X.M., Zhang, T.F., Sampson, H., Zou, Z.M., Beyer, K., Wen, M.C. & Schofield, B. (2004). The potential use of Chinese herbal medicines in treating allergic asthma. *Annals of Allergy, Asthma and Immunology*, 93, PP. (S35-S44).

Lorenzi, H. & Abreu-Matos, F.J. (2008). *Plantas Medicinais no Brasil – nativas e exóticas, (2a ed)*, Instituto Plantarum de Estudos da Flora Ltda, São Paulo, Brasil.

Lucas, V. & Machado, O. (1946). Contribuição ao estudo das plantas medicinais brasileiras - Saião. *Revista da Flora Medicinal*, 77, PP. (1-39).

Muñoz, V., Sauvain, M., Bourdy, G., Callapa, J., Rojas, I., Vargas, L. & Deharo, E. (2000). The search for natural bioactive compounds through a multidisciplinar approach in Bolivia: Part II. Antimalarial activity of some plants used by mosetane Indians. *Journal of Ethnopharmacology*, 69, pp. (139-155).

Muzitano, M.F., Cruz, E.A., Almeida, A.P., Da Silva, S.A., Kaiser, C.R., Guette, C., Rossi-Bergmann, B. & Costa, S.S. (2006a). Quercitrin: an antileishmanial flavonoid glycoside from *Kalanchoe pinnata*. *Planta Medica*, 72, pp. (81–83).

Muzitano, M.F., Tinoco, L.W., Guette, C., Kaiser, C.R., Rossi-Bergmann, B. & Costa, S.S. (2006b). Assessment of antileishmanial activity of new and unusual flavonoids from *Kalanchoe pinnata*. *Phytochemistry*, 67, pp. (2071-2077).

Muzitano, M.F., Bergonzi M.C., De Melo, G.O., Lage, C.L.S., Bilia A.R., Vincieri F.F., Rossi-Bergmann, B. & Costa, S.S. (2011). Influence of cultivation conditions, season of collection and extraction method on the content of antileishmanial flavonoids from *Kalanchoe pinnata*. *Journal of Ethnopharmacology*, 133, pp. (132–137).

Muzitano, M.F., Falcão, C.A.B., Cruz, E.A., Bergonzi M.C., Bilia A.R., Vincieri F.F., Rossi-Bergmann, B. & Costa, S.S. (2009). Oral Metabolism and Efficacy of Flavonoids in a Murine Model of Cutaneous Leishmaniasis. *Planta Medica*, 75, pp. (307-311).

Nakamura, R., Nakamura, R., Watanabe, K., Oka, K., Ohta, S., Mishima, S. & Teshima, R. (2010). Effects of propolis from different areas on mast cell degranulation and identification of the effective components in propolis. *International Immunopharmacology*, 10, pp. (1107–1112).

Nassis, C. Z., Haebisch, E.M. & Giesbrecht, A.M. (1992). Antihistamine activity of *Bryophyllum calycinum*. *Brazilian Journalof Biological Research*, 25, pp. (929-936).

Neves, J.S., Coelho, L.P., Cordeiro, R.S.B., Veloso, M.P., Silva, P.M.R.E, Dos Santos, M.H. & Martins, M.A. (2007). Antianaphylactic properties of 7-epiclusianone, a tetraprenylated benzophenone isolated from Garcinia brasiliensis. *Planta Medica*, 73, 7, pp. (644-649).

Newman, D.J. & Cragg, G.M. (2007). Natural products as sources of new drugs over the last 25 years. *Journal of Natural Products*, 70, pp. (461-477).

Okpo, S.O. & Adeyemi, O.O. (2002). The antianaphylactic effects of Crinum glaucum aqueous extract. *Journal of Ethnopharmacology*, 81, 2, pp. (187-190).

Plangger, N., Rist, L., Zimmermann, R. & Von Mandach, U. (2006). Intravenous tocolysis with *Bryophyllum pinnatum* is better tolerated than beta-agonist application. *European Journal of Obstetrics & Gynecology and Reproductive Biology*, 124, pp. (168–172).

Rossi-Bergmann, B., Costa, S.S., Borges, M.B.S., Da-Silva, S.A., Noleto, G.R., Souza, M.L.M & Moraes, V.L.G. (1994). Immunosuppressive effect of the aqueous extract of Kalanchoe pinnata in mice. *Phytotherapy Research*, 8, pp. (399–402).

Sforcin, J.M. (2007). Propolis and the immune system: a review. *Journal of Ethnopharmacology*, 113, pp. (1–14).

Shams, K.A. & Schmidt, R. (2007). Lipid fraction constituents and evaluation of anti-anaphylactic activity of Prunus mahaleb L. kernels. *African Journal of Traditional Complementary and Alternative Medicines*, 4, 3, pp. (289-293).

Siddiqui, S., Fazi, B.S. & Sultana, N. (1989). Triterpenoids and phenanthrenes from leaves of *Bryophullum pinnatum*. *Phytochemistry*, 28, pp. (2433-2438).

Sousa, P.J.C., Rocha, J.C.S., Pessoa, A.M., Alves, L.A.D. & Carvalho, J.C.T. (2005). Estudo preliminar da atividade antiinflamatória de *Bryophillum calycinum* Salisb. *Revista Brasileira de Farmacognosia*, 15, pp. (60-64).

Supratman, U., Fujita, T., Akiyama, K., Hayashi, H., Murakami, A., Sakai, H., Koshimizu, K. & Ohigashi, H. (2001). Anti-tumor promoting activity of bufadienolides from *Kalanchoe pinnata* and *K. daigremontiana* X tubiflora. *Bioscience Biotechnology and Biochemistry*, 65, 4, pp. (947-949).

Torres-Santos, E.C., Da-Silva, S.A.G, Santos, A.P.P.T., Almeida, A.P., Costa, S.S. &, Rossi-Bergmann, B. (2003). Toxicological analysis and effectiveness of oral Kalanchoe pinnata on a human case of leishmaniasis. *Phytotherapy Research* 17, pp. (801–803).

Ueda, Y., Oku, H., Iinuma, M. & Ishiguro, K. (2005). Antianaphylactic and antipruritic effects of the flowers of Impatiens textori MiQ. *Biological & Pharmaceutical Bulletin*, 28, 9, pp. (1786-1790).

Venkatesh, P., Mukherjee, P.K., Mukherjee, D., Bandyopadhyay, A., Fukui, H. & Mizuguchi, H. (2010). Potential of Baliospermum montanum against compound 48/80-induced systemic anaphylaxis. *Pharmaceutical Biology*, 48, 11, pp. (1213-1217).

Westfall, T.C. & Westfall, D.P. (2006). Adrenergic agonists and antagonists, In: *Goodman & gilman´s the basis of pharmacological therapeutics.* Brunton, L.L., Lazo, J.S., Parker, K.L., (11a ed.), pp. (237-295), McGraw-Hill, New York.

Yadav, N.P. & Dixit, V.K. (2003). Hepatoprotective activity of leaves of *Kalanchoe pinnata* Pers. *Journal of Ethnopharmacology*, 86, 2-3, pp. (197-202).

Yamagishi, T., Haruna, M., Yan, X.Z., Chang, J.J. & Lee, K.H. (1989). Antitumor agents, 110 1,2, Bryophilin B, a novel potent cytotoxic bufadienolide from *Bryophullum pinnatum*. *Journal of Natural Products*, 52, pp. (1071-1079).

Youssouf, M.S., Kaiser, P., Tahir, M., Singh, G.D., Singh, S., Shanna, V.K., Satti, N.K., Haque, S.E. & Johri, R.K. (2007). Anti-anaphylactic effect of Euphorbia hirta. *Fitoterapia*, 7-8, pp. (535-539).

24

Cissampelos sympodialis (Menispermaceae): A Novel Phytotherapic Weapon Against Allergic Diseases?

M.R. Piuvezam, C.R. Bezerra-Santos,
P.T. Bozza, C. Bandeira-Melo, G. Vieira and H.F. Costa
Federal University of Paraiba, PB,
Oswaldo Cruz Foundation, Rio de Janeiro, RJ,
Federal University of Rio de Janeiro, RJ,
Brazil

1. Introduction

Allergic diseases affect millions of people around the world. Enhanced prevalence and the chronic characteristics of these illnesses represent an important public health problem. Most prevalent allergic diseases are classified as immediate-type reactions such as urticaria, allergic conjuctivitis, food allergy, allergic rhinitis, anaphylaxis and asthma (Sicherer & Leung, 2004; Fonacier et al., 2010; Sicherer, 2011). The immediate-type reaction terminology is applied to allergic reactions because the symptoms develop few minutes after allergen contact. The immune mechanisms responsible for the initiation of these reactions depend on the production of immunoglobulins (IgG1 and/or IgE) that activate cells such as mast cells, eosinophils and basophils. Once activated, these cells are responsible for release of inflammatory mediators, contributing to the exacerbation and maintenance of the allergic processes (Lampinen et al., 2004). Urticaria is characterized by pruritic, edematous and erythematous lesions that affect 15% to 25% of individuals during their lives. Most of the cases are acute but about 30% of patients present symptoms for more than six weeks and are considered as having chronic disease. Women are more susceptible (75%) than men and only 1% to 5% of the cases are related to IgE-dependent reaction while most of the cases are considered to be induced by physical stimuli or of idiopathic nature, including autoimmune urticaria (Antunez et al., 2006). Allergic urticaria depends on skin mast cell activation which delivers preformed mediators, mainly histamine, few minutes after allergen exposure. On the other hand activated mast cells also produce and deliver neo-formed mediators, i.e., prostaglandin D2 (PGD_2) and cisleukotrienes (*cis*LT) that stimulate inflammatory responses mediated by neutrophils, basophils, eosinophils and T lymphocytes (Funk, 2001; Harizi et al., 2008; Kambe et al., 2010). Another allergic disease of great importance in public health is allergic conjunctivitis. Allergic conjuctivities prevalence in the United States was estimated to affects about 40 million people. Allergic conjunctivitis is marked by the presence of eosinophil cells in conjunctiva mucosa (Bezerra & Santos, 2010). Food allergy, another allergic disorder, is related to the genetic susceptibility of individuals to eggs, peanuts, seafood (e.g. shrimp, lobsters, crabs, squids and mussels milk and others). Oral sensitization with shrimp tropomyosin induces in mice allergen-specific IgE, T cell response and systemic anaphylactic reactions (Capobianco et al, 2008). Food allergy has been reported in some cohort studies which describe variable rates of food allergy prevalence in the United States, Canada, the United Kindom, Singapore and the Philippines (Berin & Mayer, 2009). Approximately 1% of food allergic patients develop signs and symptoms characterized by intense diarrhea, urticaria and anaphylaxis. There are divergences about the period of exposition to food allergens and development of disease symptoms. Studies showed that allergenic food ingested during pregnancy increases the risk of higher prevalence of allergic response in infants (Sausenthaler et al., 2011). In contrary to the aforementioned, other studies suggested that earlier exposure to food allergens may promote a protective response to allergic conditions. Serologic diagnosis of patients with food allergies have demonstrated high levels of specific IgE. The pathological immune response observed in these patients depended on: (i) the presence of an adjuvant responsible for stimulating inflammatory response which is considered one necessary step to initiate lymphocyte responses, (ii) allergen doses which can induce classical or alternative mechanisms of allergic process in response to food as seen in cutaneous sensitization to food allergens and (iii) the types of mediators delivered which can lead to systemic allergic reactions such as anaphilaxis (Berin & Mayer, 2009; Sicherer & Leung, 2011). In addition, asthma, which probably may be the most important allergic disorder, affects about 300 million people in the world and causes an estimated 250,000 deaths annually. This illness is characterized by a reversible lower airway inflammation, airway hyperresponsivenss, mucus hypersecretion, leukocyte recruitment to lung tissue and airway remodeling that might cause respiratory deficits. Increased prevalence and difficulties in asthma control are responsible for the elevated costs to health systems around the world (Busse & Lemanski, 2001; Mayr et al., 2003; Bateman et al., 2008).

During asthmatic crises, patients develop an intense breathing difficulty called airway hyperreactivity (AHR). This response occurs as a consequence of the exposure of the inhaled route to the environmental allergen, thereby increasing the respiratory pause. An array of inflammatory mediators such as histamine, *cis*LT, PGs, cytokines, chemokines and others present in the lung tissue elicit smooth muscle cell contraction, mucus production, lung inflammation and airway remodeling. Mucus hypersecretion and bronchiole obstructions are important features of asthmatic patients. These effects of the inflammatory mediators may worsen the respiratory functions. In the last decade studies have shown the involvement of some mediators in stimulating the mucus production by cells named globlet cells. Concomitant to lung enhanced respiratory pause and lung obstruction, recruitment of inflammatory leukocytes to bronchoalveolar space initiates a cellular response that might become a destructive response to the lung tissue architecture in a chronic phase of the disease. Different leukocytes participate in the inflammatory process in the lung, i.e., neutrophils, mononuclear cells and mainly eosinophil cells (Cowden et al., 2010). Similar cellular and molecular immunological mechanisms related to asthma are described in allergic rhinitis demonstrating a strong correlation between these two allergic disorders with the same etiology. Rhinitis is an upper airway allergic inflammation and is considered co-morbidity to asthma as several studies have suggested that upper and lower airway inflammations are a unique entity. The prevalence of this disease has been increasing in many countries and an association between asthma and allergic rhinitis has been shown. Although asthma and allergic rhinitis show certain particularities, both present similar pathophysiology with IgE-dependent allergic reactions. Another severe IgE-dependent allergic reaction is the anaphylactic shock triggered by allergens such as bee venom, domiciliary dust, cockroaches, food, pollen, and/or medicines after mast cell sensitization and activation (Bateman et al., 2008). The term 'anaphylaxis' was used for the first time by Richet and Portier (1902) to describe a potentially fatal reaction that may affect different organs and systems and the process by which all the symptoms derived from pharmacologic mediators, i.e. histamine, are released by blood leukocytes as eosinophils and basophils. Mortality rate of anaphylaxis have been increasing around the world in the last decades and at least twenty people die every year in UK due to anaphylactic reactions representing one death in three million habitants a year. Although the majority of the cases of anaphylactic reactions are related to high levels of IgE and histamine, some patients do not present these serum biologic markers, suggesting in these cases an IgE-independent mechanisms (Pumphrey, 2004; Moneret-Vautrin & Mertes, 2010; Seidel et al., 2010).

2. Immune mechanisms for the initiation of allergic reactions

The allergen sensitization phase is related to multiple factors including gene polymorphisms of HLA, FcεRI-β and IL-4 family, environmental factors like vaccination for prevention of diseases, pollutants present indoors and outdoors and viral infections. IgE is a critical participant in the onset of the effector phase of allergies due to its affinity to receptors (FcεRI) present on the surface of mast cells, basophils and/or eosinophils. The cross-linking between two IgE molecules and the allergen is responsible for cellular activation and subsequent release of preformed mediators, i.e., histamine from the cytoplasmic granules as well as neo-formed mediators such as eicosanoids (leukotrienes, prostaglandins and thromboxane) (Maddox & Schwartz, 2002). These mediators increase vascular permeability, induce smooth muscle contraction causing difficulty in breathing as well as the proliferation of fibroblasts and smooth muscle cells (Kanaoka & Boyce, 2004). The IgE production by allergen-specific B cells is associated with Th2 cell profile with IL-4, IL-5 and IL-13 productions. The IL-4 and IL-13 induce in B cells the production of allegen-specific- IgE (Munitz et al., 2008) and IL-5 induces the production, activation and differentiation of bone marrow-derived eosinophil (Takatsu & Nakajima, 2008). Among the cell types mentioned above, mast cells are of fundamental importance in the first phase of allergic disease due to their wide distribution throughout the body including skin, lungs and gastrointestinal tract (Maurer & Metz, 2005). Recently, some scientific work showed that mast cells are able to migrate to the smooth muscles of the airways of asthma patients, corroborating the interaction between mediators released by mast cells and smooth muscle response in the asthmatic lung (Brightling et al., 2003).

Another important cell population in the pathophysiology of asthma is the eosinophil. This cell participates in the late phase of the inflammatory response and it was initially described as a component of defense against intestinal parasites (Gleich et al., 1993; Weller, 1997; Rothenberg, 1998). However, there are several lines of evidence that contradicts this view, and demonstrate the eosinophils as multifunctional cells involved in the initial processes and propagation of various inflammatory diseases. They are also involved in the regulation of innate and adaptive immune responses (Rothenberger & Hogan, 2006). Eosinophils can respond to different stimuli as nonspecific tissue injury, viral infections, allograft, allergens, and tumors. Additionally, these cells release cationic proteins stored in granules as eosinophil peroxidase (EPO), major basic protein (MBP), eosinophil cationic protein (ECP) and eosinophil derived neurotoxin (EDN). Eosinophils also release a range of cytokines including the Th2 profile as well as chemokines RANTES, eotaxin 1 and MIP-1α (Rothenberger & Hogan, 2006). Eosinophils participate in many pathological processes such as parasite infections, gastrointestinal disorders and allergic processes such as asthma. Several studies have revealed the presence of high levels of MBP in bronchoalveolar lavage (BAL) of asthmatic patients that induces cytotoxicity to various body tissues, especially the airway epithelium (Rothenberg, 1998). Additionally, MBP increases the reactivity of airway smooth muscle to cause dysfunction of the muscarinic M2 vagal nerve, known to contribute to the development of airway hyperreactivity, a key feature of asthma (Jacoby et al., 1993). Several studies have demonstrated that eosinophil activation in inflammatory reactions is associated with increasing number of lipid bodies (LBs) (Bozza et al., 2011). The LBs are defined as cytoplasmatic organelles rich in lipids, surrounded by a phospholipid monolayer, posses high amounts of enzymes that produce eicosanoids such as PLA2, 5-LO, 15-LO, COX, LTC_4 and PGE synthases and also cytokines, chemokines and several kinases related with signal transductions. However LBs are found in small quantities in non-activated cells, they are associated with a wild range of pathological conditions such as cancers, infectious and inflammatory diseases like asthma (Bozza et al., 2009). Several inflammatory mediators are able to induce the leukocyte LB formation as platelet activator factor (PAF) (De Assis et al., 2003). In eosinophils other stimuli such as prostaglandin D2 (PGD_2) (Mesquita-Santos et al., 2006), IL-5 (Bozza et al., 1998), RANTES and eotaxin also induced the LB formation (Vieira-de-Abreu et al., 2005). In addition, in the allergic inflammation, the new LBs are observed and this process is mediated mainly by a *cross-talk* between eotaxin/RANTES via chemokine receptors (CCR3) with MAPK, PI3K and tyrosine kinases activation and PGD2 via an unknown receptor. The main site of *cis*LT generation in eosinophils is the LBs in the pulmonary allergic inflammation (Bozza et al., 2009). Moreover, the regulation of allergic reactions is carried out by T cells called Th1 cells (Teixeira et al., 2005), which secret cytokines such as IL-2 and INF-γ, and by the Th17 cells that produce IL-17. Both profiles can reduce the eosinophil onset in the lung and the bronchial hyperreactivity (Schnyder-Candrian, et al. 2006) (Figure 1).

3. Conventional treatment of allergic diseases

A wide variety of medicines are used to treat allergic diseases. The β2-adrenergic agonist therapy is widely used as first choice for addressing the crisis of asthma (O'Byrne, 2009). Phenoterol and salbutamol are members of this group and are largely used to reverse bronchoconstriction by binding directly to β2-receptors of lung smooth muscle cells and inducing breathing relieve due to bronchodilatation. *In vitro* studies showed these drugs are responsible for increasing the levels of cAMP described as a regulatory second messenger of intracellular calcium-dependent mechanisms. Calcium is one of several molecules responsible for the smooth muscle contraction during acute phase of asthma crises (Mahn et al., 2010). Of note, side effects are observed in patients under β2-agonists therapy, mainly cardiac frequency increases in response to activation of cardiac β1-receptors. Potent anti-inflammatory steroid therapy is also used to control asthma manifestations. These medicines are indicated to block lung inflammation mediated by inflammatory leukocytes such as neutrophils, eosinophils, basophils and lymphocytes that contribute to exacerbation of inflammatory response (Jarjour et al., 2006). As consequence of inflammation, lung tissue might present a cell phenotype change, referred to as 'remodeling' which impairs the physiological lung function causing respiratory deficiency and death in some of asthmatic patients.

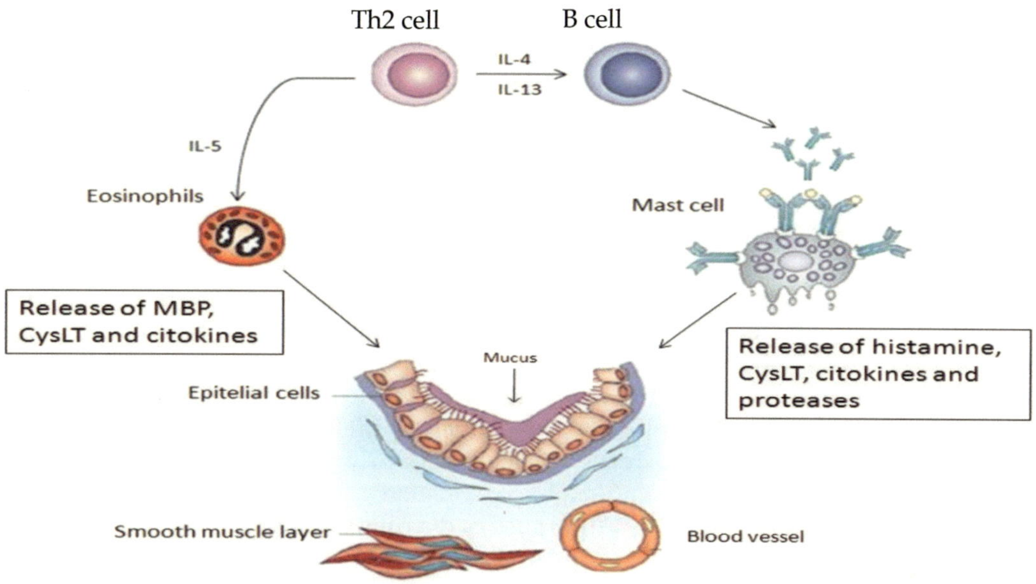

Fig. 1. Mechanism of immediate allergic reactions. Immediate allergic reactions are orchestrated by Th2 lymphocytes and its major cytokines (IL-4, IL-5 and IL-13) responsible for inducing B cell activation and IgE secretion. Mast cell sensitization depends on IgE cross-linking and binding with FcεRI, subsequent cellular activation, histamine and leukotrienes releases that are crucial to bronchospasm induction. Concomitantly, eosinophils migrate to bronchoalveolar cavity by an IL-5 (and others) dependent mechanism. Lung damage and airway remodeling are caused by cationic proteins delivered by eosinophils and matrix extracellular protein deposition.

Steroidal anti-inflammatory drugs are able to control these pathologic responses in airways by inhibition of lymphocyte functions and mainly inducing apoptosis in eosinophils, which is considered the major component of lung tissue damage. Steroids also can induce a variety of side effects like endocrine alterations, cardiovascular disturbances, psychotic crises and cancers (Belvisi, 2004). Combinations of β2-agonists and steroids are commonly used to control asthma. Another class of antiasthmatic drug that was developed about 10 years ago, the antileukotrienes (Montelukast® and derivatives). These drugs present both bronchodilator and anti-inflammatory properties. *cis*LT are known pro-inflammatory mediators and they induce vascular permeability, lung smooth muscle cell contraction/bronchospasm and leukocyte activation and chemotaxis (Funk, 2001). Previous studies reported *cis*-LT as the major bronchoconstrictor mediators in an asthmatic lung, causing sustained smooth muscle contraction. The anti-leukotriene drugs block leukotriene receptors in lung tissue, reversing bronchospasm in asthmatic patients. Additionally, leukotriene modifiers like zileutron act by blocking the 5-lipooxygenase enzyme (5-LO), thus inhibiting the leukotriene generation. Therefore, anti-leukotriene therapies strongly impair airway inflammatory response and ameliorate respiratory function (Terashima, et al. 2002; Angelova-Fischer & Tsankov, 2005). Antagonists of the enzyme phosphodiesterase, aminophylline and theophylline as well as muscarinic blockers also occupy space in the therapeutic arsenal.

3.1 Immunotherapy of asthma

Immunotherapy with anti-IgE has also contributed to the treatment of asthma patients who do not have a good response to conventional therapies (Lazaar & Panettieri, 2004; Foster et al., 2011). Despite anti-IgE therapy, which represents a major breakthrough in the treatment of asthma, the high cost of this therapy remains the major obstacle.

4. Botanical and pharmacological study with *Cissampelos sympodialis*

In northeastern Brazil, diseases such as asthma, influenza, bronchitis and rheumatism are traditionally treated with infusions of the root bark of *Cissampelos sympodialis* Eichl (Menispemaceae), popularly known in the region as milona, abuteira or orelha de onça (Correa, 1984). The Menispermaceae family was described by AL Jussieu (1789). This term is an allusion to the morphology of the seed that looks like the fourth form of the moon. This species belongs to the order Ranunculales, subdivided by Diels (1910) into eight tribes, three subtribes, 72 genera and approximately 400 species. These species are found on all continents, especially in tropical and subtropical regions. In Brazil, the Menispermaceae family is represented by 12 genera and 106 species distributed mostly in the Amazon forest (Barroso, 2004).

The genus *Cissampelos* belongs to the tribe Cocculeae, and subtribe Cissampelinae and comprises 19 species of which nine occur in Brazil (Rhodes, 1975). This genus is one of the few among the angiosperms that shows diversity and uniformity. The diversity can be seen in vegetative habitat and leaves. The uniformity is found in the sexual expression of simple flowers, pistils and small flowers. In the state of Paraiba the genus *Cissampelos* is represented by three species: *Cissampelos ovalifolia* DC, *Cissampelos glaberrima* St. Hill and *Cissampelos sympodialis* Eichl. These species are found in different types of habitat, soil and vegetation, occurring mainly in rainforests on the Atlantic coast and hills (Barbosa-Filho et al., 1997). The species *Cissampelos sympodialis* is endemic in Brazil and is found in the Northeast and Southeast, from Ceara to Minas Gerais states. This species often occurs in open areas as shrubs in sandy soil and can be distinguished mainly by the shape of the deltoid leaves (Barbosa-Filho et al., 1997). The roots of *Cissampelos sympodialis* are widely used by Indian tribes and in folk medicine to treat various diseases such as diarrhea, diseases of the genitourinary tract and especially in respiratory tract diseases such as asthma (Corrêa, 1984). Both alcoholic fraction of roots (AFR) and of leaves (AFL) and some of the chemical components (bisbenzylisoquinolinic type alkaloids) isolated from these extracts have been studied. These alkaloids have been shown to have paralytic effect, cytotoxic activity (Kupchan et al., 1965), to stimulate the central nervous system (Sur & Pradhan, 1964), to prevent hypersecretion of reactive products from neutrophils and macrophages (Castranova et al., 1991), to inhibit the inflammatory cytokine production by peripheral blood mononuclear cells (Onai et al. , 1995) and bronchodilator activity (Thomas et al., 1995). Thomas et al (1995) showed that the AFR had a relaxing effect on smooth muscle of trachea and increased the cyclic adenosine monophosphate (cAMP) levels from alveolar leukocytes in guinea pigs in a manner similar to aminophylline which antagonizes bronchial muscle contractions. Similarly, studies of AFL showed inhibition of histamine and ovalbumin (OVA)-induced bronchospasm in guinea pigs (Thomas et al., 1997a), synthesis of phosphodiesterase (PDE) IV and V in the lungs of mice and induced increased levels of cAMP in guinea pig trachea muscle cells (Thomas et al. 1997b). Also AFL had an antidepressant effect probably associated with the phosphodiesterases inhibition in rat brain

(Almeida et al., 1998), inhibited human neutrophils degranulation (Thomas et al., 1999) and induced contraction of vascular smooth muscle (Freitas et al., 2000).

5. Phytochemical study of *Cissampelos sympodialis*

Chemical studies of *Cissampelos sympodialis* led to the isolation of different alkaloids (Barbosa-Filho et al., 1997) such as bisbenzylisoquinolinic (warifteine, methilwarifteine, roraimine and simpodialine); morfinic (milonin); aporfinic (laurifolin) and oxoaporfinic (liriodenine) which have allowed for a more accurate immunopharmacological studies (Freitas et al., 1996, De Lira et al., 2002) (Table 1). Analysis of quality control of *Cissampelos sympodialis* extracts by thermogravimetry test showed that both AFL and AFR present alkaloids as major compounds and also both extracts showed the same kinetic behavior of bisbenzylisoquinolinic alkaloids (Aragão et al., 2002). Among these alkaloids warifteine showed spasmolytic activity by modifying various regulatory processes involving intracellular calcium channels and cAMP levels, which are essential for muscle contraction (Somlyo & Somlyo, 1994; Freitas et al., 1996). Therefore the purpose of our scientific study has been to develop a herbal medicine from the leaf extract of *Cissampelos sympodialis* to treat asthma as an alternative therapy.

6. Current stage of knowledge of *Cissampelos sympodialis*

6.1 Immunological study of *Cissampelos sympodialis*

Since the relaxant effect of *Cissampelos sympodialis* extracts (roots and leaves) on bronchial smooth muscle cells (Thomas et al. 1995), inhibition of phosphodiesterases (PDE) IV and V in the lung with increased levels of cAMP in muscle cells of the trachea (Thomas et al. 1997b), biological effects that corroborate with the anti-asthmatic activity of the plant were demonstrated, we began the immunological studies. Our research group, with laboratory complex located in the Laboratory of Pharmaceutical Technology (LTF), Federal University of Paraíba (UFPB), and in collaboration with Federal University of Rio de Janeiro and the Oswaldo Cruz Foundation/Rio, Brazil, has systematically studied the immunomodulatory effect of *Cissampelos sympodialis* since 1997. *In vivo* and *in vitro* tests have been conducted to understand the mechanisms of action of AFL as well as the isolated alkaloid warifteine in experimental models of allergy and inflammation.

6.2 Toxicological study of *Cissampelos sympodialis*

Several parameters can be analyzed to demonstrate the toxic potential of a plant (extracts or compounds) such as loss of weight, death, anorexia, and change of behavior. Therefore toxicological studies showed that the use of AFL in acute treatment was considered nontoxic with no deaths among rats after administration at dose of 5 g/kg orally (po) or of 2 g/kg intraperitoneally (ip) (Diniz et al., 2004). However AFL chronic treatment caused an anorexic effect in female rats and behavioral changes (Almeida et al., 2005).

The alkaloids warifteine and milonine isolated from *C. sympodialis* showed cytotoxicity in fibroblast cell line (V79) derived from hamster and in hepatocytes of Wistar rats (Melo et al., 2003). Given the mixed results of acute and chronic treatments in rats, our research group began studying the effect of chronic oral treatment (more than 15 days) with AFL into inbred BALB/c mice. We observed that this treatment induced weight gain throughout the treatment, suggesting lack of toxicity in these experimental animals (Bezerra-Santos et al., 2004).

Structure	Compound name	References
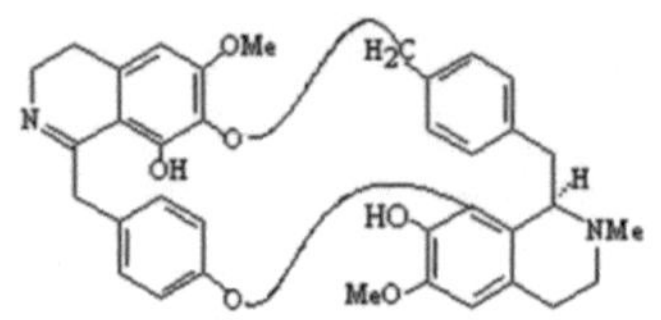	Warifteine	Barbosa et al., 1997
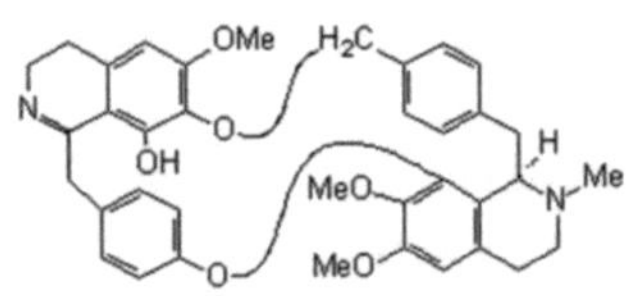	Methilwarifteine	Barbosa et al., 1997
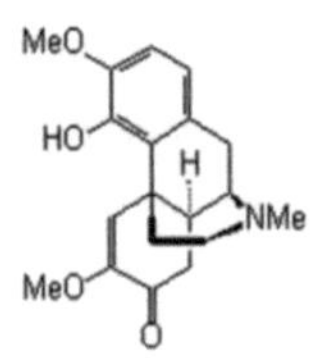	Milonine	Barbosa et al., 1997
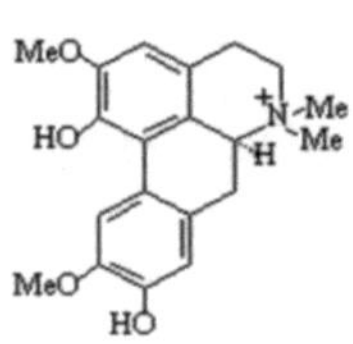	Laurifoline	Alencar, 1994
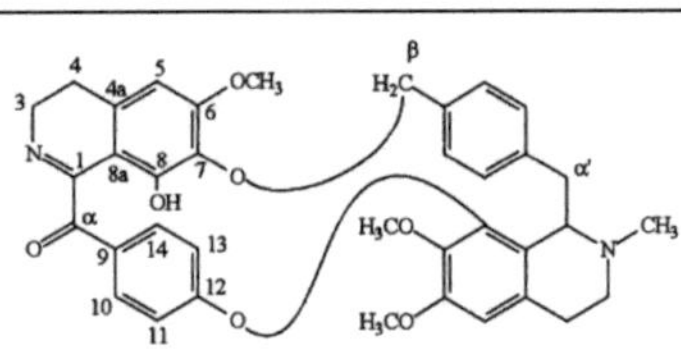	Roraimine	De Lira et al., 2002
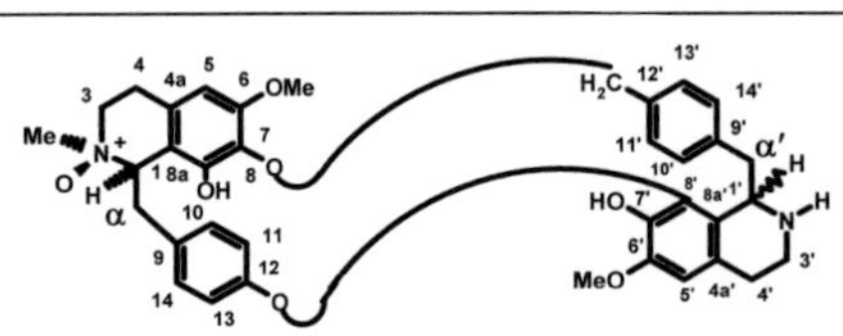	Simpodialine β-*N*-oxide	Alencar, 1994
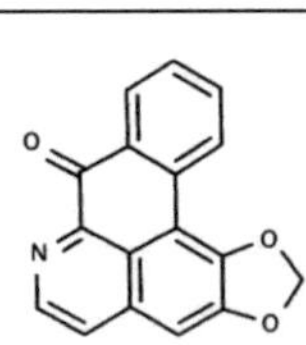	Liriodenine	De Lira et al., 2001

Table 1. Alkaloids of *Cissampelos sympodialis* Eichl.

6.3 Anti-inflammatory activity of *Cissampelos sympodialis*

The inflammatory process is a complex program of intracellular signal transduction and transcription events driven by multiple pro-inflammatory mediators and cytokines (Sherwood & Toliver-Kinsky, 2004). The acute inflammation is characterized by exudation of protein-rich fluid, edema, vasodilation and cell migration, primarily of neutrophils, into the site of injury (Sherwood & Toliver-Kinsky, 2004). Investigations on the anti-inflammatory activity of AFL were performed in experimental models of acute inflammation using phlogistic agents in Swiss mice or rats. Prophylactic treatments (before the phlogistic administration) demonstrated an AFL inhibitory effect on the ear edema formation induced by either TPA (12-O-tetradecanoyl phorbol-13-acetate) or capsaicin in Swiss mice (Batista-Lima et al., 2001). The experimental model of edema induced by TPA involves the activation of phospholipase A2 and production of prostaglandins and leukotrienes while the edema induced by capsaicin involves the release of substance P, histamine and eicosanoids such as serotonin and prostaglandins. These mediators are produced and released mainly by inflammatory cells such as mast cells, basophils, eosinophils and macrophages (Funk, 2001). Based on the anti-inflammatory effect of AFL, we inferred that the plant acts on the inflammatory cells by modulating the production of mediators. Corroborating this hypothesis was the observation that prophylactic treatment of experimental animals (rats) with AFL also showed inhibition of neutrophil migration into the intraperitoneal cavity induced by carrageenan (Batista-Lima et al., 2001). The migration of neutrophils into the peritoneal cavity of rats induced by carrageenan is dependent on the release of eicosanoids and chemotactic agents such as leukotriene B4 and/or IL-8, respectively, produced by mast cells and/or resident macrophages (Lefebvre et al., 2010, Nakagome & Nagata, 2011). Taken together the results support the hypothesis that AFL treatment is modulating cytokines as well as antiinflammatory mediator effects.

7. Immunomodulatory activity of *Cissampelos sympodialis*

7.1 Effect of *Cissampelos sympodialis* on IL-10 and NO production

Although eicosanoids and chemotactic agents produced by inflammatory cells are responsible for triggering the inflammatory process, these cells are also responsible for producing cytokines which control inflammation. IL-10 produced by mononuclear cells has been described as a potent regulatory molecule in the inflammatory process (Moore et al., 2001). Surprisingly, *in vitro* studies showed, for the first time, that the inhibitory effect of AFL on the proliferative response of BALB/c mice spleen cells stimulated with the mitogen concanavalin A was associated with the production of IL-4 and IL-10 by these cells (Piuvezam et al., 1999). Macrophages are cells that produce IL-10 and from this perspective, we investigated the effect of AFL on murine resident and elicited (sodium thioglycollate) macrophages. The experimental model used for this purpose was the infection of macrophages with trypomastigote form of *Trypanosoma cruzi*. The AFL treatment induced an increase in the release of trypomastigote forms by the cells with increase in IL-10 production. This phenomenon was shown in both types of macrophages (resident or elicited). The AFL was also able to increase the production of IL-10 even in the absence of the parasite. In addition, AFL inhibited the NO synthesis induced by interferon-gamma (IFN-γ) and lipopolysaccharide (Ding, et al., 1988; Alexandre-Moreira et al., 2003). Therefore these results confirm the effect of AFL in modulating the microbicidal activity of macrophages by increasing the IL-10 production as well as inhibition of NO synthesis.

7.2 Effect of *Cissampelos sympodialis* on the immunoglobulin production

B cells are responsible for the production of immunoglobulins (Ig) after antigen recognition and activation (Snapper & Paul, 1987; Wong & Koh, 2000). Asthma reaction is an immediate-type reaction mediated mainly by IgE (Busse & Lemanski, 2001; Mayr, et al., 2003). The release of mediators associated with the inflammatory cells to the reaction site induces the clinical symptoms of asthma (Maddox & Schwartz, 2002) such as bronchocontraction, mucus production and the strangling sensation (Funk, 2001). Based on the asthma symptoms and the fact that Brazilian folk medicine has systematically used *Cissampelos sympodialis* to prevent asthma symptoms, several studies have been conducted using the experimental model of asthma to demonstrate the AFL effect. The strain of inbred BALB/c mice is hypersensitive to ovalbumin (OVA) with the production of OVA-specific IgE, pulmonary hyperactivity and mucus production after sensitization and challenge with OVA. The chronic oral treatment (15 days before OVA sensitization) with AFL inhibited the total OVA-specific IgE production and increased the production of IFN-γ by spleen cells of these mice (Bezerra-Santos et al., 2004). Alexandre-Moreira and co-workers (2003) demonstrated that AFL inhibited activated B cell function through an increase in intracellular cAMP levels. Several studies have identified cAMP as an antagonist of B cell proliferation induced by mitogens (Cohen & Rothstein, 1989). Also it was demonstrated that cAMP is a second messenger that plays an important role in the regulation of B cell apoptosis (Myklebust et al., 1999). In general, an increase in cAMP levels is associated with anti-inflammatory and immunosuppressive effects (Cohen & Rothstein, 1989; Wong & Koh, 2000; Torgersen et al., 2002). Finally, the finding that AFL inhibited immunoglobulin secretion suggests a therapeutic use for the *Cissampelos sympodialis* extract in conditions associated with up regulation of B cell function and enhanced immunoglobulin secretion such as allergic diseases as well as autoimmune disease.

7.3 Activity of *Cissampelos sympodialis* in anaphylactic shock reaction

Anaphylaxis is a severe allergic reaction and is often fatal. It is mediated by IgE antibodies, mast cells and their mediators such as histamine. Medicines, insect bites and certain foods can trigger anaphylactic shock in genetically predisposed individuals (Teo et al., 2009; Dybendal et al., 2003). To have a better understanding of the effect of AFL treatment in allergic reactions, we evaluated the therapeutic potential of the acute treatment (five days before sensitization) in experimental model of anaphylactic shock using ovalbumin (OVA) challenge. The results demonstrated that AFL treatment was able to inhibit up to 70% death of OVA-sensitized mice after 1 hour of the OVA challenge. However, the same treatment was not able to inhibit the anaphylactic shock induced by compound 48/80. These data show that the effect of the extract is dependent on mechanisms involving IgE production (Bezerra-Santos et al., 2005).

7.4 Eosinophil lipid body inhibition by *Cissampelos sympodialis*

LBs are specialized organelles in the synthesis and storage of arachidonic acid derivatives such as prostaglandins and leukotrienes, and are present in the cytoplasm of various leukocytes and activated eosinophils (Bozza & Viola, 2010). A single treatment with AFL inhibited the formation of lipid bodies in eosinophils from mice sensitized and challenged with OVA. These results suggest that the extract is capable of modulating the synthesis of inflammatory mediators important in the chemotaxis of inflammatory cells to the lungs during asthma attacks, as well as contraction mediators that cause bronchospasm.

8. Warifteine, a bisbenzylisoquinoline alkaloid from *Cissampelos sympodialis*

Warifteine is a major bisbenzylisoquinolinic alkaloid found in AFR as well as AFL. The isolated compound is an amorphous yellow crystal and the chemical name is (R)-2,8,13,13a,14,15,16,25-Octahydro- 18,30- dimethoxy-14 -methyl -4,6:9,12:21,24 -trietheno-3H pyrido (3',2':14,15) (1,11) dioxacycloeicosino (2,3,4- ij) isoquinoline-5,19-diol with molecular weight of 592.68084 g/mol. Warifteine is insoluble in polar solvents but in acidic conditions becomes a water-soluble salt, allowing its *in vivo* and *in vitro* analysis without addition of other toxic solvents. Warifteine becomes an important compound marker for the extract standardization of the plant as well as a candidate for a phytomedicine (Cerqueira-Lima et al., 2010).

8.1 Warifteine inhibits the histamine release

Allergic reactions trigger organic changes according to body region affected as atopic dermatitis (skin), hay fever or rhinitis (upper respiratory tract), asthma (lower respiratory tract), food allergy (digestive tract), anaphylactic shock (systemic reaction) (Cavalher-Machado et al., 2004; Sicherer & Leung, 2011). All of these conditions are consequence of sensitized mast cell degranulation which releases several mediators (histamine, CisLT or prostaglandins) that cause smooth muscle contraction. Histamine is also of fundamental importance in triggering the allergic symptoms such as swelling (Baroody & Naclerio, 2000), itching (Davidson & Giesler, 2010), bronchospasm (Larsen, 2001) and anaphylactic shock (Valent et al., 2011). Warifteine effect in mast cell degranulation was then investigated. Initial findings came from *in vitro* assays which showed that warifteine was able to relax smooth muscle independently of endothelium, i.e., it did not only control the tone muscle in vessels but also relaxed the bronchioles muscles (Freitas et al., 1996). Warifteine then becomes an important tool in attempting to prevent or reverse the respiratory distress occurring during asthmatic attacks (Priel et al., 1994). To evaluate the alkaloid activity on mast cell degranulation we used several experimental models. At first OVA-sensitized mice were orally treated with warifteine then OVA-challenged in their paws. An inhibition of edema formation was observed (Costa et al., 2008). Passively IgE anti-DNP/BSA-sensitized-paw of rats were treated with warifteine and challenged with DNP/BSA and the results demonstrated that the treatment inhibited the hyperalgesia reaction, showing modulation among mast cells, vessels and nerves. Mimicking a local allergic reaction like a bee sting, the intra dermal administration of the secretagogue compound 48/80 in mice induces mast cell degranulation with histamine release and consequently induction of scratching behavior (Inagaki et al., 2002). We demonstrated that warifteine treatment inhibited the itching, indicating a direct effect in mast cell degranulation (Costa et al., 2008). Mast cells from dorsal subcutaneous tissue and peritonea from OVA sensitized rats were cultured with warifteine and after OVA challenge the histamine release was measured. The warifteine inhibited significantly the histamine release from tissue and peritoneal mast cells in a similar manner to sodium cromoglycate (CGS) (Costa et al., 2008). These data indicate that warifteine is inhibiting the mast cell degranulation and histamine release.

8.2 Warifteine inhibits the B cell functions

Several models have been employed for analyzing B cell response *in vitro*. Anti-IgM antibodies (Ab) have been used as a model for studying signals induced by binding to B cell surface Ig (Mond et al., 1995) and also T-independent type 2 antigens (TI-2), which activate B cells through a broad cross-linking of their Toll-like receptors (TLR) (Vos et al., 2000; Peng, 2005). Warifteine was then analyzed on B cells. It was observed that warifteine inhibited both B cell proliferation and Ig secretion induced by TLR ligands (LPS, Pam3Cys and CpG oligodeoxynucleotide) or anti-IgM Ab. These effects were not due to a toxicity since warifteine neither induced alteration in propidium iodide labeling of fresh spleen B cells or modified XTT metabolization by the B cell line A20. Also the inhibitory effect of B cell activated with TLR activators or anti-IgM Ab did not modify the total protein phosphorylation pattern, however it attenuated the rise in intracellular calcium levels, the phosphorylation of mitogen-activated protein kinase (MAPK) ERK and the intracellular levels of transcription factor NFκB. Warifteine also increased the cAMP level. *In vivo* study showed that pre-treatment with warifteine inhibited the anti-TNP-ficoll titles in BALB/c mice immunized with TI-2 antigen TNP-ficoll (Rocha et al., 2010). Taken together, the data showed that the alkaloid present in the AFL of *Cissampelos sympodialis* is one of the compounds responsible for the B cell modulatory effect.

8.3 Warifteine inhibits the eosinophil activity

A characteristic feature of asthma is a chronic inflammation with degeneration of bronchial epithelium in an eosinophil-dependent mechanism. Eosinophils release cationic proteins, chemotactic agents (eotaxin) and eicosanoids (*cis*-LT) (Ono et al., 2008). The treatments with warifteine or AFL inhibited eosinophil migration into the pleural and bronchoalveolar cavities of OVA sensitized BALB/c mice. Both warifteine and AFL were also capable of inhibiting the secretion of *cis*-LT and eotaxin, suggesting a role for AFL and its alkaloid in controlling the inflammatory process, thus corroborating the belief of an alternative treatment for diseases associated with eosinophil activity.

9. Cellular and molecular therapeutic targets for *Cissampelos sympodialis*

Studies performed for 15 years have contributed to the unraveling of part of the immunopharmacological mechanisms involved in *Cissampelos sympodialis* and warifteine effects. Figure 2 presents different cellular and molecular therapeutic targets for the plant extract and its alkaloid.

10. Relevance of the proposal for new herbal medicine

Some allergic diseases of major public health concerns are classified as immediate-type hypersensitivity, atopic dermatitis, food allergy, rhinitis, allergic asthma and anaphylactic shock. The incidence of allergic asthma is increasing at an alarming rate in developing countries like Brazil where around 35% of the population experience allergic diseases including asthma (Brazilian Association of Allergy and Immunopathology. 2007). Asthma is considered a public health problem. A significant variety of medicines such as bronchodilators and potent anti-inflammatory drugs that mitigate the crisis is used to treat asthma but with undesirable side effects. Our research group, with multidisciplinary profile, has been studying in a systematic way, the plant extracts of *Cissampelos sympodialis* and its components on

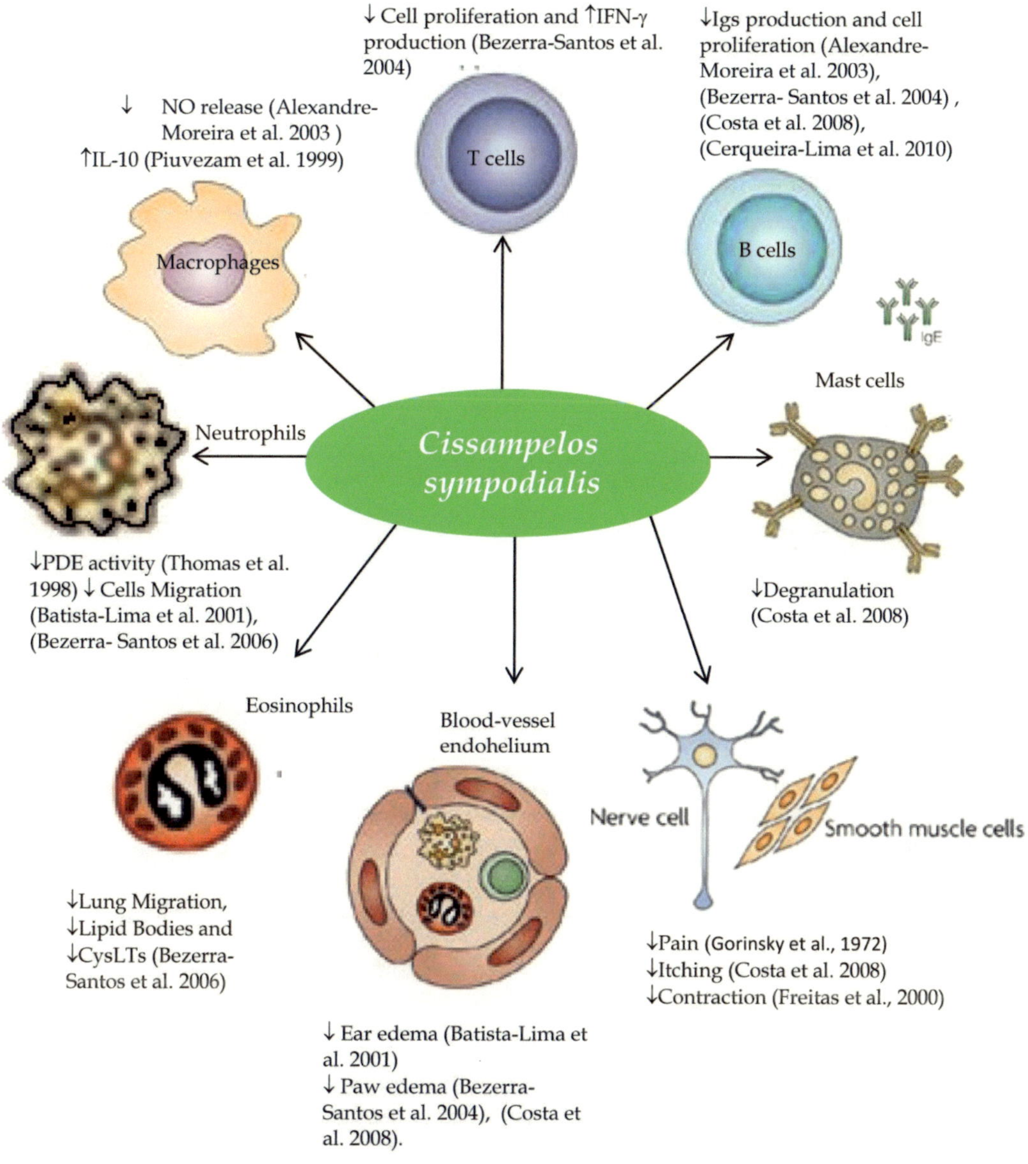

Fig. 2. Therapeutic targets for *Cissampelos sympodialis*. *In vitro* and *in vivo* studies showed that *C. sympodialis* induces IL-10 production by macrophages and IFN-γ production by splenocytes from OVA-sensitized mice. Oral treatment with AFL and warifteine inhibited OVA-specific IgE serum titer and mononuclear cell proliferation. Also both AFL as well as warifteine inhibited neutrophil and eosinophil migration and activation (PDE activity, leukotriene generation and lipid body formation) to the pleura and bronchoalveolar cavity induced by flogistic stimulus or allergens. Additionally, warifteine inhibited histamine delivery by mast cell and attenuated hyperalgesic reaction in rats.

experimental models of inflammation and allergy. The accumulated data showed that the extracts and its major alkaloid, warifteine, present potent anti-inflammatory effects, prolong the time of onset of anaphylactic shock reaction with reduction in allergen-specific IgE production, inhibit the inflammatory cell recruitment to the airways, relax airway smooth muscle in guinea pigs as well as modulate the production and release of inflammatory mediators such as histamine and cytokines. In addition, the great similarity in chemical structure among the alkaloids warifteine and milonine of *Cissampelos sympodialis* with drugs traditionally used in therapy: tubocurarine (potent muscle relaxant) and codeine (analgesic, antitussive and narcotic) respectively, (Figure 3), justified the popular use of the plant to treat respiratory diseases and the effort to produce an herbal medicine from this Brazilian plant.

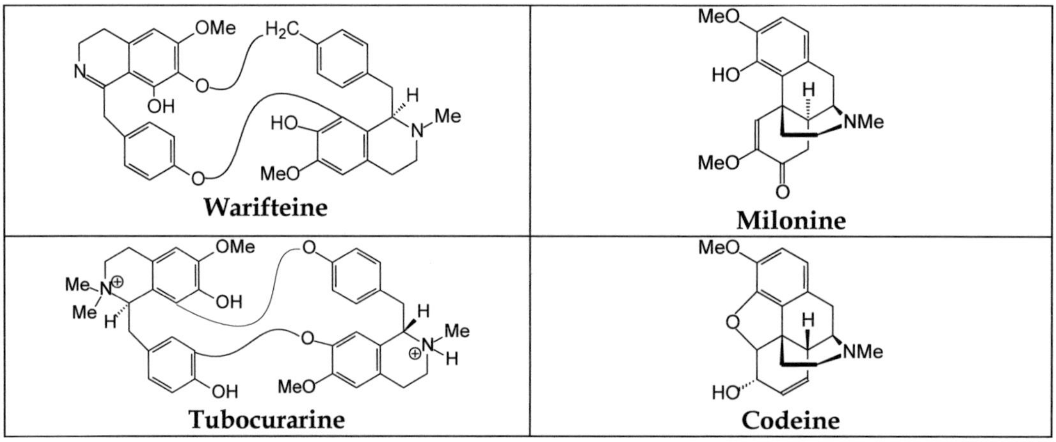

Fig. 3. Warifteine and tubocurarine are alkaloids that have the same chemical skeleton and belong to the class of bisbenzylisoquinoline. Milonine and codeine are alkaloids that have the same chemical skeleton and belong to the class of Morphinans.

11. Why *Cissampelos sympodialis* has potential as a herbal medicine?

1. *Cissampelos sympodialis* is used in folk medicine and by Indian tribes, in Northeast Brazil, for the treatment of disorders of airways such as asthma and rhinitis.
2. The preclinical data showed low or no toxicity on oral administration of the extract depending on the animal model used.
3. Studies of mechanisms of action of the extract have demonstrated efficacy in reduction of pathophysiological characteristics of allergic diseases associated with chronic inflammations such as asthma.
4. The leaf extract of the plant presents milonine, which is a morphinic alkaloid with a codeine-like chemical structure. Codeine is a classic drug with antitussive and analgesic properties.
5. Warifteine, one of the major alkaloids of the plant, presented similar effect of the extract in reducing asthma pathological profile.
6. Chemical structure of warifteine is similar to the tubocurarine chemical structure. Tubocurarine is a classic drug with muscle relaxant property.
7. Warifteine can be used as a molecular marker for the standardization of herbal medicine.

12. Acknowledgment

We thank Prof. Dr. José Maria Barbosa-Filho for the chemical expertise and for supplying the alkaloids for the immunomodulatory studies. The authors are indebted to the technical personnel of the UFPB/UFRJ/CNPq and FIOCRUZ foundation for the collaboration in the initial experiments.

13. References

Alexandre-Moreira, M.S.; Freire-De-Lima, C.G.; Trindade, M.N.; Castro-Faria-Neto, H.C.; Piuvezam, M.R. & Pecanha, L.M. (2003). *Cissampelos sympodialis* Eichl (Menispermaceae) leaf extract induces interleukin-10-dependent inhibition of Trypanosoma cruzi killing by macrophages. *Brazilian Journal of Medical and Biological Research* , VOL. 36, pp. 199-205, 0100-879X

Alencar, J. L. (1994). Isolamento e estudos das atividades relaxantes em musculatura lisa e esquelética de novos alcalóides de *Cissampelos sympodialis* Eichl.. Master's thesis (Graduate Program in Natural and Synthetic Bioactive Products) - Laboratório de Tecnologia Farmacêutica, Federal University of Paraiba, Brazil.

Almeida, R.N.; Melo-Diniz, M.F.; Medeiros, I.A.; Quintans-Junior, L.J.; Navarro, D.S.; Falcao, A.C.; Duarte, J.C. & Barbosa-Filho, J.M. (2005). Anorectic and behavioural effects of chronic *Cissampelos sympodialis* treatment in female and male rats. *Phytotherapy Research*, VOL. 19, pp. 121-124, 0951-418X

Almeida, R.N.; Navarro, D.S.; De Assis, T.S.; De Medeiros, I.A. & Thomas, G. (1998). Antidepressant effect of an ethanolic extract of the leaves of *Cissampelos sympodialis* in rats and mice. *Journal of ethnopharmacology*, VOL. 63, pp. 247-252, 0378-8741

Angelova-Fischer, I. & Tsankov, N. (2005) Successful treatment of severe atopic dermatitis with cysteinyl leukotriene receptor antagonist montelukast. *Acta Dermatovenerologica Alpina, Panonica et Adriatica,* VOL. 14, pp. 115-119, 1581-2979

Antunez, C.; Blanca-Lopez N.; Torres, M.J.; Mayorga, C.; Perez-Inestrosa, E.; Montañez, M.I.; Fernandez, T. & Blanca, M. (2006). Immediate allergic reactions to cephalosporins: Evaluation of cross-reactivity with a panel of penicillins and cephalosporins. *Journal of Allergy and Clinical Immunology*, Vol. 117, pp. 404-410, 0091-6749

Aragão, C.F.S.; Souza, F.S.; Barros, A.C.S.; Veras, J.W.E.; Barbosa-Filho, J.M. & Macedo, R.O. (2002). Aplicação da Termogravimetria (TG) no controle de qualidade da milona (*Cissampelos sympodialis* Eichl.) Menispermaceae. *Brazilian Journal of Pharmacognosy*, VOL. 12, pp. 60-61, 0102-695X

Barbosa-Filho, J.M.; Agra, M.F. & Thomas, G. Botanical, chemical and pharmacological investigation on *Cissampelos sympodialis* species from Paraíba (Brazil). (1997). *Ciência e Cultura*, VOL. 49, pp. 386-394, 0009-6725

Baroody, F.M. & Naclerio, R.M. (2000). Antiallergic effects of H1-receptor antagonists. *Allergy*, VOL. 55, pp.17-27, 0105-4538.

Barroso, G.M. (2004). *Sistemática de angiospermas do Brasil*, UFV, ISBN 85-7269-127-8, Minas Gerais, Brasil

Bateman, E. D.; Hurd S. S.; Barnes P. J.; Bousquet, J.; Drazen J. M.; Fitzgerald, M.; Gibson P. ; Ohta K.; O'byrne P.; Pedersen S. E.; Pizzichini E.; Sullivan, S. D.; Wenzel, S. E. & Zar, H. J. (2008). Global strategy for asthma management and prevention: GINA executive summary. *European Respiratory Journal* VOL. 31, pp. 143-178, 0903-

1936Batista-Lima, K.V.; Ribeiro, R.A.; Balestieri, F.M.P.; Thomas, G. & Piuvezam, M.R. (2001). Anti-inflammatory activity of *Cissampelos sympodialis* Eichl. (Menispermaceae) leaf extract. *Acta Farmaceutica Bonaerense,* VOL. 20, pp. 275-279, 0326-2383.

Berin, M.C. & Mayer, L. (2009). Immunophysiology of experimental food allergy. *Mucosal Immunology,* VOL. 2, pp. 24-32, 1933-0219

Bezerra, H.L. & Santos, G.I.V. Tracoma em pacientes com conjuntivite alérgica. (2010). *Arquivos Brasileiros de Oftalmologia,* VOL. 73, pp. 235-239, 0004-2749

Bezerra-Santos, C.R.; Balestieri, F.M.; Rossi-Bergmann, B.; Pecanha, L.M. & Piuvezam, M.R. (2004). *Cissampelos sympodialis* Eichl. (Menispermaceae): oral treatment decreases IgE levels and induces a Th1-skewed cytokine production in ovalbumin-sensitized mice. *Journal of Ethnopharmacology,* VOL. 95, pp. 191-197, 0378-8741

Bezerra-Santos, C.R.; Peçanha, L.M.T. & Piuvezam, M.R. (2005) *Cissampelos sympodialis* Eichl. (Menispermaceae) inhibits anaphylactic shock reaction in murine allergic model. *Brazilian Journal of Pharmacognosy,* VOL. 15, pp. 287-291, 0102-695X

Bezerra-Santos, C.R.; Vieira-De-Abreu, A.; Barbosa-Filho, J.M.; Piuvezam, M.R. & Bozza, P.T. (2006). Anti-Allergic properties of *Cissampelos sympodialis* and its isolated alkaloid warifteine. *International Immunopharmacology,* VOL. 6, pp. 1152-1160, 1567-5769.

Belvisi, M.G. (2004). Regulation of inflammatory cell function by corticosteroids. *Proceedings of the American Thoracic Society,* VOL. 1, pp. 207-214, 1546-3222

Brazilian Association of Allergy and Immunopathology (2007) General Information, 10/02/2007, Available from: http://www.sbai.org.br/duvidas. htm.

Brightling, C.E.; Symon, F.A.; Holgate, S.T.; Wardlaw, A.J.; Pavord, I.D. & Bradding, P. (2003). Interleukin-4 and -13 expression is co-localized to mast cells within the airway smooth muscle in asthma. *Clinical and Experimental Allergy* , VOL. 33, pp. 1711-1716, 0954-7894.

Bozza, P.T.; Bakker-Abreu, I.; Navarro-Xavier, R.A. & Bandeira-Melo, C. (2011). Lipid body function in eicosanoid synthesis: An update. *Prostaglandins, Leukotrienes and Essential Fatty Acids,* doi:10.1016/j.plefa.2011.04.020, 0952-3278

Bozza P. T., Magalhães K. G. & Weller, P. F. (2009). Leukocyte lipid bodies — Biogenesis and functions in inflammation. *Biochimica et Biophysica Acta.* VOL. 1791, pp. 540–551, 1388-1981

Bozza, P.T. & Viola, J.P.B. (2010). Lipid droplets in inflammation and cancer. *Prostaglandins, Leukotrienes and Essential Fatty Acids,* VOL. 82, pp. 243–250, 0952-3278

Bozza, P.T.; Yu, W.; Cassara, J. & Weller, P.F. (1998). Pathways for eosinophil lipid body induction: differing signal transduction in cells from normal and hypereosinophilic subjects. *Journal of Leukocyte Biology,* VOL. 64, pp.563-569, 0741-5400

Busse, W.W. & Lemanske, R.F.(2001). Asthma. *The New England Journal of Medicine,* VOL. 344, pp. 350-362, 0028-4793.Capobianco, F.; Butteroni, C.; Barletta, B.; Corinti, S.; Afferni, C.; Tinghino, R.; Boirivant, M. & Di Felice, G. (2008). Oral sensitization with shrimp tropomyosin induces in mice allergen-specific IgE, T cell response and systemic anaphylactic reactions. *International Immunology,* VOL. 20, pp. 1077-1086, 0953-8178

Castranova, V.; Kang, J.H.; Ma, J.K.; Mo, C.G.; Malanga, C.J.; Moore, M.D.; Schwegler-Berry, D. & Ma, J.Y. (1991). Effets of bisbenzylisoquinoline alkaloids on alveolar macrophages: Correlation between binding, affinity, inhibitory pontency, and antifibrotic potential. *Toxicology and Applied Pharmacology*, VOL. 108, pp. 242-252, 0041-008X

Cavalher-Machado, S.C.; De Lima, W.T.; Damazo, A.S.; De Frias Carvalho, V.; Martins, M.A.; Silva, P.M. & Sannomiya, P. (2004). Down-regulation of mast cell activation and airway reactivity in diabetic rats: role of insulin. *The European Respiratory Journal*, VOL. 24, pp. 552-558, 0903-1936

Cerqueira-Lima, A.T.; Alcântara-Neves, N.M.; de Carvalho, L.C.; Costa, R.S.; Barbosa-Filho, J.M.; Piuvezam, M.; Momtchilo, R.; Barboza, R.; de Jesus Oliveira, E.; Marinho, A. & Figueiredo, C.A. (2010). Effects of *Cissampelos sympodialis* Eichl. and its alkaloid, warifteine, in an experimental model of respiratory allergy to Blomia tropicalis. *Current Drug Targets*, VOL. 11, pp. 1458-1467, 1389-4501

Cohen, D.P. & Rothstein, T.L. (1989). Adenosine 3',5'-cyclic monophosphate modulates the mitogenic response of murine B lymphocytes. *Cellular Immunology*, VOL. 121,pp. 113-119, 0008-8749

Corrêa, M.P. (1984). *Dicionário de Plantas Úteis do Brasil e das Exóticas Cultivadas* (1). Instituto Brasileiro de Defesa Florestal, Rio de Janeiro, Brasil.

Costa H.F.; Bezerra-Santos, C.R.; Barbosa-Filho, J.M.; Martins, M.A. & Piuvezam M.R. (2008). Warifteine, a bisbenzylisoquinoline alkaloid, decreases immediate allergic and thermal hyperalgesic reactions in sensitized animals, *International Immunopharmacology* VOL.8, pp. 519-525, 1567-5769.

Cowden, J.M.; Riley, J.P.; Ma J.Y.; Thurmond R.L. & Dunford P.J. (2010). Histamine H4 receptor antagonism diminishes existing airway inflammation and dysfunction via modulation of Th2 cytokines. *Respiratory Research*, VOL. 11, pp. 1-12, 1465-9921

Davidson, S. & Giesler, G.J. (2010). The multiple pathways for itch and their interactions with pain. *Trends in Neurosciences*, VOL.33, pp.550-558, 0166-2236

De Assis, E.F.; Silva, A.R.; Caiado, L.F.; Marathe, G.K.; Zimmerman, G.A.; Prescott, S.M.; Mcintyre, T.M.; Bozza, P.T. & De Castro-Faria-Neto, H.C. (2003). Synergism between platelet-activating factor-like phospholipids and peroxisome proliferator-activated receptor gamma agonists generated during low density lipoprotein oxidation that induces lipid body formation in leukocytes. *The Journal of Immunology*, VOL. 171, pp.2090-2098, 0022-1767

De Lira, G.A.; De Andrade, L.M.; Florencio, K.C.; Da Silva, M.S.; Barbosa-Filho, J.M. & Leitao Da-Cunha, E.V. (2002). Roraimine: a bisbenzylisoquinoline alkaloid from *Cissampelos sympodialis* roots. *Fitoterapia*, VOL. 73, pp. 356-358, 0367-326X

Dybendal, T.; Guttormsen, A.B.; Elsayed, S.; Askeland, B.; Harboe, T. & Florvaag, E. (2003). Screening for mast cell tryptase and serum IgE antibodies in 18 patients with anaphylactic shock during general anaesthesia. *International Archives of Allergy and Immunology*, VOL. 47, pp. 1211-1218, 1018-2438

Ding, A.H.; Nathan, C.F. & Stuehr, D.J. (1988). Release of reactive nitrogen intermediates and reactive oxygen intermediates from mouse peritoneal macrophages. Comparison of activating cytokines and evidence for independent production. *The Journal of Immunology*, VOL. 141, pp. 2407-2412, 0022-1767

Diniz, M.F.F.M.; Melo, A.F.M.; Santos, H.B.; Silva, V.B. & Medeiros, I.A. (2004). Pre-clinical toxicological acute assays with the leaves of *Cissampelos sympodialis* Eichl in mice. *Revista Brasileira de Ciências da Saúde*, VOL. 8, pp. 135-142, 1415-2177

Freitas, M.R.; Cortes, S.F.; Thomas, G. & Barbosa Filho, J.M. (1996). Modification of Ca2+ metabolism in the rabbit aorta as a mechanism of spasmolytic action of warifteine, a bisbenzylisoquinoline alkaloid isolated from the leaves of *Cissampelos sympodialis* Eichl. (Menispermaceae). *The Journal of Pharmacy and Pharmacology*, VOL. 48, pp. 332-336, 0022-3573

Freitas, M.R.; Lemos, V.S.; Queiroga, C.E.; Thomas, G.; Medeiros, I.A. & Cortes, S.F. (2000). Mechanisms of the contractile effect of the hydroalcoholic extract of *Cissampelos sympodialis* Eichl. in the rat aorta. *Phytomedicine*, VOL. 7, pp. 63-67, 0944-7113.

Fonacier, L. S.; Dreskin S.C. & Leung D.Y.M. (2010). Allergic skin diseases. *Journal of Allergy and Clinical Immunology*, VOL. 125, pp.138-149, 1528-4050

Foster, B.; Foroughi, S.; Yin, Y.; Prussin, C. (2011). Effect of anti-IgE therapy on food allergen specific T cell responses in eosinophil associated gastrointestinal disorders. *Clinical and Molecular Allergy*. VOL. 9, pp.1-8.

Funk, C.D. Prostaglandins and Leukotrienes: Advances in Eicosanoid Biology. (2001). *Science,*VOL. 294, pp. 1871- 1875, 0036-8075

Gleich, G.J.; Adolphson C.R. & Leiferman, K.M. (1993). The biology of the eosinophilic leukocyte. *Annual Review of Medicine*, VOL.44, pp.85–101, 0066-4219

Gorinsky, C.; Luscombe, D.K. & Nicholls, P.J. (1972). Neuromuscular blocking and local anaesthetic activities of warifteine hydrochloride, an alkaloid isolated from Cissampelos ovalifolia D.C. *The journal of Pharmacy Pharmacology*. VOL. 24, pp.147-148, 0022-3573

Harizi, H.; Corcuff, J.B. & Gualde, N. (2008). Arachidonic-acid-derived eicosanoids: roles in biology and immunopathology. *Trends in Molecular Medicine* VOL. 14, pp. 461-469, 1471-4914

Inagaki, N.; Igeta, K.; Kim, J.F.; Nagao, M.; Shiraishi, N.; Nakamura, N. & Nagai, H. (2002). Involvement of unique mechanisms in the induction of scratching behavior in BALB/c mice by compound 48/80. *European Journal of Pharmacology*, VOL. 448, pp. 175– 183, 0014-2999

Jacoby, D.B.; Gleich, G.J. & Fryer, A.D. (1993). Human eosinophil major basic protein is an endogenous allosteric antagonist at the inhibitory muscarinic M2 receptor. The *Journal of Clinical Investigation*, VOL. 91, pp. 1314-1318, 0021-9738.

Jarjour N.N.; Wilson S.J., Koenig S.M.; Laviolette, M.; Moore W. C.; Davis, W.B.; Doherty, D.E.; Hamid, Q.; Israel, E.; Kavuru M.S.; Ramsdell, J.W.; Tashkin, D. P.; Reilly, D.S.; Yancey S.W.; Edwards, L.D.; Stauffer, J.L.; Dorinsky, P. M. & Djukanovic, R. (2006). Control of airway inflammation maintained at a lower steroid dose with 100/50 mg of fluticasone propionate/salmeterol. *Journal of Allergy and Clinical Immunology*, VOL. 118, pp. 44-52, 0091-6749.

Kambe, N.; Nakamura, Y.; Saito, M. & Nishikomori, R. (2010). The Inflammasome, an Innate Immunity Guardian, Participates in Skin Urticarial Reactions and Contact Hypersensitivity. *Allergology International*, VOL. 59, pp. 105-113, 1323-8930

Kanaoka, Y. & Boyce, J.A. Cysteinyl leukotrienes and their receptors: cellular distribution and function in immune and inflammatory responses. (2004). T*he Journal of Immunology*, VOL. 173, pp. 1503-1510, 0022-1767

Kupchan, S.M.; Patel, A.C. & Fujita, E. (1965). Tumor inhibitors. VI. Cissampareine, new cytotoxic alkaloid from *Cissampelos pareira*. Cytotoxicity of bisbenzylisoquinoline alkaloids. *Journal of Pharmaceutical Sciences*, VOL. 54, pp. 580-583, 0022-3549

Lampinen, M.; Carlson, M.; Hakansson, L.D. & Venge, P. (2004). Cytokine-regulated accumulation of eosinophils in inflammatory disease. *Allergy*, VOL. 59, pp. 793-805, 0105-4538.

Larsen, J.S. (2001). Do antihistamines have a role in asthma therapy? *Pharmacotherapy*, VOL. 21, pp. 28-33, 0277-0008

Lazaar, A.L. & Panettieri, R.A. (2004). Pathogenesis and treatment of asthma. Recent advances. *Drug Discovery Today: Disease Mechanisms*, VOL. 1, pp. 111-116, 1740-6765.

Lefebvre, J.S.; Marleau, S.; Milot, V.; Lévesque, T.; Picard, S.; Flamand, N. & Borgeat P. (2010). Toll-like receptor ligands induce polymorphonuclear leukocyte migration: key roles for leukotriene B4 and platelet-activating factor. *The FASEB Journal, VOL.* 24, pp. 637–647, 0892-6638

Maddox, L. & Schwartz, D.A. (2002). The pathophysiology of asthma. *Annual Review of Medicine*, VOL. 53, pp. 477-498, 0066-4219

Maurer, M. & Metz, M. (2005). The status quo and quo vadis of mast cells. *Experimental Dermatololgy*, VOL. 14, pp. 923-929, 0906-6705.

Mayr, S.I.; Zuberi, R.I. & Liu, F.T. (2003). Role of immunoglobulin E and mast cells in murine models of asthma. *Brazilian Journal of Medical and Biological Research*, VOL. 36, pp. 199-205, 0100-879X

Mahn, K.; Ojo, O.O.; Chadwick, G.; Aaronson, P.I.; Ward, J.P.T. & Lee, T.H. (2010). Ca2+ homeostasis and structural and functional remodelling of airway smooth muscle in asthma. *Thorax*, VOL. 65, pp. 547-552, 0040-6376

Melo, P.S.; De Medeiros Cavalcante, H.M.; Barbosa-Filho, J.M.; De Fatima Formiga Melo Diniz, M.; De Medeiros, I.A. & Haun, M. (2003). Warifteine and milonine, alkaloids isolated from *Cissampelos sympodialis* Eichl: cytotoxicity on rat hepatocyte culture and in V79 cells. *Toxicology Letters*, VOL. 142, pp. 143-151, 0378-4274.

Mesquita-Santos, F. P.; Vieira-De-Abreu, A.; Calheiros, A. S.; Figueiredo, I. H.; Castro-Faria-Neto, H. C.; Weller, P. F.; Bozza P. T.; Diaz, B. L. & Bandeira-Melo, C. (2006). Cutting edge: prostaglandin D2 enhances leukotriene C4 synthesis by eosinophils during allergic inflammation: synergistic in vivo role of endogenous eotaxin. *Journal of Immunology*, VOL. 176, pp. 1326-1330, 0022-1767

Mond, J.J.; Vos, Q.; Lees, A. & Snapper, C.M. (1995). T cell independent antigens. *Current Opinion in Immunology*, VOL. 3, pp. 349–354, 0952-7915.

Moneret-Vautrin, D. A.; Mertes, P. M. (2010). Anaphylaxis to general anesthetics. *Chemical Immunology and Allergy*. VOL. 95, pp. 180-189.

Moore, K. W.; De Waal R. M.; Coffman R. L. & O'garra, A. (2001). Interleukin-10 and the interleukin-10 receptor. *Annual Review of Immunology*. VOL. 19, pp.683-*765,* 0732-0582

Munitz, A.; Brandt, E. B.; Mingler, M.; Finkelman, F.D. & Rothenberg, M.E. (2008). Distinct roles for IL-13 and IL-4 via IL-13 receptor I and the type II IL-4 receptor in asthma pathogenesis. *Proceedings of the National Academy of Sciences of the United States of America*, VOL. 105, pp. 7240–7245, 0027-8424

Myklebust, J.H.; Josefsen, D.; Blomhoff, H.K.; Levy, K.; Finn, O.; Naderi, S.; Reed, J.C. & Smeland, E.B. (1999). Activation of cAMP signaling pathway increases apoptosis in human B precursor cells and is associated with down regulation of Mcl-1 expression. *Journal of Cellular Physiology*, VOL. 180, pp. 71-80, 1097-4652

Nakagome, K. & Nagata, M. (2011). Pathogenesis of airway inflammation in bronchial asthma. *Auris Nasus Larynx*, VOL. 38, pp. 555–563, 0385-8146

O'Byrne, P.M. Allergen-induced airway inflammation and its therapeutic intervention. (2009). *Allergy, asthma & immunology research,* VOL. 1, pp.3-9, 2092-7355

Onai, N.; Tsunokawa, Y.; Suda, M.; Watanabe, N.; Nakamura, K.; Sugimoto, Y. & Kobayashi, Y. (1995). Inhibitory effects of bisbenzylisoquinoline alkaloids on induction of proinflammatory cytokines, interleukin-1 and tumor necrosis factor-alpha. *Planta Medica*, VOL. 61, pp. 497-501, 0032-0943.

Ono, E.; Taniguchi M.; Mita H.; Higashi N.; Fukutomi Y.; Tanimoto H.; Sekiya K.; Oshikata C.; Tsuburai, T.; Tsurikisawa, N.; Otomo M.; Maeda, Y.; Matsuno O.; Miyazaki E.; Kumamoto, T. & Akiyama, K. (2008). Increased urinary leukotriene E4 concentration in patients with eosinophilic pneumonia. *European Respiratory Journal*, VOL. 32, pp. 437–442, 0903-1936

Peng, S.L. Signaling in B cells via Toll-like receptors. (2005). *Current Opinion in Immunology* VOL. 17, pp. 230–236, 0952-7915

Piuvezam, M.R.; Pecanha, L.M.; Alexander, J. & Thomas, G. (1999). *Cissampelos sympodialis* Eichl. leaf extract increases the production of IL-10 by concanavalin-A-treated BALB/c spleen cells. *Journal of Ethnopharmacology*, VOL. 67, pp. 93-101, 0378-8741

Priel, B.; Heimer, D.; Rabinowitz, B. & Hendler, N. (1994). Perceptions of asthma severity: the role of negative affectivity. *The Journal of Asthma*, VOL. 31, pp. 479-484, 0277-0903

Pumphrey, R. Anaphylaxis: can we tell who is at risk of a fatal reaction? (2004). *Current Opinion in Allergy and Clinical Immunology*, VOL. 4, pp.285-290, 1528-4050

Rhodes, D.G. (1975). A revision of the genus Cissampelos. *Phytologia*, VOL. 30, pp. 415-485, 0031-9430.

Rocha, J.D.B.; Decoté-Ricardo, D.; Redner, P.; Lopes, U.G.; Barbosa-Filho J.M.; Piuvezam, M.R.; Arruda- Hinds, L. & Peçanha, L.M.T. (2010). Effect of the alkaloid warifteine purified from *Cissampelos sympodialis* on B lymphocyte function *in vitro. Planta Medica,* VOL. 76 (4), pp.325-330.

Rothenberg, M.E. (1998). Eosinophilia. *The New England journal of medicine*, VOL. 338, pp. 1592-1600, 0028-4793.

Rothenberg, M.E. & Hogan, S.P. (2006). The Eosinophil. *Annual Review of Immunology*, VOL. 24, pp.147-74. 0732-0582.

Sausenthaler. S.; Heinrich, J. & Koletzko, S. (2011). Early diet and the risk of allergy: what can we learn from the prospective birth cohort studies GINIplus and LISAplus? *The American Journal of Clinical Nutrition. ajcn.001180; First published online May 4, 2011.*

Seidel, S.; Voller, B.; Geusau, A. & Wöhrl, S. (2010). Severe anaphylaxis to hymenoptera stings: does the basal serum tryptase concentration really matter? *Annals of Allergy, Asthma and Immunology*. VOL. 105, pp. 185-187.

Schnyder-Candrian, S.; Togbe, D.; Couillin, I.; Mercier, Isabelle.; Brombacher, F.; Quesniaux, V.; Fossiez, F. ; Ryff, B. & Schnyder, B. (2006). Interleukin-17 is a negative regulator of established allergic asthma. The *Journal of Experimental Medicine*, VOL. 203, pp. 2715-2725, 0022-1007.

Sherwood, E. R. & Toliver-Kinsky, T. Mechanisms of the inflammatory response. (2004). *Best Practice & Research Clinical Anaesthesiology*, VOL.18, pp. 385–405, 1521-6896

Sicherer, S.H. Epidemiology of food allergy. (2011). *Journal of Allergy and Clinical Immunology*, VOL. 127, pp.594-602, 1528-4050

Sicherer, S.H. & Leung, D.Y. (2004). Advances in allergic skin disease, anaphylaxis, and hypersensitivity reactions to foods, drugs, and insect stings. *Journal of Allergy and Clinical Immunology*, VOL. 114, pp. 118-124, 0091-6749.

Sicherer, S.H. & Leung, D.Y. (2011). Advances in allergic skin disease, anaphylaxis, and hypersensitivity reactions to foods, drugs, and insects in 2010. *Journal of Allergy and Clinical Immunology*, VOL. 137, pp. 326-335, 0091-6749.

Snapper, C.M. & Paul, W.E. (1987). B cell stimulatory factor-1 (interleukin-4) prepares resting murine B cells to secrete IgG1 upon subsequent stimulation with bacterial lipopolysaccharide. *The Journal of Immunology*, VOL. 139, pp. 10-17, 0022-1767

Somlyo, A.P. & Somlyo, A.V. (1994). Smooth muscle: excitation-contraction coupling, contractile regulation, and the cross-bridge cycle. *Alcoholism: clinical and experimental research*, VOL. 18, pp. 138-143, 0145-6008

Sur, R.N. & Pradhan, S.N. (1964). Studies on Cissampelos Alkaloids. I. Action of Hayatin Derivatives on the Central Nervous System of Cats and Dogs. *Archives Internationales de Pharmacodynamie et de Therapie* , VOL. 152, pp. 106-114, 0003-9780

Takatsu K. & Nakajima H. IL-5 and eosinophilia. (2008). *Current Opinion in Immunology*, VOL.20, pp.288–294, 0952-7915

Teixeira, L.K.; Fonseca, B.P.; Barboza, B.A. & Viola, J.P. (2005). The role of interferon-gamma on immune and allergic responses. *Memórias do Instituto Oswaldo Cruz*, VOL. 100, pp. 137-144, 0074-0276

Terashima, T.; Amakawa, K.; Matsumaru, A.; Yamaguchi, K. (2002). Correlation between cysteinyl leukotriene release from leukocytes and clinical response to a leukotriene inhibitor. *Chest*, VOL. 122, pp. 1566-1570, 0012-3692

Teo, S–L.; Gerez, I.F.A. & Ang, E.Y. (2009) Food-dependent Exercise-induced Anaphylaxis – A Review of 5 Cases. *Annals of the Academy of Medicine, Singapore.* VOL. 38, pp. 905-909, ISSN

Thomas, G.; Araújo, C.C.; Duarte, J.C.; De Souza, D.P. (1997a). Bronchodilator activity of an aqueous fraction of an ethanol extract of the leaves of *Cissampelos sympodialis* Eichl. (Menispermaceae) in the guinea pig. *Phytomedicine*, VOL. 4, pp. 233-238, 0944-7113.

Thomas, G.; Araújo, C.C.; Agra, M.F. & Diniz, M.F.F. (1995). Preliminary studies on the hydroalcoholic extract of the root of *Cissampelos sympodialis* Eichl in guinea-pig tracheal strips and bronchoalveolar leukocytes. *Phytotherapy Research*, VOL. 9, pp. 473-477, 0951-418X.

Thomas, G.; Burnes, F.; Pyne, S. & Pyne, N.J. (1997b). Characterization of the extract from the leaves of *Cissampelos sympodialis* Eichl. (Menispermaceae) on spontaneous tone of isolated trachea, cyclic nucleotide phosphodiesterase activity and intracellular cAMP. Phytotherapy research, VOL. 11, pp. 496-499, 0951-418X.

Thomas, G.; Selak, M. & Henson, P.M. (1999). Effects of the aqueous fraction of the ethanol extract of the leaves of *Cissampelos sympodialis* Eichl. in human neutrophils. Phytotherapy research, VOL. 13, pp. 9-13, 0951-418X.

Torgersen, K.M.; Vang, T.; Abrahamsen, H.; Yaqub, S. & Tasken, K. (2002). Molecular mechanisms for protein kinase-A mediated modulation of immune function. *Cellular Signalling*, VOL. 14, pp. 1-9, 0898-6568

Vos, Q.; Lees, A.;Wu, Z.Q.; Snapper, C.M. & Mond, J.J. (2000) B cell activation by T cell independent type 2 antigen as an integral part of the humoral immune response to pathogenmicroorganisms. *Immunological Reviews*; VOL. 176, pp. 154–170, 0105-2896

Valent, P.; Horny, H.P.; Triggiani, M. & Arock. M. (2011). Clinical and Laboratory Parameters of Mast Cell Activation as Basis for the Formulation of Diagnostic Criteria. *International Archives of Allergy and Immunology* VOL. 156, pp. 119–127, 1018-2438

Vieira-De-Abreu, A.; Assis, E.F.; Gomes, G.S.; Castro-Faria-Neto, H.C.; Weller, P.F.; Bandeira-Melo, C. & Bozza, P.T. Allergic challenge-elicited lipid bodies compartmentalize in vivo leukotriene C4 synthesis within eosinophils. (2005). *American Journal of Respiratory Cell and Molecular Biology*, VOL. 33, pp. 254-261, 1044-1549

Weller, P.F. Human eosinophils. (1997). *Journal of Allergy and Clinical Immunology*, VOL. 100, pp.283–287, 0091-6749.

Wong, W.S.F. & Koh, D.S.K. (2000). Advances in immunopharmacology of asthma. *Biochemical Pharmacology*, VOL. 59, pp. 1323-1355, 0006-2952

25

Derived Products of Helminth in the Treatment of Inflammation, Allergic Reactions and Anaphylaxis

C.A. Araujo[1] and M.F. Macedo-Soares[2]
[1]*Department of Immunology, St Jude Children's Research Hospital, Memphis, TN,*
[2]*Laboratory of Immunopathology, Butantan Institute, Sao Paulo, SP,*
[1]*USA*
[2]*Brazil*

1. Introduction

Anaphylaxis is a life-threatening and systemic disorder that involves several organs and may lead to death. It is believed to be mostly triggered by release of mediators from activated mast cells, basophils and macrophages after allergen exposure. There are two major types of anaphylactic mechanisms: classical and alternative anaphylactic pathways. Classical anaphylactic pathway is triggered by cross-linking of IgE bound to FcεRI, high affinity IgE receptors, on mast cell and basophil surfaces to release pre-formed vasoactive amines (e.g. histamine), lipid mediators and neutral proteases from secretory granules upon allergen exposure. The alternative anaphylactic pathway is an IgE-independent mechanism and involves basophils and macrophages. Upon allergen exposure, IgG-immune complexes binds to FcγRIII, low affinity activating IgG receptor, and subsequent release PAF (platelet activating factor), but not histamine as major mediator. The understanding of immune mechanisms on triggering anaphylaxis is crucial for understanding how to manipulate the immune system to find better therapeutic interventions.

Helminth infection and their products have been demonstrated as potential therapeutic interventions in inflammatory disorders. Helminths use several imunomodulatory strategies to evade and/or modify the host immune response in order to survive in the host, including suppression or inactivation of host antigen-specific immune response. The modulation of the immune system has been considered beneficial for both host and parasites since it could avoid helminth eradication and protect the host from inflammatory responses which may damage host's tissues and organs. Several helminth immunomodulatory molecules and strategies have been identified and reported, such as eotaxin metalloproteinase, calreticulin, antioxidants and neutrophil inhibitory factor. They interfere with antigen processing and presentation, cell proliferation, cause T cell death, decrease IgE responses, reduce B cell activation and stimulate regulatory T cells. Therefore, these immunomodulatory factors can affect both the inductive and effector immune response, being suitable to modulate the inflammatory, allergic and anaphylactic responses.

Our studies have been focused in the immunossuppressive responses induced by roundworms *Ascaris suum* infection and a protein secreted by these worms named PAS-1 (protein from *Ascaris suum*). We have demonstrated that PAS-1 suppresses LPS-induced inflammation due to stimulating the secretion of IL-10 and TGF-β. Furthermore, PAS-1 was demonstrated suppressing B and T cell responses against OVA. Besides playing a down-modulatory effect in inflammatory responses induced by unrelated antigens, PAS-1 suppresses the acute and chronic lung allergic inflammation induced by APAS-3 (allergenic protein from *Ascaris suum)*. In OVA/alum lung inflammation model, PAS-1 down-modulates the lung inflammatory response due CD4+CD25+FoxP3+ cells and CD8+γδTCR+ cells, which secretes IL-10/TGF-β and IFN-γ, respectively. In chronic lung inflammation model using OVA/alum or alum/APAS-3, besides inhibiting the inflammation into the lungs, PAS-1 also inhibits the airway remodeling by decreasing the activity of metaloproteinases and the production of angiogenic factors (IL-13 and VEGF). Taken together, these findings demonstrated that PAS-1 inhibits both acute and chronic lung inflammation in mouse models.

The understanding of immune modulatory mechanisms that control anaphylactic responses is critical to investigate therapeutic interventions for anaphylactic inflammatory disorders. The purpose of this chapter is to discuss the mechanisms triggered by allergic and anaphylactic reactions and potential therapeutic strategies using helminth products.

2. Immune responses triggered by anaphylactic reactions

2.1 Concept of anaphylaxis

Anaphylaxis is a systemic and immediate hypersensitivity with multi-organ system involvement that can progress potentially to a life-threatening reaction causing thousands deaths in the world. The term anaphylaxis was named by Dr Charles Robert Richet, a Nobel laureate in Physiology or Medicine in 1913. In 1902, Richet and his colleague Paul Portier reported that dogs immunized with non-lethal dose of sea anemone venom display fatal reactions to the second injection of the venom even in small doses. Shibasaburo Kitasato and Emil von Behring had previously demonstrated that animals immunized with bacterial toxins are able to produce anti-toxins (neutralizing antibodies). Since then, this phenomenon was named **anaphylaxis,** which term is derived from the Greek words "a-" (against) and "-phylaxis" (protection).

Anaphylaxis can occur following exposure to several allergen sources including food allergens, aeroallergens, venoms, drugs and vaccination. The most common symptoms include itching, erythema and urticaria after the exposure to allergens. The most severe cases of anaphylaxis involve cardiovascular and respiratory system with drop of cardiac pressure, bronchoconstriction, laryngeal edema and shock (Brown, 2004). The gastrointestinal system may be also involved featuring vomiting, abdominal pain and diarrhea. The central nervous system can be affected leading to a felling of impending doom and lack of consciousness related to hypotension and hypoxia. Once the anaphylactic reactions occur rapidly, an effective treatment (usually epinephrine injection) may avoid the occurrence of severe symptoms (Simons et al., 2003). Thus, it is crucial to understand the molecular mechanisms involved on anaphylactic reactions for strategically managing the risk and preventing recurrence.

2.2 Types of anaphylactic reactions

Anaphylaxis occurs due to release of vasoactive and inflammatory mediators from mast cells, basophils and macrophages upon allergen exposure. When antigens cross-link FcεRI-bound IgE or bind to IgGs, which are found as IgG-immune complexes attached to FcγRs, mainly FcγRIII, a signaling cascade is trigger to promote release of mediators which cause smooth muscle contraction and increase vascular permeability, leading to laryngeal edema (which may cause respiratory difficulty), hypotension, urticaria, abdominal muscular contraction, diarrhea (Ewan, 1998). It is reported that anaphylactic reactions in rodent models are induced by two different pathways: classical and alternative anaphylactic pathways (Figure 1).

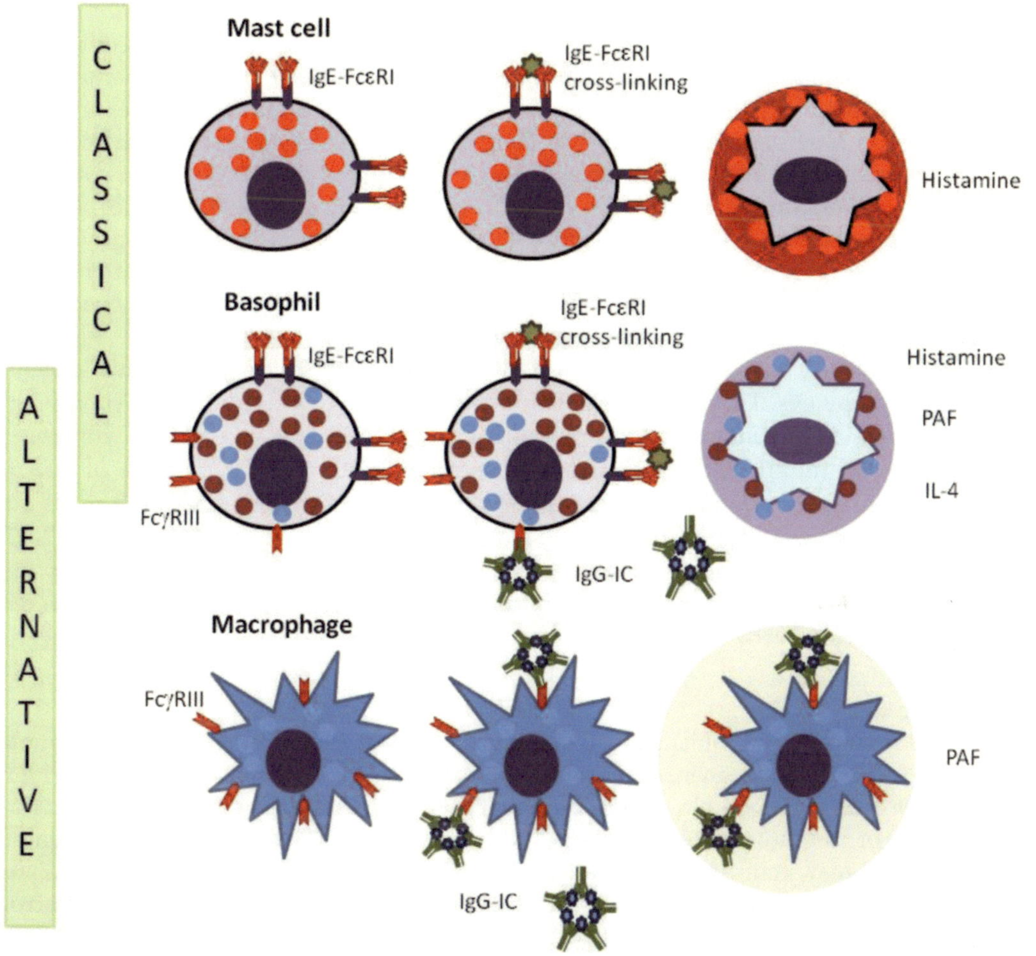

Fig. 1. Classical and alternative anaphylactic pathways. In the classical anaphylactic pathway, cross-linking among IgE-bound FcεRI and specific antigen leads to mast cell and basophil degranulation and secretion of histamine as major mediator. In the alternative anaphylactic pathway, IgG-immune complexes bind to FcγRIII on basophil and macrophage surfaces, triggering the secretion of PAF as major mediator. Basophils also secrete IL-4 that is crucial for IgE class-switching.

Classical anaphylactic pathway is triggered by cross-linking of antigen and antigen-specific IgE bound to FcεRI on mast cell and basophil surfaces, which stimulates these cells to degranulate and release histamine, serotonin, lipid mediators (such as leukotrienes) and cytokines (such as IL-4, TNFα, IL-1, VEGF) (Kumar & Sharma, 2010). Strait et al. (2003) have demonstrated that IgE-mediated anaphylaxis depends on IL-4/IL-4Rα, mast cells, FcεRI, IgE, histamine and H1 receptor but does not depend on macrophages, serotonin and leukotrienes. Alternative anaphylactic pathway is triggered by IgG-immune complexes bound to FcγRIII on basophils and macrophages, causing release of PAF (Mukai et al., 2009).

2.3 Cells involved in anaphylactic reactions

2.3.1 Mast cells

Mast cells were identified by Paul Ehrlich in 1879 (reviewed in Beaven, 2009) as cells present in connective tissues that reacts metachromatically with aniline dyes. He named them *Mastzellen* due the presence of granules that he believed to have a nutritional role on this cell type (the word *mast* denotes fattening in German). Mast cells are generated from bone marrow immature cells that migrate to skin and intestine and differentiate into connective tissue mast cells and mucosal mast cells, respectively (Arinobu et al., 2005; Galli et al., 2005). Stem cell factor (SCF or c-kit ligand) and c-kit play an important role in the growth and differentiation of mast cells, which express c-kit constitutively at all stages of differentiaton (Hu et al., 2007). They serve as important effector cells of the innate immune system along with other cell types (i.e. macrophages, dendritic cells, neutrophils, NK cells).

In anaphylactic reactions, mast cells are the effector cells in triggering the classical anaphylactic pathways. They express constitutively FcεRI, high affinity IgE receptor, which are usually bound to monomeric IgE upon antigen exposure. This receptor-IgE complex is cross-linked with multivalent antigens that consequently stimulate the release of effector mediators such as histamine, lipid mediators, and cytokines, which are pre-formed and stored in secretory granules of mast cells (Kumar & Sharma, 2010; Kemp & Lockey, 2002). These mediators act on many cellular types, including vascular endothelial cells and bronchial smooth muscle, inducing anaphylactic manifestations such as hypotension and dyspnea (Winbery & Lieberman, 2002).

2.3.2 Basophils

Similarly to mast cells, basophils were identified as cells that present metachromatic granules in the cytoplasm. Unlike human, mouse basophils are exceptionally rare (Urbina et al., 1981). They are the least common circulating cells that comprise less than 1% of total circulating granulocytes and are not normally present in tissues although are recruited to inflammatory sites. Basophils may contribute to IgE-mediated allergic inflammation and IgG1-mediated systemic anaphylaxis (Mukai et al., 2005; Tsujimura et al, 2008). They arise from bone marrow progenitors and complete their terminal differentiation in bone marrow (Arinobu et al., 2005).

Basophils constitutively express FcεRI, high affinity IgE receptor, and upon cross-linking of FcεRI-bound IgE with specific antigen, they release effector mediators such as histamine, leucotrienes, PAF and Th2 cytokines (IL-4, IL-5, IL-13) and TSLP (thymic stromal lymphopoietin) in response to protease allergens, causing immediate type hypersensitivity (Min, 2008). Mukai et al. (2009) have reported basophils as one of the major players in the IgG- but not IgE-mediated systemic anaphylaxis although basophils may function as initiator of allergic inflammation. Experiments from Tsujimura et al. (2008) demonstrated that mice passively transferred with anti-PenicillinV (PenV) monoclonal IgG1 antibody and challenged with PenV-conjugated BSA as allergen presented high drop of body temperature in both mast cell sufficient or deficient mice. They found that mainly basophils captured IgG1-immune complexes (they possessed highest amount of allergen per cell in comparison with other cell types), the binding was greatly inhibited by treatment with anti-FcγRIIb/FcγRIII antibody (against low affinity FcγRs), and they secrete high amount of PAF when stimulated by IgG1-immune complexes, indicating basophils as a good candidate to trigger IgG1-mediated anaphylatic reactions.

Besides their function as effector cells in IgG1-mediated anaphylaxis, basophils play a crucial role as early secretor of IL-4 that is essential to the development of anaphylactic reactions due to promoting class-switching to IgE. Sokol et al. (2008) have demonstrated that basophils are crucial for the initiation of Th2 cells in response to papain, a cystein protease, which activity is commonly found in most allergenic proteins. In addition, other findings reported that naïve CD4+ T cells stimulated with peptide-pulsed DCs could develop into Th2 cells when co-cultured with basophils from wild type mice but not IL-4-deficient mice (Oh et al, 2007), enforcing the role of basophils as early source of IL-4 in the immune responses.

2.3.3 Macrophages

Macrophages are long lived cells that function as a first line of defense in the body. These cells serve as early detector of invading pathogens through PAMPs, as antigen-presenting cells which initiate the immune responses, as effector cytotoxic cells to kill directly pathogens and also they play a role as regulatory and suppressor cells in parasitic infections and tumor-bearing hosts (Gordon, 2003). They arise from monocytes which are released in the blood stream and migrate to tissues to differentiate in macrophages or dendritic cells according to the stem cell factors milieu (Geissmann et al., 2010).

Macrophages have been involved in the development of IgG-dependent anaphylactic pathway (Oettgen et al., 1994; Miyajima et al., 1997; Strait et al., 2002). Passive immunization with allergen-specific monoclonal IgG1 antibody induce systemic anaphylaxis upon allergen exposure but this effect can be neutralized by treatment with anti-FcγRIIb/FcγRIII monoclonal antibodies (against low affinity FcγRs) and after depletion of macrophages with gadolinium (Strait et al, 2002), indicating the participation of macrophages in triggering IgG1-mediated anaphylactic reactions. Although platelets and neutrophils have been implicated in IgG-dependent anaphylaxis (Pinckard et al., 1977; Kimura et al., 1997), Strait et al. (2002) found in their studies that the techniques used for platelets and neutrophil depletion may inhibit IgE-independent anaphylaxis by producing immune complexes that desensitize macrophages, mimicking these cells as contributors of FcγRIII-dependent anaphylaxis.

Macrophages along with basophils also contribute to IgG-mediated anaphylaxis by releasing PAF upon antigen exposure. It has been demonstrated that the injection of anti-FcγRIIb/FcγRIII stimulates macrophages to release PAF by cross-linking FcγRIII on these cells and also inhibits IgG-dependent anaphylactic responses to antigen by blocking IgG-immune complex activation of macrophages through FcγRIII (Ujike et al., 1999; Strait et al., 2002).

2.4 Mediators involved in classical and alternative anaphylactic reactions

2.4.1 IgE and FcεRI

Ishizaka & Ishizaka (1976) discovered a new class of antibodies capable of transferring sensitivity to allergens. IgE antibodies are considered major players in allergic disorders such as anaphylaxis, asthma, atopic dermatitis, food allergy (Oettgen & Geha, 1999). It is considered the only antibody involved in classical anaphylactic reactions. It is also associated with protective immunity to parasitic infections (Capron et al., 1982). IgE consists of two identical heavy chains and two light chains with variable (V) and constant (C) regions and no hinge region which makes IgE to be less flexible. The ε-heavy chains contain one variable heavy chain and four constant region domains (Cε1-4) (Williams & Barclay, 1988) and are highly glycosylated (Arnold et al., 2007). IgE is the less abundant antibody class in serum with normal concentration of 50-200 ng/mL in nonallergic individuals (Gould et al., 2003). Even during helminth infections or allergic reactions, human serum IgE levels are lower than serum IgG levels; IgG peaks at around 30 μg/mL whereas IgG4 peaks at around 680 μg/mL (Bell, 1996). IgE has the shortest half-life of all immunoglobulins. Its half-life is about 3 days in serum (Iio et al., 1987), 16 hours on cells in suspension (Ishizaka & Ishizaka, 1971) and 2 weeks in tissues when is receptor-bound on cell surfaces (Geha et al., 1985). Its production requires class-switching from IgM, often via IgG to IgE by somatic recombination of germline genes in B cells", which depends on Th2 cytokines (IL-4/IL-13) and CD40 ligation (Poulsen & Hummelshoj, 2007).

It has been identified three IgE receptors in human (FcεRI(αβγ2 and αγ2), galectin-3 and FcεRII) and four receptors in mice (FcεRI(αβγ2 and αγ2), galectin-3, FcεRII and FcεRIV). Most of IgE bind to high affinity IgE receptor (FcεRI) that is present in mast cells, basophils (Gould et al., 2003) and antigen-presenting cells e.g. Langerhans cells (Bieber et al., 1992). FcεRI has a central role in mediating the allergic disorders (Kinet, 1999). Cross-linking of FcεRI associated to IgE with specific antigens induces the release of preformed mediators, newly formed lipid mediators and de novo synthesis of cytokines that potentially mediate anaphylactic reactions or prolonged allergic inflammation. FcεRI shares a common oligomeric structure, comprising a ligand binding immunoglobulin-like α-subunit associated to a β-subunit and two γ-subunits (Daeron, 1997). It binds stably monomeric IgE on mast cell surface (Kd ~ 10^{-10} M). The extracellular domain of α-subunit is glycosilated which seem to be crucial to appropriate maturation during FcεRI traffic through endoplasmic reticulum (Fiebiger et al., 2005) although is not required for monomeric IgE binding (Garman et al., 1999). The β- and γ-subunits bear ITAM (immunoreceptor tyrosine-based activation motif) that is phosphorylated in tyrosine residues by Lyn after cross-linking of FcεRI (Honda et al., 2000). The β-subunit possesses four transmembrane domains and the C-terminal domain has an ITAM motif. The γ-subunit belongs to T cell receptor (TCR) (gene family and is associated to Fc receptors including FcγRI, FcγRIIA, FcαRI (Takai, 2005). Other variant of FcεRI is constituted only by three chains (one α-subunit and two γ-subunits) that are expressed in monocytes, macrophages and neutrophils (Gould & Sutton, 2008). The low affinity IgE receptor (FcεRII) or CD23 is expressed in several cell types including B cells, activated T cells, monocytes, eosinophils, platelets, follicular dendritic cells, and thymic epithelial cells. CD23 facilitates the antigen presentation to T cells upon binding to IgE-antigen complex and also plays a role as negative regulator of IgE production (Gould & Sutton, 2008). Another IgE receptor is galectin-3 or ε-binding protein, which has been reported to be involved in neutrophil activation (Truong et al., 1993). In mice, it has been found a fourth type of IgE receptor, FcγRIV, which binds IgE-immune complexes on macrophage surface, inducing lung inflammation (Mancardi et al., 2008).

2.4.2 IgG and FcγRIII

IgG antibodies were identified by Tiselius and Kabat in 1939. They immunized rabbits with ovalbumin and fractionated the immune serum by electrophoresis into albumin, α-globulin, β-globulin and γ-globluin fractions. The fact that this rabbit serum binds to ovalbumin γ-globulin fraction named the immune factor present in rabbit sera as immunoglobulin(Ig) or IgG (Tiselius & Kabat, 1939). Classically, there are four types of IgG subclasses in humans (IgG1-IgG4) and mice (IgG1, IgG2a, IgG2b, and IgG3). They are the most predominant antibody isotype (70-75% of total IgG) in the blood and extravascular compartiments. Four different types of FcγRs have been identified in mice (FcγRI, FcγRIIb, FcγRIII, and FcγRIV). The human and primates FcγRs have several allelic variants that codify six types of FcγRs: FcγRI, FcγRIIa, FcγRIIc, FcγRIIb, FcγRIIIa, FcγIIIb.

Traditionally, these receptors belong to two different categories - they are classified in high or low affinity FcγRs according IgG affinity to them, and in activating or inhibitory FcγRs if the type of signaling pathway is triggered by ITAMs (immunoreceptor tyrosine-based activation motif) or ITIMs (immunoreceptor tyrosine-based inhibitory motif). Then, FcγRI is high affinity, activating FcγRs in both mice and humans; FcγRIII and FcγRIV (in mice) and FcγRIIa, FcγRIIc, FcγRIIIa, FcγRIIIb (in human) are categorized as low affinity, activating FcγRs; and FcγRIIb is the only low affinity, inhibitory FcγR in mice and humans. IgGs antibodies bind with different affinity and specificity to different FcγRs (Dijstelbloem et al., 2001). In general terms, monomeric IgG binds predominantly to high affinity FcγRs (FcγRI) and IgG-immune complexes binds to low affinity FcγR. These receptors are widely expressed in haematopoietic cells (except T cells), endothelial cells, osteoclasts, and mesangial cells. In mice, monocytes and macrophages express all activating and inhibitory FcγRs (FcγRI-IV), neutrophils express mainly FcγRIII, FcγRIV and FcγRIIb, dendritic cells express FcγRI, FcγRIII, FcγRIIb, NK cells only express FcγRIII and B cells only have FcγRIIb (Nimmerjhan & Ravetch, 2008).

IgG antibodies and FcγRIII have been implicated in triggering alternative anaphylaxis pathway. Mice lacking mast cells, IgE or FcεRI alpha chain still develop systemic anaphylactic responses upon antigen exposure (Jacoby et al., 1984; Oettgen et al., 1994; Dombrowicz et al., 1997) whereas FcRγ deficient mice that lack the expression of Fc(RI and activating Fcγ (receptors FcγRI, FcγRIII, FcγRIV) have no apparent signal of systemic anaphylaxis (Miyajima et al., 1997). Furthermore, it has been found that mice passively transferred with allergen-specific monoclonal IgG, particularly monoclonal IgG1, developed systemic anaphylaxis upon allergen exposure; when these mice were pre-treated with anti-FcγRIIb/FcγRIII, FcγRIV monoclonal antibodies, the systemic anaphylaxis was inhibited, indicating the role of FcγRIII in IgG-mediated anaphylaxis (Strait et al., 2002).

2.4.3 Histamine and H1 receptor

Histamine is an autacoid, also referred as 2-(1H-imidazol-4-yl)ethanamine, that modulates the cellular function in several tissues including dermis, small intestine, stomach, lungs and brain (Jones & Kearns, 2011). Its synthesis depends on histidine decarboxylase (HDC) that removes of carboxylic acid residue on the histidine side chain in the Golgi apparatus. It is stored basically in mast cells and basophils although it has been demonstrated that other cell types (e.g. neutrophils, lymphocytes, monocytes, dendritic cells, platelets, gastric cells and brain histaminergic cells) express HDC (MacGlashan, 2003). The release of histamine occurs in response to cross-link of antigen-specific IgE on mast cells and basophils surfaces upon antigen exposure during systemic anaphylaxis and the early phase of allergic responses. Large quantities of histamine (10^{-5} to 10^{-3} mol/L) are released within 30 minutes after allergen exposure (Simons, 2003). Histamine and other released mediators such as leukotrienes and prostaglandins produce the acute symptoms including pruritus of nasal mucosa, eyes, skin and increased vascular permeability, vasodilatation and edema resulting in nasal congestion, rhinorrea and conjuntival edema and erythema (Clough et al., 1998). Histamine can cause bronchoconstriction due to mucus accumulation by activated globet cells in the lung (Golightly & Greos, 2005) and may be involved in airway remodeling (Kunzmann et al, 2007). Histamine is responsible for mast cell activation by stimulating the secretion of cytokines and chemokines from T and B lymphocytes which up-regulates adhesion molecules in epithelial cells (Akdis & Blaser, 2003).

Histamine binds to four major receptors (H1, H2, H3 and H4) which belong to G-protein seven transmembrane receptor family. H1 receptor has been widely discussed in anaphylactic disorders. Histamine binds to H1R that activates inositol-1, 4, 5 pathway, mobilizing intracellular calcium which induces the vascular endothelium to release nitric oxide and stimulate guanyl cyclase to increase the production of cyclic GMP in vascular endothelial cells. This cascade promotes vasodilatation, erythema, vascular permeability and edema (Li et al, 2003). Activation of H1R produces direct effect in bronchial smooth muscle leading to bronchoconstriction. H1 and H2 receptors are overexpressed in patients with asthma in contrast to patients with rhinitis only (Botturi et al, 2010). The H2 receptor is expressed on gastric mucosa, vascular smooth muscle, brain, adipocytes and immune cells. Activation of H2 results in relaxation of smooth muscle in the airway and vasculature (Akdis & Simons, 2006). The stimulation of H3 receptor is been involved in pruritus (Sugimoto et al, 2004) and H4 receptor may play a role in inflammatory processes by inducing chemotaxis and calcium influx in bone marrow-derived and tracheal mast cells migration from connective tissue toward epithelium (Thurmond et al, 2004).

2.4.4 Platelet activation factor (PAF)

The term PAF was first used to describe the factors that aggregate and activate platelets (Benveniste et al., 1972). PAF is a potent proinflammatory phospholipid synthesized from the cleavage of glycerophospholipids by phospholipase A2 that binds to PAF receptor, a G-protein coupled seven-transmembrane receptor. It is active at concentration as low as 10^{-12}M (Stafforini et al, 2003). Since its discovery, pleiotropic effects of PAF have been demonstrated, including its role in bronchoconstriction, hypotension, vascular permeability, chemotaxis, degranulation of eosinophils and neutrophils (Hanahan, 1986). PAF is released from mast cells, basophils and macrophages upon antigen stimulation in human and experimental anaphylactic reactions (Vadas et al., 2008; Finkelman, 2007). Histamine, which can be secreted by mast cells and basophils, effectors cells in classical anaphylactic pathway, is a potent agonist for PAF synthesis by human endothelial cells (McIntyre et al., 1985). Circulating levels of PAF are controlled by the activity of PAF acetylhydrolase, enzyme that rapidly degrades PAF, making its half-life very short; it ranges from 3 to 13 minutes (Karasawa, 2006).

Vadas et al. (2008) have found that PAF levels positively correlate with the severity of anaphylaxis and may be pivotal for anaphylaxis outcome. Serum PAF levels is significantly elevated in allergic patients with severe anaphylaxis than those with milder manifestations of anaphylaxis. PAF has been identified as relevant vascular leak mediator in anaphylaxis (Camerer et al., 2009). The deletion of PAF receptor impairs anaphylactic responses in genetically manipulated mice (Ishii et al., 1998). In addition, recombinant PAF acetylhydrolase is protective and reduces mortality in experimental models of anaphylaxis (Fukuda et al., 2000; Gomes et al., 2006). Furthermore, PAF stimulate NO (nitric oxide) production by enhancing the activity of NOS (constitutive nitric oxide synthase), instead of iNOS (inducible nitric oxide synthase), which relaxes vascular smooth muscle, leading to hypotension and death (Cauwels et al., 2006).

2.4.5 IL-4 and IL-4Ralpha

IL-4 is a pleiotropic type I cytokine, recognized as signature cytokine of Th2 immune responses (Swain et al., 1990). It is produced by Th2 CD4+ T cells, basophils, mast cells, eosinophils and CD1-restricted NKT cells upon stimulation (Paul, 1997). IL-4 binds to IL-4 receptor, which is a heterodimer of IL-4 receptor α chain and common γ chain, resulting in phosphorylation of STAT6 (signal transducer and activator of transcription 6) (Nelms et al., 1999).

IL-4 exacerbates anaphylaxis through a direct effect on mast cell and basophils or through enhancing antibody production. Strait et al. (2003) have demonstrated that IL-4R signaling increase the responsiveness of mast cell- and macrophage-secreted mediators such as histamine, PAF, serotonin and leukotriene C4. IL-4 increases anaphylactic responses in a mouse model infected with *Thrichinella spiralis* by increasing histamine and PAF, but also enhances anaphylaxis at doses lower than those produced by helminth infections (Conrad et al., 1990). The contribution of IL-4/IL-4Rα in the anaphylaxis is also associated to their role in antibody production. IL-4 promotes class-switching to IgE antibodies (Finkelman et al., 1988) but it does not seem crucial to IgG1 production since high IgG1 levels is found in mice treated with anti-IL-4, and in IL-4 or STAT-6 deficient mice (Finkelman et al., 1989; Kuhn et al., 1991; Shimoda et al., 1996).

3. Helminth infections as predisposed factors to allergic and anaphylactic reactions

Helminths are known to cause widespread infections, mainly in tropical and subtropical areas in the developing world where the water suply and sanitation conditions are not adequate (De Silva et al., 2003). Although they did not cause high mortality, they tend to cause chronic infections in populations that live in endemic area, leading to iron-deficiency anemia and malnourishment and interfering with physical and mental growth in children (Stephenson et al., 2000).

The immune response against helminth infections is associated with high production of IgE levels and tissue infiltration of eosinophils, mast cells and Th2 cells which secrete IL-4, -5 and -13 (Fallon & Mangan, 2007). Th2 immune responses are believed to mediate protective immunity against these parasites (Anthony et al., 2007). Certain parasites such as *Schistosome mansoni* produce a strong Th2 immune response that is correlated with the formation of Th2 granuloma around schistosoma eggs (Wilson et al., 2007).

Several studies have demonstrated that helminth infection may increase allergic inflammation. Individuals exposed to helminthes for a short time often have allergic-like manifestations (Cooper, 2009). Lynch and collaborators (Lynch et al., 1984, 1987, 1992, 1997) have shown that the intensity of helminth transmission determines the effect of helminth infection on allergic reactivity - in high income urban areas where the transmission is low, the allergic reactivity is high whereas in urban and rural areas where people are chronically infected by helminthes, the allergic reactivity is low. Geohelminth parasite with pulmonary larval stages, such as *Ascaris lumbricoides, Necator americanus, Ancylostoma duodenale* and *Strongyloides stercoralis,* are found to cause Loeffler's syndrome which is characterized by eosinophilic infiltrate into the lungs after parasitic infection (Loefller, 1959).

Corroborating with Lynch's studies, it has been reported high association between dust mites and parasitic diseases in tropical allergies (Caraballo & Acevedo, 2011). Mites are important source of allergens in tropical areas (Fernandez-Caldas et al., 1993, 2008). The warm temperatures and high humidity facilitate the proliferation of dust mites such as *Blomia tropicalis* and *Dermatophagoides pteronyssinus* (Puerta et al., 1993). Likewise, nematodes are highly prevalent in tropical areas. *Ascaris lumbricoides* is the most prevalent, affecting around 1.5 million people worldwide (McSharry et al., 1999) by oral contamination with embryonated eggs that differentiate in migratory larvae, compromising intestine, liver, and lungs (Bradley & Jackson, 2004). Cross-reactivity between mites and *Ascaris* could explain why there is a positive correlation between allergies caused by dust mites and nematode infections in tropical areas. Acevedo et al. (2009) found cross-reactivity of specific IgE and tropomyosin from *B. tropicalis, D. pteronyssinus* and *A. lumbricoides* in asthmatic patients. It is postulated that high prevalence of specific IgE to mites in a tropical environment may be influenced by cross-reactivity with *Ascaris* spp. allergens (Acevedo et al., 2011). Another study also suggested that nematode infections may induce reactivity to tropomyosin in atopic individuals. Santiago et al. (2011) have demonstrated that there is 72% of amino acid identity between tropomyosin from *D. pteronyssinus* (Der p10) and *Onchocerca volvulus* in sera from *O. volvulus*-infected and non-infected atopic individuals and the prevalence of Der p10-specific IgE and IgG was increased in *O. volvulus*-infected individuals. Besides *Ascaris* infection, HDM (house dust mite) sensitization is strongly associated to wheeze symptoms in individuals from urban areas than in rural areas that had *Trichuris* infection (Scrivener et al., 2001).

Cooper (2009) and Smits et al. (2010) have listed four factors that may determine the effect of helminthic infections in promoting allergic responses (Figure 2): 1) **Timing** - periodic helminth infections in adult age (acute infections) may induce allergic manifestations whereas long-lasting helminthic infections in early age (childhood) (chronic infections) may suppress allergic inflammation due to inducing an immunomodulatory environment. 2) **Intensity of infection** – light parasite burden may induce allergic manifestations and heavy parasite burdens may induce down-modulation of allergic symptoms. 3) **Host genetics** – atopic individuals may be more likely to develop allergic manifestations than non-atopic individuals. 4) **Parasite** – different helminthes have different effects on atopy and allergies, parasites with larvae stages in the lung and skin than in other organs/tissues may be more predisposed to allergic manifestations.

4. Helminths and their products as anti-inflammatory modulators for allergic and anaphylactic disorders

Despite inducing strong Th2 and being considered predisposing factor to allergic manifestations, helminth infections can induce suppression of allergic diseases. Smits et al. (2010) related that chronic helminth infections may protect against allergic diseases by stimulating regulatory B and T cells and modulating dendritic cell functions. The immunosuppressive effect of helminthes and their products in the immune response have been widely reported in the literature (Smits et al., 2010; Hewitson et al., 2009; Soares & Araujo, 2008; Harnett & Harnett, 2008; Maizels et al., 2004). Helminth molecules can degrade some host molecules such as eotaxin and antibodies, inhibit the formation of reactive oxygen and nitrogen intermediates, interfere with macrophage activaction, down-modulate the antigen presentation by dendritic cell and macrophages, and mimic cytokines such as IFN-γ, TGF-β and MIF.

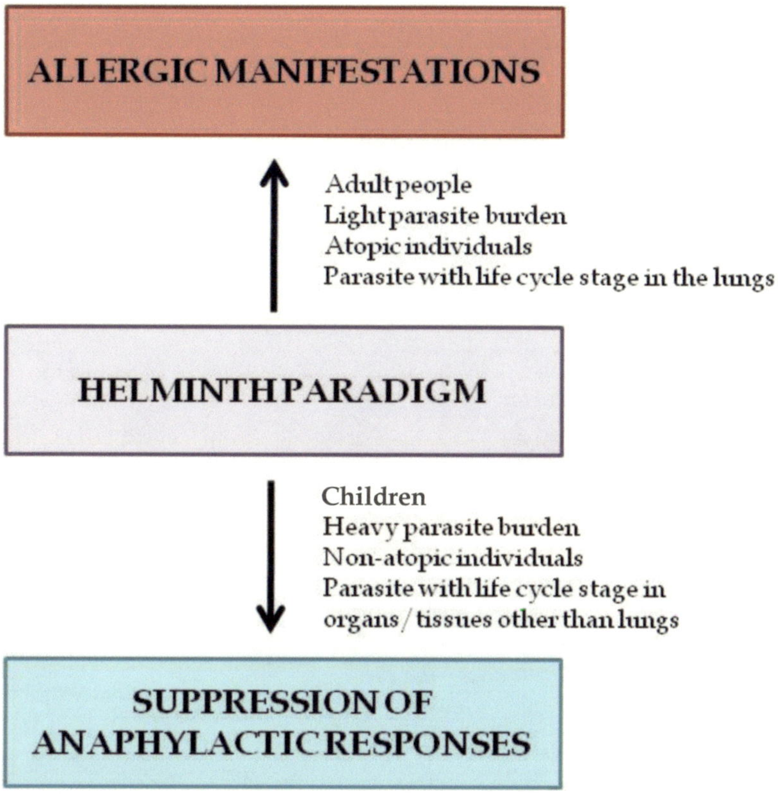

Fig. 2. Helminth paradigm. Helminthes can stimulate allergic manifestations or suppress inflammatory/anaphylactic responses depending on time and intensity of the infection, host genetic background and parasite life cycle.

Helminth infections can impair immune response toward heterologous antigen (Stewart et al., 1999), allografts (Liwski et al., 2000), viral infections (Actor et al., 1993) and other helminth infections (Jenkins, 1975). Helminths employ several immunomodulatory strategies in order to evade and/or modify the host immune response and, consequently, perpetuate their survival in the host (Playfair, 1982), including inactivation and/or modulation of the host protective immune response. The immunomodulation has been considered beneficial both to the host and the parasites since it could avoid helminth erradication and protect the host from inflammatory responses that may damage the host´s tissue (van Riet et al., 2007).

It has been identified several immunomodulatory molecules and strategies by which the helminths evade the host immune system, permitting that the parasites subvert the host protective responses. Some of these molecules include eotaxin metalloproteinase (Culley et al., 2000), calreticulin (Pritchard et al., 1999), antioxidants (Brophy et al., 1995) and neutrophil inhibitory factor (Moyle et al., 1994). They can interfere with antigen processing and presentation (Dainichi et al., 2001), cell proliferation (Allen & MacDonalds, 1998), cause T cell death (Semnani et al., 2003), decrease IgE responses (Langlet et al., 1984), reduce B cell activation (Deehan et al., 1997) and stimulate regulatory T cells (Belkaid et al., 2006). In this section, we will discuss about some helminth products and their immunomodulatory effect in the immune system (Figure 3).

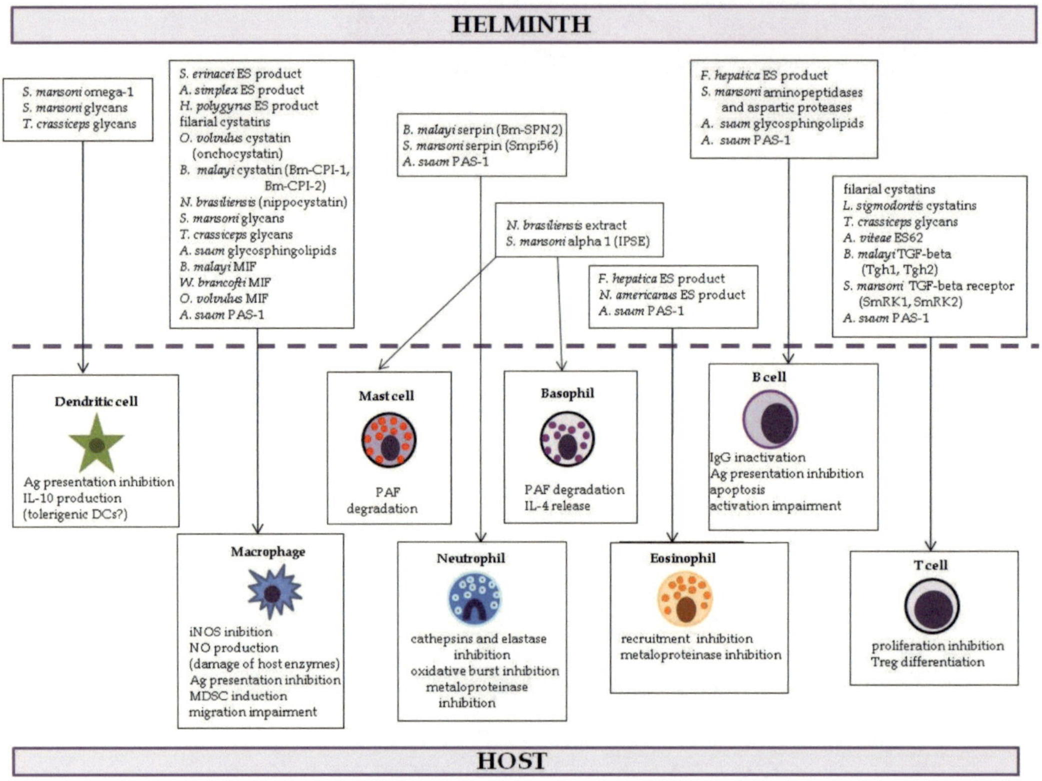

Fig. 3. Some immunosuppressive products secreted by helminthes that may be used as therapeutic strategies for anaphylactic disorders. Helminth can secrete molecules that possess down-modulatory effect on the host's immune system. The upper panel show some molecules secreted by helminthes and the lower panel show the cell targets of the helminth-secreted products. Abs, antibodies; Ag, antigen; ES, excretory/secretory products; MIF, macrophage-migration inhibition factor; MDSC, myeloid-derived suppressor cells; NO, nitric oxide; iNOS, inducible nitric oxide synthase; PAF, platelets-activating factor; PAS-1, protein from *Ascaris suum*; Treg, regulatory T cells.

4.1 Helminth products and their strategies to immunomodulate the host immune responses

4.1.1 Cleavage of host immune system molecules

It has been described several helminth defense mechanisms that can block host immune system by cleaving immune factors. The adult stage of *Nippostrongylus brasiliensis* releases in *in vitro* culture a product with acetylhydrolase activity that promotes cleavage of platelet-activating factor (PAF), promoting bronchoconstriction and increasing vascular permeability (Blackburn & Selkirk, 1992). Excretory/secretory (ES) products from hookworm *Necator americanus* cleave eotaxin (Culley et al., 2000), and in this way inhibit the recruitment of eosinophils, pivotal cells in development of the late phase of allergic responses.

Helminth serpins can also interfere in the immune response by cleaving immune factors. Serpins are an extensive family of serine proteinase inhibitors which regulate a wide variety of proteinase-dependent physiological functions, such as blood coagulation, fibrinolysis, activation of complement, and the inflammatory response (Potempa et al., 1994). A serpin produced by microfilarial stage of *Brugia malayi*, Bm-SPN-2, inhibits the enzymatic activity of serine proteinases, cathepsin G and elastase from human neutrophils (Zang et al., 1999). In addition, Smpi56, a serpin from *Schistosoma mansoni*, inhibits the neutrophil elastase (Ghendler et al., 1994), protecting the parasite from activated neutrophils during inflammation.

Besides promoting the cleavage of PAF, eotaxin and inactivation of neutrophil enzymes, helminth products also can cleave host antibody. Antibody cleavage is critical for the parasite evasion because it inhibits ADCC (antibody-dependent cell cytotoxity) and promotes IgG degradation, which blocks FcγR-mediated cytokine release. For instance, ES products from *Fasciola hepatica* cleave all human IgG subclasses at the hinge region (Berasain et al., 2000). In addition, *S. mansoni* schitosomula produces a trypsine-like proteinase or aminopeptidase that cleave Fab fragment when Fc receptor of the worm binds IgG (Auriault et al., 1981). Recombinant schistosome aspartic proteases from *S. japonicum* cleave specifically human IgG, suggesting that these proteases may play a role in the degradation of host serum proteins ingested as part of the schistosome bloodmeal (Verity et al., 2001).

4.1.2 Modulation of nitric oxide production

Nitric oxide (NO) is a potent microbicidal agent that plays a role in host defense against parasites. This effect has been demonstrated toward several helminthes. It has been found that ES products from parasites such as *Spirometra erinacei* (Fukumoto et al., 1997), *Anisakis simplex* (Cuellar et al., 1998), *Heligmosomoides polygyrus* (Rzepecka et al., 2006) suppress the expression of iNOS in LPS-activated macrophages in a dose dependent manner. However, filarial nematode cystatins (Hartmann et al., 2002) up-regulate NO production from IFN-γ-activacted macrophages. In spite of the susceptibility of parasites to NO, its stimulation in the host by helminth products is critical to promote nitration and oxidation of host´s molecules and damage several biological processes. Moreover, in filariasis murine model NO production was associated with suppression of T cell proliferation (O'Connor et al., 2000), suggesting that the secretion of NO is linked to microfilariae killing and T cell response inhibition.

4.1.3 Interference with antigen presentation and T cell responses

Helminth cystatins are thought to be the most important molecules that interfere with antigen presentation. Cystatins constitute a family of cysteine protease inhibitors that are widely distributed and play essential roles in a spectrum of physiological processes (Barrett, 1986). Nematode cystatins could lead to severe changes in antigen processing and inhibit efficient generation of peptide-MHC class II molecule, decreasing the antigen presentation by APC. These molecules target cysteine proteases such as cathepsins, which play a role in two catalytic processes (Hartmann & Lucius, 2003). First, cysteine proteases degrade proteins within the endosomal-lysosomal compartment of APC. Second, cysteine proteases are involved in the cleavage of the MHC class II-associated invariant chain, which leads to the formation of MHC molecules associated to CLIP (class II-associated invariant chain peptide). Then, synthesized CLIP molecules allow the binding of peptides to MHC class II molecules to promote antigen presentation. The invariant chain cleavage is promoted by cathepsins S in B cells and dendritic cells (Riese et al., 1996), cathepsins L in thymus epithelial cells (Nakagawa et al., 1998) and cathepsin F in macrophages (Shi et al., 2000).

Nematode cystatins are homologous to mamalian cystatin C, which are highly expressed by immature dendritic cells and are down-regulated during dendritic cells maturation process to permit the transport of MHC II molecules to cell surface. Parasite cystatins maintain dendritic cells in immature state, preventing the antigen presentation by these cells and also down-regulate *in vitro* cellular proliferation (Pierre & Mellman, 1998). The first described parasite cystatin was onchocystatin, derived from *Onchocerca volvulus* (Lustigman et al., 1992), that down-regulates the HLA-DR expression by human monocytes after 72 hours of co-culture (Hartman et al., 1997). *Brugia malayi* nematodes secrete two homologues cystatins (Schonemeyer et al., 2001; Manoury et al., 2001): Bm-CPI-1, which is selectively expressed by L2 and L3 stage into the mosquito vector and Bm-CPI-2, which is constitutively expressed during the parasite life and interferes with two classes of proteases in the MHC class II antigen presentation: cathepsins B, L and S and asparagine endopeptidase. Also, Bm-CPI-2 blocks the presentation of peptide derived from tetanus toxoid by human B cells. Nippocystatin, a cysteine protease inhibitor found in ES products from *N. brasiliensis*, modulate the antigen processing and interfere with antigen presentation due to inhibiting multiple cysteine protease activities found in endosomes/lysosomes of B cells (Dainichi et al., 2001). In addition, *Litomosoides sigmodontis* cystatins upregulate the production of tumor necrosis factor alpha (TNF-α) and decrease antigen-specific proliferation of spleen cells in mice (Pfaff et al., 2002). Besides inhibiting proteases from MHC classe II pathway, cystatins can also down-modulate T cell proliferation and up-regulate IL-10 production (Hartmann et al., 1997; Schonemeyer et al., 2001). ES62, a phosphorylcholine-bearing filarial product, secreted by *Acanthocheilonema viteae*, desensitizes LPS-stimulated mouse peritoneal macrophages to produce IFN-γ (Goodridge et al., 2001). ES-62 also reduces lymphocyte proliferation and stimulates anti-inflammatory properties (Harnett & Harnett, 2001). Phosphorylcholine(PC)-containing glycosphingolipids from *Ascaris suum* are immunomodulatory molecules due to the fact that they inhibit BCR-mediated B cell proliferation by causing apoptosis, inhibit LPS-induced activation of B cells by decreasing Erk phosphorylation, modulate IL-12p40 production in LPS/IFN-γ-induced peritoneal macrophages (Deehan et al., 2002) indicating the PC moiety is important to induce the immunomodulatory effect. In addition, lysophosphatidylserine from *S. mansoni* can specifically target the immune system via TLR-2, interacts to dendritic cells and induce IL-10-producing regulatory T cells involved in immunosuppression (van der Kleij et al., 2002).

4.1.4 Stimulation of myeloid-derived suppressor cells

Several carbohydrate components derived from helminthes also modulate the immune response by stimulating myeloid-derived suppressor cells (MDSC) (Reyes & Terazas, 2007) These cells are a heterogeneous population of cells that express CD11b and Gr-1 and consists of early myeloid progenitors and immature myeloid cells (macrophages, granulocytes and dendritic cells) at different stages of differentitation (Gabrilovich & Nagaraj, 2009). The basic concept about suppressor cells is based on the findings of Gordon's group who observed a direct in vitro effect of IL-4 on the expression of mannose receptor in macrophages (reviewed in Gordon, 2003). This observations lead to macrophages being categorized in classically-activated (CA) macrophages which are NO- and IFN-γ-dependent (Kusmartsev et al., 2000) and alternatively-activated (AA) macrophages which are IL-4- or IL-13-dependent (Kreider et al., 2007; Goerdt et al., 1999). In this regard, Mantovani et al. (2004) proposed that macrophages can be polarized in inflammatory (M1) or anti-inflammatory (M2) conditions. Besides, M2 macrophages can be classified into subpopulations M2a (which are AA macrophages) and M2b (which are IL-10-secreting cells upon immune complex activation), and M3c (which are IL-10-induced deactivated macrophages). All these type of macrophages (and other suppressor cells) can be found in several different of immunological situations, including tumors, autoimmunity, intracellular pathogen infections, helminthic infections.

Two glycans derived from *Schistosoma* eggs, lacto-N-fucopentaose III and lacto-N-neotetraose, have been related to induce IL-10 production, suppressing T cell proliferation (Terrazas et al., 2001). Soluble egg antigens (SEA) from *S. mansoni*, which are rich in lacto-N-fucopentaose III, suppress the LPS-induced inflammation by inducing Th2 responses (Pearce & MacDonald, 2002), by enhancing production of IL-10 and impairing dendritic cell (DC) activation. This latter property is due to the fact that SEA inhibit MyD88-independent, but not dependent-, pathways which result in IL-10 production (Kane et al., 2004), suggesting that SEA regulate multiple signaling pathways downstream and may target the initiation signaling in DC. The suppression of DC activation could be through the ligation of mannose receptor or DC-SIGN (DC-specific intercellular adhesion molecule-grabbing non-integrin) that results in inhibition of DC to secrete IL-12 in response to TLR ligands (Nigou et al., 2001). DC-SIGN ligation leads to IL-10 production, which has been implicated in suppression of DC function (Geijtenbeek et al., 2001). It has been found that lacto-N-fucopentaose III presents an anti-inflammatory effect due to inducing Th2 response and functioning as an adjuvant (Okano et al., 2001). High levels of IL-4, IL-5, IL-10, but not IFN-γ, are secreted by nasal lymphocytes from mouse immunized with human serum albumin conjugated to lacto-N-fucopentaose III. Lacto-N-fucopentaose III is also able to expand peritoneal macrophages that bear Gr1+ marker and act as suppressor cells, inhibiting CD4+ T cell proliferation via NO- and IFN-γ-dependent mechanisms (Atochina et al., 2001).

Carbohydrate components from *Taenia crassiceps* also favor Th2 responses, stimulating IgG1 and polyclonal IgE responses, IL-4, IL-5, IL-10 production to a bystander antigen and are critical to induce gene expression in AA macrophages (Gomes-Garcia et al., 2006), indicating that these components enhance Th2 responses as an adjuvant and trigger anti-inflammatory responses by stimulating AA macrophages. Glycans from *Taenia crassiceps* in their conformational structure recruit F4/80+ Gr1+ peritoneal exudate cells and suppresses proliferation of CD90+ cells (T cells) via cell-to-cell contact, not via IFN-γ and NO (Gomes-Garcia et al., 2005). Moreover, *T. crassiceps* glycans did not activate F4/80+ Gr1+ cells (M2a macrophages) through TLR-4 as has been proposed to synthetic and natural glycoconjugates (Terrazas et al., 2001; Atochina et al., 2001). In addition, the treatment of intact glycans with sodium periodate, which removes glycosilation, decrease M2a macrophages indicating that intact glycans are essential to recruit F4/80+ Gr1+ cells.

4.1.5 Inititation of Th2 immune responses

S. mansoni eggs secrete two proteins that have been implicated in Th2 differentiation: alpha-1 and omega-1. Alpha-1 is a dimer that cross-link IgE-FcεRI complex on basophils, in an antigen-dependent manner, hence being named IL-4 inducing principle of schistosoma eggs (IPSE). It induces the degranulation of mouse and human basophils and releases of IL-4 release (Schramm et al., 2003, 2007), initiating Th2 differentiation. Omega-1 is a ribonuclease also secreted by schistosoma eggs which is necessary to egg transit into the host tissues (Fitzsimmons et al., 2005). It is believed to be involved in Th2 responses by conditioning human monocyte-derived dendritic cells to drive Th2 polarization (Everts et al., 2009; Steinfelder et al., 2009).

4.1.6 Mimicry of cytokines and other mediators

Helminthes can produce homologous proteins to immune system mediators/receptors, such as TGF-β, IFN-γ, TNF-αR and histamine that play a role in regulating anti-parasite responses. Parasite-encoded TGF-β molecules have been characterized in filarial nematodes *Brugia malayi* and *B. pahrangi*. They are two TGF-β homologues that show to be differentially regulated during the filarial life cycle: tgh-1 in *Brugia malayi* and *B. pahangi* (Gomez-Escobar et al., 1997), and tgh-2 in *B. malayi* (Gomes-Escobar et al., 2000). Tgh-1 molecule is required for filarial development within the human host (Gomes-Escobar et al., 1998) and Tgh-2 is predominantly expressed in adult stages and binds to the human TGF-β receptor (Hirata et al., 2005), mimicking human TGF-β and stimulating regulatory responses in the host. In addition to *Brugia* species, TGF-β immunorective molecules have been detected at the surface of cervical bodies, in tegument and subtegumental cells of other parasite stages of *Schistosoma japonicum*, during the whole life cycle (eggs, cercariae, schistosomula and adult worms), although being distinctly regulated at each developmental stage (Davies et al., 1998).

Besides TGF-β homologues, TGF-β receptor homologues have also been described in *Brugia* and *Schistosoma* species. SmTβR1 or SmRK1, a homologue of type I TGF-β receptor and a type of TGF-β family of receptor serine/threonine kinase, have been shown in *Schistosoma mansoni* surface following its entry into the mammalian host (Forrester et al., 2004). In addition to expressing SmRK1, *S. mansoni* expresses another type I TGF-β receptor, SmRK2, from schistosomula and adult stages and it is located predominantly to the tegumental surface of parasite (Grencis & Entwistle, 1997). Type I TGF-β receptor (Bp-trk-1) has been also isolated from the filarial parasitic nematode *Brugia pahangi* in the three main stages of its life cycle: microfilariae, infective larvae and adults; although the ligand remains unknown, it may likely act as a receptor for host TGF-β rather than for parasite ligands (Gomes-Escobar et al., 2000).

Helminths also produce homologues that mimic IFN-γ. *Trichuris muris*-derived molecules share cross reactive epitopes with the host IFN-γ. Moreover, these molecules can be shown to bind to IFN-γ receptor and induce change in lymphoid cells similar to those induced by murine IFN-γ (Calandra & Bucala, 1997). Thus, it possible that the host immune system produces IL-4 to expulse the worms, the IFN-γ homologue production may perpetuate the parasite survival into the host.

Other types of molecules that mimic the host cytokines are macrophage-migration inhibition factors (MIFs), which are produced by several nematodes. Mammalian MIFs are small proteins produced by non-haematopoietic cells that act as pro-inflammatory cytokines and induce TNF production by macrophages in acute settings, such as septic shock (Pastrana et al, 1998). The first MIF homologue to be characterized from a nematode was BM-MIF-1 identified in the filarial parasite *Brugia malayi*, but *Wuchereria bancrofti* and *O. volvulus* also encode MIF family proteins (Reyes & Terrazas, 2007). It may play multiple roles in host-parasite interaction due being located in several tissue types and being found in both cell-associated and secreted forms. Possibly, helminthes may secrete MIF molecules down-modulate the inflammatory response, mainly by stimulating myeloid-derived suppressor cells that has been found to play down-regulatory functions in helminth infections, such as T cell proliferation inhibition and IL-10 and TGF-β release.

5. PAS-1, an anti-inflammatory protein from *Ascaris suum*

Our research group has been investigating the effect of *Ascaris suum* infection and secreted products in the inflammatory response. We have been demonstrated that components from *Ascaris suum* body extract modulate the antibody response and the cell-mediated response in mice. Soares et al. (1987) have demonstrated that, besides inhibiting the IgE production, *A. suum* extract suppresses the IgG1 and IgG2a antibody production. Ferreira et al. (1995) have shown that DBA/2 mice immunized subcutaneouly with OVA + *A. suum* extract and challenged with OVA in the footpad present suppression of immediate (3 hour after challenge) and late (24 hours after challenge) type IV hypersensitivity reaction. The isolation of protein fractions from *A. suum* extract by Sephacryl S-300 gel filtration chromatography yields three peaks (PI, PII, and PIII). PI is constituted by high weight components that suppress anti-OVA IgE antibody production in mice immunized with OVA + PI (Soares et al., 1992; Faquim-Mauro & Macedo, 1998). Thus, the suppressive effect observed in *A. suum* extract is due to high molecular weight components. PI protein fraction was used to obtain the monoclonal antibody MAIP-1, which recognizes one of the suppressive components in the *A. suum* extract; it is a 200-kDa-protein named PAS-1 (protein from *Ascaris suum*) (Oshiro et al., 2004).

PAS-1 suppresses the LPS-induced leukocyte migration and pro-inflammatory (IL-1β, IL-6 and TNF-α) cytokines production in air pouches exudates and macrophage culture supernatant; moreover, it stimulates the production of IL-10 and TGF-β (Oshiro et al., 2005), indicating that the modulatory effect of PAS-1 in LPS-induced inflammation is likely due to these two cytokine. Furthermore, PAS-1 was demonstrated modulating the humoral and cellular immune response against OVA. It inhibits the production of IgM, IgG1, IgG2a, IgE and anaphylactic IgG1 toward T-dependent but not T-independent, antigens and anti-OVA type IV hypersensitivity reaction in mouse footpad injected with carrageenan (Oshiro et al., 2006), suggesting that PAS-1 suppresses B and T cell responses.

PAS-1 also down-modulates antibody production, Th2 cytokine secretion, cellular recruitment and airway hyperesponsiveness induced by APAS-3, allergenic protein from *A. suum* (Itami et al., 2005). We have demonstrated that regulatory T CD4+CD25+ cells and T CD8+ cells secrete IL-10/TGF-β and IFN-γ, respectively and they are involved in the mechanisms by which PAS-1 down-modulate the acute lung allergic inflammation in mice since OVA-induced inflammation is reverted when PAS-1-primed regulatory T CD4+CD25+ cells or T CD8+ cells are adoptively transferred to OVA-immunized mice (Araujo et al., 2008; De Araujo et al., 2010). Besides playing an immunosuppressive role in the acute lung inflammation, we recently found that PAS-1 decreases the airway remodeling and angiogenesis in a mouse chronic lung inflammation model induced by OVA or APAS-3 by inhibiting metaloproteinases (MMP-2, MMP-9, ADAM-33) and angiogenic factors (VEGF and IL-13) (Araujo et al., manuscript in preparation).

6. Conclusion

In conclusion, anaphylaxis is a life-threatening and systemic disorder that involves two different pathways: classical anaphylactic pathway which is IgE-dependent mechanism triggered by IgE-FcεRI signaling on mast cell and basophils to secrete histamine, and alternative anaphylactic pathway which is IgG-dependent triggered by IgG-immune complex bound to FcγRIII on basophils and macrophages to secrete PAF. The understanding of molecular and cellular mechanisms involved in the anaphylactic disorders is crucial to investigate terapeuthic strategies for preventing anaphylaxis risk and recurrence.

Helminths secrete several immmunomodulatory factors that can modulate inflammatory response. Some helminth products can cleave host molecules, such as chemokines, antibodies, and enzymes; modulate the NO production; interfere with antigen presentation and T cell responses by down-modulating DC functions; mimic cytokines such as IFN-γ and TGF-β and MIF. Other potent immunodulatory molecule from helminth is PAS-1, a protein from *A. suum*, that down-modulate acute inflammatory responses and chronic lung allergic inflammation, decreasing IgG1 and IgE production, eosinophil infiltrate, and Th2 cytokines and interfering with metaloproteinase activity and production of angiogenic factors. Thus, due to their capacity to induce immunomodulation, these helminth products may be useful for therapeutic interventions in inflammatory, allergic and anaphylactic disorders.

7. References

Acevedo, N.; Sanchez, J.; Erler, A.; Mercado, D.; Briza, P; Kennedy, M; Fernandez, A; Gutierrez, M; Chua, KY; Cheong, N; Jimenez, S; Puerta, L & Caraballo, L. (2009). IgE cross-reactivity between Ascaris and domestic mites: the role of tropomyosin and the nematode polyprotein ABA-1. *Allergy*, Vol.64, No. 11, (November 2009), pp. 1635-1643, ISSN0105-4538

Acevedo, N.; Erler, A.; Briza, P.; Puccio, F.; Ferreira, F. & Caraballo, L. (2011). Allergenicity of Ascaris lumbricoides tropomyosin and IgE sensitization among asthmatic patients in a tropical environment. *International Archives of Allergy and Immunology*, Vol.154, No.3, (September 2011), pp.195-206, ISSN1018-2438

Actor, J.K.; Shirai, M.; Kullberg, M.C.; Buller, R.M.; Sher, A. & Berzofsky, J.A. (1993). Helminth infections results in decreased virus-specific CD8+ cytotoxic T cell and Th1 cytokine responses as well as delayed virus clearance. *Proceedings of the National Academy of Sciences USA*, Vol.90, No.3, (February 1993), pp.948-952, ISSN0027-8424

Akdis, C.A. & Blaser, K. (2003). Histamine in the immune regulation of allergic inflammation. *Journal of Allergy and Clinical Immunology*, Vol.112, No.1, (July 2003), pp.15-22, ISSN0091-6749

Akdis, C.A. & Simons, F.E. (2006). Histamine receptors are hot in immunopharmacology. *European Journal of Pharmacology*, Vol.533, No.1-3, (March 2006), pp.69-76, ISSN0014-2980

Allen, J.E. & MacDonalds, A.J. (1998). Profound suppression of cellular proliferation mediated by the secretions of nematodes. *Parasite Immunology*, Vol.20, No.5, (May 1998), pp.241-247, ISSN0141-9838

Anthony, R.M.; Rutitzky, L.I.; Urban, J.F. Jr; Stadecker, M.J. & Gause, W.C. (2007). Protective immune mechanisms in helminth infection. *Nature Reviews Immunology*, Vol.7, No.12, (December 2007), pp.975-987, ISBN1474-1733

Araujo, C.A.; Perini, A.; Martins, M.A.; Macedo, M.S. & Macedo-Soares, M.F. (2008). PAS-1, a protein from Ascaris suum, modulates allergic inflammation via IL-10 and IFN-gamma, but not IL-12. *Cytokine*, Vol.44, No.3, (December 2008), pp.8308-8314, ISSN1043-4666

Arinobu, Y.; Iwasaki, H.; Gurish, M.F.; Mizuno, S.; Shigematsu, H.; Ozawa, H.; Tenen, D.G.; Austen, K.F. & Akashi, K. (2005) Developmental checkpoints of the basophils/mast cell lineages in adult murine hematopoiesis. *Proccedings of the National Academy of Science USA*, Vol.102, No.50, (December 2005), pp.18105-18110, ISSN0027-8424

Arnold, J.N.; Wormald, M.R.; Sim, R.B.; Rudd, P.M. & Dwek R.A. (2007). The impact of glycosilation on the biological function and structure of human immunoglobulins. *Annual Reviews of Immunology*, Vol.25, (2007), pp.21-50, ISSN0732-0582

Atochina, O.; Daly-Engel, T.; Piskorska, D.; McGuire, E. & Harn, D.A Jr. (2001). A schistosome-expressed immunomodulatory glycoconjugate expands peritoneal Gr1(+) macrophages that suppress naïve CD4(+) T cell proliferation via an IFN-gamma and nitric oxide mechanism. *Journal of Immunology*, Vol.167, No.8, (October 2001), pp.4293-4302, ISSN0022-1467

Auriault, C.; Ouaissi, M.A.; Torpier, G.; Eisen, H.; Capron, A. (1981). Proteolytic cleavage of IgG bound to the Fc receptor of Schistosoma mansoni schistosomula. *Parasite Immunology*,Vol.3, No.1, (Spring 1981), pp.33-44, ISSN0141-9838

Barrett, A.J. (1986). The cystatins: a civerse superfamily of cysteinase peptidadase inhibitors. *Biomedica Biochimica Acta*,Vol.45, No.11-12, (1986), pp.1363-1374, ISSN0232-766X

Beaven, M.A. (2009). Our perception of the mast cell from Paul Ehrlich to now. *European Journal of Immunology*, Vol.39, No.1, (January 2009), pp.11-25, ISSN0014-2980

Belkaid, Y.; Sun, C.M. & Bouladoux, N. (2006). Parasites and immunoregulatory T cells. *Current Opinion in Immunology*, Vol.18, No.4, (August 2006), pp.406-412, ISSN0952-7915

Bell, R.G. (1996). IgE, allergies and helminth parasites: a new perspective on an old conundrum. *Immunology and Cell Biology*, Vol.74, No.4, (August 1996), pp.337-345, ISSN0818-9641

Benveniste, J.; Henson, P.M & Cochrane, C.G. (1972). Leukocyte dependent histamine release from rabbit platelets. The role of IgE, basophils, and a platelet-activating factor. *Journal of Experimental Medicine*, Vol.136, No.6, (December 1972), pp.1356-1377, ISSN0022-1007

Berasain, P.; Carmona, F.; Frangione, B.; Dalton, J.P. & Goni, F. (2000). Fasciola hepatica: parasite-secreted proteinases degrade all human IgG subclasses: determination of the specific cleavage sites and identification of the immunoglobulin fragments produced. *Experimental Parasitology*, Vol.94, No.2, (February 2000), pp.99-110, ISSN0014-4894

Bieber, T.; De La Salle, H.; Wollenberg, A.; Hakimi, J.; Chizzonite, R.; Ring, J.; Hanau, D. & De la Salle, C. (1992). Human epidermal Langerhans cells express the high affinity receptor for immunoglobulin E (Fc epsilon RI). *Journal of Experimental Medicine*, Vol.175, No.5, (May 1992), pp.1285-1290, ISSN0022-1007

Blackburn, C.C. & Selkirk, M.E. (1992). Inactivation of platelet-activation factor by a putative acetylhydrolase from the gastrointestinal nematode parasite Nippostrongylus brasiliensis. *Immunology*, Vol,75, No.1, (January 1992), pp.41-46, ISSN0019-2805

Botturi, K.; Lacoeuille, Y.; Vervloet, D.;& Magnan A. (2010). Histamine induces Th2 activation through the histamine receptor 1 in house dust mite rhinitic but asmathic patients. *Clinical and Experimental Allergy*, Vol.40, No.5, (May 2010), pp.755-762, ISSN0954-7894

Bradley, J.E & Jackson, J.A. (2004). Immunity immunoregulation and the ecology of trichuris and ascariasis. *Parasite Immunology*, Vol.26, No.11-12, (November-December 2004), pp.429-441, ISSN0141-9838

Brophy, P.M.; Patterson, L.H.; Brown, A. & Pritchard, D.I. (1995). Glutathione S-transferase (GST) expression in the human hookworm Necator americanus: potential roles for excretory-secretory forms of GST. *Acta Tropica*, Vol.59, No.3, (June 1995), pp.259-263, ISSN0001-706X

Brown, S.G. (2004). Clinical features and severity grading of anaphylaxis. *Journal of Allergy and Clinical Immunology*, Vol.114, No.2, (August 2004), pp.371-376, ISSN0091-6749

Calandra, T. & Bucala, R. (1997) Macrophage migration inhibitory factor (MIF): a glucocorticoid counter-regulator within the immune system. *Critical Reviews in Immunology*, Vol.17, No.1, (1997), pp.77-88, ISSN1040-8401

Camerer, E.; Regard, J.B.; Cornelissen, I.; Srinivasan, Y.; Duong, D.N.; Palmer, D.; Pham, T.H.; Wong, J.S.; Pappu, R. & Coughlin, S.R. (2009). Sphingosine-1 phosphate in the plasma compartment regulates basal and inflammation-induced vascular lead in mice. *Journal of Clinical Investigation*, Vol.119, No.7, (July 2009), pp.1871-1879, ISSN0021-9738

Caraballo, A. & Acevedo, N. (2011). Allergy in the tropics: the impact of cross-reactivity between mites and Ascaris. *Frontiers in Bioscience*, Vol. E3, (January 2011), pp.51-64, ISSN1093-9946

Capron, A.; Dessaint, J.P.; Haque, A. & Capron, M. (1982). Antibody-dependent cell-mediated cytotoxicity against parasites. *Progress in Allergy*, Vol. 31, (1982), pp.234-267, ISSN0079-6034

Cauwels, A.; Janssen, B.; Buys, E.; Sips, P. & Brouckaert, P. (2006). Anaphylactic shock depends on PI3K and eNOS-derived NO. *Journal of Clinical Investigation*, Vol.116, No.8, (August 2006), pp.2244-2251, ISSN0021-9738

Clough, G.F.; Bennett, A.R. & Church, M.K. (1998). Effects of H1 antagonist on the cutaneous vascular response to histamine and bradykinin: a study using scanning laser Doppler imaging. *British Journal of Dermatology*, Vol.138, No.5, (May 1998), pp.806-814, ISSN0007-0963

Conrad, D.H.; Ben-Sasson, S.Z.; Le Gros, G.; Finkelman, F.D. & Paul, W.E. (1990). Infection with Nippostrongylus brasiliensis or injection of anti-IgD antibodies markedly enhances Fc-receptor-mediated interleukin 4 production by non-B, non-T cells. *Journal of Experimental Medicine*, Vol.171, No.5, (May 1990), pp.1497-1508, ISSN0022-1007

Cooper, P.J. (2009). Interactions between helminth parasites and allergy. *Current Opinion in Allergy and Clinical Immunology*, Vol.9, No.1, (February. 2009), pp.29-37, ISSN1528-4050

Cuellar, C.; Pertequer, M.J. & de Las Heras, B. (1998). Effect of Anisakis simplex on nitric oxide production in J774 macrophages. *Scandinavian Journal of Infectious Diseases*, Vol.30, No.6, (1998), pp.603-606, ISSN0300-9475

Culley, F.J.; Brown, A.; Conroy, D.M.; Sabroe, I.; Pritchard, D.I. & Williams, T.J. (2000). *Journal of Immunology*, Vol.165, No.11, (December 2000), pp.6447-6453, ISSN0022-1767

Daeron M. (1997). Fc receptor biology. *Annual Reviews of Immunology*, Vol.15, (1997), pp.203-234, ISSN0732-0582

Dainichi, T.; Maekawa, Y.; Ishii, K.; Zhang, T.; Nashed, B.F.; Sakai, T.; Takashima, M. & Himeno, K. (2001). Nippocystatin, a cystein protease inhibitor from Nippostrongylus brasiliensis, inhibits antigen processing and modulates antigen-specific immune responses. *Infecion and Immunity*, Vol.69, No.12, (December 2001), pp.730-7386, ISSN0019-9567

Davies, S.J.; Shoemaker, C.B. & Pearce, E.J. (1998). A divergent member of the transforming factor beta receptor family from Schistosoma mansoni is expressed on the parasite surface membrane. *Journal of Biological Chemistry*, Vol.273, No.18, (May 1998), pp.11234-11240, ISSN1178-6264

De Araujo, C.A.; Perini, A.; Martins, M.A.; Macedo, M.S. & Macedo-Soares, M.F. (2010). PAS-1, an Ascaris suum protein, modulates allergic airway inflammation via CD8+γδTCR+ and CD4+CD25+FoxP3+ T cells. *Scandinavian Journal of Immunology*, Vol.72, No.6, (December 2010), pp.491-503, ISSN0300-9475

Deehan, M.R.; Harnett, M.M. & Harnett, W. (1997). A filarial nematode secreted product differentially modulates expression and activation of protein kinase C isoforms in B lymphocytes. *Journal of Immunology*, Vol.159, No.12, (December 1997), pp.6105-6111, ISSN0022-1767

Deehan, M.R.; Goodridge, H.S.; Blair, D.; Lochnit, G.; Dennis, R.D.; Geyer, R.; Harnett, M.M. & Harnett, W. (2002). Immunomodulatory properties of Ascaris suum glycosphingolipids - phosphorylcholine and non-phosphorylcholine- dependent effects. *Parasite Immunology*, Vol.24, No.9-10, (September-October 2002), pp.463-469, ISSN0141-2980

De Silva, N.R.; Brooker, S.; Hotez, P.J.; Montresor, A.; Engels, D. & Savioli, L. (2003). Soil-transmitted helminth infections: updating the global picture. Trends of Parasitology, *Vol.19, No.12, (December* 2003), pp.547-551, ISSN1471--4906

Dijstelbloem, H.M.; van de Winkel, J.G. & Kallenberg, C.G. (2001). Inflammation in autoimmunity: receptors for IgG revisited. *Trends in Immunology*, Vol..22, No.9, (September 2001), pp.510-516, ISSN1471-4906

Dombrowicz, D.; Flamand, V.; Miyajima, I.; Ravetch, J.V.; Galli, S.J. & Kinet, J.P. (1997) Absence of Fc epsilon RI alpha chain results in upregulation of Fc gamma RIII-dependent mast cell degranulation and anaphylaxis. Evidence of competition between Fc epsilon RI and Fc gamma RIII for limiting amounts of FcR beta and gamma chains. *Journal of Clinical Investigation*, (March 1997), Vol.99, No.5, pp.915-922, ISSN0021-9738

Everts, B.; Perona-Wright, G.; Smits, H.H.; Hokke, C.H.; van der Ham, A.J.; Fitzsimmons, C.M.; Doenhoff, M.J.; van der Bosch, J.; Mohrs, K.; Haas, H.; Mohrs, M.; Yazdanbakhsh, M. & Schramm, G. (2009). Omega-1, a glycoprotein secreted by Schistosoma mansoni eggs, drives Th2 responses. *Journal of Experimental Medicine*, Vol.206, No.8, (August 2009), pp.1673-1680, ISSN0022-1007

Ewan, P.W. (1998). ABC of Allergies-Anaphylaxis. *BMJ*, Vol.316, No.7142, (May 1998), pp.1442-1445, ISSN0958-8146

Fallon, P.G. & Mangan, N.E. (2007). Suppression of Th2 type allergic reactions by helminth infections. *Nature Reviews Immunology*, Vol.7, (March 2007), pp. 220-230, ISSN1474-1733

Faquim-Mauro, E.L. & Macedo, M.S. (1998). The immunosuppressive activity of Ascaris suum is due to high molecular weight components. *Clinical and Experimental Immunology*, Vol.114, No.2, (November 1998), pp.245-251, ISSN0009-9104

Fernandez-Caldas, E.; Puerta, L.; Mercado, D.; Lockey, R.F. & Caraballo, L.R. (1993). Mite fauna, Der p1, Der f1 and Blomia tropicalis allergen levels in a tropical environment. *Clinical and Experimental Allergy*, Vol.23, No.4, (April 1993), pp.292-297, ISSN0954-7894

Fernandez-Caldas, E.; Puerta, L.; Caraballo, L. & Lockey, R.F. (2008). Mite allergens. *Clinical Allergy and Immunology*, Vol.21, (2008), pp.161-182, ISSN1075-7910

Ferreira, A.P.; Faquim-Mauro, E.S.; Abrahamsohn, I.A. & Macedo, M.S. (1995). Immunization with Ascaris suum extract impairs T cell functions in mice. *Cellular Immunology*, Vol.162, No.2, (May 1995), pp.202-210, ISSN0008-8749

Fiebiger, E.; Tortorella, D.; Jouvin, M.H.; Kinet, J.P. & Ploegh, H.L. (2005). Cotranslational endoplasmic reticulum assembly of FcεRI controls the formation of functional IgE-binding receptors. *Journal of Experimental Medicine*, Vol.201, No.2, (January 2005), pp.267-277, ISSN0022-1007

Finkelman, F.D.; Katona, I.M.; Urban, J.F. Jr; Holmes, J.; Ohara, J.; Tung, A.S.; Sample, J.V. & Paul, W.E. (1988). IL-4 is required to generate and sustain in vivo IgE responses. *Journal of Immunology*, Vol.141, No.7, (October 1988), pp.2335-2341, ISSN0022-1767

Finkelman, F.D.; Holmes, J.; Urban, J.F. Jr; Paul, W.E. & Katona, I.M. (1989). T help requirements for the generation of an in vivo IgE response: a late acting form of T cell help other than IL-4 is required for IgE but not for IgG1 production. *Journal of Immunology*, Vol.142, No.2, (January 1989), pp.403-408, ISSN0022-1767

Finkelman, F.D. (2007). Anaphylaxis: lessons from mouse models. *Journal of Allergy and Clinical Immunology*, Vol.120, No.3, (September 2007), pp.506-515, ISSN0091-6749

Fitzsimmons, C.M.; Schramm, G.; Jones, F.M.; Chalmers, I.W.; Hoffman, K.F.; Grevelding, C.G.; Wuhrer, M.; Hokke, C.H.; Haas, H.; Doenhoff, M.J. & Dunne, D.W. (2005). *Molecular and Biochemical Parasitology*, Vol.144, No.1, (November 2005), pp.123-127, ISSN0166-6851

Forrester, S.G.; Warfel, P.W. & Pearce, E.J. (2004). Tegumental expression of a novel type II receptor serine/threonine kinase (SmRK2) in Schistosoma mansoni. *Molecular and Biochemical Parasitology*, Vol.136, No.2, (August 2004), pp.149-156, ISSN0166-6851

Fukuda, Y.; Kawashima, H.; Saito, K.; Inomata, N.; Matsui, M. & Nakanishi, T. (2000). Effect of human plasma-type platelet-activating factor acetylhydrolase in two anaphylactic shock models. *European Journal of Pharmacology*, Vol.390, No.1-2, (February 2000), pp.203-207, ISSN0021-8219

Fukumoto, S.; Hirai, K.; Tanikata, T.; Ohmori, Y.; Stuehr, D.J. & Hamilton, T.A. (1997). Excretory/secretory products from plerocercoids of Spirometra erinacei reduce iNOS and chemokine mRNA levls in peritoneal macrophages stimulated with cytokines and/or LPS. *Parasite Immunology*, Vol.19, No.7, (July 1997), pp.325-332, ISSN0141-2980

Gabrilovich, D.I. & Nagaraj, S. (2009). Myeloid-derived suppressor cells as regulators of the immune system. *Nature Reviews Immunology*, Vol.9, No.3, (March 2009), pp.162-174, ISSN1474-1733

Galli, S.J.; Kalesnikoff, J.; Grimbaldeston, M.A.; Piliponsky, A.M.; Williams, C.M. & Tsai, M. (2005). Mast cells as "tunable" effector and immunoregulatory cells: recent advances. *Annual Reviews of Immunology*, Vol.23, (2005), pp.749-786, ISSN0732-0582

Garman, S.C.; Kinet, J.P. & Jardetzky, T.S. (1999). The crystal structure of the human high affinity IgE receptor (FcεRI α). *Annual Reviews of Immunology*, Vol.17, (1999), pp.973-976, ISSN0732-0582

Geijtenbeek, T.B.; Kroosshoop, D.J.; Bleijs, D.A.; van Vliet, S.J.; Koppel, E.A.; van Duijnhoven, G.C.; Alon, R.; Figdor, C.G .& van Kooyk, Y. (2001). DC-SIGN-ICAM-2 interaction mediates dendritic cell trafficking. *Journal of Experimental Medicine*, Vol.193, No.6, (March 2001), pp.671-678, ISSN0022-1007

Geha, R.S.; Helm, B. & Gould, H. (1985). Inhibition of the Prausnitz-Kustner reaction by an immunoglobulin epsilon-chain fragment synthesized in E. coli. *Nature*, Vol. 315, No.6020, (June 1985), pp.577-578, ISSN0028-0836

Geissmann, F.; Manz, M.G.; Jung, S.; Sieweke, M.H.; Merad, M. & Ley, K. (2010). Development of monocytes, macrophages and dendritic cells. *Science*, Vol.327, No.5966, (February 2010), pp.656-661, ISSN0272-4634

Ghendler, Y.; Arnon, R. & Fishelson, Z. (1994). Schistosoma mansoni: isolation and characterization of Smpi56, a novel serine protease inhibitor. *Experimental Parasitology*, Vol.78, No.2, (March 1994), pp.121-131, ISSN0014-4894

Goerdt, S.; Politz, O.; Schledzewski K.; Birk, R.; Gratchev, A.; Guillot, P.; Hakiy, N.; Klembe C.D.; Dippel, E.; Kodelja, V. & Orfanos, C.E. (1999). Alternative versus classical activation of macrophages. *Pathobiology*, Vol.67, No.5-6, (1999), pp.222-226, ISSN1015-2008

Golightly, L.K. & Greos, L.S. (2005). Second generation antihistamines: actions and efficacy in the management of allergic disorders. *Drugs*, Vol.65, No.3, (2005), pp.341-384, ISSN0012-6667

Gomes, R.N.; Bozza, F.A.; Amancio, R.T.; Japiassu, A.M.; Vianna, R.C.; Larangeira, A.P.; Gouveia, J.M.; Bastos, M.S.; Zimmerman, G.A.; Stafforini, D.M.; Prescott, S.M.; Bozza, P.T. & Castro-Faria-Neto, H.C. (2006). Exogenous platelet-activating factor acetylhydrolase reduces mortality in mice with systemic inflammatory response syndrome and sepsis. *Shock*, Vol.26, No.1, (July 2006), pp.41-49, ISSN1073-2322

Gomez-Escobar, N.; van der Biggelaar, A. & Maizels, R. (1997). A member of the TGF-beta receptor gene family in the parasitic nematode Brugia parangi. *Gene*, Vol.199, No.1-2, (October 1997), pp.101-109, ISSN0378-1119

Gomez-Escobar, N.; Lewis, E. & Maizels, R.M. (1998). A novel member of the transforming growth factor-beta (TGF-beta) superfamily from the filarial nematodes Brugia malayi and B. parangi. *Experimental Parasitology*, Vol.88, No.3, (March 1998), pp.200-209, ISSN0014-4894

Gomez-Escobar, N.; Gregory, W.F. & Maizels, R.M. (2000). Identification of tgh-2, a filarial nematode homolog of Caenorhabditis elegans daf-7 and human transforming growth factor beta, expressed in microfilarial and adult stages of Brugia malayi. *Infection and Immunity*, Vol.68, No.11, (November 2000), pp.6402-6410, ISSN0019-9567

Gomez-Garcia, L.; Lopez-Marin L.M.; Saavedra, R.; Rodriguez-Sosa, M. & Terrazas, L.I. (2005). Intact glycans from cestode antigens are involved in innate activation of myeloid suppressor cells. *Parasite Immunology*, Vol.27, No.10-11, (October-November 2005), pp.395-405, ISSN0141-2980

Gomez-Garcia, L.; Rivera-Montoya, I.; Rodriguez-Sosa, M. & Terrazas, L.I. (2006). Carbohydrate components of Taenia crassiceps metacestodes display Th2-adjuvant and anti-inflammatory properties when co-injected with bystander antigen. *Parasitology Research*, Vol.99, No.4, (September 2006), pp.440-448, ISSN0932-0113

Goodridge, H.S.; Wilson, E.H.; Harnett, W.; Campbell, C.C.; Harnett, M.M. & Liew, F.Y. (2001). Modulation of macrophage cytokine production by ES-62, a secreted product of the filarial nematode Acanthocheilonema viteae. *Journal of Immunology*, Vol.167, No.2, (July 2001), pp.94-945, ISSN0022-1767

Gordon S. (2003). Alternative activation of macrophages. *Nature Reviews Immunology*, Vol.3, No.1, (January 2003), pp.23-35, ISSN1474-1733

Gould, H.J.; Sutton, B.J.; Beavil, A.J.; Beavil, R.L.; McCloskey, N.; Coker, H.A.; Fear, D. & Smuthwaite, L. (2003). The biology of IgE and the basis of allergic diseases. *Annual Reviews of Immunology*, Vol.21, (2003), pp.579-628, ISSN0732-0582

Gould, H.J. & Sutton, B.J. (2008). IgE in allergy and asthma today. *Nature Reviews Immunology*, Vol. 8, No.3, (March 2008), pp.205-217, ISSN1474-1733

Grencis, R.K. & Entwistle, G.M. (1997). Production of an interferon-gamma homologue by an intestinal nematode: functionally significant or interesting artifact? *Parasitology*, Vol.115, No. Suppl, (1997), pp.S101-106, ISSN0031-1820

Hanahan, D.J. (1986). Platelet activating factor: a biologically active phosphoglyceride. *Annual Reviews of Biochemistry*, Vol.55, (1986), pp.483-509, ISSN0066-4154

Harnett, W. & Harnett, M.M. (2001). Modulation of the host immune system by phosphorylcholine-containing glycoproteins secreted by parasitic filarial nematodes. *Biochimica et Biophysica Acta*, Vol.1539, No.1-2, (May 2001), pp.7-15, ISSN0006-3002

Harnett W & Harnett MM. (2008). Parasitic nematode modulation of allergic disease. *Current Allergy and Asthma Reports*, Vol.8, No.5, (September 2008), pp.392-397, ISSN1529-7322

Hartmann, S.; Kyewski, B.; Sonnenburg, B. & Lucius, R. (1997). A filarial cysteine protease inhibitor down-regulates T cell proliferation and enhances interleukin-10 production. *European Journal of Immunology*, Vol.27, No.9, (September 1997), pp.2253-2260, ISSN0014-2980

Hartmann, S.; Schonemeyer, A.; Sonnenburg, B.; Vray, B. & Lucius, R. (2002). Cystatins of filarial nematodes up-regulate the nitric oxide production of interferon-gamma activated murine macrophages. *Parasite Immunology*, Vol.24, No.5, (May 2002), pp.253-262, ISSN0141-9838

Hartmann, S. & Lucius, R. (2003). Modulation of hsot immune responses by nematode cystains. *International Journal of Parasitology*, Vol.30, No.11, (September 2003), pp.1291-1303, ISSN0020-7519

Hewitson, J.P.; Grainer, J.R. & Maizels, R.M. (2009). Helminth immunoregulation: the role of parasite secreted proteins in modulating host immunity. *Molecular and Biochemical Parasitology*, Vol.167, No.1, (September 2009), pp.1-11, ISSN0166-6851

Hirata, M.; Hirata, K.; Hara, T.; Kawabuchi, M. & Fukuma, T. (2005). Expression of TGF-beta-like molecules in the life cycle of Schistosoma japonicum. *Parasitology Research*, Vol.95, No.6, (April 2005), pp.367-373, ISSN0932-0113

Honda, Z.; Suzuki, T.; Kono, H.; Okada, M.; Yamamoto, T.; Ra, C.; Morita, Y. & Yamamoto, K. (2000). Sequential requirements of the N-terminal palmytoylation site and SH2 domain of Src family kinases in the initiation and progression of FcεRI signaling. *Molecular and Cellular Biology*, Vol.20, No.5, (March 2000), pp.1759-1771, ISSN0270-7306

Hu, Z.Q.; Zhao, W.H. & Shimamura, T. (2007). Regulation of mast cell development by inflammatory factors. *Current Medicinal Chemistry*, Vol.14, No. 28, (2007), pp.3044-3050, ISSN0929-8673

Iio, A.; Waldmann, T.A. & Strober, W. (1987). Metabolic study of human IgE: evidence for an extravascular catabolic pathway. *Journal of Immunology*, Vol.120, No.5, (May 1987), pp.1696-1701, ISSN0022-1767

Ishii, S.; Kuwaki, T.; Nagase, T.; Maki, K.; Tashiro, F.; Sunaga, S.; Cao, W.H.; Kume, K.; Fukuchi, Y., Ikuta, K.; Miyazaki, J.; Kumada, M. & Shimizu, T. (1998). *Journal of Experimental Medicine*, Vol.187, No.11, (June 1998), pp.1779-1788, ISSN0022-1007

Ishizaka, K. & Iszhizaka, T. (1971). Mechanism of reaginic hypersensitivity: a review. *Clinical Allergy*, Vol. 1, No.1, (March 1971), pp.9-25, ISSN0009-9090

Ishizaka, K. & Ishizaka, T. (1976). Identification of gamma-E-antibodies as a carrier of reaginic activity. *Journal of Immunology*, Vol.99, No.6, (1976), pp.1187-1198, ISSN0022-1767

Itami, D.M.; Oshiro, T.M.; Araújo, C.A.; Perini, A.; Martins, M.A.; Macedo, M.S. & Macedo-Soares, M.F. (2005). Modulation of murine experimental asthma by Ascaris suum components. *Clinical and Experimental Allergy*, Vol.35, No.7, (July 2005), pp.873-879, ISSN0954-7894

Jacoby, W.; Cammarata, P.V.; Findlay, S. & Pincus, S.H. (1984). Anaphylaxis in mast cell-deficient mice. *Journal of Investigative Dermatology*, Vol.83,No.4, (October 1984), pp.302-304, ISSN0022-202X

Jenkins, D.C. (1975). The influence of Nematospiroides dubius on subsequent Nippostrongylus brasiliensis infections in mice. *Parasitology*, Vol.71, No.2, (October 1975), pp.349-355, ISSN0031-1820

Jones BL & Kearns GL. (2011). Histamine: new thoughts about a familiar mediator. *Clinical Pharmacology and Therapeutics*, Vol.89, No.2, (February 2011), pp.189-197, ISSN0009-9325

Kane, C.M.; Cervi, L; Sun, J; McKee, A.S.; Masek, K.S.; Shapira, S.; Hunter, C.A. & Pearce, E.J. (2004). Helminth antigens modulate TLR-initiated dendritic cell activation. *Journal of Immunology*, Vol.173, No.12, (December 2004), pp.7454-7461, ISSN0022-1767

Karasawa, K. (2006). Clinical aspects of plasma platelets-activating factor- acetylhydrolase. *Biochimica et Biophysica Acta*, Vol.1761, No.11, (November 2006), pp.1359-1372, ISSN0006-3002

Kemp, S.F. & Lockey, R.F. (2002). Anaphylaxis: a review of causes and mechanisms. *Journal of Allergy and Clinical Immunology*, Vol. 110, No. 3, (September 2002), pp.341-348, ISSN0091-6749

Kumar, V. & Sharma, A. (2010). Mast cells; emerging sentinel innate immune cells with diverse role in immunity. *Molecular Immunology*, Vol.48, No.1-3, (November-December 2010), pp.14-25, ISSN0161-5890

Kimura, S; Nagata, M.; Takeuchi, M.; Takano, K. & Harada, M. (1997). Anti-granulocyte antibody suppression of active and passive anaphylactic shock in WBB6F1-W/Wv mice. *Cellular and Molecular Life Sciences*, Vol.53, No.8, (August 1997), pp.663-669, ISSN1420-682X

Kinet, J.P. (1999). The high –affinity IgE receptor (FcεRI): from physiology to pathology. *Annual Reviews of Immunology*, Vol.17, (1999), pp.931-972, ISSN0732-0582

Kreider, T.; Anthony, R.M.; Urban Jr, J.F.& Gause, W.C. (2007). Alternativelly activated macrophages in helminth infections. *Current Opinion in Immunology*, Vol.19, No.4, (August 2007), pp.448-453, ISSN0952-7915

Kuhn, R.; Rajewsky, K. & Muller, W. (1991). Generation and analysis of interleukin-4 deficient mice. *Science*, Vol.254, No.5032, (November 1991), pp.707-710, ISSN0272-4634

Kunzmann, S.; Schmidt-Weber, C.; Zingg, J.M.; Azzi, A.; Kramer, B.W.; Blaser, K.; Akdis, C.A. & Speer, C.P. (2007). Connective tissue growth factor expression is regulated by histamine in lung fibroblast: potential role of histamine in airway remodeling. *Journal of Allergy and Clinical Immunology*, Vol.119, No.6, (June 2007), pp.15-22, ISSN0091-6749

Kusmartsev, S.A.; Li, Y.& Chen, S.H. (2000). Gr-1+ myeloid cells derived from tumor-bearing mice inhibit prmary T cell activation induced through CD3/CD28 costimulation. *Journal of Immunology*, Vol.165, No.2, (July 2000), pp.779-785, ISSN0022-1767

Langlet, C.; Mazingue, C.; Dessaint, J.P. & Capron, A. (1984). Inhibition of primary and secondary IgE response by a schistosome-derived inhibitory factor. *International Archives of Allergy and Applied Immunology*, Vol.73, No.3, (1984), pp.225-230, ISSN0020-5915

Li, H.; Burkhardt, C.; Heinrich, U.R.; Brausch, I.; Xia, N. & Forstermann, U. (2003). Histamine upregulates gene expression of endothelial nitric oxide synthase in human vascular endothelial cells. *Circulation*, Vol.107, No.18, (May 2003), pp.2348-2354, ISSN0009-7322

Liwski, R.; Zhou, J.; McAlister, V.& Lee, T.D. (2000). Prolongation of allograft survival by Nippostrongylus brasiliensis is associated with decreased allospecific cytotoxic T lymphocyte activity and development of T cytotoxic cell type 2. *Transplantation*, Vol.69, No.9, (May 2000), pp.1912-1922,ISSN0041-1337

Loffler, W. (1956). Transient lung infiltrations with blood eosinophilia. *International Archives of Allergy and Applied Immunology*, Vol.8, No.1-2,(1956), pp.54-59, ISSN0020-5915

Loke, P.; MacDonald, A.S. & Allen, J.E. (2000). Antigen-presenting cells recruited by Brugia malayi induce Th2 differentiation of naïve CD4(+) T cells. *European Journal of Immunology*, Vol.30, No.4, (April 2000), pp.1127-1135, ISSN0014-2980

Lustigman, S.; Brotman, B.; Huima, T.; Prince, A.M. & McKerrow, J.H. (1992). Molecular cloning and characterization of onchocystatin, a cysteine proteinase inhibitor of Onchoceerca volvulus. *Journal of. Biological Chemistry*, Vol.267, No.24, (August 1992), pp.17339-17146, ISSN1178-6264

Lynch, N.R.; Medouze, L.P.F.; DiPrisco-Fuenmayor, M.C.; Verde, O.; Lopez, R.I. & Malave, C. (1984). Incidence of atopic disease in a tropical environment: partial independence from intestinal helminthiasis. *Journal of Allergy and Clinical Immunology*, Vol.73, No.2, (February 1984), pp.229-233, ISSN0091-6749

Lynch, N.R.; Lopez, R.I.; Di Prisco-Fuenmayor, M.C.; Hagel, I.; Medouze, L.; Viana, G.; Ortega, C. & Prato, G. (1987). Allergic reactivity and socio-economic level in a tropical environment. *Clinical Allergy*, Vol.17, No.3, (May 1987), pp.199-207, ISSN0009-9090

Lynch, N.R.; Hagel, I.; Perez, M.; DiPrisco, M.; Alvarez, N. & Rojas, E. (1992). Bronchoconstriction in helminthic infection. *International Archives of Allergy and Immunology*, Vol. 98, No.1, (1992), pp.77-79, ISSN1018-2438

Lynch, N.R.; Palenque, M.; Hagel, I. & DiPrisco, M.C. (1997). Clinical improvement of asthma after antihelminthic treatment in a tropical situation. *American Journal of Respiratory and Critical Care*, Vol.156, No.1, (July 1997), pp.50-54, ISSN1073-449X

MacGlashan, D. Jr. (2003). Histamine: a mediator of inflammation. *Journal of Allergy and Clinical Immunology*, Vol.112, No.4, (October 2003), pp.S53-S59, ISSN0091-6749

Maizels, R.M.; Balic, A.; Gomez-Escobar, N.; Nair, M.; Taylor, M.D. & Allen, J.E. (2004). Helminth parasites: masters of regulation. *Immunological Reviews*, Vol.201, (October 2004), pp. 89-116, ISSN0105-2896

Mancardi, D.A.; Iannascoli, B.; Hoos, S.; England, P.; Daeron, M. & Bruhns, P. (2008). FcgammaRIV is a mouse IgE receptor that resembles macrophage FcepsilonRI in human and promotes IgE-induced lung inflammation. *Journal of Clinical Investigation*, Vol.118, No.11, (November 2008), pp.3738-3750, ISSN0021-9738

Manoury, B.; Gregory, W.F.; Maizels, R.M. & Watts, C. (2001). Bm-CPI-2, a cystatin homolog secreted by the filarial parasite Brugia malayi, inhibits classII MHC-restricted antigen processing. *Current Biology*, Vol11, No.6, (March 2001), pp.447-451, ISSN0960-9822

Mantovani, A.; Sica, A.; Sozzani, S.; Allavena, P.; Vechii, A. & Locati, M. (2004). The chemokine system in diverse forms of macrophage activation and polarization. *Trends in Immunology*, Vol.25, No.12, (December 2004), ISSN1471-4906

McIntyre, T.M.; Zimmerman, G.A.; Satoh, K. & Prescott, S.M. (1985). Cultured endothelial cells synthesize both platelet-activating factor and prostacyclin in response to histamine, bradykinin, and adenosine triphosphate. *Journal of Clinical Investigation*, Vol.76, No.1, (July 1985), pp.271-280, ISSN0021-9738

McSharry, C.; Xia, Y.; Holland, C.V. & Kennedy, M.W. (1999). Natural immunity to Ascaris lumbricoides with immunoglobulin E antibody to ABA-1 allergen and inflammation indicators in children. *Infection and Immunity*, Vol.67, No.2, (February 1999), pp.484-489, ISSN0019-9567

Min, B. (2008). Basophils: what they "can do" versus what they "actually do". *Nature Immunology*, Vol.9, No.12, (December 2008), pp.1333-1339, ISSN1529-2908

Miyajima, I.; Dombrowicz, D.; Martin, T.R.; Ravetch, J.V.; Kinet, J.P. & Galli, S.J. (1997). Systemic anaphylaxis in the mouse can be mediated largely through IgG1 and FcgammaRIII. Assessment of cardiopulmonary changes, mast cell degranulation, and death associated with active or IgE- or IgG1-dependent passive anaphylaxis. *Journal of Clinical Investigation*, Vol. 99, No.5, (March 1997), pp.901-914, ISSN0021-9738

Moyle, M.; Foster, D.L.; McGrath, D.E, Brown, S.M.; Laroche, Y.; De Meutter, J.; Stanssens, P.; Bogowitz, C.A.; Fried, V.A. & Ely, J.A. (1994). A hookworm glycoprotein that inhibits neutrophil functions is a ligandof the integrin CD11b/CD18. *Journal of Biological Chemistry*,Vol.269, No.13, (April 1994), pp.10008-10015, ISSN1178-6264

Mukai, K.; Matsuoka, K.; Taya, C.; Suzuki, H.; Yokozeki, H.; Nishioka, K.; Hirokawa, K.; Etori, M.; Yamashita, M.; Kubota, T.; Minegishi, Y.; Yonekawa, H.; Karasuyama, H. (2005). Basophils play a critical role in the development of IgE-mediated chronic allergic inflammation independently of T cells and mast cells. *Immunity*, Vol. 23, No. 2, (August 2005), pp.191-202, ISSN1074-7613

Mukai, K.; Obta, K.; Tsujimura, Y. & Karasuyama, H. (2009). New insights into the roles for basophils in acute and chronic allergy. *Allergology International*, Vol.58, No.1, (March 2009), pp.11-19, ISSN1323-8930

Nakagawa, T.; Roth, W.; Wong, P.; Nelson, A.; Farr, A.; Deussing, J.; Villadangos, J.A.; Ploegh, H.; Peters, C. & Rudensky, A.Y. (1998). Cathepsin L: critical role in Ii degradation and CD4 T cell selection in the thymus. *Science*, Vol.280,No.5362, (April 1998), pp.450-453, ISSN0272-4634

Nelms, K.; Keegan, A.D.; Zamorao, J.; Ryan, J.J. & Paul, W.E. (1999). The IL-4 receptor: signaling mechanisms and biologic functions. *Annuals Reviews of Immunology*, Vol.17, (1999), pp.701-738, ISSN0732-0582

Nigou, J.; Zelle-Rieser, C.; Gilleron, M.; Thurnher, M. & Puzo, G. (2001). Mannosylated lipoarabinomannans inhibit IL-12 production by human dendritic cells: evidence for a negative signal delivered through the mannose receptor. *Journal of Immunology*, Vol.166, No.12, (June 2001), pp.7477-7485, ISSN0022-1767

Nimmerjahn, F. & Ravetch, J.V. (2008). Fcγ receptors as regulators of immune responses. *Nature Reviews of Immunology*, Vol.8, No.1, (January. 2008), pp.34-47, ISSN1474-1733

O´Connor, R.A.; Jenson, J.S. & Devaney, E. (2000). No contributes to proliferative suppression in a murine model of filariasis. *Infection and Immunity*, Vol.68, No.11, (November 2000), pp.6101-6107, ISSN0019-9567

Oettgen, H.C.; Martin, T.R.; Wynshaw-Boris, A.; Deng, C.; Drazen, J.M. & Leder, P. (1994). Active anaphylaxis in IgE-deficient mice. *Nature*, Vol.370, No.6488, (August 1994), pp.367-370, ISSN0028-0836

Oettgen, H.C. & Geha, R.S. (1999). IgE in asthma and atopy: cellular and molecular connections. Journal of Clinical Investigation, Vol.104, No.7, (October 1999), pp.829-835, ISSN0021-9738

Oh, K.; Shen, T.; Le Gros, G. & Min, B. (2007). Induction of Th2 type immunity in a mouse system reveals a novel immunoregulatory role of basophils. *Blood*, Vol. 109, No.7, (April 2007), pp.2921-2927, ISSN0006-4971

Okano, M.; Satoskar, A.R.; Nishizaki, K. & Harn, D.A Jr. (2001). Lacto-N-fucopentaose III found on Schistosome mansoni egg antigens functions as adjuvant for proteins by inducing Th2-type response. *Journal of Immunology*, Vol.167, No.1, (July 2001), pp.442-450, ISSN0022-1767

Oshiro, T.M.; Rafael, A.; Enobe, C.S.; Fernandes, I. & Macedo-Soares, M.F.(2004). Comparison of different monoclonal antibodies against immunosuppressive proteins of Ascaris suum. *Brazilian Journal of Medical and Biological Research*, Vol.37, No.2, (February 2004), pp.223-226, ISSN0100-879X

Oshiro, T.M.; Macedo, M.S. & Macedo-Soares, M.F. (2005). Anti-inflammatory activity of PAS-1, a protein component of Ascaris suum. *Inflammation Research*, Vol.54, No.1, (January 2005), pp.17-21, ISSN1023-3830

Oshiro, T.M.; Enobe, C.S.; Araújo, C.A.; Macedo, M.S. & Macedo-Soares, M.F. (2006). PAS-1, a protein affinity purified from Ascaris suum worms, maintain the ability to modulate the immune response to a bystander antigen. *Immunology and Cell Biology*, Vol.84, No.2, (April 2006), pp.138-144, ISSN0818-9641

Paul, W.E. (1997). Interleukin 4: signaling mechanisms and control of T cell differentiation. *Ciba Foundation Symposium*, Vol.204, (1997), pp.208-216, ISSN0300-5208

Pastrana, D.V.; Raghavan, N.; FitzGerald, P.; Eisinger, S.W.; Metz, C.; Bucala, R.; Schleimer, R.P.; Bickel, C & Scott, A.L. (1998). Filarial nematode parasites secrete a homologue of the human cytokine macrophage migration inhibitory factor. *Infection and Immunity*, Vol.66, No.12, (December 1998), pp.5955-5963, ISSN0019-9567

Pearce, E.J. & MacDonald A.S. (2002). The immunobiology of schistosomiasis. *Nature Reviews Immunology*, Vol.2, No.7, (July 2002), pp.499-511, ISSN1474-1733

Pfaff, A.W.; Schulz-Key, H.; Soboslay, P.T.; Taylor, D.W.; MacLennan, K. & Hoffmann, H.W. (2002). Litomosoides sigmodontis cystain acts as an immunomodulator during experimental filariasis. *International Journal of Parasitology*, Vol.32, No.2, (February 2002), pp.171-178, ISSN0020-7519

Playfair, J.H.L. (1982). Immunity to malaria. *British Medical Bulletin*, Vol.38, No.2, (May 1982), pp.153-159, ISSN0007-1420

Pierre, P. & Mellman, I. (1998). Developmental regulation of invariant chain proteolysis controls MHC classII trafficking in mouse dendritic cells. *Cell*,Vol.93, No.7, (June 1998), pp.1135-1145, ISSN0092-8674

Pinckard, R.N.; Halonen, M.; Plamer, J.D.; Butler, C.; Shaw, J.O. & Henson, P.M. (1977). Intravascular aggregation and pulmonary sequestration of platelets during IgE-induced systemic anaphylaxis in the rabbit: abrogation of lethal anaphylactic shock by platelet depletion. *Journal of Immunology*, Vol. 119, No.6, (December 1977), pp. 2185-2193, ISSN0022-1767

Potempa, J.; Korzus, E. & Travis J. (1994).The serpin superfamily of proteinase inhibitors: structure, function and regulation. *Journal of Biological Chemistry*, Vol.269, No.23, (June 1994), pp.15957-15960, ISSN1178-6264

Poulsen, L.K. & Hummelshoj, L. (2007). Triggers of IgE switching and allergy development. *Annals of Medicine*, Vol.39, No.6, (July 2007), pp.440-456, ISSN0785-3890

Pritchard, D.I.; Brown, A.; Kasper, G.; McElroy, P.; Loukas, A.; Hewitt, C.; Berry, C.; Füllkrug, R. & Beck, E. A hookworm allergen which strongly resembles calreticulin. *Parasite Immunology*, Vol.21, No.9, (September 1999), pp.439-450, ISSN0141-9838

Puerta, L.; Fernandez-Caldas, E.; Lockey, R.F. & Caraballo, L.R. (1993). Mite allergy in the tropics: sensitization to six domestic mite species in Cartagena, Colombia. *Journal of Investigational Allergology and Clinical Immunology*, Vol. 3, No.4, (July-August 1993), pp.198-204, ISSN1018-9068

Reyes, J.L. & Terrazas, L.I. (2007). The divergent roles of alternatively acitvated macrophages in helminthic infections. *Parasite Immunology*, Vol.29, No.12, (December 2007), pp.609-619, ISSN0141-9838

Riese, R.J.; Wolf, P.R.; Bromme, D.; Natkin, L.R.; Villadangos, J.A.; Ploegh, H.L. & Chapman, H.A. (1996). Essential role for cathepsin S in MHC classII-associated invariant chain processing and peptide loading. *Immunity*, Vol.4, No.4, (April 1996), pp.357-366, ISSN1074-7613

Rzepecka, J.; Lucius, R.; Dolegalska, M.; Beck, S.; Rausch, S. & Hartmann, S. (2006). Screening for immunomodulatory proteins of the intestinal parasitic nematode Heligmosomoides polygyrus. *Parasite Immunology*, Vol.28, No.9, (September 2006), pp.463-472, ISSN0141-9838

Santiago, H.C.; Bennuru, S.; Boyd, A.; Eberhard, M. & Nutman, T.B. (2011). Structural and immunological cross-reactivity among filarial and mite tropomyosin: implications for the hygiene hypothesis. *Journal of Allergy and Clinical Immunology*, Vol. 127, No. 2, (February 2011), pp.479-486, ISSN0091-6749

Schramm, G.; Mohrs, K.; Wodrich, M.; Doenhoff, M.J.; Pearce, E.J., Haas, H. & Mohrs, M. (2007). IPSE/alpha-1, a glycoprotein from *Schistosoma mansoni* eggs, induces IgE-dependent, antigen-independent IL-4 production by murine basophils in vivo. *Journal of Immunology*, Vol.178, No.10, (May 2007), pp.6023-6027, ISSN0022-1767

Schramm, G.; Falcone, F.H.; Gronow, A.; Haisch, K.; Mamat, U.; Doenhoff, M.J.; Oliveira, G.; Galle, J.; Dahinden, C.A. & Haas, H. (2003). Molecular characterization of an interleukin-4-inducing factor from Schistosoma mansoni eggs. *Journal of Biological Chemistry*, Vol.278, No.20, (May 2003), pp.18384-18392, ISSN1178-6264

Schönemeyer, A.; Lucius, R.; Sonnenburg, B.; Brattig, N.; Sabat, R.; Schilling, K.; Bradley, J. & Hartmann S. (2001). Modulation of human T cell responses and macrophage functions by onchocystatin, a secreted protein of the filarial nematode Onchocerca volvulus. *Journal of Immunology*, Vol.167, No.6, (September 2001), pp.3207-3215, ISSN0022-1767

Scrivener, S.; Yemaneberhan, H.; Zebenigus, M.; Tilahun, D.; Girma, S.; Ali, S.; McElroy, P.; Custovic, A.; Woodcock, A.; Pritchard, D.; Venn, A. & Britton, J. (2001). Independent effects of intestinal parasite infection and domestic allergen exposure on risk of wheeze in Ethiopia: a nested case-control study. *Lancet*, Vol.358, No.9292, (November 2001), pp.1493-1499, ISSN0099-5355

Semnani, R.T.; Liu, A.Y.; Sabzevari, H.; Kubofcik, J.; Ahou, J.; Gilden, J.K. & Nutman, T.B. Brugia malayi microfilariae induce cell death in human dendtric cells, inhibit their ability to make IL-12 and IL-10, and reduce their capacity to activate CD4+ cells. *Journal of Immunology*, Vol.171, No.4, (August 2003), pp.1950-1960, ISSN0022-1767

Shi, G.P.; Bryant, R.A.; Riese, R.; Verhelst, S.; Driessen, C.; Li, Z.; Bromme, D.; Ploegh, H.L. & Chapman, H.A. Role for cathepsin F in invariant processing and major histocompatibility complex classII peptide loading by macrophages. *Journal of Experimental Medicine*, Vol.19, No.7, (April 2000), pp.1177-1186, ISSN0022-1007

Shimoda, K.; van Deursen, J.; Sangster, M.Y.; Sarawar, S.R.; Carson, R.T.; Tripp, R.A.; Chu, C.; Quelle, F.W.; Nosaka, T.; Vignali, D.A.; Doherty, P.C.; Grosveld, G.; Paul, W.E. & Ihle, J.N. (1996). Lack of IL-4 induced Th2 response and IgE class switching in mice with disrupted Stat6 gene. *Nature*, Vol.380, No.6575, (April 1996), pp.630-633, ISSN0028-0836

Simons, F.E.; Frew, A.J.; Ansotegui, I.J.; Bochner, B.S.; Golden, D.B.; Finkelman, F.D.; Leung, D.Y.; Lotvall, J.; Marone, G.; Metcalfe, D.D.; Muller, U.; Rosenwasser, L.J.; Sampson, H.A.; Schwartz, L.B.; van Hage, M. & Walls, A.F. (2007). Risk assessement in anaphylaxis: current and future approaches. *Journal of Allergy and Clinical Immunology*, Vol. 120, No. 1, (July. 2007), pp.S2-24, ISSN0091-6749

Simons, F. (2003). H1-antihistamines: more relevant than ever in the treatment of allergic disorders. *Journal of Allergy and Clinical Immunology*, Vol.112, No.4(Suppl), (October 2003), pp.S42-52, ISSN 0091-6749

Smits, H.H.; Everts, B.; Hartgers, F.C. & Yazdanbakhsh, M. (2010). Chronic helminth infections protect against allergic diseases by active regulatory processes. *Current Allergy and Asthma Reports*, Vol.10, No.1, (January 2010), pp.3-12, ISSN1529-7322

Soares, M.F.M.; Macedo, M.S. & Mota, I. Suppressive effect of an Ascaris suum extract on IgE and IgG antibody responses in mice. *Brazilian Journal of Medical and Biological Research*, Vol., No.2, (1987), pp.203-211, ISSN0100-879X

Soares, M.F.M.; Mota, I. & Macedo, M.S. Isolation of Ascaris suum components which suppress IgE antibody responses. *International Archives of Allergy and Immunology*, Vol.97, No.1, (1992), pp.37-43, ISSN1871-5281

Soares MFM & Araujo CA. Helminth products as a potential therapeutic strategy for inflammatory diseases. *Inflammation and Allergy Drug Targets*, Vol.7, No.2, (June 2008), pp.113-118, ISSN1871-5281

Sokol, C.L.; Barton, G.M.; Farr, A.G. & Medzhitov, R. (2008). A mechanism for the initiation of allergen-induced T helper type 2 responses. *Nature Immunology*, Vol.9, No.3, (Mar 2008), pp.310-8, ISSN1529-2908

Stafforini, D.M.; McIntyre, T.M.; Zimmermann, G.A. & Prescott, S.M. (2003). Platelet-activating factor, a pleiotrophic mediator of physiological and pathological processes. *Critical Reviews in Clinical Laboratory Sciences*, Vol.40, No.6, (2003), pp.643-672, ISSN1040-8363

Steinfelder, S.; Andersen, J.F.; Cannons, J.L.; Feng, C.G.; Joshi, M.; Dwyer, D.; Caspar, P.; Schwartzberg, P.L.; Sher, A. & Jankovic, D. (2009) The major component in schistosome eggs responsible for conditioning dendritic cells for Th2 polarization is a T2 ribonuclease (omega-1). *Journal of Experimental Medicine*, Vol.206, No.8, (August 2009), pp.1681-1690, ISSN0022-1007

Stephenson, L.S.; Latham, M.C. & Ottesen, E.A. (2000). Global malnutrition. Parasitology, *Vol.121, (*2000), pp.S5-22, ISSN0031-1820

Stewart, G.R.; Boussinesq, M.; Coulson, T.; Elson, L.; Nutman, T. & Bradley, J.E. (1999). Onchocerciasis modulates the immune response to mycobacterial antigens. *Clinical and Experimental Immunology,*Vol.117, No.3, (September 1999), pp.571-523, ISSN0009-9104

Strait, R.T.; Morris, S.C.; Yang, M.; Qu, X.W. & Finkelman, F.D. (2002). Pathways of anaphylaxis in the mouse. *Journal of Allergy and Clinical Immunology*, Vol.109, No.4, (April 2002), pp.658-668, ISSN0091-6749

Strait, R.T.; Morris, S.C.; Smiley, K.; Urban, J.F. Jr & Finkelman, F.D. (2003). IL-4 exarcebates anaphylaxis. *Journal of Immunology*, Vol.170, No.7, (April 2003), pp.3835-3842, ISSN0022-1767

Sugimoto, Y.; Iba, Y.; Nakamura, Y.; Kayasuga, R. & Kamei, C. (2004). Pruritus-associated response mediated by cutaneous histamine H3 receptors. *Clinical and Experimental Allergy*, Vol.34, No.3, (March 2004), pp.456-459, ISSN0954-7894

Swain, S.L.; Weinberg, A.D.; English, M. & Huston, G. (1990). IL-4 directs the development of Th2 like helper effectors. *Journal of Immunology*, Vol.145, No.11, (December 1990), pp.3796-3806, ISSN0022-1767

Takai, T. (2005). Fc receptors and their role in immune regulation and autoimmunity. *Journal of Clinical Immunology*, Vol. 25, No.1, (January 2005), pp.1-18, ISSN0271-9142

Terrazas, L.I.; Walsh, K.L.; Piskorska, D.; McGuire, E.& Harn, D.A Jr. (2001). The schistosome oligosaccharide lacto-N-neotetraose expands Gr1(+) cells that secrete anti-inflammatory cytokinse and inhibit proliferation of naive CD4(+) cells: a potential mechanism for immune polarization in helminth infections. *Journal of Immunology*, Vol.167, No.9, (September 2001), pp.5412-5416, ISSN0022-1767

Tiselius A & Kabat EA. (1939). An eletrophoretic study of immune sera and purified antibody preparations. *Journal of Experimental Medicine*, Vol.69, No.1, (January 1939), pp.119-131, ISSN0022-1007

Thurmond, R.L.; Desai, P.J.; Dunford, P.J.; Fung-Leung, W.P.; Hofstra, C.L., Jiang, W.; Nguyen, S.; Riley, J.P.; Sun, S.; Williams, K.N.; Edwards, J.P. and Karlsson, L. (2004). A potent and selective histamine H4 receptor antagonist with anti-inflammatory properties. *Journal of Pharmacology and Experimental Therapeutics*, Vol.309, No.1, (April 2004), pp.401-413, ISSN0022-3565

Truong, M.J.; Gruart, V.; Kusnierz, J.P.; Papin, J.P.; Loiseau, S.; Capron, A. & Capron M. (1993). Human neutrophils express immunoglobulin E (IgE)-binding proteins (Mac-2/epsilon BP) of the S-type lectin family: role in IgE-dependent activation. *Journal of Experimental Medicine*, Vol.177, No.1, (January 1993), pp.243-248, ISSN0022-1007

Tsujimura, Y.; Obata, K.; Mukai, K.; Shindou, H.; Yoshida, M.; Nishikado, H.; Kawano, Y.; Minegishi, Y.; Shimizu, T. & Karasuyama, H. (2008). Basophils play a pivotal role in immunoglobulin-G-mediated but not immunoglobulin-E-mediated systemic anaphylaxis. *Immunity*, Vol.28, No.4, (April 2008), pp.581-589, ISSN1074-7613

Ujike, A.; Ishikawa, Y.; Ono, M.; Yuasa, T.; Yoshino, T.; Fukumoto, M.; Ravetch, J.V. & Takai, T. (1999). Modulation of immunoglobulin(Ig)E-mediated systemic anaphylaxis by low-affinity Fc receptor for IgG. *Journal of Experimental Medicine*, Vol.189, No.10, (May 1999), pp.1573-1519, ISSN0022-1007

Urbina, C.; Ortiz, C. & Hurtado, I. (1981). A new look at basophil in mice. *International Archives of Allergy and Applied Immunology*, Vol. 66, No.2, (1981), pp.158-160, ISSN0020-4793

Vadas, P.; Gold, M.; Perelman, B.; Liss, G.M.; Lack, G.; Blyth, T.; Simons, F.E.; Simons, K.J.; Cass, D. & Yeung, J. (2008). Platelet-activating factor, PAF acetylhydrolase, and severe anaphylaxis. *New England Journal of Medicine*, Vol.358, No.1, (January 2008), pp.28-35, ISSN0028-4793

van der Kleij, D.; Latz, E.; Brouwers, J.F.; Kruize, Y.C.; Schmitz, M.; Kurt-Jones, E.A.; Espervik, T.; de Jong, E.C.; Kapsenberg, M.L.; Golenbock, D.T.; Tielens, A.G. & Yazdanbakhsh, M. (2002). A novel host-parasite lipid cross-talk. Schistosomal lyso-phosphatideylserine activates toll-like receptor 2 and affects immune polarization. *Journal of Biological Chemistry*, Vol.277, No.50, (December 2002), pp.48122-48129, ISSN1178-6264

van Riet, E.; Hartgers, F.C. & Yazdanbakhsh, M. (2007). Chronic helminth infections induce immunomodulation: consequences and mechanisms. *Immunobiology*, Vol.212, No.6, (April 2007), pp.475-490, ISSN0175-2985

Verity, C.K.; Loukas, A.; McManus, D.P. & Brindley, P.J. (2001). Schistosoma japonicum cathepsin D aspartic protease cleaves human IgG and other serum components. *Parasitology*, Vol.122, No.4, (April 2001), pp.415-421, ISSN0031-1820

Williams, A.F. & Barclay, A.N. (1998). The immunoglobulin superfamily - domains for cell surface recognition. *Annual Reviews of Immunology*, Vol.6, (1988), pp.381-405, ISSN0732-0582

Wilson, M.S.; Mentink-Kane, M.M.; Pesce, J.T.; Ramalingam, T.R.; Thompson, R. & Wynn, T.A. (2007). Immunopathology of schistosomiasis. *Immunology and Cell Biology*, Vol.85, No.2, (February-March. 2007), pp.148-154, ISBN0818-9641

Winbery, S.L. & Lieberman, P.L. (2002). Histamine and antihistamines in anaphylaxis. *Clinical Allergy and Immunology*, Vol. 17, (2002), pp. 287-317, ISSN1075-7910

Zang, X.; Yazdanbakhsh, M.; Jinag, H.; Kanost, M.R & Maizels, R.M. (1999). A novel serpin expressed by blood-borne microfilariae of the parasitic nematode Brugia malayi inhibits human neutrophil serine proteinase. *Blood*, Vol.94, No.4, (August 1999), pp.1418-1428, ISSN0006-4971

26

Parasite-Derived Proteins Inhibit Allergic Specific Th2 Response

Hak Sun Yu
Department of Parasitology, School of Medicine,
Pusan National University, Yangsan-si,
South Korea

1. Introduction

The prevalence of allergic disease and asthma has increased dramatically during the last 30-40 years. Atopic disorders comprise a range of allergic diseases including asthma, anaphylaxis, allergic rhinitis, and atopic dermatitis; these diseases have been seen a precipitous increase in the last four decades. Intriguingly, geographic regions with a high helminth infection burden tend to have a lower incidence of asthma (1). The effects of parasitic infections on the incidence of allergic disease has been receiving increased attention from researchers of late, with studies conducted in Ethiopia and Gabon demonstrating that parasitic infestation is associated with reduced atopic sensitization and dust mite skin test sensitivity (2-4). Children treated repeatedly for *Trichuris trichiura* and *Ascaris lumbricoides* exhibited increased dust-mite skin responses as compared with children that had not been treated for asymptomatic soil-associated helminthic infections (5). Several molecules from helminthes induce pronounced Th2 responses in a manner similar to that seen in cases of full-blown parasitic infection. Excretory-secretory (ES) glycoproteins isolated from the rodent nematode, *Nippostrongylus brasiliensis,* have been shown to evidence Th2-promoting activity on dendrite cells, however, the exact nature of the molecules involved in *N. brasiliensis* ES proteins remain to be clearly elucidated. This activity is heat-labile and protease-sensitive, thereby suggesting that the active component is proteinaceous in nature (6). Also, in schistosomiasis, the soluble extract of *Schistosoma mansoni* eggs (SEA) was shown to induce SEA-specific Th2 responses when injected into mice (7), and SEA was also demonstrated to condition human dendrite cells (DCs) to polarize Th response in a Th2 direction *in vitro* (8). When exposed to Th2 cytokines, these molecules can also activate host CD4+CD25$^+$Foxp3$^+$ T cells (regulatory T cells, T_{reg}) which subsequently release IL-10 and tumor growth factor β (TGF-β), which may be functionally involved in the suppression of the level of Th2 cytokines IL-4, IL-5, and IL-13. These parasites can establish a chronic infection, which highlights important issues (9), in that the presence of these metabolically active pathogens indicates that the immune system is being relentlessly challenged with foreign antigens; this continuous immune reactivity, if uncontrolled, could eventuate severe pathology. In addition, these pathogens may have developed evolutionary strategies by which they may evade the immune system for long-term survival in an immunocompetent host (10).

In order to ascertain, then, whether parasitic infections can reduce allergic reactions and whether their infective stage influences the immune system of the host, we have mimicked chronic infection conditions in our experiment via treatment with parasite-derived proteins for one month prior to allergen treatment. We attempted to determine whether or not these parasite-derived proteins suppressed allergy-specific Th2 reactions.

2. Immunization of parasite derived proteins inhibits allergic specific Th2 response

Long-lived parasites are highly accomplished practitioners of immune evasion and manipulation, utilizing strategies honed during their long co-evolutionary interaction with the mammalian immune system (10, 11). How is the host affected by these parasitic strategies? Although many hypotheses have been advanced, until the present time there has been little evidence to support these theories. Th2 host response as the result of parasitic infection was apparent, although this is the result of parasitic strategies to escape from the host immune system or the result of a human protective system associated with parasitic infection. Additionally, we could readily detect Th2 responses in allergic patients. Thus, until now, there has been considerable controversy regarding the relationship between parasites and allergic reactions; particularly, whether parasites can evoke some allergic-specific response or can reduce allergen-specific responses (12-14).

We have attempted to determine whether parasite-derived proteins can accelerate or reduce asthma symptoms in accordance with the treatment period (15). We have mimicked chronic infection conditions in our experiment via treatment with parasite (*Toxascaris leonina* adult worm)-derived proteins [ES protein (Tl-ES) and total proteins (Tl-TP)] for one month prior to the administration of allergen treatment. We mentioned this group as Immunized group; also Challenged with OVA group were mentioned which were administrated Tl-ES and Tl-TP at the same challenge days in airway allergic reaction procedure. As results, the immunized Tl-ES and Tl-TP groups evidenced a thinning of the bronchial epithelial and muscle layer, a disruption and shedding of the epithelial cells, a reduction in the number of goblet cells as compared to the OVA-challenged groups (Fig. 1). When the airway functions of these mice were monitored, we detected that the Penh values by methacholine treatment (from 2.5 mg/ml to 25 mg/ml) were significantly higher in the OVA-inhalation mice than those of Tl-TP and Tl-ES immunized group (Fig. 2A). The numbers of most inflammatory cells (macrophages, eosinophils, lymphocytes and neutrophils) in the BAL fluids were significantly increased in all of the OVA-challenged groups (Fig. 2B & 2C). The administration of Tl-ES and Tl-TP prior to asthma induction (immunized group) and the Tl-ES and Tl-TP with OVA challenge (challenged with OVA groups) evidenced inhibited recruitment of inflammatory cells into the airway (Fig. 2B & 2C). In particular, neutrophils and lymphocytes were significantly reduced by the parasite proteins at any administration time (p value < 0.05). The total number of eosinophils of the immunized and OVA-challenged group were slightly reduced; however, this reduction was not statistically significant (P value > 0.05).

Although some articles have previously asserted that nematodes can induce allergic reactions during their larval migration period (16, 17), many articles have reported that parasitic infections, particularly chronic parasitism, help to reduce host allergic reactions and to modulate host immune responses (14, 18, 19). We have determined that immunization with *T. leonina* adult worm ES and total proteins induces a down-regulation of asthma-associated cytokines, including IL-4 and IL-5, in the bronchial alveolar lavage (BAL) fluids (Fig. 3). However, these proteins did not significantly influence allergic airway inflammation response as the result of simultaneous OVA challenge, as compared to the immunization method. In particular, the Tl-ES treatment with OVA challenge group exhibited more severe lung inflammation than was observed in the immunized group. We believe that certain allergens or proteases might be included in the ES proteins, and parasitic proteases have also been identified as allergens (20-23). Sokol *et al.* previously suggested that a host-derived sensor of proteolytic activity might involve cleavage via parasite or allergic proteases. This sensor, once cleaved, activates the cells of the innate immune system to induce a Th2 response (13).

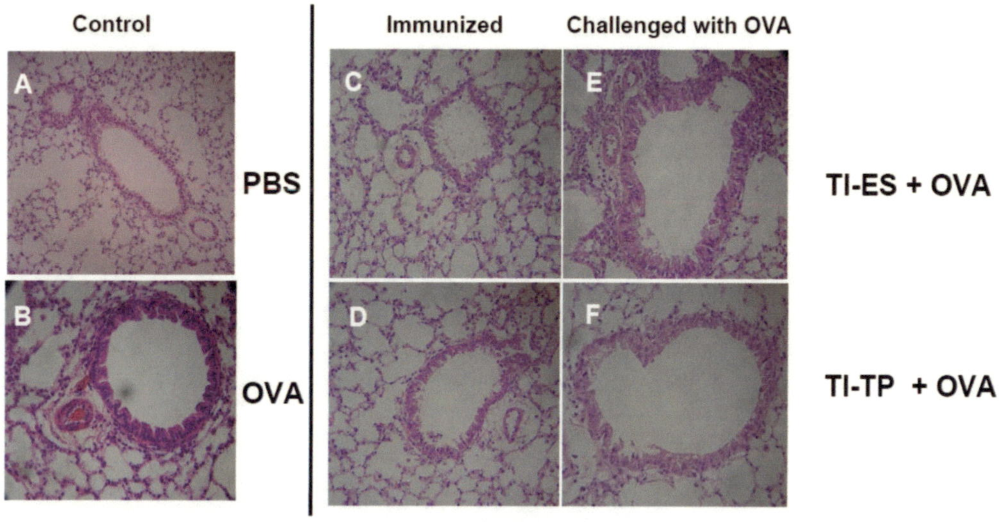

Fig. 1. **Histological findings of airway inflammation in ova-challenged control mice and the effect of immunization and challenge with OVA groups.** Female and 6 weeks of age mice were induced airway allergic reaction using intraperitoneally (I.P.) sensitizing with 75 ug of ovalbumin (OVA, Sigma, Grade V) and 2 mg of aluminium hydroxide gel, on days 0 and 7. One week after the final sensitization, the mice were intra nasal challenged with 50 ug of OVA on 4 consecutive days (days 13, 14, 19, and 20). We mentioned "Immunized group" that were injected by I.P. with 100 ul of 10 ug/ml *Toxascaris leonina* excretory-secretory (Tl-ES) and *T. leonina* total protein (Tl-TP), respectively, on 7 and 14 days before airway allergic reaction procedure. Also "Challenged with OVA" group were mentioned which were injected by I.P. with 100 ul of 10 ug/ml of Tl-ES and Tl-TP respectively at the same challenge days in airway allergic reaction procedure. The negative control group was challenged with PBS (I.N.) on the same challenge day in airway allergic reaction procedure. A; PBS-treated, B-F; OVA+ alum-treated (induced asthma), (C) immunized Tl-ES protein, (D) immunized Tl-TP, (E) Tl-ES protein treatment with OVA challenge, (F) Tl-TP protein with OVA challenge.

IL-4 has been demonstrated to regulate isotype class switching in B cells to IgE synthesis, and IL-5 stimulates eosinophil growth, activates these cells, and prolongs eosinophil survival. *T. leonina*-derived proteins could inhibit increases in the levels of IL-4 and IL-5 from OVA challenge. In particular, the level of IL-4 in the BAL fluid in the immunized group was almost half of that observed in the OVA-only challenge group. This result was consistent with the results regarding the IgE concentration in the blood (15). Although levels of the IL-5 cytokine of *T. leonina* ES and total protein-immunized mice were lower than those observed in asthma control mice, this effect was not remarkable. Also, the total number of eosinophils was not substantially reduced as the result of immunization. Eosinophils and IgE proved vitally important in allergy-induced Th2 response; additionally, the elevation of the numbers of these cells and IgE levels were identified as specific responses to parasite infection and this response was shown to be elicited only by treatment with parasite total proteins (24, 25).

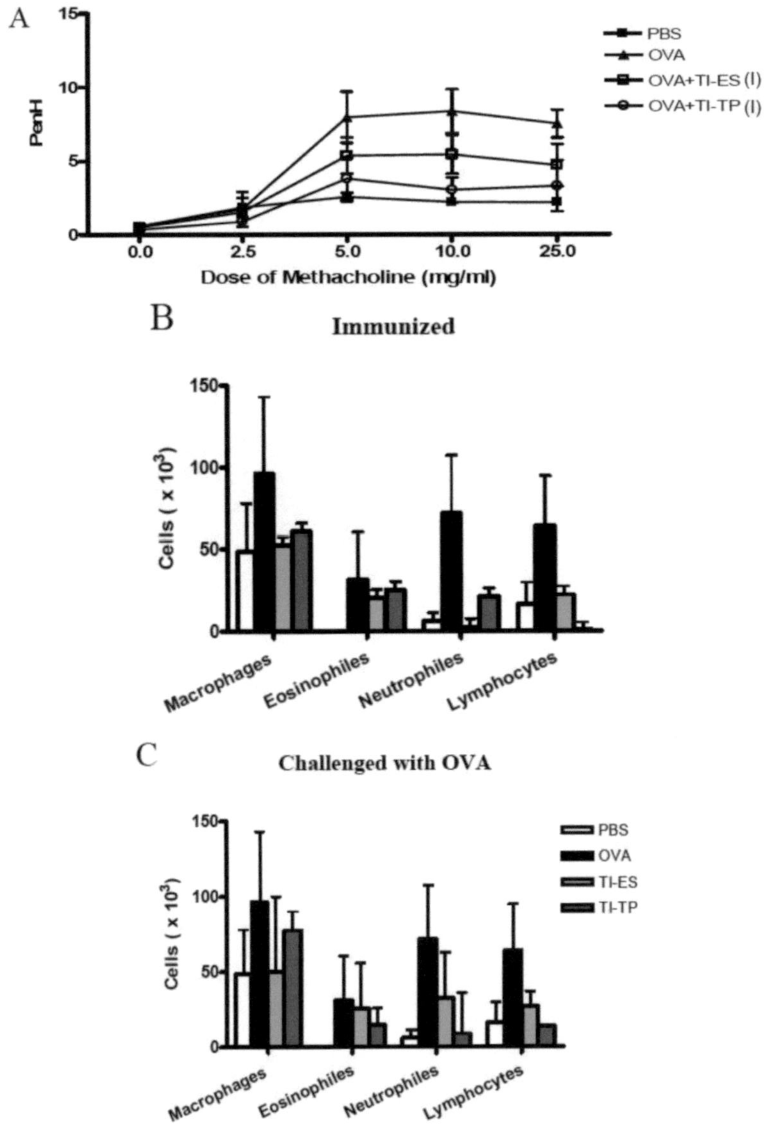

Fig. 2. **Airway hyperresponsiveness measurements and comparison of differential cell counts obtained via airway inflammation in ova-sensitized PBS mice and the effects in immunized and OVA-challenged groups**. Total protein of *T. leonina* immunization group [Tl-TP (I)] has lower penh value than those of OVA challenge group (A). The numbers of inflammatory cells were significantly lower in the parasite-derived protein-treated mice (B & C). The data were expressed as the means ± SD of individual mice.

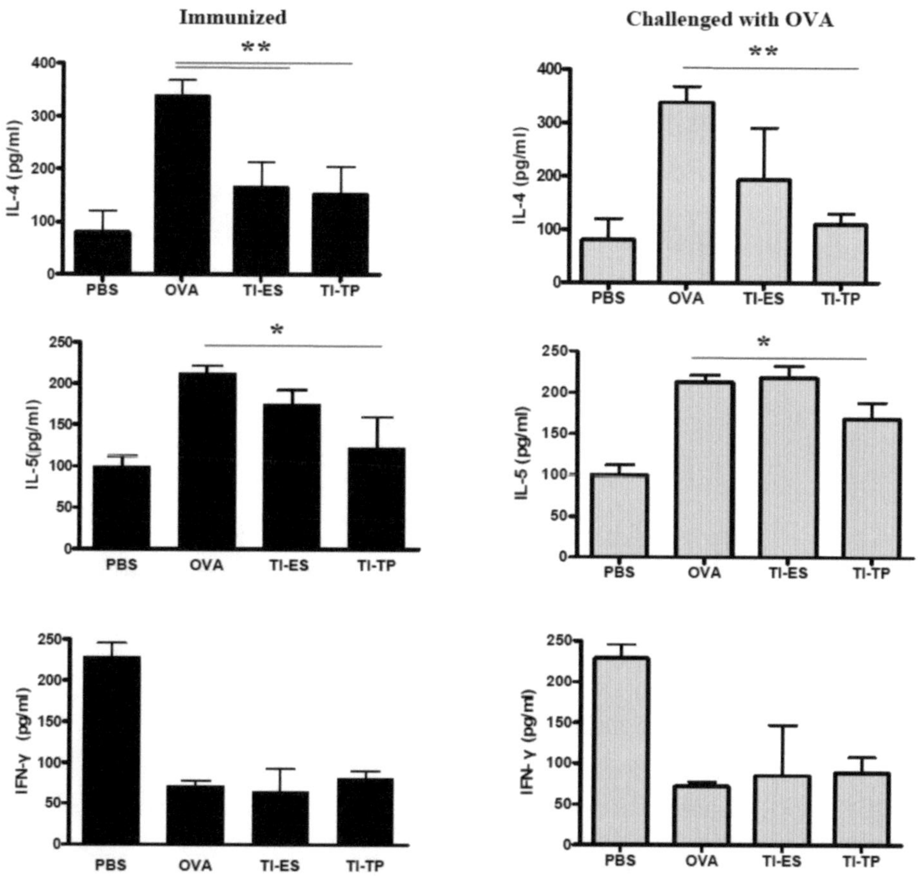

Fig. 3. **Th1 and Th2 cytokines levels in the BAL fluids of Tl-ES and Tl-TP treated mice.** The levels of all Th2 cytokines of the immunized group were contrasted with those of the OVA-challenged control mice. The data were expressed as the means ± SD of individual mice (* ; p value <0.05, **; p value <0.01).

How does helminth infection protect against allergy? Many hypotheses have been advanced thus far regarding this theme. One of these hypotheses is that non-specific IgE generated as the result of helminthic infection may inhibit allergen-specific IgE binding sites on mast cells or basophils. Although Jarrett suggested in 1980 that parasite-induced 'nonspecific' IgE does not protect against host allergic reactions (26). However, other scientists have suggested that nonspecific IgE can modulate host immune responses, as in the case of insulin-dependent diabetes, as well as Th2 response by allergens (25, 27-29). The other hypothesis states that helminth parasites stimulate the production of immunoregulatory mediators, which are likely to perform a function in the maintenance of the chronicity of infection, with no marked induction of pathology. In particular, elevated IL-10 levels have been associated previously with protection against allergic diseases in helminth-infected African children (4). Helminth infections can induce T_{reg} cells from hosts, and these cells secrete IL-10 and suppress the proliferation of other CD4+ T cells (30-32). We also found that parasite proteins could also induce the IL-10 cytokine, particularly in the Tl-TP immunized group (Fig. 4).

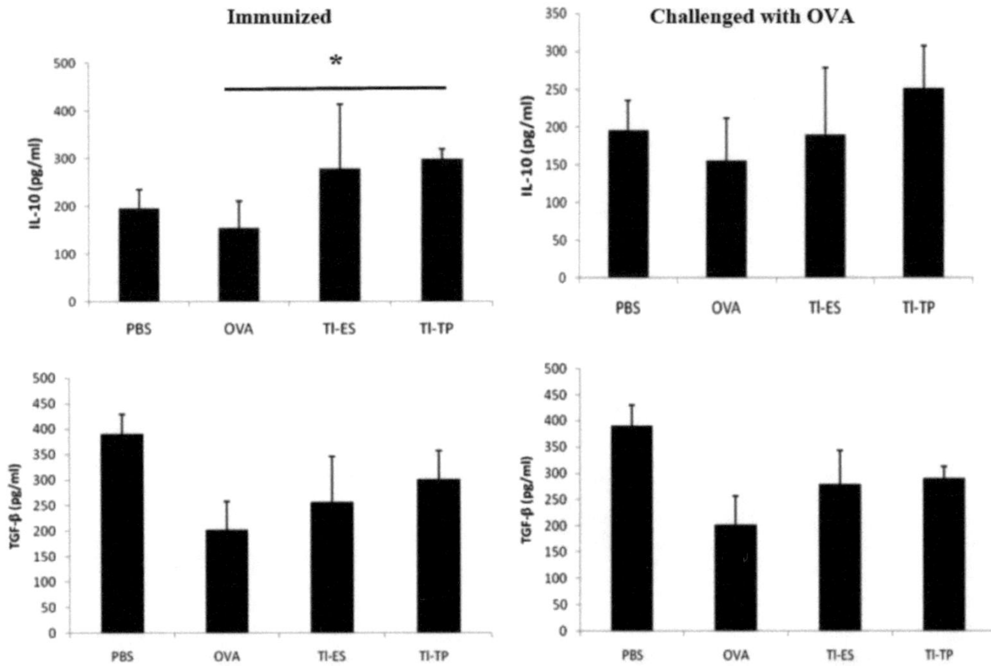

Fig. 4. **T_{reg} cell related cytokines levels in the BAL fluids of Tl-ES and Tl-TP treated mice.** The data were expressed as the means ± SD of individual mice (* ; p value <0.05, **; p value <0.01).

Finally, the data presented herein demonstrate that *T. leonina*-derived proteins may perform a crucial function in resistance against Th2 immune responses. We suggested that this inhibition may be related to the IL-10 cytokine, which was induced by parasite proteins. Further steps are currently being taken in an effort to gain a greater understanding of the molecular basis of immune evasion by nematodes. Thus, we are attempting to gain new insights into the immune regulation strategies of nematodes, and the growing number of new strategies employed by parasites to exert their marked down-regulatory effects.

3. Macrophage migration inhibitory factor homologues of parasite suppress Th2 response in allergic airway inflammation model via T_{reg} cell recruitment

A number of parasite-derived proteins, glycoconjugates, and small lipid moieties have been demonstrated to perform known or hypothesized functions in immune interference. Other researchers have already isolated several other immune downregulatory molecules from parasites, and these molecules have been identified as mammal cytokine homologues, protease inhibitors, abundant larval transcript antigens, glyco-networks, and venom allergen-like proteins (33-39). The cytokine network is a crucial component of host defense against pathogens. It is not, therefore, surprising to find that one of the immune evasion strategies utilized by infectious organisms is the generation of mammalian cytokine homologues, including TGF-β and the macrophage migration inhibitory factor (MIF) (40, 41).

MIF was described initially as one of the earliest cytokines to be derived from activated T-cells, and was believed to prevent the random migration of macrophages (42). MIF has also been demonstrated to be generated abundantly by monocytes/macrophages and to function in an autocrine/paracrine manner in the upregulation and sustenance of the activation of diverse cell types (43). The profile of the activities of MIF, both *in vivo* and *in vitro,* is reflective of a role for MIF in the pathogenesis of a variety of inflammatory diseases, including rheumatoid arthritis, inflammatory bowel disease, ankylosing spondylitis, and psoriasis (44). MIF performs a crucial function in airway inflammation and airway hyper-responsiveness in asthma (45).

Recently, several MIF homologues have been isolated from parasitic nematodes. Two types of MIF homologues have thus far been identified in nematodes (34). The type 1 MIF homologues bear a greater amino acid similarity with the mammalian MIFs than do the type 2 MIF homologues (46). The type 1 MIF homologues isolated from *Brugia malayi* (Bm-MIF1) induce eosinophil recruitment, and alternatively activated macrophage recruitment *in vivo* when injected into the peritoneal cavities of mice. Mutation of the conserved proline residue induces the abrogation of this activity (47). This ability of parasite MIF homologues was similar to those of mammalian MIF. However, recently Cho et al. reported that hookworm MIF (structurally type 2 MIF) functions differently from mammalian MIF (48, 49).

We have cloned another type 2 MIF homologue (As-MIF) from *Anisakis simplex* (whale worm) 3rd stage larva, which causes anisakidosis in humans (50). Recombinant As-MIF (rAs-MIF) proved highly effective with regard to the inhibition of goblet cell hyperplasia and inflammatory responses in the airways of OVA-induced asthma model mice (Fig. 5). Increasing concentrations of rAs-MIF induced an increase in the anti-inflammatory effects on asthma model mice. Additionally, the function of rAs-MIF was antagonized as compared to the function of host MIF (59).

How does As-MIF suppress allergy responses in mice? There have been many reports demonstrating that Th2-type effector responses may be regulated by T_{reg} cells (51-53). Additionally, nematode infections can induce and expand naturally occurring T_{reg} cells in both humans and mice (4, 54), thereby suggesting a role for these T_{reg} cells in the helminth-induced modulation of inflammatory diseases (55, 56). In particular, the clinical symptoms of allergic airway inflammation in the mouse model was clearly modulated by T_{reg} cell mediated immune suppression, which was itself activated by helminth infection or antigen treatment (57, 58). We could determine the increase in T_{reg} cells as the result of rAs-MIF treatment in OVA-alum asthma-induced mice (Fig. 6).

IL-10 and TGF-β were produced primarily by T_{reg} cells, and they are known to suppress immune response effects. The IL-10 and TGF-β levels measured in BALFs from rAs-MIF-treated asthma-induced mice were higher than those of the asthma-induced mice; the IL-10 and TGF-β levels occurred in accordance with their treated concentrations (59). The helminthic parasites stimulate the production of immunoregulatory mediators, which likely perform a function in the maintenance of the chronicity of infection, without any marked induction of pathology. In particular, elevated IL-10 levels have been associated with responses against allergic diseases in helminth-infected individuals (4). Also, Nagler-Anderson *et al.* showed that in mice sensitized with peanut plus cholera toxin, anti-IL-10 treatment abrogated the ability of helminths to protect against allergic symptoms and to downregulate allergen-specific IgE. IL-10, which is referred to as the cytokine synthesis inhibitory factor, is an anti-inflammatory cytokine, which is capable of inhibiting the synthesis of pro-inflammatory cytokines (60). The IL-10 requirement is critical to several important human diseases, including schistosomiasis, wherein marked increases in host morbidity and mortality are observed when IL-10 levels are low or absent (61). In cases of murine *S. mansoni* infection, IL-10 attenuates the hepatocyte damage induced by the eggs of the parasite. IL-10 is also essential for the maintenance of non-lethal chronic infections, in addition to the inhibition of inappropriate immune responses in experimental models (62). TGF-β1 is also a strong candidate for immune suppression by T_{reg} cells from helminth-infected mice, and has already been recognized to alleviate experimental airway allergy symptoms (63) and to instruct peripheral T cells to develop their regulatory capacities (64). Thus, the inhibition of asthma response by rAs-MIF may be associated with the principal T_{reg} cell–associated downregulatory cytokines, including TGF-β1 and IL-10.

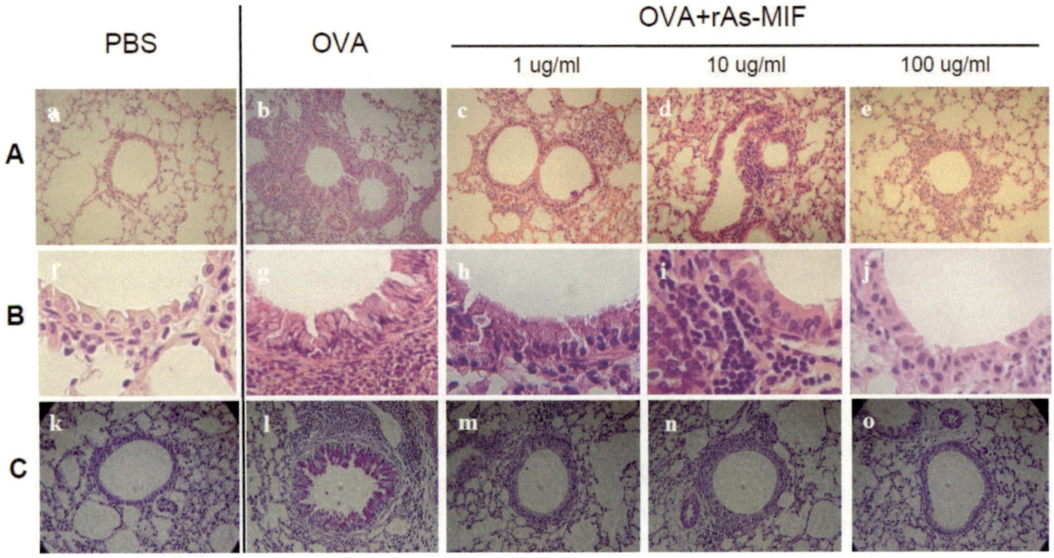

Fig. 5. **Histologic appearance of lungs after challenge with PBS, OVA, and rAs-MIF by concentration (H-E stain).** (A; x 100, B; x 600; C; PAS stain), C; **a**, **f**, and **k**; phosphate-buffered saline (PBS) treated, **b-e**, **g-j**, and **l-o**; OVA plus alum-treated (induced asthma), **c**, **h** and **m**; challenged with 1 μg/ml rAs-MIF, **d**, **i**, and **n**; challenged with 10 μg/ml rAs-MIF. **e**, **j**, and **o**; challenged with 100μg/ml rAs-MIF. In asthma-induced mice, a massive peri-bronchial infiltration with immune-related cells and hyperplasia of bronchial epithelial cells were observed. Upon challenge with 1μg/ml rAs-MIF treatment (**c**, **h** and **m**), asthma-induced mice evidenced thinner bronchial epithelial cells than were observed in the asthma-induced mice (**b**, **g**, and **l**). Mice challenged with treatment with 10 and 100μg/ml rAs-MIF evidenced thinner than normal bronchial epithelial cells and decreased numbers of immune-related cells. Goblet cells and immune-related cells in the airway walls of mice exposed to PBS, OVA and OVA challenge with 1, 10, and 100 μg/ml rAs-MIF. In asthma-induced mice (g), a massive peri-bronchial infiltration of inflammatory cells and hyperplasia of bronchial epithelial cells were detected. However, goblet cell hyperplasia was reduced in the bronchial epithelial cells of the rAs-MIF-treated mice (h-j).

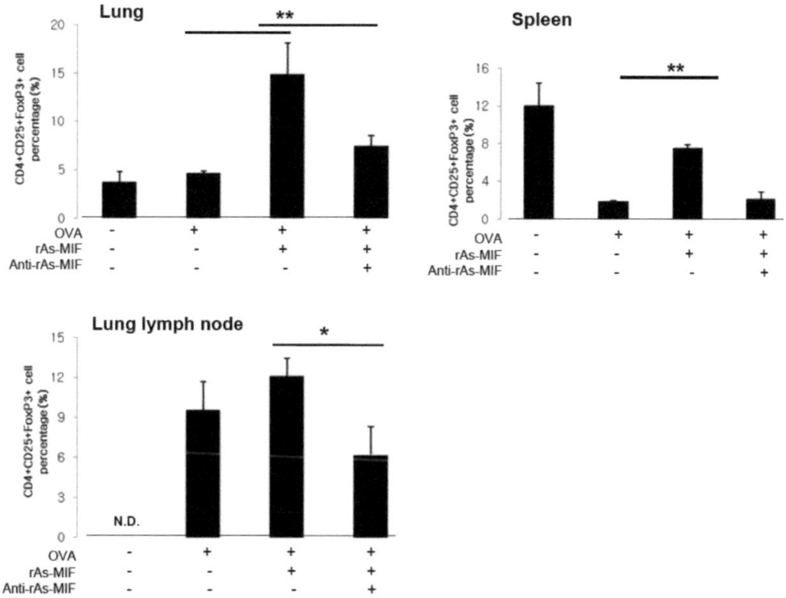

Fig. 6. T_{reg} cell production could be induced by rAs-MIF treatment. T_{reg} cell populations in the lungs and spleen were significantly increased by rAs-MIF treatment, but this effect was inhibited by rAnti-As-MIF. (*; $p < 0.05$, **; $p < 0.01$, $n = 5$ mice per group, 3 independent experiments).

4. Conclusion

We showed that parasite derived proteins may perform a crucial function in resistance against allergic airway inflammation via IL-10 cytokine induction and Treg cell recruitment. Parasites regulate or suppress their host immune response, maintaining their parasitism for a prolonged period, using unknown molecules. As-MIF might be one of the molecules that affect host immune regulation. The further characterization of parasite derived proteins might ultimately result in the design of novel therapeutic intervention strategies for the treatment of asthma.

5. References

[1] Zaccone, P., Z. Fehervari, J. M. Phillips, D. W. Dunne, and A. Cooke. 2006. Parasitic worms and inflammatory diseases. *Parasite immunology* 28:515-523.

[2] Scrivener, S., H. Yemaneberhan, M. Zebenigus, D. Tilahun, S. Girma, S. Ali, P. McElroy, A. Custovic, A. Woodcock, D. Pritchard, A. Venn, and J. Britton. 2001. Independent effects of intestinal parasite infection and domestic allergen exposure on risk of wheeze in Ethiopia: a nested case-control study. *Lancet* 358:1493-1499.

[3] Dagoye, D., Z. Bekele, K. Woldemichael, H. Nida, M. Yimam, A. Hall, A. J. Venn, J. R. Britton, R. Hubbard, and S. A. Lewis. 2003. Wheezing, allergy, and parasite

infection in children in urban and rural Ethiopia. *Am J Respir Crit Care Med* 167:1369-1373.

[4] van den Biggelaar, A. H., R. van Ree, L. C. Rodrigues, B. Lell, A. M. Deelder, P. G. Kremsner, and M. Yazdanbakhsh. 2000. Decreased atopy in children infected with Schistosoma haematobium: a role for parasite-induced interleukin-10. *Lancet* 356:1723-1727.

[5] van den Biggelaar, A. H., L. C. Rodrigues, R. van Ree, J. S. van der Zee, Y. C. Hoeksma-Kruize, J. H. Souverijn, M. A. Missinou, S. Borrmann, P. G. Kremsner, and M. Yazdanbakhsh. 2004. Long-term treatment of intestinal helminths increases mite skin-test reactivity in Gabonese schoolchildren. *J Infect Dis* 189:892-900.

[6] Balic, A., Y. Harcus, M. J. Holland, and R. M. Maizels. 2004. Selective maturation of dendritic cells by Nippostrongylus brasiliensis-secreted proteins drives Th2 immune responses. *Eur J Immunol* 34:3047-3059.

[7] MacDonald, A. S., A. D. Straw, B. Bauman, and E. J. Pearce. 2001. CD8- dendritic cell activation status plays an integral role in influencing Th2 response development. *J Immunol* 167:1982-1988.

[8] de Jong, E. C., P. L. Vieira, P. Kalinski, J. H. Schuitemaker, Y. Tanaka, E. A. Wierenga, M. Yazdanbakhsh, and M. L. Kapsenberg. 2002. Microbial compounds selectively induce Th1 cell-promoting or Th2 cell-promoting dendritic cells in vitro with diverse th cell-polarizing signals. *J Immunol* 168:1704-1709.

[9] Allen, J. E., and R. M. Maizels. 1996. Immunology of human helminth infection. *Int Arch Allergy Immunol* 109:3-10.

[10] Behnke, J. M., C. J. Barnard, and D. Wakelin. 1992. Understanding chronic nematode infections: evolutionary considerations, current hypotheses and the way forward. *Int J Parasitol* 22:861-907.

[11] Maizels, R. M., D. A. Bundy, M. E. Selkirk, D. F. Smith, and R. M. Anderson. 1993. Immunological modulation and evasion by helminth parasites in human populations. *Nature* 365:797-805.

[12] Demirturk, N., E. Kozan, T. Demirdal, F. Fidan, O. C. Aktepe, M. Unlu, and Z. Asci. 2007. Effect of parasitosis on allergic sensitization in rats sensitized with ovalbumin: interaction between parasitosis and allergic sensitization. *Adv Ther* 24:1305-1313.

[13] Sokol, C. L., G. M. Barton, A. G. Farr, and R. Medzhitov. 2007. A mechanism for the initiation of allergen-induced T helper type 2 responses. *Nat Immunol.*

[14] van Riet, E., F. C. Hartgers, and M. Yazdanbakhsh. 2007. Chronic helminth infections induce immunomodulation: consequences and mechanisms. *Immunobiology* 212:475-490.

[15] Lee, K. H., H. K. Park, H. J. Jeong, S. K. Park, S. J. Lee, S. H. Choi, M. K. Cho, M. S. Ock, Y. C. Hong, and H. S. Yu. 2008. Immunization of proteins from Toxascaris leonina adult worm inhibits allergic specific Th2 response. *Veterinary parasitology* 156:216-225.

[16] Kim, J. S., K. H. Kim, S. Cho, H. Y. Park, S. W. Cho, Y. T. Kim, K. H. Joo, and J. S. Lee. 2005. Immunochemical and biological analysis of allergenicity with excretory-

secretory products of anisakis simplex third stage larva. *Int Arch Allergy Immunol* 136:320-328.

[17] Baeza, M. L., A. Rodriguez, V. Matheu, M. Rubio, P. Tornero, M. de Barrio, T. Herrero, M. Santaolalla, and J. M. Zubeldia. 2004. Characterization of allergens secreted by Anisakis simplex parasite: clinical relevance in comparison with somatic allergens. *Clin Exp Allergy* 34:296-302.

[18] Flohr, C., L. N. Tuyen, S. Lewis, R. Quinnell, T. T. Minh, H. T. Liem, J. Campbell, D. Pritchard, T. T. Hien, J. Farrar, H. Williams, and J. Britton. 2006. Poor sanitation and helminth infection protect against skin sensitization in Vietnamese children: A cross-sectional study. *The Journal of allergy and clinical immunology* 118:1305-1311.

[19] Wang, C. C., T. J. Nolan, G. A. Schad, and D. Abraham. 2001. Infection of mice with the helminth Strongyloides stercoralis suppresses pulmonary allergic responses to ovalbumin. *Clin Exp Allergy* 31:495-503.

[20] Kobayashi, Y., S. Ishizaki, K. Shimakura, Y. Nagashima, and K. Shiomi. 2007. Molecular cloning and expression of two new allergens from Anisakis simplex. *Parasitology research* 100:1233-1241.

[21] Shaw, R. J., M. M. McNeill, D. R. Maass, W. R. Hein, T. K. Barber, M. Wheeler, C. A. Morris, and C. B. Shoemaker. 2003. Identification and characterisation of an aspartyl protease inhibitor homologue as a major allergen of Trichostrongylus colubriformis. *International journal for parasitology* 33:1233-1243.

[22] Furmonaviciene, R., H. F. Sewell, and F. Shakib. 2000. Comparative molecular modelling identifies a common putative IgE epitope on cysteine protease allergens of diverse sources. *Clin Exp Allergy* 30:1307-1313.

[23] Holt, D. C., K. Fischer, G. E. Allen, D. Wilson, P. Wilson, R. Slade, B. J. Currie, S. F. Walton, and D. J. Kemp. 2003. Mechanisms for a novel immune evasion strategy in the scabies mite sarcoptes scabiei: a multigene family of inactivated serine proteases. *The Journal of investigative dermatology* 121:1419-1424.

[24] Ishizaka, T., J. Urban, Jr., K. Takatsu, and K. Ishizaka. 1976. Immunoglobulin E synthesis in parasite infection. *The Journal of allergy and clinical immunology* 58:523-538.

[25] Ehigiator, H. N., A. W. Stadnyk, and T. D. Lee. 2000. Extract of Nippostrongylus brasiliensis stimulates polyclonal type-2 immunoglobulin response by inducing De novo class switch. *Infection and immunity* 68:4913-4922.

[26] Jarrett, E., S. Mackenzie, and H. Bennich. 1980. Parasite-induced 'nonspecific' IgE does not protect against allergic reactions. *Nature* 283:302-304.

[27] Imai, S., H. Tezuka, Y. Furuhashi, R. Muto, and K. Fujita. 2001. A factor of inducing IgE from a filarial parasite is an agonist of human CD40. *The Journal of biological chemistry* 276:46118-46124.

[28] Imai, S., H. Tezuka, and K. Fujita. 2001. A factor of inducing IgE from a filarial parasite prevents insulin-dependent diabetes mellitus in nonobese diabetic mice. *Biochemical and biophysical research communications* 286:1051-1058.

[29] Lynch, N. R., M. Palenque, I. Hagel, and M. C. DiPrisco. 1997. Clinical improvement of asthma after anthelminthic treatment in a tropical situation. *American journal of respiratory and critical care medicine* 156:50-54.

[30] Nagler-Anderson, C. 2006. Helminth-induced immunoregulation of an allergic response to food. *Chemical immunology and allergy* 90:1-13.

[31] Maloy, K. J., L. Salaun, R. Cahill, G. Dougan, N. J. Saunders, and F. Powrie. 2003. CD4+CD25+ T(R) cells suppress innate immune pathology through cytokine-dependent mechanisms. *The Journal of experimental medicine* 197:111-119.

[32] Mottet, C., H. H. Uhlig, and F. Powrie. 2003. Cutting edge: cure of colitis by CD4+CD25+ regulatory T cells. *J Immunol* 170:3939-3943.

[33] Gomez-Escobar, N., E. Lewis, and R. M. Maizels. 1998. A novel member of the transforming growth factor-beta (TGF-beta) superfamily from the filarial nematodes Brugia malayi and B. pahangi. *Experimental parasitology* 88:200-209.

[34] Gregory, W. F., M. L. Blaxter, and R. M. Maizels. 1997. Differentially expressed, abundant trans-spliced cDNAs from larval Brugia malayi. *Molecular and biochemical parasitology* 87:85-95.

[35] Yenbutr, P., and A. L. Scott. 1995. Molecular cloning of a serine proteinase inhibitor from Brugia malayi. *Infection and immunity* 63:1745-1753.

[36] Joseph, G. T., T. Huima, and S. Lustigman. 1998. Characterization of an Onchocerca volvulus L3-specific larval antigen, Ov-ALT-1. *Molecular and biochemical parasitology* 96:177-183.

[37] Thomas, P. G., M. R. Carter, O. Atochina, A. A. Da'Dara, D. Piskorska, E. McGuire, and D. A. Harn. 2003. Maturation of dendritic cell 2 phenotype by a helminth glycan uses a Toll-like receptor 4-dependent mechanism. *J Immunol* 171:5837-5841.

[38] Murray, J., W. F. Gregory, N. Gomez-Escobar, A. K. Atmadja, and R. M. Maizels. 2001. Expression and immune recognition of Brugia malayi VAL-1, a homologue of vespid venom allergens and Ancylostoma secreted proteins. *Molecular and biochemical parasitology* 118:89-96.

[39] Beall, M. J., S. McGonigle, and E. J. Pearce. 2000. Functional conservation of Schistosoma mansoni Smads in TGF-beta signaling. *Molecular and biochemical parasitology* 111:131-142.

[40] Gomez-Escobar, N., A. van den Biggelaar, and R. Maizels. 1997. A member of the TGF-beta receptor gene family in the parasitic nematode Brugia pahangi. *Gene* 199:101-109.

[41] Maizels, R. M., N. Gomez-Escobar, W. F. Gregory, J. Murray, and X. Zang. 2001. Immune evasion genes from filarial nematodes. *International journal for parasitology* 31:889-898.

[42] Bloom, B. R., and B. Bennett. 1966. Mechanism of a reaction in vitro associated with delayed-type hypersensitivity. *Science (New York, N.Y* 153:80-82.

[43] Baugh, J. A., and R. Bucala. 2002. Macrophage migration inhibitory factor. *Crit Care Med* 30:S27-S35.

[44] Morand, E. F. 2005. New therapeutic target in inflammatory disease: macrophage migration inhibitory factor. *Internal medicine journal* 35:419-426.

[45] Kobayashi, M., Y. Nasuhara, A. Kamachi, Y. Tanino, T. Betsuyaku, E. Yamaguchi, J. Nishihira, and M. Nishimura. 2006. Role of macrophage migration inhibitory factor in ovalbumin-induced airway inflammation in rats. *Eur Respir J* 27:726-734.

[46] Pastrana, D. V., N. Raghavan, P. FitzGerald, S. W. Eisinger, C. Metz, R. Bucala, R. P. Schleimer, C. Bickel, and A. L. Scott. 1998. Filarial nematode parasites secrete a homologue of the human cytokine macrophage migration inhibitory factor. *Infection and immunity* 66:5955-5963.

[47] Falcone, F. H., P. Loke, X. Zang, A. S. MacDonald, R. M. Maizels, and J. E. Allen. 2001. A Brugia malayi homolog of macrophage migration inhibitory factor reveals an important link between macrophages and eosinophil recruitment during nematode infection. *J Immunol* 167:5348-5354.

[48] Cho, Y., B. F. Jones, J. J. Vermeire, L. Leng, L. DiFedele, L. M. Harrison, H. Xiong, Y. K. Kwong, Y. Chen, R. Bucala, E. Lolis, and M. Cappello. 2007. Structural and functional characterization of a secreted hookworm Macrophage Migration Inhibitory Factor (MIF) that interacts with the human MIF receptor CD74. *The Journal of biological chemistry* 282:23447-23456.

[49] Vermeire, J. J., Y. Cho, E. Lolis, R. Bucala, and M. Cappello. 2008. Orthologs of macrophage migration inhibitory factor from parasitic nematodes. *Trends in parasitology* 24:355-363.

[50] Yu, H. S., S. K. Park, K. H. Lee, S. J. Lee, S. H. Choi, M. S. Ock, and H. J. Jeong. 2007. Anisakis simplex: analysis of expressed sequence tags (ESTs) of third-stage larva. *Experimental parasitology* 117:51-56.

[51] Umetsu, D. T., J. J. McIntire, O. Akbari, C. Macaubas, and R. H. DeKruyff. 2002. Asthma: an epidemic of dysregulated immunity. *Nature immunology* 3:715-720.

[52] Lisbonne, M., S. Diem, A. de Castro Keller, J. Lefort, L. M. Araujo, P. Hachem, J. M. Fourneau, S. Sidobre, M. Kronenberg, M. Taniguchi, P. Van Endert, M. Dy, P. Askenase, M. Russo, B. B. Vargaftig, A. Herbelin, and M. C. Leite-de-Moraes. 2003. Cutting edge: invariant V alpha 14 NKT cells are required for allergen-induced airway inflammation and hyperreactivity in an experimental asthma model. *J Immunol* 171:1637-1641.

[53] Araujo, L. M., J. Lefort, M. A. Nahori, S. Diem, R. Zhu, M. Dy, M. C. Leite-de-Moraes, J. F. Bach, B. B. Vargaftig, and A. Herbelin. 2004. Exacerbated Th2-mediated airway inflammation and hyperresponsiveness in autoimmune diabetes-prone NOD mice: a critical role for CD1d-dependent NKT cells. *European journal of immunology* 34:327-335.

[54] Kornas, S., M. Skalska, B. Nowosad, and J. Gawor. 2007. [The communities of cyathostomes (Cyathostominae) in year-old and two-year-old Pure Blood Arabian mares]. *Wiadomosci parazytologiczne* 53:325-329.

[55] Belkaid, Y., and B. T. Rouse. 2005. Natural regulatory T cells in infectious disease. *Nature immunology* 6:353-360.

[56] Anthony, R. M., L. I. Rutitzky, J. F. Urban, Jr., M. J. Stadecker, and W. C. Gause. 2007. Protective immune mechanisms in helminth infection. *Nature reviews* 7:975-987.

[57] Pacifico, L. G., F. A. Marinho, C. T. Fonseca, M. M. Barsante, V. Pinho, P. A. J. Sales, L. S. Cardoso, M. I. Araujo, E. M. Carvalho, G. D. Cassali, M. M. Teixeira, and S. C. Oliveira. 2008. Schistosoma mansoni antigens modulate experimental allergic asthma in a murine model: a major role for CD4+CD25+Foxp3+ T cells independent of IL-10. *Infection and immunity*.

[58] Kitagaki, K., T. R. Businga, D. Racila, D. E. Elliott, J. V. Weinstock, and J. N. Kline. 2006. Intestinal helminths protect in a murine model of asthma. *J Immunol* 177:1628-1635.

[59] Park, S. K., M. K. Cho, H. K. Park, K. H. Lee, S. J. Lee, S. H. Choi, M. S. Ock, H. J. Jeong, M. H. Lee, and H. S. Yu. 2009. Macrophage migration inhibitory factor homologs of anisakis simplex suppress Th2 response in allergic airway inflammation model via CD4+CD25+Foxp3+ T cell recruitment. *J Immunol* 182:6907-6914.

[60] Akbari, O., R. H. DeKruyff, and D. T. Umetsu. 2001. Pulmonary dendritic cells producing IL-10 mediate tolerance induced by respiratory exposure to antigen. *Nature immunology* 2:725-731.

[61] Rankin, E. B., D. Yu, J. Jiang, H. Shen, E. J. Pearce, M. H. Goldschmidt, D. E. Levy, T. V. Golovkina, C. A. Hunter, and A. Thomas-Tikhonenko. 2003. An essential role of Th1 responses and interferon gamma in infection-mediated suppression of neoplastic growth. *Cancer biology & therapy* 2:687-693.

[62] Hawrylowicz, C. M., and A. O'Garra. 2005. Potential role of interleukin-10-secreting regulatory T cells in allergy and asthma. *Nature reviews* 5:271-283.

[63] Hansen, G., J. J. McIntire, V. P. Yeung, G. Berry, G. J. Thorbecke, L. Chen, R. H. DeKruyff, and D. T. Umetsu. 2000. CD4(+) T helper cells engineered to produce latent TGF-beta1 reverse allergen-induced airway hyperreactivity and inflammation. *The Journal of clinical investigation* 105:61-70.

[64] Chen, W., W. Jin, N. Hardegen, K. J. Lei, L. Li, N. Marinos, G. McGrady, and S. M. Wahl. 2003. Conversion of peripheral CD4+CD25- naive T cells to CD4+CD25+ regulatory T cells by TGF-beta induction of transcription factor Foxp3. *The Journal of experimental medicine* 198:1875-1886.

27

Pharmaceutical Treatment of Asthma Symptoms in Elite Athletes – Doping or Therapy

Jimmi Elers and Vibeke Backer
Copenhagen University,
Denmark

1. Introduction

According to the World Health Organization (WHO), 300 million people suffer from asthma, a disease which is increasing in western societies, and furthermore asthma is the most common chronic disease among children, adolescents and young adults. A steady increase in the prevalence of asthma, has been seen in most countries in recent decades (Thomsen et al 2011) and the higher frequency of asthma in young people may partly explain the high frequency found in elite athletes - although both frequency of asthma symptoms and use of anti-asthmatic medication are different than expected. Moreover, the frequency of airway hyperresponsiveness (AHR) in elite athletes is higher than expected as well as the frequency of asthma-like symptoms (cough, wheeze, shortness of breath and chest tightness) which might be caused by exhaustive ventilation, but the pathogenesis is still unknown.

The frequency of asthma among the general population is around 7-10%; whereas the frequency of asthma among elite athletes is found to be higher, especially among endurance athletes (Pedersen et al 2008b). It seems as asthma is something they gain, as only one third of Olympic athletes had childhood asthma. Although asthma among the general public is a permanent phenomenon, it seems to be different in elite athletes, as asthma apparently disappeared after retiring from the sport (Fitch et al 2008).

2. Asthma among athletes

Asthma is a chronic respiratory condition classically characterised by airway inflammation and airway hyperresponsiveness (AHR) to multiple stimuli (Anderson et al 2009). AHR is defined as a pathological bronchoconstrictive response to a given stimulus . AHR to a direct stimulus (e.g. methacholine) acts through airway smooth muscles and the response is thought to be independent of airway inflammation. Whereas response to an indirect stimulus (e.g. exercise, hyperventilation, mannitol) acts through a release of inflammatory mediators, such as histamine, prostaglandins, and leukotrienes, which causes contraction of the airway smooth muscle cells. Airway inflammation in asthma is characterised by inflammatory cells, such as eosinophils, mast cells, and macrophages. The inflammation causes remodelling of the basal membrane, enlargement of the mass of smooth muscles, and disturbance of the surface area. Permanent use of controller therapy with inhaled steroids (ICS) is needed in asthma, as well as relief therapy with short-acting beta$_2$-agonists (SABA), long-acting beta$_2$-agonists (LABA) or others.

Elite athletes, with or without asthma, have asthma-like symptoms during their training season, especially cough, phlegm and shortness of breath is a dominant complain among athletes (Lund et al 2009). Furthermore, athletes are more often found with AHR to direct stimuli and less to direct stimuli than found in normal subjects thus suggesting a respiratory illness. Variation in action of the different provocative agents is related to the fact that response to an indirect challenge would reflect an ongoing inflammation better than would direct tests, and perhaps thus reflect the presence of classical asthma, whereas AHR to direct agents indicates airway smooth muscle dysfunction and, in some cases, asthma (Pedersen et al 2008a, Sue-Chu et al 2010).

The definition of asthma includes respiratory symptoms, variable airway obstruction and airway hyperresponsiveness to multiple agents. The respiratory symptoms in patients with common asthma and the elite athletes with or without asthma are similar, which leave a diagnostic problem in these cases where symptoms are the single diagnostic parameter available. Whereas, the differences between common asthma and asthma among elite athletes are predominantly related to the airway responsiveness to inhaled agents, the day-to-day variability of lung function as well as the content of the inflammatory cells which predominantly are neutrophilic cells and not eosinophilic.

3. Exercise-induced asthma and bronchoconstriction in elite athletes

Exercise-induced bronchoconstriction (EIB) is an acute, transient narrowing of the airway that occurs during and particularly after exercise. In most scientific papers, exercise-induced asthma (EIA) are defined as respiratory symptoms and a significant reduction in FEV1 after exercise, i.e. Δ $FEV_1 \geq 10\%$, whereas EIB is a significant reduction in FEV1 ($\geq$10%) when tested, independent of symptoms or not. In population samples, the prevalence of EIB (16%) is the same as the findings of AHR to histamine (16%), although only 6% had responsiveness to both test (Backer et al 1992). EIB is believed to be more specific to asthma, but less sensitive, as the number of false negative results is a problem when research and clinical situations settings are evaluated (Anderson & Kippelen 2005). The frequency of AHR is frequently found above 40%, which is higher than the frequency of asthma. Elite athletes claim that exercise is the most prominent trigger of asthma symptoms, as they very seldom complain of respiratory symptoms at rest or during the night.

The pathogenesis of asthma-like symptoms in elite athletes is multifactorial, and is not completely understood. However, deep, exhaustive ventilation during exercise brings atmospheric air which is cold and dry and this manoeuvre overcomes the ability of the upper airways to warm up and humidify the air reaching the smaller airways(Anderson & Kippelen 2005). This brings about airway narrowing due to osmotic and thermal evaporative water loss, and some vascular involvement. These airway differences, together with some degree of inflammation, lead to a respiratory condition described as EIB or sports asthma. This abnormal response is most often found in endurance sports, such as cross-country skiing , swimming, rowing, cycling, fast-track skating and long distance running.

The symptoms of exercise-induced bronchoconstriction range from mild impairment of performance with minor reduction in lung function after exercise to severe bronchospasm with large reduction in FEV_1. In athletes, however, the most common symptoms include cough, wheezing, chest tightness, dyspnoea, and fatigue. These symptoms are frequently found in healthy subjects, subjects with asthma, subjects who are not in good condition and sometimes in subjects suffering from an extrathoracal disorder such as vocal cord dysfunction (VCD).

In conclusion, the most frequent complaint among healthy and diseased athletes is respiratory symptoms during exercise. Furthermore, healthy elite athletes often have AHR with a pattern which differ from the general asthma patient. Lastly, the types of cells involved in the inflammation are different from those in normal asthmatics.

4. Diseases mimicking exercise-induced asthma

Not all that wheezes is asthma. When the diagnosis of asthma is based on respiratory symptoms alone, misdiagnosis may occur. Patients may present with respiratory distress, such as wheezy, when experiencing a low level of fitness, a psychological condition, inhalation of airborne irritants, rhinosinusitis, or gastroesophageal reflux disease. Moreover, exercise-induced symptoms can occur as periodic occurance of laryngeal obstruction (POLO) or exercise induced laryngeal obstruction (EILO) and present with asthma like symptoms. These diseases include conditions such as vocal cord dysfunction (VCD), exercise-induced paradoxical arytenoid motion (EPAM), exercise-induced laryngomalacia (EIL), exercise-induced laryngochalasia, angioedema, vocal cord tumours, and vocal cord paralysis. There seems to be a substantial overlap between EILO and EIA, at least in elite athletes. It could be of minor importance, but it could also have a major influence on the diagnostic procedure in the daily care settings of those with asthma-like symptoms. When POLO/EILO is misdiagnosed as asthma, patient are erroneously treated with anti-asthma therapy, even high doses because of "resistant disease".

These diseases are easily recognized by performing a Flow/Volume curve where a classical cutoff of the inspiratory loop is apparent. On the other hand, a specific diagnose of the actual pathology need laryngeal examination during exercise. The definitive diagnosis of laryngeal obstruction might require laryngoscopy during strenuous exercise. Heimdal et al (Heimdal et al 2006) recently published a paper describing a model for use when performing the continuous laryngoscopy exercise test (CLE). Patients with asthma should start asthma medication, and for those with satisfactory adherence who do not achieve well-controlled disease, other reasons for persistent respiratory symptoms should be explored. In such cases CLE should be performed.

5. Treatment

Treatment of elite athletes with asthma can be divided into non-pharmacological and pharmacological treatment. During the last decades the International Olympic Committee (IOC) increased their focus on the increasing use of anti-asthmatic medication by Olympic and other elite athletes. At the 1996 Olympic Games in Atlanta 3.7% of the athletes used beta2-agonists, 5.6% at the 1998 Winter Games in Nagano, and 5.7% at the Sydney Games 2000. The IOC and the World Anti Doping Agency (WADA) have had many changes in the anti-doping regulations on beta2-agonists through the years, partly due to concerns regarding ergogenic effects and partly because of health risk concerns. Due to the increased use of beta2-agonists as mentioned above the IOC introduced a criterion of demonstration of asthma by an objective measure of reversibility or bronchial airway hyperresponsiveness in order approved use of beta2-agonist. This resulted in a 27% reduction in the use of beta2-agonists in the 2004 Games in Athen.

5.1 Pharmacological treatment

Treatment of asthma and exercise-induced bronchoconstriction (EIB) in elite athletes should follow international asthma treatment guidelines like the Global Initiative for Asthma (GINA), see Figure 1 (Bateman et al 2008). The main purpose of pharmacotherapy is control of asthma symptoms, reducing airway inflammation and airway hyperresponsiveness, achieving normal lung function, and prevent exacerbations

Step1	Step2	Step3	Step4	Step5
	Asthma education	and	Environmental control	
Short-acting beta2-agonist as needed		Short-acting beta2-agonist as needed		
	Select one	Select one	Select one	Select one
	Low-dose inhaled corticosteroid	Low-dose inhaled corticosteroid + Long acting beta2-agonist	Medium or high-dose inhaled corticosteroid + Long acting beta2-agonist	Oral glucocorticosteroid
	Leukotriene modifier	Medium or high-dose inhaled corticosteroid	Leukotriene modifier	Anti-IgE treatment
		Low-dose inhaled corticosteroid + Leukotriene modifier	Theophylline	
		Low-dose inhaled corticosteroid + Theophylline		

Fig. 1. Management approach. Adapted from GINA.

5.2 Beta2-agonists

Inhaled short acting beta2-agonists (SABA), e.g. salbutamol and terbutaline, are first choice therapy for fast relief of EIB. Moreover, SABA is useful in preventing EIB if taken 15 minutes before exercise. Frequent and increased use indicates uncontrolled asthma and should result in reassessment of treatment strategies. Side effects are tremor, tachycardia, palpitations and headache, which increase in frequency and intensity with higher doses. With high systemic doses hypopotassemia and muscle convulsions can occur. Systemic use of beta2-agonists by elite athletes is entirely prohibited according to the Prohibited List, see Table 1.

Inhaled long acting beta2-agonists (LABA), e.g. salmeterol and formoterol, are used in management of uncontrolled asthma treated with inhaled corticosteroid alone. LABA is used as add-on therapy to inhaled corticosteroids, either as fixed combination or in two separate devices. LABA should never be used as monotherapy in asthma due to risk of serious adverse events with increased risk of mortality in case of exacerbation. In a review from 2005 it was concluded that combined fluticasone and salmeterol was superior to fluticasone as monotherapy in preventing EIA. Furthermore, in a randomized, double-blinded study combined budesonide/formoterol was compared with budesonide alone, asthma control was better with reduced symptoms when treated with combination of budesonide/formoterol. A new study from 2010 confirms previous findings with more efficacy when inhaled budesonide is combined with formoterol among adults and adolescents with moderate to severe asthma. These findings indicate that it is not an effect related to the specific drug, but a class effect of the combination.

I SUBSTANCES AND METHODS PROHIBITED AT ALL TIMES (IN- AND OUT-OF-COMPETITION):
S0. Non-approved substances
S1. Anabolic agents
S2. Peptide hormones, growth factors and related substances
S3. Beta2-agonists
S4. Hormone antagonists and modulators
S5. Diuretics and other masking agents
M1. Enhancement of oxygen transfer
M2. Chemical and physical manipulation
M3. Gene doping
II SUBSTANCES AND METHODS PROHIBITED IN-COMPETITION:
S0-5 and M1-3 defined above
S6. Stimulants
S7. Narcotics
S8. Cannabinoids
S9. Glucocorticosterooids
III SUBSTANCES PROHIBITED IN PARTICULAR SPORTS:
P1. Alcohol
P2. Beta-Blockers

Table 1. The 2011 Prohibited List by World Anti-Doping Agency.

It is well known that regular use of beta2-agonist could lead to development of tolerance to bronchodilation (i.e. reduced bronchodilator response during acute asthma) and bronchoprotection (i.e. reduced ability to prevent exercise-induced bronchoconstriction). Tolerance to bronchodilator develops rapidly, after only few doses, and regardless of ongoing treatment with inhaled corticosteroid. Tolerance to bronchoprotection develops after few weeks of treatment and regardless of ongoing treatment with inhaled corticosteroids. The decreased bronchoprotection might result in increased use of beta2-

agonist and higher risk of side effects. Though theoretical concerns that regular beta2-agonist treatment may lead to tolerance and failure to respond to emergency asthma treatment, there is little evidence that this is a clinical problem. However, as elite athletes exercise daily and often several times a day, use of beta2-agonists, either before exercise to prevent bronchoconstriction or during/after due to bronchoconstriction, would exceed the maximal recommend weekly use in the GINA guidelines, indicating that other treatment strategies than SABA in case of EIB are needed.

5.3 Inhaled corticosteroids

Inhaled corticosteroids (ICS) are the most used and most effective inhaled anti-inflammatory drug available. ICS improves asthma symptoms, self-reported quality of life and lung function, reduces airway inflammation and airway hyperresponsiveness and furthermore, ICS has been found to reduce number and severity of exacerbations and asthma mortality (Jeffery et al 1992, Suissa et al 2000). GINA guidelines recommend ICS when asthma is uncontrolled with non-pharmacological interventions and rescue therapy alone. Effects are observed after 7-14 days, while full effects are seen after eight weeks of treatment.

Our current knowledge about effects of ICS on exercise-induced bronchoconstriction is based on adults and children with asthma. Existing studies ranges from three weeks to two years duration of treatment, mostly conducted in a parallel design. A study with 40 adult asthmatic subjects randomized to 6 weeks treatment with placebo or 800 micrograms budesonide twice a day showed a post-exercise fall in FEV_1 of 7% in the budesonide group and to 22% in the placebo group. Similar findings are reported in asthmatic children.

5.4 Leukotriene modifiers

Leukotriene modifiers have anti-inflammatory and bronchodilatory effects. Leukotriene modifiers are administered orally and once daily for montelukast and twice daily for zileuton. Montelukast is used as add-on treatment in case of uncontrolled asthma with medium dose ICS as monotherapy(Lofdahl et al 1999). Prevention of EIA is another indication in elite athletes with asthma. Studies report a reduced post-exercise fall in FEV_1 and a reduced period of bronchoconstriction after exercise when treated with montelukast compared to placebo in non-smoking asthmatic subjects. No studies have reported development of tolerance during regular use.

5.5 Cromoglycate

In a study from 2010 treatment with sodium cromoglycate decreased the FEV_1 fall after a eucapnic voluntary hyperpnoea (EVH) challenge in elite athletes with EIB (Anderson et al 2010). This finding support that release of mast cell mediators is an important factor for the severity of EIB. However, use of cromones in asthmatic elite athletes is limited.

6. Non-pharmacological interventions

Asthmatic athletes with pollen allergy should avoid prolonged outdoor endurance exercise in areas with high pollen counts. Exercise in temperatures below minus 15 degrees Celsius should be avoided, particularly in areas with air pollution or other airway irritants.

Few studies have investigated correlation between physical warm-up and degree of EIA in asthmatic athletes and a warm-up period has been shown to induce refractoriness to

EIA without itself inducing significant bronchoconstriction. The protective effect of different types of warm-up has been compared in controlled studies, but no consensus is found. Different study protocols and designs make it difficult to compare the existing studies, but physical warm-up in some form and extent seems generally to have a protective effect on EIA, and physical warm-up should be advised for all athletes with asthma. Breathing filters may reduce EIB among those exercising in cold conditions. A study from 2000 compared response to exercise in cold air (decrease in FEV_1) in nine patients with EIA when given no treatment, given premedication with a beta2-agonist, wearing a heat-and-moisture-exchanging facemask, and given both premedication and facemask. The mean maximal change in FEV_1 was 27% with no treatment, 12% with facemask, 7% with premedication, and no change with the combination of premedication and facemask. Another study from 2006 examined effects of a heat exchanger mask, placebo mask, and premedication with a beta2-agonist. Five patients with EIA performed a treadmill exercise test while breathing cold air. It was concluded that a heat exchanger mask prevented cold exercise-induced fall in lung function as effectively as treatment with beta2 agonist before exercise in cold air.

During the last decade some research has focused on nutritional factors, especially omega-3-polyunsaturated fatty acids' influence on airway inflammation and exercise-induced bronchoconstriction. A review from 2005 concluded that omega-3-polyunsaturated fatty acid supplementation reduces the degree of exercise-induced bronchoconstriction compared with placebo in patients with EIA. The review was based on a small number of studies with limited range of clinically important outcomes. Further controlled and well-designed research is needed to establish any evidence-based recommendations.

7. Treatment or doping

As mentioned above the IOC and WADA have increased their attention on the status of beta2-agonists on the "The 2010 Prohibited List" (www.wada-ama.org). Until the end of 2009 granting of a Therapeutic Use Exemption (TUE) was necessary for use of inhaled salbutamol, terbutaline, salmeterol and formoterol. From 2010 use of inhaled salbutamol and salmeterol in therapeutic doses are allowed. From 2010 use of inhaled terbutaline and formoterol is still prohibited and requires a TUE and a reasonable explanation of why these drugs are prescribed when other equal drugs are permitted. Use of inhaled corticosteroids in therapeutic doses is permitted, except when used in a fixed combination with formoterol, which requires a TUE. Use of oral or topical antihistamines or leukotriene modifiers is permitted. Use of systemic corticosteroids is prohibited during competition. Systemic intake of beta2-agonist and clenbuterol is strictly prohibited in elite athletes. The criteria for granting a TUE, the "Prohibited List", and guidelines are available on WADA's website (www.wada-ama.org). As the anti-doping legislation and the prohibited list are continually updated, it is important to be familiar with the current regulations before prescribing asthma medication to an elite athlete with asthma. The 2011 Prohibited List is shown in Table 2. For details visit WADA´s website.

In the academic societies of sports and pulmonary medicine it is discussed whether or not beta2-agonists have any ergogenic, i.e. performance enhancing effects, and if it should be considered doping or not. According to the World Anti-Doping Agency (WADA) minimum two of three criteria must be met in order to consider a substance or method for inclusion on the Prohibited List:

1. The substance or method can be performance enhancing
2. The use of the substance or the method can endanger the athlete´s health
3. The use of the substance or method is against the spirit of sport

As it appears a substance or method can be listed without being performance enhancing. Due to health issues the IOC considers inhaled use of beta2-agonist without need unacceptable. Beta2-agonists have received much attention the last decades because of side effects, and few studies have reported and the US Food and Drug Administration have issued some concerns about beta2-agonists and side effects/serious adverse events. Regarding health issues in elite athletes using beta2-agonists the IOC is concerned about athletes using beta2-agonists without need and in supratherapeutic doses. Studies in asthmatic children have shown both significant raised and normal blood levels of myocardial stress markers after inhalation of beta2-agonists in ten times prophylactic doses. Studies with unrestrained rats have documented dose-response myocyte apoptosis after administration of the beta2-agonists formoterol and clenbuterol. Significant changes in human cardiac electrophysiological properties is seen after administration of salbutamol 5 mg as a single dose.

Several studies have investigated the ergogenic effects of inhaled and oral beta2-agonists conducted with healthy well-trained men, most studies in therapeutic doses. The extensive research on therapeutic doses of inhaled beta2-agonsits clearly rules out any ergogenic effects. Only few studies have shown ergogenic effects of inhaled salbutamol, but these are limited by enrolment of recreational subjects. It is now a common opinion that inhaled beta2-agonists in therapeutic doses has no advantageous effects in healthy athletes. However, animal and human studies, where beta2-agonists are given in systemic supra-therapeutic doses daily for few weeks, have shown evidence of improvement of muscle strength and endurance performance. Pluim et al. concluded in a systematic review and meta-analyses of randomized controlled trials on beta2-agonists and physical performance published in 2011 that there is some evidence indicating that systemic beta2-agonists may have a positive effect on physical performance in healthy subjects(Pluim et al 2011). Clenbuterol, another beta2-agonist used in veterinary medicine via prescription as a bronchodilator, cardiotonic and tocolytic agent. However used in supratherapeutic doses in animals and humans it is misused as a growth promotor with anabolic and lipolytic effects.

8. References

[1] Anderson SD, Brannan JD, Perry CP, Caillaud C, Seale JP. 2010. Sodium cromoglycate alone and in combination with montelukast on the airway response to mannitol in asthmatic subjects. *J. Asthma.* 47(4):429-33

[2] Anderson SD, Charlton B, Weiler JM, Nichols S, Spector SL, Pearlman DS. 2009. Comparison of mannitol and methacholine to predict exercise-induced bronchoconstriction and a clinical diagnosis of asthma. *Respir Res.* 10:4

[3] Anderson SD, Kippelen P. 2005. Exercise-induced bronchoconstriction: pathogenesis. *Curr. Allergy Asthma Rep.* 5(2):116-22

[4] Backer V, Ulrik CS, Hansen KK, Laursen EM, Dirksen A, Bach-Mortensen N. 1992. Atopy and bronchial responsiveness in random population sample of 527 children and adolescents. *Ann. Allergy.* 69(2):116-22

[5] Bateman ED, Hurd SS, Barnes PJ, Bousquet J, Drazen JM, FitzGerald M, Gibson P, Ohta K, O'Byrne P, Pedersen SE, Pizzichini E, Sullivan SD, Wenzel SE, Zar HJ. 2008. Global strategy for asthma management and prevention: GINA executive summary. *Eur. Respir J* 31(1):143-78

[6] Fitch KD, Sue-Chu M, Anderson SD, Boulet LP, Hancox RJ, McKenzie DC, Backer V, Rundell KW, Alonso JM, Kippelen P, Cummiskey JM, Garnier A, Ljungqvist A. 2008. Asthma and the elite athlete: summary of the International Olympic Committee's consensus conference, Lausanne, Switzerland, January 22-24, 2008. *J Allergy Clin Immunol.* 122(2):254-60, 260

[7] Heimdal JH, Roksund OD, Halvorsen T, Skadberg BT, Olofsson J. 2006. Continuous laryngoscopy exercise test: a method for visualizing laryngeal dysfunction during exercise. *Laryngoscope* 116(1):52-7

[8] Jeffery PK, Godfrey RW, Adelroth E, Nelson F, Rogers A, Johansson SA. 1992. Effects of treatment on airway inflammation and thickening of basement membrane reticular collagen in asthma. A quantitative light and electron microscopic study. *Am. Rev. Respir. Dis.* 145(4 Pt 1):890-9

[9] Lofdahl CG, Reiss TF, Leff JA, Israel E, Noonan MJ, Finn AF, Seidenberg BC, Capizzi T, Kundu S, Godard P. 1999. Randomised, placebo controlled trial of effect of a leukotriene receptor antagonist, montelukast, on tapering inhaled corticosteroids in asthmatic patients. *BMJ.* 319(7202):87-90

[10] Lund TK, Pedersen L, Anderson SD, Sverrild A, Backer V. 2009. Are asthma-like symptoms in elite athletes associated with classical features of asthma? *Br. J Sports Med.* 43(14):1131-5

[11] Pedersen L, Lund TK, Barnes PJ, Kharitonov SA, Backer V. 2008a. Airway responsiveness and inflammation in adolescent elite swimmers. *J Allergy Clin Immunol.* 122(2):322-7, 327

[12] Pedersen L, Winther S, Backer V, Anderson SD, Larsen KR. 2008b. Airway responses to eucapnic hyperpnea, exercise, and methacholine in elite swimmers. *Med. Sci. Sports Exerc.* 40(9):1567-72

[13] Pluim BM, de Hon O, Staal JB, Limpens J, Kuipers H, Overbeek SE, Zwinderman AH, Scholten RJ. 2011. beta-Agonists and physical performance: a systematic review and meta-analysis of randomized controlled trials. *Sports Med.* 41(1): 39-57

[14] Sue-Chu M, Brannan JD, Anderson SD, Chew N, Bjermer L. 2010. Airway hyperresponsiveness to methacholine, adenosine 5-monophosphate, mannitol, eucapnic voluntary hyperpnoea and field exercise challenge in elite cross-country skiers. *Br. J. Sports Med.* 44(11):827-32

[15] Suissa S, Ernst P, Benayoun S, Baltzan M, Cai B. 2000. Low-dose inhaled corticosteroids and the prevention of death from asthma. *N. Engl. J. Med.* 343(5):332-6

[16] Thomsen SF, van der SS, Kyvik KO, Skytthe A, Skadhauge LR, Backer V. 2011. Increase in the heritability of asthma from 1994 to 2003 among adolescent twins. *Respir. Med.*